Oxford Textbook of

Colorectal Cancer

OXFORD TEXTBOOKS IN ONCOLOGY

Oxford Textbook of Neuro-Oncology, 2nd Edition
Edited by Tracy Batchelor, Michael Weller

Oxford Textbook of Cancer in Children, 7th Edition
Edited by Hubert N. Caron, Andrea Biondi, Tom Boterberg, François Doz

Oxford Textbook of Cancer Biology
Edited by Francesco Pezzella, Mahvash Tavassoli, David J. Ker

Oxford Textbook of

Colorectal Cancer

EDITED BY

Rachel S. Kerr

Associate Professor of Gastrointestinal Oncology, University of Oxford and Oxford University Hospitals NHS Trust, UK

Li Yang

Department of Gastroenterology and Hepatology and Sichuan University-University of Oxford Huaxi Joint Centre for Gastrointestinal Cancer, West China Hospital, Sichuan University, China

David J. Kerr

Professor of Cancer Medicine, University of Oxford, UK

OXFORD
UNIVERSITY PRESS

OXFORD
UNIVERSITY PRESS

Great Clarendon Street, Oxford, OX2 6DP,
United Kingdom

Oxford University Press is a department of the University of Oxford. It furthers the University's objective of excellence in research, scholarship, and education by publishing worldwide. Oxford is a registered trade mark of Oxford University Press in the UK and in certain other countries.

Published in the United States of America by Oxford University Press
198 Madison Avenue, New York, NY 10016, United States of America.

British Library Cataloguing in Publication Data
Data available

Library of Congress Control Number: 2025937498

ISBN 978–0–19–284999–1

DOI: 10.1093/med/9780192849991.001.0001

Printed and bound by
CPI Group (UK) Ltd., Croydon, CR0 4YY

Preface

The opportunity to compile the *Oxford Textbook of Colorectal Cancer* represented a chance to deliver a definitive and comprehensive text detailing the evolution, biological base, and current best practice in multidisciplinary colorectal cancer care. The textbook opens with introductory chapters covering the basic science and general principles that underpin optimal approaches to oncology treatments, embracing innovations in surgery, radiotherapy, and the delivery of targeted cancer medicines, which are described by internationally recognized experts in the field. We explore the unique challenges presented by balancing population health (early detection and screening) and the needs of individual patients both during and after personalized cancer treatment.

The last decade has seen an explosion of biological knowledge and genomic data, integrated by the application of AI driven bioinformatics, which has been translated into clinically useful tests and therapies, and we believe that while the high number of research and review papers provide a continuous update on increasingly narrow and specialized topics in cancer biology, there will be always a need for a textbook such as this which enables us to catch up with the current state of art in multiple fields, within a wider contextual framework. We hope that this book will offer readers a clear understanding of what is now possible and what is still needed to take things forward into the future.

We would like to thank the contributors to this edition, our colleagues and collaborators, and the outstanding team at OUP who have helped with the preparation of this book.

Professor Rachel Kerr, Department of Oncology,University of Oxford; Professor Li Yang, Department of Gastroenterology, Huaxi Hospital, Sichuan University, Chengdu, China; Professor David Kerr, Radcliffe Department of Medicine, University of Oxford

Contents

SECTION 4

Novelty interventions and personalizing the CRC pathway

Abbreviations

4DCBT	4D cone beam CT
5-FU	5-fluorouracil
AAPM	American Association of Physicists in Medicine
ACE	Antegrade Continence Enema
ACF	aberrant crypt foci
ACS	American Cancer Society
AE	adverse event
AF	allele fraction
AFAP	attenuated familial adenomatous polyposis
AIDS	Acquired Immunodeficiency Syndrome
ALPPS	associating liver partition and portal vein ligation for staged hepatectomy
AMPK	AMP-activated protein kinase
APACC	Association pour la Prevention par l'Aspirine du Cancer Colorectal
APC	adenomatous polyposis coli
APC	Adenoma Prevention with Celecoxib trial
APC	antigen-presenting cells
APC	argon plasma coagulation
APR	abdominoperineal resection
ASCO	American Society of Clinical Oncology
ASTRO	American Society for Radiation Oncology
AUROC	area under receiver operating characteristic curve
BAcc	balanced accuracy
BCG	Bacillus Calmette Guérin
BCSP	Bowel Cancer Screening Programme (UK)
BER	base excision repair
BM	basement membrane
BMI	body mass index
BMP	bone morphogenetic protein
BRAF	V-raf Murine sarcoma viral oncogene homologue B1
BRRS	Bannayan Riley–Ruvalcaba syndrome
CACs	colorectal adenocarcinomas
CAD	computer-aided diagnosis
CADe	computer-aided detection
CAFs	cancer-associated fibroblasts
CAPP	Colorectal Adenoma/Carcinoma Prevention Programme
CBCT	cone beam CT
CC	completeness of cytoreduction
CCE	colon capsule endoscopy
CCS	Completeness of Cytoreduction Score
cCR	clinical complete response
cDC	conventional DC
CE	contrast-enhanced
CEA	carcinoma embryonic antigen
CEA	cardioembryonic antigen
CEACAM	carcinoembryonic antigen-related cell adhesion molecule
cfDNA	cell-free DNA
CHRPE	congenital hypertrophy of the retinal pigment epithelium
CI	chronic inflammation
CI	confidence interval
CIMP	CpG island methylator phenotype
CIMP-H	CpG methylator island phenotype-high
CIN	chromosomal instability
CLM	colorectal liver metastasis
cMMRd	constitutional mismatch repair deficiency syndrome
CMS	consensus molecular sub-type
CNAs	copy number alterations
CNN	convolutional neural networks
CNS	Clinical Nurse Specialist
COBRA	Colorectal BReath Analysis
COX	cyclooxygenase
CPET	cardiopulmonary exercise test
CPM	colorectal peritoneal metastasis
CRA	colorectal adenomas
CRC	colorectal cancer
CRF	cancer-related fatigue
CRM	circumferential resection margin
CRS	cytoreductive surgery
CSCs	cancer stem cells
CS	Cowden syndrome
CT	centre of the tumour
CT	computed tomography
CTC	CT colonography
CTCs	circulating tumour cells
ctDNA	circulating tumour DNA
CTLA	cytotoxic T-lymphocyte antigen
CTLs	cytotoxic T cells
DCC	deleted in colorectal cancer'
DCE	dynamic contrast enhancement
DCR	disease control rate
DCs	dendritic cells
ddPCR	droplet digital PCR
DFI	disease-free interval
DFMO	difluoromethylornithine
DFS	disease-free survival
DHA	docosahexaenoic acid 0
DL	deep learning

DLT	dose limiting toxicity
dMMR	MMR deficiency
DPD	dihydropyrimidine dehydrogenase
DR	death receptor
drTF	disease-related treatment failure
DW-MRI	diffusion-weighted MRI
EC	endometrial cancer
ECs	endothelial cells
ECM	extracellular matrix
ECOG	Eastern Cooperative Oncology Group
EGF	epidermal growth factor
EGFR	epidermal growth factor receptor
EMA	European Medicines Agency
EMR	endoscopic mucosal resection
EMT	epithelial mesenchymal transition
EMVI	extra mural venous invasion
EPA	eicosapentaenoic acid
EQD2	equivalent 2 Gy/fraction
ERK	extracellular signal-regulated kinase
ESD	endoscopic submucosal dissection
ESMO	European Society for Medical Oncology
FAP	familial adenomatous polyposis
FDA	Food and Drug Administration
FDG-PET	[18F]2-fluoro 2-deoxy-D-glucose positron emission tomography
FFPE	formalin-fixed paraffin-embedded
FGFR	fibroblast growth factor receptor
FISH	fluorescence *in situ* hybridization
FIT	faecal immunochemical testing
FMT	faecal microbiota transplantation
GDP	Guanosine 5'-diphosphate
gFOBt	guaiac faecal occult blood test
GI	gastrointestinal
GLEM	grey level entropy matrix
GPCR	G protein coupled chemokine receptor
GTP	Guanosine 5'-triphosphate
GWAS	Genome Wide Association Studies
H&E	haematoxylin and eosin
HADS	Hospital Anxiety and Depression Scale
HAI	hepatic arterial infusion
HCC	hepatocellular carcinoma
HCW	healthcare workers
HER	human epidermal growth factor receptor
HES	Hospital Episode Statistics
HGF	hepatocyte growth factor
HHT	haemorrhagic telangiectasia
HIPEC	hyperthermic intraperitoneal chemotherapy
HM	horizontal margin
HMPS	hereditary mixed polyposis syndrome
HNA	Holistic Needs Assessment
HNPCC	hereditary non-polyposis colon cancer
HPCs	hematopoietic progenitor cells
HPT	hepatopancreatobilary
HPV	human papillomavirus
HR	hazard ratio
HRD	homologous recombination deficiency
ICIs	immune checkpoint inhibitors
IDEA	International Duration Evaluation of Adjuvant
iDCs	immature DCs
IDO	indoleamine 2.3-dioxygenase
IFN	interferon
IG	Integrated Gradients
IGF	insulin growth factor
IGRT	image-guided radiotherapy
IHC	immunohistochemical/chemistry
IL	interleukin
IM	invasive margin
iMCS	immature myeloid cells
IRLM	International Registry of Lung Metastases
ISH	*in situ* hybridization
ITT	intention-to-treat
IV	intravenous
IWWD	International Watch & Wait Database
J-CAPP	Japan Colorectal Aspirin Polyps Prevention
JPS	Juvenile polyposis syndrome
JSCCR	Japanese Society for Cancer of the Colon and Rectum
KPI	key performance indicator
KRAS	Kirsten rat sarcoma viral oncogene homolog
LARC	locally advanced rectal cancer
LARS	Low Anterior Resection syndrome
LASSO	Least Absolute Shrinkage and Selection Operator
LCCRT	long-course chemoradiotherapy
LDD	Lhermitte–Duclos disease
LPS	lipopolysaccharide
LRP	layer-wise relevance propagation
LRRC	locally recurrent rectal cancer
LS	Lynch syndrome
LSECtin	liver sinusoidal endothelial cell lectin
LV	leucovorin
LVI	lymphovascular invasion
mAb	monoclonal antibody
MAMs	metastasis-associated macrophages
MANS	*MBD4*-associated neoplasia syndrome
MAP	*MUTYH*-associated polyposis
MAPK	mitogen-activated protein kinase
MCC	Matthews correlation coefficient
MCED	multi-cancer early detection
MCR	mutation cluster region
MCS	mesenchymal stromal cells
MDSCs	myeloid derived suppressor cells
MDT	multidisciplinary team
MET	mesenchymal epithelial transition
MET	metabolic equivalent task
MGMT	O6-methylguanine–DNA methyltransferase
MHC	major histocompatibility complex
MIF	migration inhibitory factor
MMP	metalloproteinase
MMPs	matrix metalloproteinases
MMR	mismatch repair
MMRd	MMR deficiency
MR	Mendelian randomization
MRF	mesorectal fascia
MRI	magnetic resonance imaging
MR-LINAC	MR imaging with a linear accelerator
MSI	microsatellite instability

MSS	microsatellite-stable
MTB	Molecular tumor boards
MWA	microwave ablation
MyD88	myeloid differentiation factor 88
NAP	*NTHL1*-associated polyposis
NAR	neoadjuvant rectal score
NCCTG	North Central Cancer Therapy Group
NCNN	National Comprehensive Cancer Network
NET	neutrophil extracellular trap
NGS	next-generation sequencing
NHS	National Health Service (UK)
NI	non-interiority
NICE	National Institute for Health and Care Excellence
NK	natural killer
NOM	non-operative management
NORCCAP	Norwegian Colorectal Cancer Prevention trial
NOS	non-specific
NPV	negative predictive value
NSAIDs	nonsteroidal anti-inflammatory drugs
NSCLC	non-small cell lung cancer
NTRK	neurotrophic tyrosine receptor kinase
OARs	organs at risk
OS	overall survival
ORR	overall response rate
PAMPs	pathogen-associated molecular patterns
PCCRC	post-colonoscopy colorectal cancer
PCI	Peritoneal Cancer Index
pCR	pathological complete response
PCR	polymerase chain reaction
PD	programmed death
pDC	plasmacytoid DC
PDE	phosphodiesterase
PDX	patient-derived xenograft
PET	positron emission tomography
PFS	progression-free survival
PG	prostaglandins
PGE_2	prostaglandin E2
PHTS	*PTEN* hamartoma tumour syndrome
PI3K	phosphatidylinositol-3 kinase
PICC	peripherally inserted central catheter
PIPAC	pressurized intraperitoneal aerosol chemotherapy
PJS	Peutz–Jeghers syndrome
PLCO	Prostate, Lung, Colorectal and Ovarian cancer screening trial (USA)
PLS	Proteus-like syndrome
PM	pulmonary metastasis
pMMR	MMR proficient
PMP	pseudomyxoma peritonei
PNI	perineural invasion
p.o.	per os (orally)
POI	premature ovarian insufficiency
POLD1	polymerase delta 1
POLE	polymerase epsilon
PPAP	polymerase proofreading-associated polyposis
PPV	positive predictive value
PRs	partial responses
PREMS	patient-reported experience measures
PROMS	patient-reported outcome measures
PS	Proteus syndrome
PSOGI	Peritoneal Surface Oncology Group International
PTV	planned target volume
PulMiCC	Pulmonary Metastasectomy versus Continued Active Monitoring in Colorectal Cancer Trial
PVE	portal vein embolization
QoL	quality of life
RCT	randomized controlled trial
rDCs	regulatory DCs
RFA	radiofrequency ablation
RFS	relapse-/recurrence-free survival
ROC	receiver operating characteristic
ROIs	region of interests
ROS	reactive oxygen species
RR	relative risk
RS	recurrence score
RT	radiotherapy
RT-PCR	reverse transcription PCR
SACT	systemic anti cancer therapy
SBRT	stereotactic body radiotherapy
SCFAs	Short-chain fatty acids
SCNS	Supportive Care Needs Survey
SCORE	Screening for Colon and Rectum trial (Italy)
scRNA-seq	single cell RNAseq
SCRT	short-course radiotherapy
sDCs	stimulatory DCs
SDF	stromal cell-derived factor
SeHCAT	Selenium homocholic acid taurine test
SG	sacituzumab govitecan
SIRT	selective internal radiation therapy
SNVs	single nucleotide variants
SOBP	spread-out Bragg peak
SOC	standard of care
SPS	serrated polyposis syndrome
STAS	spread through air spaces
STS	Society of Thoracic Surgeons
SWOG	Southwest Oncology Group
TAAs	tumour-associated antigens
TACE	transcatheter arterial chemoembolization
TAM	tumour-associated macrophage
TAN	tumour-associated neutrophil
TCGA	The Cancer Genome Atlas
TCR	T-cell receptor
TECs	tumour-associated endothelial cells
TFH	T follicular helper
TGFB	transforming growth factor B
Th	T Helper
TIDCs	tumour-infiltrating dendritic cells
TILs	tumour-infiltrating lymphocytes
TLRs	Toll-like receptors
TLSs	tertiary lymphoid structures
TMB	tumour mutational burden
TME	total mesorectal excision
TME	tumour micro-environment
TNF	tumour necrosis factor
TNM	tumour, nodes, and metastasis/tumor lymph node metastasis
TNT	total neoadjuvant therapy

Treg	regulatory T cells
TRG	tumour regression grade
TSG	tumour suppressor gene
TTF	time to treatment failure
TTR	time to recurrence
UICC	Union for International Cancer Control
USMSTF	US Multi-Society Task Force
USPSTF	US Preventive Services Task Force
VATS	video-assisted thoracoscopic surgery
VEGF	vascular endothelial growth factor
VEGFR	VEGF receptor
VIT	Vision Transformer
VM	vertical margin
VOCs	volatile organic compounds
WES	whole-exome sequencing
WGS	whole-genome sequencing
WSI	whole slide images
WW	watch and wait

Contributors

Anusha Amanullah, University of Edinburgh, UK

Elizabeth Belcher, Consultant Thoracic Surgeon, Oxford University NHS Foundation Trust, UK

Sarah Chamberlain, Dr., University of Southampton University Hospital Southampton NHS Foundation Trust Southampton, UK

Zhebin Chen, PhD, Chengdu Institute of Computer Application/Chinese Academy of Sciences, China

David N. Church, University of Oxford, UK

Håvard Danielsen, Professor, Oslo University Hospital, Norway

Amy Davies, Monash Health and Monash University, Australia

Meng Dou, PhD, Chengdu Institute of Computer Application/Chinese Academy of Sciences, China

James E. East, Professor, Translational Gastroenterology and Liver Unit and Oxford NIHR Biomedical Research Centre, University of Oxford, UK

Elena Élez, Vall d'Hebron Barcelona Hospital, Barcelona, Spain

Jesus Garcia-Foncillas, Professor, Autonomous University of Madrid, Spain

Xiaojing Gu, Postdoctoral Fellow, West China School of Medicine/West China Hospital, China

Glen R. Guerra, Consultant Colorectal Surgeon, Peter MacCallum Cancer Centre and St Vincent's Hospital, Australia

Ernest Hawk, Vice President and Division Head, Cancer Prevention and Population Sciences, The University of Texas MD Anderson Cancer Center, USA

Daniel Hughes, Speciality Trainee in HPB Surgery, University of Oxford, UK

Tarjei S. Hveem, Oslo University Hospital, Norway

Faiz Jabbar, University of Oxford, UK

Dan Jiang, Associate Professor, Department of Pathology and Sichuan University-University of Oxford Huaxi Joint Centre for Gastrointestinal Cancer, West China Hospital, Sichuan University, China

Rebecca Johnson, Oxford University Hospitals Trust, UK

Andreas Kleppe, Oslo University Hospital, Norway

Valentinos Kounnis, Oxford University Hospitals Trust, UK

Xuejiao Li, Clinician, The Affiliated Hospital of Guizhou Medical University, Guizhou Medical University, China

Knut Liestøl, Oslo University Hospital, Norway

Tong Liu, West China Hospital of Sichuan University, China

Yuzhi Liu, West China Hospital of Sichuan University, China

Zijian Lu, Pathologist, Department of Pathology, West China Hospital, Sichuan University, China.

Xiuhe Lv, West China Hospital of Sichuan University, China

Lynda McSorley, Clinical Trials Fellow, Monash Health Translational Precinct, Australia

Brendan Moran, Consultant Surgeon, Peritoneal Malignancy Unit, Basingstoke Hospital, UK

Rebecca Muirhead, Oxford University Hospitals Trust, University of Oxford, UK

Daniel Novelli, Kings College Medical School, Guys and St Thomas' NHS Trust, London, UK

Marco Novelli, Professor, UCL, London, UK

Timothy O'Brien, Research Fellow Patrick G Johnstone Cancer Research Centre Queens University Belfast, Belfast, UK

Sean M. O'Cathail, Consultant Radiation Oncologist, CUH/UCC Cancer Centre, Cork, Ireland Senior Research Fellow, University of Glasgow, Glasgow, UK

Ashley Pheely, Monash University, Australia

Alexandra Poole, Oxford University Hospitals Trust, UK

Javier Ros, Vall d'Hebron University Hospital, Barcelona, Spain

Vasanth Mark Samuel, Consultant Surgeon, Peritoneal Malignancy Unit, Basingstoke Hospital, UK

Nadia Saoudi-Gonzalez, Vall d'Hebron University Hospital, Barcelona, Spain

Eva Segelov, Professor, Monash University, Australia

Michael Shackcloth, Consultant Thoracic Surgeon, Liverpool Heart and Chest Hospital, UK

Vanessa Shearwood, Senior Colorectal Cancer Specialist Nurse, Oxford University Hospitals Trust, UK

Mike Silva, Conulstant HPB Surgeon, Oxford University Hospitals Trust, Oxford, UK

Josep Tabernero, Vall d'Hebron Institute of Oncology, Spain

Ian Tomlinson, Professor, University of Oxford, UK

Anoop Kozhippatu Varghese, Specialist Gastroenterologist, Lifeline Hospital, Abu Dhabi, United Arab Emirates

Eduardo Vilar-Sanchez, Professor, Department of Clinical Cancer Prevention, The University of Texas MD Anderson Cancer Center, USA

Jin Wang, West China Hospital of Sichuan University, China

Xin Wang, Professor of Cancer Medicine and Radiotherapy, West China Hospital, Sichuan University, China

Zijing Wang, West China Hospital of Sichuan University, China

Alex Gordon-Weeks, Consultant HPB Surgeon, Oxford, UK

Xianhong Xu, Oxford Cancer Biomarkers University of Bath, UK

Jinlin Yang, Professor, Department of Gastroenterology and Hepatology and Sichuan University-University of Oxford Huaxi Joint Centre for Gastrointestinal Cancer, West China Hospital, Sichuan University, China

Xian Zhang, Pathologist, Department of Pathology, West China Hospital, Sichuan University, China

SECTION 1
Pathology and aetiology

1

Colorectal cancer genetics

Anusha Amanullah and Ian Tomlinson

Brief history

A classic example of a Mendelian colorectal cancer (CRC) syndrome is familial adenomatous polyposis (FAP), said to be first reported by Sklifasowski in 1881 (Bülow et al., 2006), in which patients can develop hundreds or thousands of polyps and cancers in any part of the intestines, but are also predisposed to cancers of the thyroid and adrenal glands, benign fibrous desmoid tumours, and jaw cysts.

As knowledge increases, the number of different clinical features reliably associated with each CRC syndrome tends to increase over time, sometimes including tumours for which the magnitude of the increased risks is modest and/or of little clinical importance, in contrast to very high risks of CRC. Based on the clinical features of polyps, Mendelian CRC syndromes can be broadly placed into five groups: adenomatous polyposis; hamartomatous polyposis; serrated polyposis; hereditary mixed polyposis; and cancer without polyposis, otherwise known as Lynch syndrome (Tomlinson, 2015; Daca Alcarez et al., 2021). We show below that these classifiers have largely been replaced by a definition of disease defined by the identification of the gene that carries the germline mutations. There is often, nonetheless, considerable clinical heterogeneity among individuals with different, but functionally similar, mutations in the same CRC-predisposing gene. Furthermore, some germline mutations in the known genes remain undetectable with standard methods, and this can lead to diagnostic uncertainty. Finally, genetic causes have not been found for many patients with multiple colorectal polyps or early onset CRC. As a result, the old clinical classifications of inherited CRC still retain some use in patient diagnosis and management. At the time of writing (2024), cancer genetics is arguably leaving an exciting period of disease gene discovery and entering a period of different challenges, namely managing genetic cancer risk on an individual basis.

Lynch syndrome: The most common Mendelian cause of CRC, but an exception

CRC predisposition syndromes

The first family of this type was reported by Aldred Warthin in 1913. The kindred predominantly exhibited cases of uterine, stomach, and colorectal cancer, with multi-generational inheritance, suggestive of a Mendelian dominant trait (Warthin, 1913). In 1962, a similar case was encountered by Henry Lynch, who also noted the absence of multiple adenomatous polyps. The clinical features of these families, especially compared with FAP, was suggestive of a different, presumably genetic aetiology (Lynch et al., 1966). These CRC families went by various names for many years, most notably hereditary nonpolyposis colorectal cancer (HNPCC). The name Lynch syndrome (LS) has since come to be universally adopted, at least for families and individuals with a specific, identified genetic aetiology (see below).

The presence of a high proportion of tumours in the proximal colon was also observed in LS cases in 1977 (Lynch et al., 1977). However, the genetic underpinning of Lynch syndrome only started to unfold in the 1990s when microsatellite instability (MSI) was characterized in the cancers of LS-type cases (Aaltonen et al., 1993; Ionov et al., 1993; Thibodeau et al., 1993). MSI is a tendency for short repeat sequences in the cancer genome (e.g. repeats of single nucleotides or dinucleotides, known as microsatellites) to acquire short insertion or deletion mutations. Around the same time, a series of basic science experiments on lower organisms showed MSI as a hallmark of defective DNA mismatch repair (MMR) activity (Levinson & Gutman, 1987; Strand et al., 1993). Also in parallel, in 1993, the first genetic locus associated with Lynch syndrome was mapped in families to a genomic region on the short arm of chromosome 2 by linkage analysis (Peltomäki et al., 1993). After a few months, Fishel and Leach et al. mapped one of the human MMR genes, *MSH2*, to the chromosome 2 locus (2p22-21) and reported deleterious germline mutations in Lynch syndrome families (Fishel et al., 1993; Leach et al., 1993). In 1994, the second LS locus (Chr3p21–23) was found to be *MLH1*, another MMR gene (Bronner et al., 1994; Papadopoulos et al., 1994). Simultaneously, another LS MMR gene, *PMS2* (Chr7p22), was found (Nicolaides et al., 1994). In 1997, Miyaki et al. reported the pathogenic mutations of *MSH6* in the LS family with a high incidence of extracolonic tumours and suggested that LS cases might show phenotypic heterogeneity depending on the MMR gene involved (Miyaki et al., 1997). A small subset of LS cases have germline *MSH2* mutations through disruption of a distal control element that actually lies within the nearby *EPCAM* gene, and other cases with germline hypermethylation of *MSH2* or *MLH1* promoters have been found (Chan et al., 2006; Niessen et al., 2009).

The LS mutations require a second somatic (acquired) hit in normal cells to cause loss of MMR activity. MMR normally acts as part of a multi-layer safety net to repair random errors created when DNA replicates, and MMR deficiency (MMRd) thus increases the burden of random somatic mutations, resulting in a 'mutator phenotype'. Other repair systems, notably polymerase proofreading repair (see below), also act to correct replication errors, and MMR seems particularly important in correcting small insertions and deletions of bases, hence the MSI molecular phenotype. MMR defects can be reflected in specific mutational signatures, including COSMIC single base substitution signatures SBS6, SBS14, SBS15, SBS20, SBS21, SBS26, and SBS44 (Sondka et al., 2024). Since this system acts in all cells, there is quite a broad tumour spectrum in LS, including malignancies of not only the colorectum but also of the endometrium, skin, stomach, small bowel, hepatobiliary system, urinary tract, ovary, pancreas, and brain (Lynch et al., 2015; Abildgaard et al., 2023; Li et al., 2021). LS can present as early as the second decade of life, with mean ages of 45–60 years for CRC and 47–55 years for endometrial cancer (EC) (Gambini et al., 2022). A few gene carriers remain cancer-free throughout an average lifespan, particularly those with *MSH6* or *PMS2* variants (Dominguez-Valentin et al., 2020; Sidenna et al., 2022). Historically, phenotypic variants of HNPCC have been reported, namely Muir-Torre syndrome (sebaceous neoplasms of the skin) and Turcot syndrome (brain tumours), but these are now encompassed in LS. There are various genotype–phenotype associations in LS (Lynch et al., 2006; Sidenna et al., 2022), including risks by age and cancer type (Dominguez-Valentin et al., 2020; Møller et al., 2022). Cancer prevention in LS is complex, but often includes one- to two-yearly colonoscopy to remove polyps and, in some centres, chemoprevention measures (Vasen et al., 2013; Seppälä et al., 2021; Serrano et al., 2022). Surveillance of the other organs most prone to tumours is also often performed, although formal evidence of efficacy is often lacking, even though LS is a relatively common Mendelian disease.

It is now thought that LS contributes about 3% of all CRCs (Abildgaard et al., 2023). In most cases of Lynch syndrome (70%), germline mono-allelic mutations are found in *MLH1* and *MSH2*, while the rest are almost all found in *MSH6* and *PMS2* (Peltomäki, 2016). The proportion of LS mutations that are cryptic to molecular detection is unclear. There is evidence that an important proportion of LS cases is undiagnosed, and calls have been made for population testing, or at least testing of all cases with MSI-positive CRCs or ECs (McRonald et al., 2024). It is of note that about 15% of sporadic CRCs with no major genetic basis acquire MMR deficiency, mostly through *MLH1* promoter methylation (albeit occasionally through somatic *MSH2* or *MLH1* mutation), and this sub-group of CRCs has distinct clinical features, including survival and response to treatment (Sinicrope, 2010). Current clinical interest is focused on helping patients by exploiting the immune response elicited by the large number of neo-antigens thought to be produced by MMR-deficient tumours. Immune therapies for patients with these cancers are already in use, and there are plans to vaccinate LS cases to prevent cancer, based on proteins particularly to acquired mutations owing to deficient MMR (Therkildsen et al., 2021).

Constitutional mismatch repair deficiency (cMMRd) syndrome

Constitutional mismatch repair deficiency syndrome (cMMRd) is a very rare autosomal recessive syndrome. Unlike LS, which results from the presence of a monoallelic germline mutation in MMR genes, cMMRd results from homozygous or compound heterozygous germline mutations within the MMR genes. Any of the four LS genes can cause cMMRd, but it appears that *PMS2* is a particularly common culprit. Whilst cMMRd has a stronger, universal mutator phenotype than LS, there is evidence that the individual mutations found in cMMRd have weaker effects on the mutation rate than LS mutations, thus allowing the entire body to tolerate both copies of the gene being deficient (Wimmer & Etzler, 2008). cMMRd has a variable phenotype that is generally more severe than LS, with earlier onset and a larger number of tumours. It is characterized by the paediatric onset of various lesions, including malignant tumours of the brain, blood, endometrium, urinary tract, small bowel, and colorectum (occasionally with multiple adenomatous polyps) (Will et al., 2007; Rana & Syngal, 2017), in addition to café-au-lait spots, neurofibromas, and general developmental delay.

Adenomatous polyposis CRC predisposition syndromes

Although the chance that an individual (benign) colorectal adenoma will become cancerous appears low, most sporadic CRCs do result from the progression to malignancy of a colorectal adenoma (CRA) or polyp. Although CRAs are common in the general population, individuals predisposed to develop tens, hundreds, or thousands of adenomas are at greatly increased risk of CRC. There seem to be two aetiological sub-types of adenoma predisposition syndrome: (i) dominant inheritance (in the *APC* gene), in which activation of the Wnt molecular signalling pathway results from one inherited protein-inactivating mutation, followed by a spontaneous mutation in the wildtype copy of the gene that normal cells acquire at random; or (ii) an inherited deficiency in DNA repair (usually recessive, often associated with mutations in the *MUTYH* gene) that causes a genome-wide increase in a specific type of base substitution mutation. Why these two very different defects should cause similar (and sometimes indistinguishable) clinical features is unclear. We know that the somatic driver (cancer-promoting) mutations present in tumours in both types of syndromes are very similar, and it is tempting to speculate that the presence of one major mutant driver allele (e.g. *APC* loss-of-function) is roughly equivalent to the more rapid acquisition of driver mutations caused by the DNA repair defect. However, there is a limit on phenotypic severity, such that patients cannot develop too many tumours or else the bowel would be dysfunctional. We will outline the differing characteristics of these two syndromes; and also describe some of the less common polyposis syndromes.

Familial adenomatous polyposis (FAP)

The germline mutation underlying familial adenomatous polyposis (FAP), a loss-of-function variant in the *APC* gene, was first reported in 1991 (Groden et al., 1991; Nishisho et al., 1991). *APC* encodes a scaffold protein that controls Wnt signalling by, in effect, destroying the main Wnt effector protein, β-catenin. Loss of function mutations in both copies of *APC* result in constitutive activation of the Wnt signalling pathway in the cell. This occurs in about 90% of sporadic CRCs through two somatic *APC* mutations, whereas only one somatic mutation is required in FAP owing to inheritance of one aberrant copy of *APC*. FAP is thus an autosomal dominant disorder and accounts for around 1% of all CRC cases (Vasen et al., 2008). It is marked by the presence of hundreds to thousands of adenomatous polyps in the colorectum, with a high risk of transforming into a carcinoma at an early age. FAP also exhibits extra-colonic cancers, such as those of the duodenum, thyroid, pancreas, liver, adrenal cortex, and brain. Fibroblastic tumours, known as intra-abdominal desmoids, are also common, especially after surgery. Non-tumour features also occur, including a benign proliferation termed congenital hypertrophy of the retinal pigment epithelium (CHRPE), and the epidermoid cysts and dental abnormalities present in the FAP variant historically called Gardner syndrome (Panjwani et al., 2011). Turcot syndrome type 2 is another variant of FAP, characterized by brain malignancy, CRC, and multiple colorectal adenmoas (CRAs) (Leoz et al., 2015).

The severity of FAP is influenced by the location of the patient's germline *APC* mutation in the gene. This provides a classic example of genotype–phenotype association within a single gene (as opposed to a link between phenotype and predisposition gene, as occurs across the Mendelian CRC syndromes in general). Patients with germline *APC* mutations between codons 1250 and 1464 are linked to a severe form of FAP (often with thousands of colorectal polyps), while mutations before codon 157, after codon 1595, and in exon nine (codons 213–412) are associated with a milder form, comprising tens of CRAs, that is known as attenuated familial adenomatous polyposis (AFAP) (Leoz et al., 2015). Duodenal cancer is, however, more common in individuals with mutations before codon 1395 and in between codons 564 and 1493 (Nieuwenhuis & Vasen, 2007).

FAP patients require highly specialist care. AFAP can sometimes be managed by regular colonoscopy, but CRC risk in classical FAP is usually reduced by removal of most or all of the large bowel, accompanied by measures to support functioning of the residual intestines. Duodenal cancer risk requires regular upper gastrointestinal endoscopy. Desmoids remain a challenging tumour to manage and are associated with considerable morbidity. Chemoprevention has not yet achieved consistent success, but it does remain a topic of investigation.

MUTYH-associated polyposis (MAP)

The *MUTYH* gene encodes a DNA glycosylase that works in the base excision repair pathway (BER), which principally acts to correct mis-paired bases in the context of DNA damage rather than replication. *MUTYH* specifically acts by removing bases that are mismatched owing to oxidative damage. The most common mismatch is between 8-oxoguanine and adenine, which typically can cause G > T transversion mutations in *MUTYH*-deficient cells (although other mutational outcomes are possible). In 2002, biallelic germline mutations in *MUTYH* were found to cause an autosomal recessive CRA and CRC predisposition syndrome (Al-Tassan et al., 2002). This hereditary syndrome, known as *MUTYH*-associated polyposis (MAP), contributes to about 0.5% of CRC cases. The two most common germline variants associated with MAP in northern Europeans are Y165C and G382D, with different mutations over-represented in other ancestral groups (e.g. E466X and Y90X in south Asians). *MUTYH*-associated carcinogenesis is characterized by excess somatic G: C > T: A transversions throughout the genome and in driver genes such as *APC* and *KRAS*. The morphology of polyps in MAP patients mainly resembles that of attenuated FAP (Dolwani et al., 2007; Khan et al., 2017; Magrin et al., 2022). MAP cases also show extracolonic manifestations, particularly duodenal tumours and possibly cancers of other sites. MAP tumours are generally microsatellite-stable (Vanesio et al., 2012; Magrin et al., 2022). Management of MAP is otherwise similar to that of AFAP.

Polymerase proofreading-associated polyposis (PPAP)

Polymerase epsilon and delta are the main polymerases involved in replication of the leading and lagging DNA strands in all dividing cells, respectively. They each contain an exonuclease domain for proofreading activity to remove mis-paired bases on the nascent DNA strand. In 2012, Palles et al. reported dominantly inherited germline mutations in the exonuclease domains of *POLE* (Leu424Val) and *POLD1* (Ser478Asn) in families with multiple CRAs, CRC, and EC (Palles et al., 2013). Several other pathogenic and likely pathogenic genetic mutations have since been found in the exonuclease domain of *POLE* (a.a residues 268–471) and *POLD1* (a.a residues 304–533). These mutations are thought unlikely to affect the polymerase functions of these proteins, and instead selectively abrogate accurate proofreading. The mutations have functional effects in the heterozygous state, and it is unclear whether second hits are required, in contrast to LS (Sherwood et al., 2023). The syndrome, known as polymerase proofreading-associated polyposis (PPAP), may include a variety of additional cancer types, including tumours of the breast, brain, duodenum, and ovary (Palles et al., 2022). The resultant tumours have a so-called ultra-mutator phenotype and characteristic mutational signatures (principally SBS10, SBS14 ,and SBS20). Specific driver gene mutations are also found, such as *APC* p.R1114X and *TP53* p.R213X (Palles et al., 2013; Heitzer & Tomlinson, 2014; Sherwood et al., 2023). Whilst PPAP can sometimes resembles LS, microsatellite-stable (MSS) tumours and multiple CRAs are much more common in the former. Polymerase proofreading-associated syndrome accounts for approximately 0.3–0.7% of CRC and polyposis cases (Palles et al., 2013; Bellido et al., 2016; Mur et al., 2020). Somatic proofreading mutations in polymerase ε and δ are also present in ~2% of sporadic CRCs and 8% of ECs.

NTHL1-associated polyposis (NAP)

NTHL1 also belongs to the family of base excision repair (BER) genes and encodes a bifunctional glycosylase which removes oxidized pyrimidines and ring-opened purines. In 2015, Weren et al. showed that biallelic germline mutations in the *NTHL1* gene can predispose to CRAs and CRC (Weren et al., 2015). The first cases detected, from the Netherlands, carried homozygous *NTHL1* C268C > T (p.Gln90*) germline mutations. Other loss-of-function mutations have since been found across ancestral groups. The tumour spectrum in NAP is not well understood outside the colorectum, but may include duodenal, endometrial, breast, bladder, basal cell, and head-and-neck cancer (Rivera et al., 2015). The mutational profile of NAP (signature SBS30) mostly shows CA > TA and CC > TA substitutions which occur at an increased frequency in NTHL1-deficient cells (Sondka et al., 2024).

MBD4-associated neoplasia syndrome (MANS)

MBD4 encodes a BER glycosylase that repairs C > T mismatches resulting from spontaneous 5'-methylcytosine deamination. Biallelic germline loss of function variants of *MBD4* cause an autosomal recessive syndrome of colorectal polyposis and several other tumours not found in other CRC syndromes, including acute myeloid leukaemia and myelodysplasia, uveal melanoma, and schwannoma (Palles et al., 2022). The MBD4 mutations increase the somatic mutation burden and produce a CpG > TpG mutational signature very similar to the very common signature SBS1, which is thought to arise from the same mutational process that occasionally escapes repair in MBD4-proficient cells (Terradas et al., 2023). As a result, driver gene mutations in MANS tumours are often similar to those in sporadic tumours, although the overall burden of mutations is greatly increased in the former.

Hamartomatous polyposis syndromes

Hamartomatous polyps are thought to resemble a non-neoplastic growth, but are generally poorly understood. These polyps can occur as solitary, sporadic lesions, in which case there is believed to be a very low risk of malignant progression and rarely an inherited component. Here, however, we shall focus on the inherited hamartoma syndromes.

Peutz–Jeghers syndrome (PJS)

Peutz–Jeghers syndrome (PJS) is perhaps the best known hamartomatous polyposis syndrome, given its unusual classical combination of gastrointestinal polyps and freckle-like lesions on the face, buccal mucosa, and other sites. PJS cases are often identified based on family history or as a result of the freckling, but can present as children with intestinal obstruction caused by volvulus or intussusception secondary to classical polyps that are non-dysplastic, with a prominent smooth muscle core, and often a cauliflower-like macroscopic appearance. PJS can also present in adults owing to the development of tumours. PJS is an autosomal dominant syndrome caused by germline mutations in the *STK11* (*LKB1*) gene, which encodes a serine-threonine kinase that regulates energy metabolism and cellular polarity (Jelsig et al., 2024; Gorji & Albrecht, 2023). The mutation leads to the loss of STK11-AMPK regulation of the mTOR pathway, resulting in its constitutional activation. PJS increases the risk of tumours in the gastrointestinal tract and extra-intestinal tissues including the pancreas, cervix, thyroid, breast, testes, ovary, and uterus. The mucocutaneous hyperpigmentation can vary greatly and may surround the oral cavity, eyes, nostrils, and anus. The increased risk of multiple tumour types makes the preventive management of PJS patients difficult (Wagner et al., 2021; Gorji & Albrecht, 2023). Polyp and CRC risk is generally managed by one- to two-yearly colonoscopy.

Juvenile polyposis syndrome (JPS)

Juvenile polyposis syndrome (JPS) is a dominant condition leading to a predisposition to hamartomatous polyps in the gastrointestinal tract, and caused by pathogenic germline mutations in *SMAD4* and *BMPR1A*: Both genes are involved in the TGFβ/bone morphogenetic protein (BMP) signalling pathway, and the mutations are expected to reduce signalling. JPS polyps typically have a non-dysplastic, rounded appearance with large cysts and can be found in the upper and lower gastrointestinal (GI) tract. CRAs are also often present; it is unclear whether these have developed from juvenile polyps. CRC and upper GI malignancy risks are high (Brosens et al., 2007; Collins, 2024), but can probably be reduced by regular colonoscopy and upper GI endoscopy. JPS patients with *SMAD4* mutations are reported to have a greater risk of developing GI malignancies than those with *BMPR1A* mutations. JPS, particularly the *SMAD4* type, is also associated in a minority of cases with vascular malformations, including haemorrhagic telangiectasia (HHT) and pulmonary hypertension (Gallione et al., 2004; Hashimoto et al., 2020; Liu et al., 2020; Kang et al., 2021). Three sub-types of JPS are sometimes recognized (Larsen et al., 2003), although they may actually reflect a phenotypic continuum: (i) juvenile polyposis of infancy, caused by rare, contiguous deletion of *BMPR1A* and *PTEN*, which is mostly observed in children and the clinical manifestations of which include macrocephaly, digital clubbing, hypotonia, hypoproteinaemia, malnutrition, bloody diarrhoea, and sessile or pedunculated polyps throughout the GI tract; (ii) juvenile polyposis coli, which is phenotypically limited to colorectal regions and is associated with *SMAD4* and *BMPR1A* heterozygous mutations; and (iii) generalized juvenile polyposis in which polyps are found diffusely throughout the GI tract. A substantial minority of JPS cases have no detectable *SMAD4* or *BMPR1A* mutation. Both *SMAD4* and *BMPR1A* are somatic driver genes in CRCs.

PTEN hamartoma tumour syndrome (PHTS)

As the name suggests *PTEN* hamartoma tumour syndrome (PHTS) comprises a group of apparently different disorders associated with pathogenic germline mutations in the *PTEN* gene. *PTEN* is a tumour suppressor that is a key modulator in mTOR and PI3K-AKT/PKB signalling, where mutations can result in abnormal cellular regulation. PHTS commonly includes Cowden syndrome (CS), Bannayan Riley–Ruvalcaba syndrome (BRRS), Proteus syndrome (PS), and Proteus-like syndrome (PLS) (Pilarski, 2019). Cowden syndrome is a rare autosomal dominant multisystemic disorder, first reported in 1963 and later in 1997 the germline *PTEN* mutations were found in the individuals with this disorder (Lloyd & Dennis, 1963; Liaw et al., 1997). It presents a broad spectrum of clinical manifestations including hamartomatous polyps in the GI tract, macrocephaly, Lhermitte–Duclos disease (LDD), multiple mucocutaneous lesions and malignancies of the breast, thyroid, endometrium, colon, and skin (Dragoo et al., 2021). BRRS is a rare paediatric disorder and is relatively less explored. Its clinical features resemble much of CS including GI hamartomas, macrocephaly, developmental delay, vascular anomalies, and penile mucocutaneous lesions (Pilarski, 2019; Plamper et al., 2022). Proteus syndrome and Proteus-like syndrome clinically present with nervous system abnormality, structural deformity, scoliosis, ophthalmic complications, and pulmonary malformations (Plamper et al., 2022).

The intestinal cancer risk associated with *PTEN* intestinal hamartomas is unclear, although many PHTS cases are offered regular colonoscopic screening.

Serrated polyposis syndrome (SPS)

Serrated polyposis syndrome is characterized by the presence of multiple colorectal polyps with a serrated/hyperplastic morphology. Diagnostic criteria have been developed in which the diagnosis is favoured by polyps that are large and/or in the proximal colon, but this is predominantly a pragmatic classification to prevent over-screening of older individuals with low-risk polyps (e.g. small rectal hyperplastic polyps). In 2014, Gala et al. reported the germline pathogenic mutation in *RNF43* to be associated with this syndrome (Gala et al., 2014), but since then only six more *RNF43* families, mostly with dominant inheritance, have been described (Taupin et al., 2015; Buchana et al., 2017; Yan et al., 2017; Quintana et al., 2018; Mikaeel et al., 2022; Chan et al., 2024). *RNF43* acts as a tumour suppressor gene by negatively regulating the Wnt signalling pathway, and it would be expected that the polyps that develop in the SPS families would be dysplastic (e.g. serrated adenomas), rather than large hyperplastic lesions. Whilst evidence indicates that germline *RNF43* mutations do cause SPS, the phenotype and molecular genetic mechanisms behind this condition remain unclear.

Hereditary mixed polyposis syndrome (HMPS)

As the name suggests, HMPS is an autosomal dominant condition typified by polyps with mixed histological features, whether adenomatous, serrated, or hamartomatous (JP or PJ). Individual polyps may be mixed, or a patient may have polyps of different types. CRC risk is high without preventive measures, which generally take the form of one- to two-yearly colonoscopy as, uniquely, no extracolonic features are known in HMPS. Initially, HMPS shown in a set of Ashkenazi Jewish families to be caused by a non-coding 40kb duplication upstream of the BMP antagonist *GREM1* (Jaeger et al., 2012; Lieberman et al., 2017). This mutation affects regulatory elements and results in expression of *GREM1* in the colorectal epithelium, whereas it is usually expressed in the mesenchymal myofibroblasts. The upstream and downstream mechanisms are not yet known. Tumours do not require second hits at *GREM1*. More recently, other structural variants upstream of *GREM1*, including 16kb and 24kb duplications, have been associated with HMPS in non-Ashkenazi families (Venkatachalam et al., 2011; Rohlin et al., 2016).

Multiple colorectal polyps of unknown aetiology

Population bowel cancer screening and advancements in colonoscopy techniques have significantly increased the detection of multiple adenomatous and/or serrated polyps, particularly among individuals in their fifties and sixties. Concurrently, the growing awareness of the familial aspect of cancer syndromes has encouraged the integration of genetic variant identification into routine clinical practice. Interestingly, a subset of individuals is observed to show the presence of multiple polyps suggestive of familial cancer syndromes like FAP or MAP. They occasionally carry mutations in established Mendelian cancer syndrome genes in the absence of family history (e.g. MAP or other recessive conditions, *de novo* LS mutations, or mosaicism for *APC*). The majority of such cases may, however, represent chance occurrence of somatic mutations, unknown environmental exposures or individuals who carry a high burden of low-risk predisposition genes or polymorphisms (see below) (Cheng et al., 2015). The management of such cases and their families is not established. Specifically, the need for regular colonoscopy, or surveillance by methods such as faecal testing for blood, is not yet established.

Common genetic influences on CRC risk

Familial clustering and twin studies have estimated that around 35% of the variation in CRC risk can be explained by genetic factors. The Mendelian syndromes explain only some of that risk, and the remaining estimated heritability could be attributed to various factors, not all of them truly genetic.

Familial clustering of CRC outside the Mendelian syndromes is often found, and it is sometimes termed Familial Colorectal Cancer Type X (or similar). Whether this represents a real clinical or aetiological entity remains highly uncertain, but it could, in theory, result from germline variants that are a little more common than, say, LS variants, yet have moderate effects on CRC risk. To date, there exist very few genetic variants known to predispose to CRC that could be described as non-rare (population genotype frequency approximately 0.5–2%), that is, more common than the Mendelian syndromes, yet have moderate effect sizes (e.g. two- to threefold increased risk (Carmona & Tomlinson, 2016). Such variants might yet await discovery in well-powered studies, and thereby contribute to the known causes of CRC heritability. A more successful activity in the past 15 years has been Genome Wide Association Studies (GWAS) for CRC in order to identify common genetic variants (polymorphisms) that affect CRC risk in the general population. These polymorphisms typically have a high frequency (allele frequency > 5%), and modest effects on risk (typically 5% to 20% increase or decrease per allele). Over 200 polymorphisms that affect CRC risk are now known in Asian and European populations (Fernandez-Rozadilla et al., 2023). Genetic risk through common alleles is unlikely to contribute much to explaining CRC heritability, but it has two clear uses. First, polymorphism-based genetic risk generally follows a normal distribution and individuals could be offered special preventive measures if, say, they lay on the right-hand tail of that risk distribution. For example, CRC screening could begin at an earlier age. The use of polymorphisms in this way remains controversial, even when genetic and non-genetic risk factors are combined into a risk score. In part, this reflects the possible costs and acceptability of genetic testing in this setting that could outweigh the predicted modest benefits of risk scores on CRA and CRC detection.

A further insight from GWAS is mechanistic. If the gene targeted by a risk polymorphism can be identified, we can obtain valuable clues about CRC aetiology. This can be extended into methods such as Mendelian randomization (MR) that aim to establish causality, if a polymorphism is linked not only to CRC but to an 'intermediate phenotype' or risk factor that can be modified. Eventually chemoprevention strategies based on CRC risk polymorphism data could be identified.

A minor contribution to the heritability of CRC might come from causal risk factors for CRC (e.g. diabetes mellitus, inflammatory bowel disease) that themselves have a genetic component derived from polymorphisms. Such polymorphisms individually will have too weak an effect to be detected using current CRC GWAS, but they are indeed contributors to CRC heritability.

Table 1.1 A comparison of the various inherited CRC syndromes

	Nonpolyposis CRC	Adenomatous Polyposis						Hamartomatous Polyposis			Serrated Polyposis	Mixed Polyposis
Mendelian Syndrome	Lynch Syndrome	Constitutional Mismatch Repair Deficiency Syndrome (CMMRD)	Familial Adenomatous Polyposis (FAP) and Attenuated Familial Adenomatous Polyposis (AFAP)	Polymerase Proofreading Associated Polyposis (PPAP)	*MUTYH* Associated Polyposis (MAP)	*NTHL1* Associated Polyposis Syndrome (NAPS)	*MBD4* Associated Neoplasia Syndrome (MANS)	Peutz-Jeghers Syndrome (PJS)	Juvenile Polyposis Syndrome (JPS)	*PTEN* Hamartoma Tumor Syndrome (PHTS)	Serrated Polyposis Syndrome (SPS)	Hereditary Mixed Polyposis Syndrome (HMPS)
Mutated Genes	*MSH2* *MLH1* *MSH6* *PMS2* *MSH3**	*MSH2* *MLH1* *MSH6* *PMS2*	*APC*	*POLE* *POLD1*	*MUTYH*	*NTHL1*	*MBD4*	*STK11*	*BMPR1A* *SMAD4*	*PTEN*	*RNF43*	*GREM1*
Mode of Inheritance	Autosomal Dominant	Autosomal Recessive	Autosomal Dominant	Autosomal Dominant	Autosomal Recessive	Autosomal Recessive	Autosomal Recessive	Autosomal Dominant	Autosomal Dominant	Autosomal Dominant	Autosomal Dominant	Autosomal Dominant
Affected Pathways	Mismatch Repair Pathway	Mismatch Repair Pathway	Wnt Signalling Pathway	Polymerase Proofreading	Base Excision Repair Pathway	Base Excision Repair Pathway	Base Excision Repair Pathway	mTOR Signalling Pathway	TGFβ/BMP Signalling Pathway	PI3K/AKT Signalling Pathway	Wnt Signalling Pathway	BMP Signalling Pathway
Mutational Signatures	SBS6 SBS14 SBS15 SBS20 SBS21 SBS26 SBS44	SBS6 SBS14 SBS15 SBS20 SBS21 SBS26 SBS44		SBS10a SBS10b SBS10c SBS10d SBS14 SBS20	SBS36	SBS30	SBS1					

Mendelian Colorectal Cancer Syndrome: The figure illustrates various Mendelian colorectal cancer syndromes, categorised by the clinical features of polyps, which are represented in different colours. For each colorectal cancer syndrome, the associated candidate genes with germline mutations, the mode of inheritance, affected signalling pathways, and relevant mutational signatures are listed. A '*' symbol next to a gene name indicates that additional robust evidence is needed to link that gene to the disease confidently.

Molecular diagnostics

Currently, CRC risk scores based on polymorphisms and non-genetic risk factors are barely used in clinical practice, even though some decisions on patient management in the Genetics Clinic are arguably based on less solid foundations (e.g. on family history alone). Molecular analysis of CRC cases is thus generally limited to screening for the Mendelian syndromes. There is phenotypic overlap between most of the Mendelian syndromes which suggests that analysis of all genes together is worthwhile. That task that could be achieved using a 16-gene panel, or whole genome sequencing (with its greater ability to detect the more unusual mutation types). Interpretation of genetic variants is often helped, or sometimes preceded, by tumour analysis, including immunohistochemistry for MMR protein loss, *MLH1* promoter methylation, MSI or mutation signature analysis using exomes or genomes, second hits at tumour suppressor loci, and driver gene mutation spectra. This ability to put together multiple strands of evidence is likely to be increasingly important for variant interpretation.

Conclusions and future directions

Over the next decade, it is likely that colorectal cancer genetic investigation will move towards exploring more deeply the multifactorial inheritance of the vast majority of colorectal cancers. It is clear that, although it is important to identify those who have a very strong inherited cause, such as Lynch syndrome or FAP, most cancers, even in 'younger' patients, will be driven by a broader base of multiple inherited genes, each having a weak effect on risk, rather than a single driving, easily characterizable dominant genetic driver. Through mining databases, both from large clinical trials, and whole population genomic projects, and using excellent AI systems, these more common roots of multifactorial inheritance will become clear.

REFERENCES

Aaltonen, L. A., Peltomäki, P., Leach, F. S., et al. (1993). Clues to the pathogenesis of familial colorectal cancer. *Science*, *260*(5109), 812–816.

Abildgaard, A. B., Nielsen, S. V., Bernstein, I., et al. (2023). Lynch syndrome, molecular mechanisms and variant classification. *British Journal of Cancer*, *128*(5), 726–734.

Al-Tassan, N., Chmiel, N. H., Maynard, J., et al. (2002). Inherited variants of MYH associated with somatic G: C→ T: A mutations in colorectal tumors. *Nature Genetics*, *30*(2), 227–232.

Bellido, F., Pineda, M., Aiza, G., et al. (2016). POLE and POLD1 mutations in 529 kindred with familial colorectal cancer and/or polyposis: review of reported cases and recommendations for genetic testing and surveillance. *Genetics in Medicine* *18*(4), 325–332.

Bronner, C. E., Baker, S. M., Morrison, P. T., et al. (1994). Mutation in the DNA mismatch repair gene homologue hMLH 1 is associated with hereditary non-polyposis colon cancer. *Nature*, *368*(6468), 258–261.

Brosens, L. A., Van Hattem, A., Hylind, L. M., et al. (2007). Risk of colorectal cancer in juvenile polyposis. *Gut*, *56*(7), 965–967.

Buchanan, D. D., Clendenning, M., Zhuoer, L., et al. (2017). Lack of evidence for germline RNF43 mutations in patients with serrated polyposis syndrome from a large multinational study. *Gut*, *66*(6), 1170–1172.

Bülow, S., Berk, T., & Neale, K. The history of familial adenomatous polyposis. (2006). *Familial Cancer*, *5*(3), 213–220.

Carmona, L. G., & Tomlinson, I. (2016). The hunting of the snark: whither genome-wide association studies for colorectal cancer? *Gastroenterology*, *150*(7), 1528–1530.

Chan, J. M., Clendenning, M., Joseland, S., et al. (2024). Inherited BRCA1 and RNF43 pathogenic variants in a familial colorectal cancer type X family. *Familial Cancer*, *23*(1), 9–21.

Chan, T. L., Yuen, S. T., Kong, C. K., et al. (2006). Heritable germline epimutation of MSH2 in a family with hereditary nonpolyposis colorectal cancer. *Nature Genetics*, *38*(10), 1178–1183.

Cheng, T. H., Gorman, M., Martin, L., et al. (2015). Common colorectal cancer risk alleles contribute to the multiple colorectal adenoma phenotype, but do not influence colonic polyposis in FAP. *European Journal of Human Genetics*, *23*(2), 260–263.

Collins, P. (2024). Inherited gastrointestinal cancer syndromes. *Medicine*, *52*(5), 268–270.

Daca Alvarez, M., Quintana, I., Terradas, M., et al. (2021). The inherited and familial component of early-onset colorectal cancer. *Cell*, *10*(3), 710.

Dolwani, S., Williams, G. T., West, K. P., et al. (2007). Analysis of inherited MYH/(MutYH) mutations in British Asian patients with colorectal cancer. *Gut*, *56*(4), 593.

Dominguez-Valentin, M., Sampson, J. R., Seppälä, T.T., et al. (2020). Cancer risks by gene, age, and gender in 6350 carriers of pathogenic mismatch repair variants: findings from the Prospective Lynch Syndrome Database. *Genetics in Medicine*, *22*(1), 15–25.

Dragoo, D. D., Taher, A., Wong, V. K., et al. (2021). PTEN hamartoma tumor syndrome/Cowden syndrome: genomics, oncogenesis, and imaging review for associated lesions and malignancy. *Cancers*, *13*(13), 3120.

Fernandez-Rozadilla, C., Timofeeva, M., Chen, Z., et al. (2023). Deciphering colorectal cancer genetics through multi-omic analysis of 100,204 cases and 154,587 controls of European and east Asian ancestries. *Nature Genetics*, *55*(1), 89–99.

Fishel, R., Lescoe, M. K., Rao, M. R., et al. (1993). The human mutator gene homolog MSH2 and its association with hereditary nonpolyposis colon cancer. *Cell*, *75*(5), 1027–1038.

Gala, M. K., Mizukami, Y., Le, L. P., et al. (2014). Germline mutations in oncogene-induced senescence pathways are associated with multiple sessile serrated adenomas. *Gastroenterology*, *146*(2), 520–529.

Gallione, C. J., Repetto, G. M., Legius, E., et al. (2004). A combined syndrome of juvenile polyposis and hereditary haemorrhagic telangiectasia associated with mutations in MADH4 (SMAD4). *The Lancet*, *363*(9412), 852–859.

Gambini, D., Ferrero, S., & Kuhn, E. (2022). Lynch syndrome: from carcinogenesis to prevention interventions. *Cancers*, *14*(17), 4102.

Gorji, L., & Albrecht, P. (2023). Hamartomatous polyps: diagnosis, surveillance, and management. *World Journal of Gastroenterology*, *29*(8), 1304.

Groden, J., Thliveris, A., Samowitz, W., et al. (1991). Identification and characterization of the familial adenomatous polyposis coli gene. *Cell*, *66*(3), 589–600.

Hashimoto, Y., Yokoyama, K., Kumagai, H., et al. (2020). Juvenile polyposis syndrome-hereditary hemorrhagic telangiectasia associated with a SMAD4 mutation in a girl. *Clinical Journal of Gastroenterology*, *13*(6), 1096–1101.

Heitzer, E., & Tomlinson, I. (2014). Replicative DNA polymerase mutations in cancer. *Current Opinion in Genetics & Development*, *24*, 107–113.

Ionov, Y., Peinado, M. A., Malkhosyan, S., et al. (1993). Ubiquitous somatic mutations in simple repeated sequences reveal a new mechanism for colonic carcinogenesis. *Nature*, *363*(6429), 558–561.

Jaeger, E., Leedham, S., Lewis, A., et al. (2012). Hereditary mixed polyposis syndrome is caused by a 40-kb upstream duplication that leads to increased and ectopic expression of the BMP antagonist GREM1. *Nature Genetics*, *44*(6), 699–703.

Jelsig, A. M., Qvist, N., Brusgaard, K., et al. (2014). Hamartomatous polyposis syndromes: a review. *Orphanet Journal of Rare Diseases*, *9*(1), 101.

Kang, B., Hwang, S. K., Choi, S., et al. (2021). Case report of juvenile polyposis/hereditary hemorrhagic telangiectasia syndrome: first report in Korea with a novel mutation in the SMAD4 gene. *Translational Pediatrics*, *10*(5), 1369.

Khan, N., Lipsa, A., Arunachal, G., et al. (2017). Novel mutations and phenotypic associations identified through APC, MUTYH, NTHL1, POLD1, POLE gene analysis in Indian Familial Adenomatous Polyposis cohort. *Scientific Reports*, *7*(1), 2214.

Kinzler, K. W., Nilbert, M. C., Su, L. K., et al. (1991). Identification of FAP locus genes from chromosome 5q21. *Science*, *253*(5020), 661–665.

Larsen, H. J., MacFarland, S. P., & Howe, J. R. Juvenile polyposis syndrome. 13 May 2003 [updated 3 Feb 2022]. GeneReviews®[Internet]. *University of Washington, Seattle*. https://www.ncbi.nlm.nih.gov/books/NBK1469/

Leach, F. S., Nicolaides, N. C., Papadopoulos, N., et al. (1993). Mutations of a mutS homolog in hereditary nonpolyposis colorectal cancer. *Cell*, *75*(6), 1215–1225.

Leoz, M. L., Carballal, S., Moreira, L., et al. (2015). The genetic basis of familial adenomatous polyposis and its implications for clinical practice and risk management. *The Application of Clinical Genetics*, *8*, 95–107.

Levinson, G., & Gutman, G. A. (1987). High frequencies of short frameshifts in poly-CA/TG tandem repeats borne by bacteriophage M13 in Escherichia coli K-12. *Nucleic Acids Research*, *15*(13), 5323–5338.

Li, X., Liu, G., & Wu, W. (2021). Recent advances in Lynch syndrome. *Experimental Hematology and Oncology*, *10*(1), 37.

Liaw, D., Marsh, D. J., Li, J., et al. (1997). Germline mutations of the PTEN gene in Cowden disease, an inherited breast and thyroid cancer syndrome. *Nature Genetics*, *16*(1), 64–67.

Lieberman, S., Walsh, T., Schechter, M., et al. (2017). Features of patients with hereditary mixed polyposis syndrome caused by duplication of GREM1 and implications for screening and surveillance. *Gastroenterology*, *152*(8), 1876–1880.

Liu, J. R., Liu, H., Wang, B., et al. (2020). Case report of hereditary hemorrhagic telangiectasia in children and literature review. *Zhonghua er ke za zhi = Chinese Journal of Pediatrics*, *58*(8), 674–678.

Lloyd, K. M., II, & Dennis, M. (1963). Cowden's disease: a possible new symptom complex with multiple system involvement. *Annals of Internal Medicine*, *58*(1), 136–142.

Lynch, P. M., Lynch, H. T., & Harris, R. E. Hereditary proximal colonic cancer. (1977). *Diseases of the Colon & Rectum*, *20*(8), 661–668.

Lynch, H. T., Boland, C. R., Gong, G., et al. (2006). Phenotypic and genotypic heterogeneity in the Lynch syndrome: diagnostic, surveillance and management implications. *European Journal of Human Genetics*, *14*(4), 390–402.

Lynch, H. T., Shaw, M. W, Magnuson, C. W., et al. (1966). Hereditary factors in cancer: study of two large midwestern kindreds. *Archives of Internal Medicine*, *117*(2), 206–212.

Lynch, H. T., Snyder, C. L., Shaw, T. G., et al. (2015). Milestones of Lynch syndrome: 1895–2015. *Nature Reviews Cancer*, *15*(3), 181–194.

Magrin, L., Fanale, D., Brando, C., et al. (2022). MUTYH-associated tumor syndrome: the other face of MAP. *Oncogene*, *41*(18), 2531–2539.

McRonald, F. E., Pethick, J., Santaniello, F., et al. (2024). Identification of people with Lynch syndrome from those presenting with colorectal cancer in England: baseline analysis of the diagnostic pathway. *European Journal of Human Genetics*, *32*, 529–538.

Mikaeel, R. R., Young, J. P., Li, Y., et al. (2022). RNF43 pathogenic Germline variant in a family with colorectal cancer. *Clinical Genetics*, *101*(1), 122–126.

Miyaki, M., Konishi, M., Tanaka, K., et al. (1997). Germline mutation of MSH6 as the cause of hereditary nonpolyposis colorectal cancer. *Nature Genetics*, *17*(3), 271–272.

Møller P., Seppälä T., Dowty J. G., et al. (2022). Colorectal cancer incidences in Lynch syndrome: a comparison of results from the prospective Lynch syndrome database and the international mismatch repair consortium. *Hereditary Cancer in Clinical Practice*, *20*(1), 36.

Mur, P., García-Mulero, S., Del Valle, J., et al. (2020). Role of POLE and POLD1 in familial cancer. *Genetics in Medicine*, *22*(12), 2089–2100.

Nicolaides, N. C., Papadopoulos, N., Liu, B., et al. (1994). Mutations of two P/WS homologues in hereditary nonpolyposis colon cancer. *Nature*, *371*(6492), 75–80.

Niessen, R. C., Hofstra, R. M., Westers, H., et al. (2009). Germline hypermethylation of MLH1 and EPCAM deletions are a frequent cause of Lynch syndrome. *Genes, Chromosomes and Cancer*, *48*(8), 737–744.

Nieuwenhuis, M. H., & Vasen, H. F. (2007). Correlations between mutation site in APC and phenotype of familial adenomatous polyposis (FAP), a review of the literature. *Critical Reviews in Oncology/Hematology*, *61*(2), 153–161.

Nishisho, I., Nakamura, Y., Miyoshi, Y., et al. (1991). Mutations of chromosome 5q21 genes in FAP and colorectal cancer patients. *Science*, *253*(5020), 665–669.

Palles, C., Cazier, J. B., Howarth, K. M., et al. (2013). Germline mutations affecting the proofreading domains of POLE and POLD1 predispose to colorectal adenomas and carcinomas. *Nature Genetics*, *45*(2), 136–144.

Palles, C., Martin, L., Domingo, E., et al. (2022). The clinical features of polymerase proof-reading associated polyposis (PPAP) and recommendations for patient management. *Familial Cancer*, *21*(2), 197–209.

Palles, C., West, H. D., Chew, E., et al. (2022). Germline MBD4 deficiency causes a multi-tumor predisposition syndrome. *The American Journal of Human Genetics*, *109*(5), 953–960.

Panjwani, S., Bagewadi, A., Keluskar, V., et al. (2011). Gardner's syndrome. *Journal of Clinical Imaging Science*, 1, 65.

Papadopoulos, N., Nicolaides, N. C., Wei, Y. F., et al. (1994). Mutation of a mutL homolog in hereditary colon cancer. *Science*, *263*(5153), 1625–1629.

Peltomäki, P. (2016). Update on Lynch syndrome genomics. *Familial Cancer*, *15*(3), 385–393.

Peltomäki, P., Aaltonen, L. A., Sistonen, P., et al. (1993). Genetic mapping of a locus predisposing to human colorectal cancer. *Science*, *260*(5109), 810–812.

Pilarski, R. (2019). PTEN hamartoma tumor syndrome: a clinical overview. *Cancers*, *11*(6), 844.

Plamper, M., Gohlke, B., & Woelfle, J. (2022). PTEN hamartoma tumor syndrome in childhood and adolescence—a comprehensive review and presentation of the German pediatric guideline. *Molecular and Cellular Pediatrics*, *9*(1), 3.

Quintana, I., Mejías-Luque, R., Terradas, M., et al. (2018). Evidence suggests that germline RNF43 mutations are a rare cause of serrated polyposis. *Gut*, *67*(12), 2230–2232.

Rana, H. Q., & Syngal, S. (2017). Biallelic mismatch repair deficiency: management and prevention of a devastating manifestation of the Lynch syndrome. *Gastroenterology*, *152*(6), 1254–1257.

Rivera, B., Castellsagué, E., Bah, I., et al. (2015). Biallelic NTHL1 mutations in a woman with multiple primary tumors. *New England Journal of Medicine*, *373*(20), 1985–1986.

Rohlin, A., Eiengård, F., Lundstam, U., et al. (2016). GREM 1 and POLE variants in hereditary colorectal cancer syndromes. *Genes, Chromosomes and Cancer*, *55*(1), 95–106.

Seppälä, T. T., Latchford, A., Negoi, I., et al. (2021). European guidelines from the EHTG and ESCP for Lynch syndrome: an updated third edition of the Mallorca guidelines based on gene and gender. *British Journal of Surgery*, *108*(5), 484–498.

Serrano, D., Patrignani, P., Stigliano, V., et al. (2022). Aspirin colorectal cancer prevention in Lynch syndrome: recommendations in the era of precision medicine. *Genes*, *13*(3), 460.

Sherwood, K., Ward, J. C., Soriano, I., et al. (2023). Germline de novo mutations in families with Mendelian cancer syndromes caused by defects in DNA repair. *Nature Communications*, *14*(1), 3636.

Sidenna, M., Khodjet-El-khil, H., Al Mulla, H., et al. (2022). Prevalence and genotype-phenotype correlation of Lynch syndrome in a selected high-risk cohort from Qatar's population. *Genes*, *13*(11), 2176.

Sinicrope, F. A. (2010). DNA mismatch repair and adjuvant chemotherapy in sporadic colon cancer. *Nature Reviews Clinical Oncology*, *7*(3), 174–177.

Sondka, Z., Dhir, N. B., Carvalho-Silva, D., et al. (2024). COSMIC: a curated database of somatic variants and clinical data for cancer. *Nucleic Acids Research*, *52*(D1), D1210–D1217.

Strand, M., Prolla, T. A., Liskay, R. M., et al. (1993). Destabilization of tracts of simple repetitive DNA in yeast by mutations affecting DNA mismatch repair. *Nature*, *365*(6443), 274–276.

Taupin, D., Lam, W., Rangiah, D., et al. (2015). A deleterious RNF43 germline mutation in a severely affected serrated polyposis kindred. *Human Genome Variation*, *2*(1), 1–3.

Terradas, M., Gonzalez-Abuin, N., García-Mulero, S., et al. (2023). MBD4-associated neoplasia syndrome: screening of cases with suggestive phenotypes. *European Journal of Human Genetics*, *31*(10), 1185–1189.

Therkildsen, C., Jensen, L. H., Rasmussen, M., et al. (2021). An update on immune checkpoint therapy for the treatment of Lynch syndrome. *Clinical and Experimental Gastroenterology*, *14*, 181–197.

Thibodeau, S. N., Bren, G., & Schaid, D. (1993). Microsatellite instability in cancer of the proximal colon. *Science*, *260*(5109), 816–819.

Tomlinson, I. (2015). The Mendelian colorectal cancer syndromes. *Annals of Clinical Biochemistry*, *52*(6), 690–692.

Vasen, H. F., Blanco, I., Aktan-Collan, K., et al. (2013). Revised guidelines for the clinical management of Lynch syndrome (HNPCC), recommendations by a group of European experts. *Gut*, *62*(6), 812–823.

Vasen, H. F., Moeslein, G., Alonso, A., et al. (2008). Guidelines for the clinical management of familial adenomatous polyposis (FAP). *Gut*, *57*(5), 704–713.

Venesio, T., Balsamo, A., D'Agostino, V., et al. (2012). MUTYH-associated polyposis (MAP), the syndrome implicating base excision repair in inherited predisposition to colorectal tumors. *Frontiers in Oncology*, *2*, 83.

Venkatachalam, R., Verwiel, E. T., Kamping, E. J., et al. (2011). Identification of candidate predisposing copy number variants in familial and early-onset colorectal cancer patients. *International Journal of Cancer*, *129*(7), 1635–1642.

Wagner, A., Aretz, S., Auranen, A., et al. (2021). The management of Peutz–Jeghers syndrome: European hereditary tumour group (EHTG) guideline. *Journal of Clinical Medicine*, *10*(3), 473.

Warthin, A. S. (1913). Heredity with reference to carcinoma: as shown by the study of the cases examined in the pathological laboratory of the University of Michigan, 1895–1913. *Archives of Internal Medicine*, *12*(5), 546–555.

Weren, R. D., Ligtenberg, M. J., Kets, C. M., et al. (2015). A germline homozygous mutation in the base-excision repair gene NTHL1 causes adenomatous polyposis and colorectal cancer. *Nature Genetics*, *47*(6), 668–671.

Will, O., Carvajal-Carmona, L. G., Gorman, P., et al. (2007). Homozygous PMS2 deletion causes a severe colorectal cancer and multiple adenoma phenotype without extraintestinal cancer. *Gastroenterology*, *132*(2), 527–530.

Wimmer, K., & Etzler, J. (2008). Constitutional mismatch repair-deficiency syndrome: have we so far seen only the tip of an iceberg? *Human Genetics*, *124*(2), 105–122.

Yan, H. H., Lai, J. C., Ho, S. L., et al. (2017). RNF43 germline and somatic mutation in serrated neoplasia pathway and its association with BRAF mutation. *Gut*, *66*(9), 1645–1656.

2

Lifestyle factors and the third healthcare revolution

Amy Davies, Lynda McSorley, Ashley Pheely, and Eva Segelov

Introduction

Colorectal cancer (CRC) is one of the three most common cancers and a leading cause of cancer-related death. The global burden is increasing, with 1.8 million estimated new diagnoses in 2020 and stark variation across countries and regions (Sung et al. 2021). Most CRC is sporadic, with only 5% typically related to inherited conditions such as Lynch syndrome or familial adenomatous polyposis (see Chapter 1). More recently, an increase in diagnoses in younger adults (under 50) has been observed, the cause of which is unclear, but diet and obesity are thought to be implicated (Liu et al. 2019; Hofseth et al. 2020).

In recent years there has been considerable focus on the contribution of diet and lifestyle, particularly exercise, to the carcinogenesis of all primary cancers, as well as in the pathogenesis of recurrent and metastatic disease. For CRC, it has been estimated that up to 55% can be attributed to lifestyle and environmental factors (Parkin et al., 2011), with sedentary lifestyle and obesity established as risk factors for primary CRC (Martínez et al. 1997; Larsson and Wolk 2007; Wolin et al. 2009). Certain foods and physical activity have been demonstrated to prolong disease-free survival (DFS) and overall survival (OS) in patients with stage III colon cancer (Cheng et al. 2022). The importance of diet and exercise remains key along the entire CRC continuum, from prevention through to management of advanced disease.

The importance of modifiable risk factors links to the key foundations of the third healthcare revolution, one that strives to consider health not merely as absence of disease but as a positive concept of a full, capable, and long life (Breslow 2004). This evolution has been driven by immense changes in technology and knowledge generation and dispersal, alongside changes in attitudes of the general population, with a desire to control their own healthcare choices (Laing 2004). Profound changes in how care is provided for cancer patients (e.g. telehealth) enhance how patients engage with their own healthcare; one important statistic being that the majority of current patients with CRC use social media platforms (Lopez 2022; Patel, 2022).

This chapter explores the contribution of modifiable risk factors in CRC carcinogenesis and disease recurrence. Links are drawn with the third healthcare revolution and its impact from patient and provider perspectives within the contemporary medical and sociopolitical landscape.

Lifestyle factors and their influence on the pathway to primary CRC

Ascertaining evidence

Despite the complex methodology and other challenges involved in undertaking clinical trials of diet and lifestyle modification, many studies have been performed. Dietary studies are typically conducted using self-reported questionnaires or diaries, with significant limitations including recall bias (Tual et al. 2022). Regarding studying lifestyle interventions, significant biases that weaken the internal validity of studies are difficult to avoid (Piraux et al. 2022). These include recruitment or ascertainment bias in those willing to consent, inability to conduct allocation blinding, and potential for contamination by drop-out and off-protocol adoption of the intervention being tested by controls (Steins Bisschop et al. 2015; Gal et al. 2019).

One strategy to minimize bias is to implement a pilot or feasibility study, prior to a randomized controlled trial (RCT). This can inform recruitment potential, test study processes, and provide preliminary adherence data (particularly in control group) as well as understanding of participant experience and barriers/enablers (El-Kotob and Giangregorio 2018).

Factors associated with increased risk

Red and processed meats

Consumption of red meat has been widely studied to establish this as a risk factor for CRC development, whereas no increase has been found with white meat such as pork, chicken, and fish (Norat et al. 2002; Larsson and Wolk 2006; Carr et al. 2016). The seminal study described a relative risk (RR) increasing approximately 10% with every 100 gram (g) per day (equal to a small adult palmful) increase in red and processed meats (Vieira et al. 2017). However, no proportionate risk increase was seen in a meta-analysis of 27 prospective trials evaluating intake of red meat (including only beef, pork, lamb, and some processed meats) (Alexander et al. 2015). Further, in a pooled meta-analysis of eight studies (6,620 cases), there was no dose–response relationship with red meat amount (relative risk [RR] 1.12; 95% confidence interval [CI] 1.00–1.25) (World Cancer Research Fund 2018). Nevertheless, red meat is considered a likely causative factor in CRC, given persistent positive associations even though these are not always statistically significant in all studies, according to many national and international bodies (World Health Organization 2015; World Cancer Research Fund 2018; National Health Service 2021).

The case for increased risk from processed meats (ham, bacon, sausages, cured or preserved meat) remains more convincing. A meta-analysis of 18 prospective studies demonstrated 18% increased risk of CRC development with every 50 g (approximately seven slices) per day intake (95% CI 1.10–1.28, p = 0.00, heterogeneity [I^2] 12%) (Chan et al. 2011). Whilst the exact mechanism is unclear, proposed mechanisms include cooking processes (heat causing production of polycyclic aromatic hydrocarbons and heterocyclic amines) (Sugimura et al. 2004; Cross et al. 2010), nitrites used in processing (Joosen et al. 2009), and higher levels of heme iron (Bastide et al., 2011). In a large study, a 124-item food frequency questionnaire was used in 300,000 unselected Americans with an incident rate of CRC approximately 2,700 at 7 years follow-up (Cross et al. 2010). Higher levels of heme iron (hazard ratio [HR] 1.13, 95% CI 0.99–1.29), nitrates (HR 1.16, 95% CI 1.02–1.32), and heterocyclic amines (HR 1.19; 95% CI 1.05–1.34) were positively associated with CRC (Cross et al. 2010).

In considering the race disparity of CRC incidence and the role that traditional diets may play, a subset analysis of the Women's Health Initiative study found African American patients had a poorer outcome of invasive CRC compared to White participants (HR 1.11, 95% CI 0.94–1.29) when stratified for dietary factors (total energy, red meat, fruits, and vegetables) (Women's Health Initiative study 1992). This disparity was not seen with Hispanic, Native American, or Asian participants (Simon et al. 2011). In another study of Asian participants, traditional risk factors held true, with higher CRC rates associated with increased intake of red and processed meats (Azeem et al. 2015).

Alcohol

There is a strong relationship between CRC risk and alcohol consumption. Globally, CRC contributes 20% of disability-adjusted life years of all alcohol-attributable cancer (World Health Organization 2019). In a meta-analysis of 57 studies a positive dose-response was found, where no additional risk in light drinkers (< one drink/day; RR 1.00, 95% CI 0.95–1.05) increased to 1.21 in moderate drinkers (two to three drinks/day; 95% CI 1.13–1.28) and 1.52 in heavy drinkers (> four drinks/day) (95% CI 1.27–1.81) (Fedirko et al. 2011). There is no relationship between type of alcohol and CRC risk (Cho et al. 2004).

The underlying mechanism of alcohol as a carcinogen is unclear and not purely related to ethanol or its main metabolite acetaldehyde. Broadly, alcohol is thought to cause oxidative stress and potentially directly damage DNA via acetaldehyde. Other mechanisms involve risk according to genotype of various folate metabolism genes, particularly *MTHFR 677TT* homozygotes (Sharp and Little 2004). Early data also suggest damage via induction of CYP2EI in colon cells (Linhart et al., 2014).

Obesity

In a seminal review of eight meta-analyses or systematic reviews (with varying definition of obesity, from body mass index (BMI) > 25 mg/m^2 in Asian populations and > 30 kg/m^2 in Caucasians) the incidence of CRC was higher in obese men (RR ranging 1.37 to 1.95), with less impact in women (RR 1.12 per 5 mg/m^2 increase in BMI) (Bardou et al., 2013). The pattern of distribution of body fat also seems important, with increased risk seen with central adiposity across both genders (MacInnis et al. 2006a, 2006b). Obesity has also been associated with larger size of premalignant colon adenomas, particularly in the distal colon (Giovannucci et al. 1996).

Mechanisms are thought to be multifactorial but underpinned by metabolic changes related to increased adipose tissue, such as chronic hyperinsulinemia with associated risk of type II diabetes mellitus and increased growth hormone and insulin-like growth factor 1 (IGF1) production (Calle and Kaaks 2004; McTiernan 2008). Pre-clinical data has shown that excessive insulin causes direct DNA damage to colon cancer cells (Othman et al., 2013). To date there is no evidence of a link between obesity and any particular molecular subtype of CRC (Carr et al. 2018).

In contrast, the impact of weight loss on CRC risk reduction was shown in a prospective control-matched study evaluating the effect of bariatric surgery on mortality. Whilst not powered for analysis of cancer, and not isolating CRC, there was a risk reduction of death of 40% in women who underwent this surgery (Sjöström et al. 2009). This risk reduction was not seen for men. The sustained weight change in men and women who underwent surgery was 19.9 kg at 15 years follow-up. In the control group the mean weight change was an increase of 1.3 kg (Sjöström et al. 2009).

Factors associated with decreased risk

Exercise

Exercise is typically defined as planned, structured, and repeated physical activity (Yang et al. 2021). Multiple international authorities recommend exercise as a primary CRC prevention strategy, with varying prescriptions of type, duration, and frequency (Table 2.1). Challenges in recommending exercise include overcoming the significant contribution of social, economic, and cultural influences that determine an individual's body weight (Rock et al. 2020). Access to healthy eating, recreational activities, and transport are some of the many confounders which are compromised for those with lower income and disadvantage, including people with disability and remote place of residence (Rock et al. 2020).

In clinical trials, exercise amount is generally quantified using metabolic equivalent task (MET) hours per week (Matthews et al. 2020). This allows for comparison across different types of activity, often coupled with assessment of effort (strenuous versus non-strenuous activity (Matthews et al. 2020; Díaz-Balboa et al. 2021).

The American Society of Clinical Oncology (ASCO) 2018 guidelines recommend 150 minutes of moderate intensity exercise (e.g. walking, dancing) or 75 minutes of high-intensity exercise (e.g. jogging, running, cycling) per week to reduce the risk of all cancers, including CRC (LoConte et al. 2018). This translates into

Table 2.1 Recommendations for exercise as primary prevention of cancer from leading authorities

Authority	Recommendation	Reference
National Cancer Institute of USA	1. 150 to 300 minutes of moderate-intensity aerobic activity, 75 to 100 minutes of vigorous aerobic activity, or an equivalent combination of each intensity each week 2. Muscle-strengthening activities at least two days a week 3. Balance training, in addition to aerobic and muscle-strengthening activity	National Cancer Institute (2020). https://www.cancer.gov/about-cancer/causes-prevention/risk/obesity/physical-activity-fact-sheet accessed 12 May 2022
American Cancer Society	1. Adults should get 150–300 minutes of moderate intensity or 75–150 minutes of vigorous intensity activity each week 2. Children and teens should get at least 1 hour of moderate or vigorous intensity activity each day. 3. Limit sedentary behaviour such as sitting, lying down, watching TV, and other forms of screen-based entertainment.	American Cancer Society (2020). https://www.cancer.org/healthy/eat-healthy-get-active/acs-guidelines-nutrition-physical-activity-cancer-prevention/guidelines.html accessed 12 May 2022
Cancer Council Australia	1. 60 minutes of moderate activity or 30 minutes of vigorous activity every day	Cancer Council. https://www.cancer.org.au/cancer-information/causes-and-prevention/diet-and-exercise/move-your-body accessed 12 May 2022
World Cancer Research Fund	1. 150 minutes of moderate intensity activity per week 2. 75 minutes of vigorous activity per week	World Cancer Research Fund (2018). https://www.wcrf.org/wp-content/uploads/2021/02/Colorectal-cancer-report.pdf accessed 12 May 2022

recommendations for adults to walk briskly for 2.5 to 5 hours, or run for 1.5 hours, per week.

Exercise recommendations have been informed by convincing data demonstrating the potential to reduce the colon cancer risk (Wolin et al. 2009; Boyle et al. 2012). However, many studies are non-randomized and/or observational studies, inducing bias. One meta-analysis of 18 studies (nine case-control, nine prospective cohort studies) did not support exercise for risk reduction in individuals at higher risk, such as first-degree relatives (Shaw et al. 2018). The result may reflect selection bias by only including studies which had stratified CRC by risk group.

Mechanistically, preclinical data demonstrates rises in certain inflammatory cytokines (IL-6, IL-8, TNF-a) for up to two hours after high-intensity exercise (Devin et al. 2019). Patient-derived xenograft models have shown tumour growth inhibition, potentially via nucleotide and mitochondrial metabolism, in mice running on a wheel (Lu et al. 2018). Immunocompetent mice with transplanted murine CRC organoids were less likely to develop distant metastases if provided access to a running wheel, but primary tumour growth was similar between exercise versus no exercise groups (Wijler et al. 2022).

Fibre

Dietary fibre (defined as foods with high amounts of fibre or diets with high intake of vegetables, grains or fruits) has been associated with a reduction in risk of CRC development with an odds ratio of 0.57 (Trock et al., 1990). Legume-derived fibre has an RR of 0.62, compared to cereal-derived fibre with RR 0.90 (Aune et al. 2011). The risk seems proportionate, with a 20% reduced RR with each 10 g daily increase in fibre (whole grain) (Vieira et al. 2017).

However, the data are not straightforward. Due to significant heterogeneity, the certainty of the association was considered low in a recent review of observational studies in an average-risk population (Chapelle et al. 2020).

Calcium and vitamin D

Observational data about the protective effect of diets high in calcium and vitamin D are also mixed. Several case-control (Zhang et al. 2020) and cohort studies (Um et al. 2019) suggest risk reduction high dietary intake (~20%) as well as supplementation (~15%), but another large case-control study found the association not statistically significant in multivariate analysis (Vallès et al. 2018). A meta-analysis of five RCTs demonstrated a 24% RR in CRC-specific mortality with supplementation of vitamin D for a period ranging from 400 to 4000 international units per day (Vaughan-Shaw et al. 2020).

Lifestyle factors important in initial adenoma formation

A prospective observational study of asymptomatic participants undergoing initial colonoscopy, showed a higher risk of polyps in obese individuals (OR 2.94 in BMI > 30) (Khan and Arfin 2021). Smoking, alcohol intake, obesity, and family history of CRC were associated with greater risk of serrated polyps and conventional adenomas in a subset analysis of the Nurses Health Study, but vitamin D and omega-3 fatty acids appeared to lower this risk (He et al. 2018). Interestingly, in a cross-sectional study of Chinese people there was a strong association with preserved (pickled) vegetable consumption and prevalence of colonic polyps (Wu et al. 2022). xyz[67]. It has also been reported that adolescents with excessive sugar and sugar-sweetened drink intake have an associated risk of adenoma development (Joh et al. 2021).

Lifestyle factors and CRC recurrence after completion of treatment

For the early stages of CRC, despite increasingly effective definitive and adjuvant treatments, there remains a risk of local and distant relapse and death. A recent pooled analysis of six phase 3 RCTs of Stage III and high risk Stage II patients demonstrated relapse-free survival (RFS) rates nearing 80% at five years (André et al. 2020). Minimizing cancer recurrence is a key priority for patients and

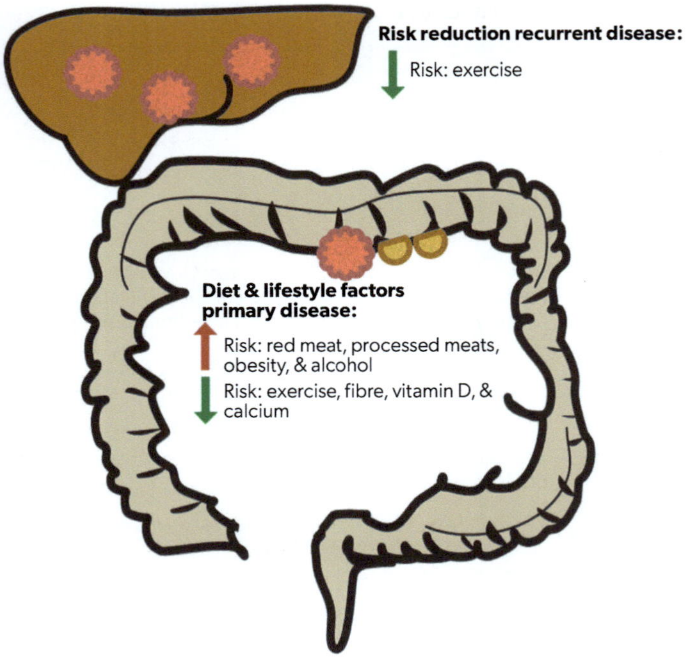

Figure 2.1 Summary of lifestyle factors and their impact upon the risk of CRC.

healthcare systems. Many patients feel empowered by actions they can personally undertake and control to reduce cancer recurrence risk, and exercise is a key activity which also has benefits for their cardiovascular and mental health and general well-being (Ziegler et al. 2022).

RCTs investigating the secondary prevention effect of diet and exercise have been undertaken for many tumour types, including CRC. Challenges include that formal specialty oncology follow-up usually finishes at five years. However, general practitioners, endoscopists, and surgeons as well as specialized survivorship clinics are well placed to institute or continue long-term studies of lifestyle factors and take advantage of 'teachable moments' for education and monitoring of modifiable risk factors (Fig. 2.1) (Argilés et al. 2020).

Exercise

A meta-analysis of seven studies of CRC survivors who engaged in high levels of post-diagnosis exercise documented a 40% reduced risk of CRC-related death (Schmid and Leitzmann 2014). A prospective cohort study of 800 survivors of stage III colon cancer demonstrated improved disease-free survival (DFS) with more METs per week, even when adjusted for sex, age, and number of positive lymph nodes. In those who undertook 18 to 27 MET hours per week compared to only three METs, the HR was 0.51 (95% CI 0.26–0.97) (Meyerhardt et al. 2006). Although of course direct comparisons cannot be made, the magnitude of impact is interesting when considering the reasonably minimal impact of adjuvant chemotherapy for many CRC substages. In any case, exercise should be used complementarily with other adjuvant therapies.

In a recent sub analysis of a trial evaluating adjuvant chemotherapy there was a greater DFS in patients adopting positive diet and exercise behaviours (Cheng et al. 2022). In a cohort of 1,024 patients with stage III CRC enrolled in a trial of two different adjuvant chemotherapy regimens (5-flurouracil and leucovorin vs irinotecan, 5-flurouracil, and leucovorin), self-reported diet and exercise demonstrated an additional improved five-year DFS of 6.3% in those with good risk clinicopathological features, 21% for average risk, and 42% for poor risk (Cheng et al. 2022). As with diet, it is important to consider potential influences of ascertainment bias.

Regarding potential mechanisms, RCT data demonstrated a reduction in circulating tumour cells in cancer patients after a six-month exercise programme was initiated (Brown et al. 2018a). Further, it has been reported that CRC survivors (stages I–III) who engage in low and high dose exercise programmes, (comparing 150 and 300 minutes per week respectively) demonstrate lower levels of intracellular adhesion molecules, which are implicated in the growth of existing micrometastases and generation of new disease (Brown et al. 2018b). There are also data showing that a six-week exercise programme in CRC survivors alters epigenetic markers of methylation (Hwang et al. 2022). Taken together, these studies give biological plausibility to exercise exerting a physiological effect on patients with active cancer and in cancer survivors, although there is much more remaining to be understood.

Diet

The role of diet in increasing DFS after CRC is less clear than for primary prevention. Data suggest poorer survival with high intake of sugar-sweetened drinks, for example the study by Zoltick et al. (2021) but in a systematic review of seven RCTs there lacked a clear signal of impact from any individual diet or BMI factors, owing to the heterogeneity of included studies (Aubrey et al. 2019). Despite this, international guidelines generally recommend CRC survivors to adopt a healthy diet. Adherence to these practices has been shown to improve health-related quality of life; patients with high fibre intake have better physical functioning in the two years after diagnosis (van Veen et al. 2019; Kenkhuis et al., 2022).

The third healthcare revolution and how it may impact upon CRC care

History

It is important to contextualize the current healthcare revolution with respect to the first and second revolutions in order to appreciate the influence these accelerated periods had in the otherwise gradual evolution of healthcare. The first healthcare revolution occurred during the nineteenth century, as a consequence of the Industrial Revolution. Mass population shifts into towns and cities led to overcrowding, poor sanitation, and inadequate nutrition, and set a breeding ground for communicable diseases that ultimately threatened workforce reliability and economic productivity (Breslow 2004). Rapid urbanization occurred in a vacuum of administration, planning, and governance structures, with no effective coordination of healthcare and welfare (Szreter 2003). A workforce in increasingly fragile health created a burgeoning impetus to improve public health through sanitation, law reform, and vaccination. This secured a stable workforce which then drove the Industrial Revolution forward (Szreter 2003).

With this progress came changes in daily living, many with negative health benefits, including smoking, decreased physical activity, and increase in low-quality food (Breslow 2004). However, the first healthcare revolution resulted overall in improvements in life expectancy; paradoxically this foreshadowed the emergence of chronic diseases associated with older age (Breslow 2004).

The twentieth century saw a significant shift in cause of mortality from communicable to non-communicable diseases in the industrialized world (although these remain predominant in low- and middle-income countries) (Breslow 2004). This resulted in cardiovascular diseases, chronic obstructive pulmonary disease, and cancer becoming the commonest causes of death, a legacy that continues (World Health Organization 2020). Characterized as an era of global confidence, the second healthcare revolution was inspired and driven by seemingly limitless scientific discoveries. Dramatic improvements in population health resulted from increased availability of diagnostics, interventions, and therapies. Procedures as diverse as prosthetic hip replacements, chemotherapy, and medication for chronic conditions such as diabetes, hypertension, and asthma resulted in significantly improved life expectancy and reductions in infant, child, perinatal, and peripartum mortality.

In essence, the first healthcare revolution strived to tackle communicable diseases and the second, non-communicable diseases. The immense progress from both is still felt to this day, with people in industrialized countries having record longevity, with a considerable reduction in morbidity.

Definition of the third healthcare revolution

The current (third) healthcare revolution is being driven by information technology and knowledge, as resource-rich countries reach the limits of benefit from the second healthcare revolution. Technology has become a revolutionary force, changing not only how healthcare is delivered but evolving the approach of clinical and public health relationships from a paternalistic model to a patient-centred paradigm. This change has also been driven by the repositioning of perspectives of citizens towards health, defined now not merely as the absence of disease but as a positive concept affecting everyday life, encompassing physical, mental, and social wellbeing (World Health Organization 1986).

Central to this revolution is the interest of individual citizens in their own personal health and the adoption by healthcare workers (HCWs) of a holistic approach (Breslow 2004; Creaney 2019). This has been underpinned by increasing patient awareness and access to education, decreasing social barriers between HCWs and patients, and, most profoundly, the impact of the digital era on disseminating knowledge, evidence, and opinion (Laing, 2004). The patient has evolved from a passive recipient to active participant and, in fact, to director of their own healthcare.

Technology and the digital age are fulfilling their vast potentials to transform the healthcare landscape positively in high-income countries. At the same time, this widens the gap of disparity in healthcare provision and outcomes in low- and middle-income countries, as well as in disadvantaged populations within wealthy countries. The birth of movements such as 'Global Oncology' are responses to data reporting healthcare access and outcomes across geographical regions and different populations (Segelov 2020; Davies 2021).

The 'Moonshot' programme of the US government, focusing on controlling cancer through a 'technocentric, high-cost research strategy', has been countered with a 'Groundshot' initiative, aiming to improve the lives of patients with cancer in the next two decades through initiatives such as global human papillomavirus (HPV) vaccination to target one of the most preventable causes of cancer death (Gyawali 2018). Strategies include repurposing drugs and locally affordable innovations or modifications (e.g. generics and biosimilars) as well as cost-effective modifications of treatment paradigms (e.g. hypofractionation schedules for radiotherapy). Despite billions of US dollars of investment, it is likely that the Moonshot initiative (aiming to speed up implementation of cancer research into clinical practice) may benefit only a modest number of patients, if the total global cohort is considered.

Artificial intelligence

The development of artificial intelligence (AI) and computer learning has contributed to advances in screening and diagnosis of cancer, with CRC as a key example (Mitsala 2021). Technologies ranging from low-cost, sensitive methods for detecting clinically actionable gene mutations through to virtual endoscopy to machine learning to analyse and assimilate large volumes of data to generate 'procedure companions' providing real-time support to increase detection rates of polyps (Liu 2022; Hardy 2021; Mitsala 2021). Examples are growing exponentially and are too numerous to list in detail but several excellent reviews are recommended (Wang et al. 2020b; Bhinder et al. 2021; Elemento et al. 2021).

Digital technology and social media

This major part of the third healthcare revolution has allowed significant advances but also raised challenges, as discussed below with reference particularly to CRC. Each has had a profound impact on the experience of patients and caregivers, HCWs, and the general community.

Apps

A plethora of apps of various degrees of sophistication have been developed to assist clinicians and patients with cancer in multiple aspects: keeping track of diagnosis, stage, treatments, symptoms, appointments, medical questions; interacting with in-app support groups, accessing resources, and options to post questions to the app's community; mindfulness and, more recently, providing real-time feedback on treatment toxicity in the form of patient-reported outcome measures and patient-reported experience measures (PROMs and PREMs). These empower active participation in the cancer journey and provide a practical interface between HCWs and patient. A recent study demonstrated that an app to encourage CRC screening using virtual human technology provided accessible, clear, and impartial information; multiple studies have shown the utility of various cancer apps (Griffin 2019). Examples include the Fight Colorectal Cancer app (Fight Colorectal Cancer 2022) and bowel cancer app' (Bowel Cancer Australia 2022). Regulation of apps continues to present challenges (Wicks 2015).

Social media

The uptake of social media amongst patients with cancer has been widespread. Although the majority of content currently is based on an individual's subjective experience or opinion, this gives deep insight into the concerns of various cancer populations (Patel et al., 2022). One study reported use of social media by over two-thirds of patients with CRC, with many using it as a form of support, to share experiences and gain knowledge (Pellino 2017). Patel et al. looked at tweets pertaining to CRC during 2020–2021, showing the majority came from individuals (44%) (Patel et al., 2022). However, organizations such as the Cancer Council, Cancer Research UK, and the CRC Alliance had the largest impressions, with over a million users reading their tweets (Patel et al. 2022). This study also demonstrated that social media influencers made the largest overall mean impressions, lending weight to the strategy of partnering with influential individuals to highlight public health campaigns (Patel et al. 2022).

Although social media should not necessarily replace established population-based educational initiatives, it has been shown to be useful in promoting healthy behaviours, including diet and lifestyle measures, as well as cancer screening that was not restricted by demographics (Pellino et al. 2017).

Misinformation and limitations

Alongside the benefits exists the very real detriments of misinformation and the potential for harm and isolation from personal support and interaction with HCWs. There is a lack of mandatory regulation surrounding the creation and use of digital technology and social media in cancer care (Böhme et al. 2018). A 2017 study using a rating tool to assess the content of cancer apps found that nearly half were 'deficient' or 'insufficient' with regards to the sources of information used, actual purpose of the app, and ability to distinguish between advertisements/promotions and scientific evidence (Bohme et al. 2018).

Particularly in the absence of guidance from HCWs, patients in the third healthcare revolution use other sources of support including social media, print media, and even pharmaceutical company advertising, to name a few (Finney Rutten 2005; Muusses 2012). Control of content and access through legislation has proven difficult in all jurisdictions and competes with rights of privacy and freedom of speech. Legislation such as the Online Safety Bill has been proposed in the United Kingdom, attempting to make companies accountable for delivering harmful misinformation (Department of Digital, Culture, Media & Sport UK 2021).

Creating an informed population is critical to the delivery of safe, functional healthcare (Gigerenzer and Muir Gray 2011). Government, non-government organizations (NGOs), and institutional websites are increasingly providing resources but a major challenge is keeping up to date with rapid changes and removing outdated information.

Impact on clinician–patient relationships

Information technology increasingly represents the third 'person' in the room, before, during, and after HCW interaction. As the third healthcare revolution progresses, recommending online resources or apps to patients will become routine. Clinicians have been shown to play a vital role in suggesting reliable sources of digital information and social media (Böhme et al. 2018). This necessitates HCWs having sufficient training and expertise to assess the reliability, appropriateness and quality of technology platforms.

Knowledge and education

An OECD (Organisation for Economic Co-Operation and Development) report on patient safety and engagement highlighted the involvement of patients as a key stakeholder in healthcare as one of critical means of ensuring safe healthcare delivery (Slawomirski 2017). This approach needs to be taken at a national, regional, health service, and individual facility level.

A tension exists between the abundance of information available and any individual's ability and willingness to assess this information to make better informed decisions. This landscape is characterized by the patient cohort who, despite exposure to an abundance of health-related information from multiple sources, remains relatively poorly informed regarding the potential risks, possible benefits, and expected success rates of any given procedure; chemotherapy toxicity is a common example. The situation is eloquently summarized as the 'seven sins' of twentieth-century healthcare and the argument has been put forward that educating the patient will provide the most tangible benefits in value-added health interventions in twenty-first-century healthcare (Gigerenzer 2011).

In attempting to create a more integrated approach for both HCW and patient, it is important to cater for the differing perspectives that exist despite the common goal of maintaining or improving the patient's health. Timeliness is another major factor, with the instant access to answers from the digitized world competing with overburdened traditional healthcare services with increasing delays in access.

Governance of healthcare technology and information is an issue to be navigated as the third healthcare revolution progresses. In a competitive environment, those sections of healthcare that champion patient engagement as an integral component of service delivery are likely to predominate.

Knowledge transparency

The improvements in chronic disease burden as a consequence of the second healthcare revolution have in no small part occurred due to the evolution of the multidisciplinary team (Gray 2021). Many patients now encounter a plethora of HCWs, even for one condition. An important aspect of the third healthcare revolution is thus recognition that the only constant is the patient themself (Gray 2021). Digital technology has thus become increasingly important in reliable and integrated use of patient data to facilitate consistent, high-quality care (Awad 2021; Gray 2021).

Gathering statistics to track diseases was an important revelation in the second healthcare revolution and continues to be of significant public health importance, as the COVID-19 pandemic strikingly demonstrates (Breslow 2004). Data are a key foundation of twenty-first-century healthcare (Gray 2021). However, with the third healthcare revolution, the concept of health measurement has ventured into new grounds, such as the collection of personalized health data from wearables and remote monitors, amongst many new technologies, with the concept broadened to includes wide-ranging factors that contribute to health, such as social, educational, environmental (e.g. climate, air quality), economic, and cultural inputs (Breslow 2004).

Telehealth

The increase in incidence of cancer, as well as prolonged survivorship resulting from dramatically improved outcomes from screening, early intervention, and improved therapies and monitoring have the consequence of greatly increasing the demand for cancer services. Concurrently, the modern patient rightly demands to be well-informed across all care options, to be able to contribute and actually drive decisions regarding their care. In oncology, as for many specialties, additional complexities are the growing decentralization of care within geographical regions; sub-specialization across all craft groups (from imaging through to surgery, radiation and medical oncology, and palliative care); and rapid evolution in treatments, including those that can be delivered at home.

Considerable adaptations have occurred relatively quickly, in particular a shift away from purely in-hospital care. The COVID-19 pandemic by necessity inspired immense innovation in an extraordinarily short period, normalizing and standardizing remote forms of communication through telehealth across the world (Segelov et al., 2020; Burbury et al., 2021; Seivert et al., 2021). The widespread implementation of telemedicine has improved access to complex cancer care, including for rare cancers and access to clinical trials and for rural and regional as well as under-served communities (Lee et al., 2020; Lopez et al. 2022). The importance of evidence-based frameworks and the involvement of government, clinicians, and patients in successfully implementing teletrials of healthcare provision was shown to be paramount (Sabesan et al. 2022).

Health inequities can counterintuitively be increased by telehealth, particularly for vulnerable populations (Lopez et al. 2022). Poor financial and social circumstances hamper access to appropriate digital equipment; some demographics, such as the elderly, those with disability, and persons who communicate in a second language find telehealth more challenging (Lopez et al. 2022).

Overall, telehealth has been shown to enhance cancer patient care by decreasing the burden of appointments (travel time, absence from work, parking costs, etc.), increasing access and improving continuity of care (Lopez et al. 2022). Strategies to reduce disparities are essential (Lopez et al. 2022).

Self-management and its part in cancer care

Modern society has seen a vast change from the concept of health promotion first outlined by the World Health Organization in the 1980s, which focused heavily on the healthcare sector being responsible for the physical, mental, and social well-being of individuals in the industrialized world (World Health Organization 1986). In the twenty-first century, there are enormous, highly profitable, private and publicly funded industry sectors who have 'skin in the game'. This includes wide-ranging products and services, from nutrition and dietary supplements, fitness, alternative therapies, and wellness resources to genetic testing, devices, and provision of HCW labour (Kickbusch 2003).

Guidelines for cancer care now puts considerable emphasis on wellness, with diligence being paid to aspects of care such as physical and emotional well-being after a cancer diagnosis and treatment; lifestyle adaptations; consideration of financial impact of a cancer diagnosis ('financial toxicity' now recognized as a category of side effects) and the importance of support networks (Cancer Council Australia 2021). Regarding the third healthcare revolution and cancer 'wellness', the focus for many patients is on prevention and survivorship (Rushton 2015). For those on treatment, remaining as well as possible for as long as possible, is usually top priority (Rushton 2015).

With continued improvements in survival rates, cancer is increasingly considered a chronic disease. Alongside the shift to self-empowerment and engagement by patients and the relocation of many services outside hospital settings, the importance of appropriately equipping patients with the knowledge and skills to manage certain aspects of their health has become paramount.(Howell et al. 2020) Effective self-management requires a patient who is not only willing but able to engage with interventions. Wholistic consideration of the patient's circumstances and competencies is required, including comorbidities, cancer status, literacy, cognitive impairment, mental health, and sociocultural diversity (Howell et al. 2020).

Given the complexity of cancer patients, self-management programmes need to be tailored to relevant scenarios and within them, appropriate individuals. Despite evidence of successful self-management programmes in low-risk cancer populations, survivorship and symptom monitoring, the prevailing culture still considers cancer care as a heavily medicalized domain (Howell et al. 2020). Integration and involvement of patients and carers from the start of their journey is key to changing this culture (Howell et al. 2020).

Realistic medicine

The traditional sole prerogative of the physician was the welfare of the patient sitting in front of them. In twenty-first century healthcare, responsibilities have expanded considerably to include the wider and emerging healthcare requirements of communities and regions and increasingly encompass a global perspective. Health economics (ensuring cost-effectiveness), balancing longer-term goals and competing priorities of the healthcare institutions, budgeting, equity, and multiple other 'non-patient' factors all must be considered in delivering care. Equally, as discussed, the patient's prerogative has also changed, where strong care preferences may exist prior to HCW engagement.

To reign in soaring healthcare costs and promote evidence-based care, various education programmes tailoring clinical decision-making have gained widespread traction. Though not specifically focused on oncology, one study found that rates of rehospitalization and healthcare outcomes were equal between patients whose doctors order more versus fewer investigations (Tsugawa 2017). The 'Choosing Wisely' campaign (www.choosingwisely.org) has a three-pronged approach to educate individual HCWs, patients and carers, and finally healthcare providers and stakeholders about unnecessary tests and interventions. Another example is the on-going 'Realistic Medicine' campaign launched in Scotland in 2015, to support innovation of healthcare whilst emphasizing the importance of shared decision-making, informed consent, reduction of waste, reducing harm of over- and under- provision, and reducing unwarranted variation (Realistic Medicine 2021).

Precision medicine

A major focus of the third healthcare revolution brought about by astonishing technological advances, particularly in multi-omic analyses (molecular medicine), is the concept of precision (less accurately called personalized) medicine. This holds great promise, not only for rare diseases and small cohorts but in understanding inter-person variation of normal and abnormal human physiology. The expanding cost and demand of research and then translation into practice must be married with the realism of caring for growing numbers of increasingly complex patients (Tsugawa et al. 2017). Advances in therapies based on precision diagnoses and targeted treatments have greatly benefitted many patients, but once again this has increased disparity with communities and across the globe, in large part due to the expense of precision tests and therapies.

Patient experience

Patient experiences now plays a considerable role in shaping how healthcare systems operate, evolve, and are assessed for quality. The patient's perspective in designing and improving healthcare systems is imperative in meeting the goals of the third healthcare revolution. Substantial weighting is given by accreditation and funding bodies not only to 'hard' morbidity and mortality outcomes but also measures of impact on quality of life and patient experience, extending to include family and carers.

Often, patient opinions are gathered through institution-administered questionnaires, which are in essence satisfaction surveys only. The validation of such forms of evaluation has itself become a subject of research. Selva et al. (2021) found that the majority of questionnaires used to evaluate patient experience and satisfaction associated with bowel screening were in fact not validated. Furthermore, these often lack consideration of aspects such as cross-cultural adaptation, socio-cultural differences, and gratitude bias (Selva et al. 2021). A true study of PREMS, which itself is a burgeoning academic field, involves repeated measures with validated scales; their use should be approached with the rigour of academic methodology. An essential yet practical aspect of PREMS is the means to respond to issues raised in a way visible to the patient so that the same (negative) experiences are not reported repeatedly, as this will undermines the importance of the measurement and reduces morale and motivation to participate.

REFERENCES

Alexander, D. D., Weed, D. L., Miller, P. E., et al. (2015). Red meat and CRC: a quantitative update on the state of the epidemiologic science. *Journal of the American College of Nutrition, 34*, 521–543.

André, T., Meyerhardt, J., Iveson, T., et al. (2020). Effect of duration of adjuvant chemotherapy for patients with stage III colon cancer (IDEA collaboration): final results from a prospective, pooled analysis of six randomised, phase 3 trials. *Lancet Oncology, 21*, 1620–1629.

Argilés, G., Tabernero, J., Labianca, R., et al. (2020). Localised colon cancer: ESMO Clinical Practice Guidelines for diagnosis, treatment and follow-up. *Annals of Oncology, 31*, 1291–1305.

Aubrey, V., Hon, Y., Shaw, C., et al. (2019). Healthy eating interventions in adults living with and beyond CRC: a systematic review. *Journal of Human Nutrition and Diet, 32*, 501–511.

Aune, D., Chan, D. S. M., Lau, R., et al. (2011). Dietary fibre, whole grains, and risk of CRC: systematic review and dose-response meta-analysis of prospective studies. *British Medical Journal, 343*. doi: 10.1136/bmj.d6617.

Awad, A., Trenfield, S. J., Pollard, T. D., et al. (2021). Connected healthcare: improving patient care using digital health technologies. *Advanced Drug Delivery Reviews, 178*(2021), 113958.

Azeem, S., Gillani, S. W., Siddiqui, A., et al. (2015). Diet and CRC risk in Asia—a systematic review. *Asia Pacific Journal of Cancer Prevention, 16*, 5389–5396.

Bardou, M., Barkun, A. N., & Martel, M. (2013). Obesity and CRC. *Gut, 62*, 933–947.

Bastide, N. M., Pierre, F. H. F., & Corpet, D. E. (2011). Heme iron from meat and risk of CRC: a meta-analysis and a review of the mechanisms involved. *Cancer Prevention Research, 4* 177–184.

Bhinder, B., Gilvary, C, Madhukar, NS., et al. (2021). Artificial intelligence in cancer research and precision medicine. *Cancer Discovery, 11*, 900–915.

Böhme, C., Osthoff, M. B., & Frey, K. (2018). Qualitative evaluation of mobile cancer apps with particular attention to the target group, content, and advertising. *Journal of Cancer Research and Clinical Oncology, 144* 173–181.

Bowel Cancer Australia. (2020). Bowel Cancer App. https://www.bowelcanceraustralia.org/previous-campaigns#app accessed 14 May 2022.

Boyle, T., Keegel, T., Bull, F., et al. (2012). Physical activity and risks of proximal and distal colon cancers: a systematic review and meta-analysis. *Journal of the National Cancer Institute, 104*, 1548–1561.

Breslow, L. The third revolution in health. (2004). *Annual Review of Public Health, 25*. doi: 10.1146/annurev.pu.25.022604.100011.

Brown, J. C., Rhim, A. D., Manning, S. L., et al. (2018a). Effects of exercise on circulating tumor cells among patients with resected stage I-III colon cancer. *PLoS One, 13*, e0204875.

Brown, J. C., Troxel, A. B., Ky, B., et al. (2018b). Dose-response effects of aerobic exercise among colon cancer survivors: a randomized phase II trial. *Clinical CRC, 17*, 32–40.

Burbury, K., Wong, Z. W., Yip, D., et al. (2021). Telehealth in cancer care: during and beyond the COVID-19 pandemic. *Internal Medicine Journal, 51*(1), 125–133.

Calle, E. E., & Kaaks, R. (2004).Overweight, obesity and cancer: epidemiological evidence and proposed mechanisms. *Nature Reviews Cancer, 4*, 579–591.

Cancer Council Australia. (2021). Living Well After Cancer. https://www.cancervic.org.au/living-with-cancer/life-after-treatment/wellness-and-life-after-cancer accessed 14 March 2022.

Cancer Council Australia. (2022). Meat and Cancer Risk. https://www.cancer.org.au/cancer-information/causes-and-prevention/diet-and-exercise/meat-and-cancer-risk accessed 11 May 2022.

Carr, P. R., Alwers, E., Bienert, S., et al. (2018). Lifestyle factors and risk of sporadic CRC by microsatellite instability status: a systematic review and meta-analyses. *Annals of Oncology, 29*, 825–834.

Carr, P. R., Walter, V., Brenner, H., et al. (2016). Meat subtypes and their association with CRC: Systematic review and meta-analysis. *International Journal of Cancer, 138*, 293–302.

Chan, D. S. M., Lau, R., Aune, D., et al. (2011). Red and processed meat and CRC incidence: meta-analysis of prospective studies. *PLoS One, 6*, e20456.

Chapelle, N., Martel, M., Toes-Zoutendijk, E., et al. (2020). Recent advances in clinical practice: CRC chemoprevention in the average-risk population. *Gut, 69*, 2244–2255.

Cheng, E., Ou, F.-S., Ma, C., et al. (2022). Diet- and lifestyle-based prediction models to estimate cancer recurrence and death in patients with stage III colon cancer (CALGB 89803/Alliance). *Journal of Clinical Oncology, 40*, 740–751.

Cho, E., Smith-Warner, S. A., Ritz, J., et al. (2004). Alcohol intake and CRC: a pooled analysis of 8 cohort studies. *Annals of Internal Medicine, 140*, 603–613.

Cross, A. J., Ferrucci, L. M., Risch, A., et al. (2010). A large prospective study of meat consumption and CRC risk: an investigation of

potential mechanisms underlying this association. *Cancer Research, 70*, 2406–2414.
Davies, A., Gurney, J., & Garvey, G. (2021). Cancer care disparities among Australian and Aotearoa New Zealand Indigenous peoples. *Current Opinion in Supportive and Palliative Care, 15*(3), 162–168.
Department for Digital, Culture, Media & Sport. (2021). Draft Online Safety Bill. https://www.gov.uk/government/publications/draft-online-safety-bill accessed 10 May 2022.
Devin, J. L., Hill, M. M., Mourtzakis, M., et al. (2019). Acute high intensity interval exercise reduces colon cancer cell growth. *Journal of Physiology, 597*, 2177–2184.
Díaz-Balboa, E., González-Salvado, V., Rodríguez-Romero, B., et al. (2021). A randomized trial to evaluate the impact of exercise-based cardiac rehabilitation for the prevention of chemotherapy-induced cardiotoxicity in patients with breast cancer: ONCORE study protocol. *BMC Cardiovascular Disorders, 21*, 165.
Elemento, O., Leslie, C., Lundin, J., et al. (2021). Artificial intelligence in cancer research, diagnosis and therapy. *Nature Reviews Cancer, 21*, 747–752.
El-Kotob, R., & Giangregorio, L. M. (2018). Pilot and feasibility studies in exercise, physical activity, or rehabilitation research. *Pilot and Feasibility Studies, 4*, 137.
Fedirko, V., Tramacere, I., Bagnardi, V., et al. (2011). Alcohol drinking and CRC risk: an overall and dose-response meta-analysis of published studies. *Annals of Oncology, 22*, 1958–1972.
Fight Colorectal Cancer. (2022). Fight Colorectal Cancer App. https://fightcolorectalcancer.org/resources/icancerhealth-app/ accessed 14 May 2022.
Finney Rutten, L. J., Arora, N. K, Bakos, A. D., et al. (2005). Information needs and sources of information among cancer patients: a systematic review of research (1980–2003) *Patient Education and Counselling, 57*(3), 250–261 doi: 10.1016/j.pec.2004.06.006.
Gal, R., Monninkhof, E. M., van Gils, C. H., et al. (2019). The Trials within Cohorts design faced methodological advantages and disadvantages in the exercise oncology setting. *Journal of Clinical Epidemiology, 113*, 137–146.
Gigerenzer, G., & Gray, M. (Eds.). (2011). *Better doctors, better patients, better decisions*. The MIT Press.
Giovannucci, E., Colditz, G. A., Stampfer, M. J., et al. (1996). Physical activity, obesity, and risk of colorectal adenoma in women (United States). *Cancer Causes Control, 7*, 253–263.
Gray, M. (2021). Reducing the Burden of Treatment in the Third Healthcare Revolution. https://www.iwgc.org/post/8-reducing-the-burden-of-treatment-in-the-third-healthcare-revolution accessed 1 March 2022.
Griffin, L., Lee, D., Jaisle, A., et al. (2019). Creating an mHealth App for CRC screening: user-centered design approach. *JMIR Human Factors, 6*(2), e12700. https://doi.org/10.2196/12700.
Gyawali (2018). Cancer groundshot: going global before going to the moon. *Lancet Oncol*, Mar;19(3):288–290. doi: 10.1016/S1470-2045(18)30076-7.
Hardy, N. P., Mac Aonghusa, P., Neary, P. M., et al. (2021). Intraprocedural artificial intelligence for CRC detection and characterisation in endoscopy and laparoscopy. *Surgical Innovation, 28*(6), 768–775.
He, X., Wu, K., Ogino, S., et al. (2018). Association between risk factors for CRC and risk of serrated polyps and conventional adenomas. *Gastroenterology, 155*, 355–373.e18.
Hofseth, L. J., Hebert, J. R., Chanda, A., et al. (2020). Early-onset CRC: initial clues and current views. *Nature Reviews Gastroenterology & Hepatology, 17*, 352–364.
Howell, D., Mayer, D. K., Fielding, R., et al. (20. (2021). Management of cancer and health after the clinic visit: a call to action for self-management in cancer care. *Journal of the National Cancer Institute, 113*(5), 523–531.
Hwang, S.-H., Kang, D.-W., Lee, M.-K., et al. (2022). Changes in DNA methylation after 6-week exercise training in CRC survivors: a preliminary study. *Asia Pacific Journal of Clinical Oncology, 18*, 52–60.
Joh, H.-K., Lee, D. H., Hur, J., et al. (2021). Simple sugar and sugar-sweetened beverage intake during adolescence and risk of CRC precursors. *Gastroenterology, 161*, 128–142.e20.
Joosen, A. M. C. P., Kuhnle, G. G. C., Aspinall, S. M., et al. (2009). Effect of processed and red meat on endogenous nitrosation and DNA damage. *Carcinogenesis, 30*, 1402–1407.
Khan, M. N., & Arfin, M. S. (2021). Increased BMI, sedentary lifestyle & metabolic syndrome as independent risk factors for development of colorectal adenomas: A prospective study. *European Journal of Preventative Medicine*. doi: 10.11648/j.ejpm.20210906.13.
Kenkhuis, M.-F., van Duijnhoven, F. J. B., van Roekel, E. H., et al. (2022). Longitudinal associations of fiber, vegetable, and fruit intake with quality of life and fatigue in CRC survivors up to 24 months posttreatment. *American Journal of Clinical Nutrition, 115*, 822–832.
Kickbusch, I., & Payne, L. (2003). Twenty-first century health promotion: the public health revolution meets the wellness revolution. *Health Promotion International, 18*(4), 275–278.
Laing, A., Hogg, G., & Winkleman, D. (2004). Healthcare and the information revolution: re-configuring the healthcare service encounter. *Health Services Management Research, 17*(3), 188–199.
Larsson, S. C., & Wolk, A. (2006). Meat consumption and risk of CRC: a meta-analysis of prospective studies. *International Journal of Cancer, 119*, 2657–2664.
Larsson, S. C., & Wolk, A. (2007). Obesity and colon and rectal cancer risk: a meta-analysis of prospective studies. *American Journal of Clinical Nutrition, 86*, 556–565.
Lee, J. J., Burbury, K., Underhill, C., et al. (2020). Exploring Australian regional cancer patients' experiences of clinical trial participation via telemedicine technology. *Journal of Telemedicine and Telecare, 13*, 508–516.
LoConte, N. K., Gershenwald, J. E., Thomson, C. A., et al. (2018). Lifestyle modifications and policy implications for primary and secondary cancer prevention: diet, exercise, sun safety, and alcohol reduction. *American Society of Oncology of Clinical Oncology Education Book, 38*, 88–100.
Linhart, K., Bartsch, H., & Seitz, H. K. (2014). The role of reactive oxygen species (ROS) and cytochrome P-450 2E1 in the generation of carcinogenic etheno-DNA adducts. *Redox Biology, 3*, 56–62.
Liu, Z., Guo, C., Dang, Q., et al. Integrative analysis from multi-center studies identities a consensus machine learning derived lncRNA signature for stage II/III CRC eBioMedicine 2022;75:103750 https://doi.org/10. 1016/j.ebiom.2021.103750
Liu, P.-H., Wu, K., Ng, K., et al. (2019). Association of obesity with risk of early-onset CRC among women. *JAMA Oncology, 5*, 37–44.
Lopez, A. M., Lam, K., Thota, R. (2021). Barriers and facilitators to telemedicine: can you hear me now? *American Society of Oncology of Clinical Oncology education book.*
Lu, M., Sanderson, S. M., Zessin, A., et al. (2018). Exercise inhibits tumor growth and central carbon metabolism in patient-derived xenograft models of CRC. *Cancer & Metabolism, 6*, 14.
MacInnis, R. J., English, D. R., Haydon, A. M., et al. (2006a). Body size and composition and risk of rectal cancer (Australia). *Cancer Causes Control, 17*, 1291–1297.
MacInnis, R. J., English, D. R., Hopper, J. L., et al. (2006b). Body size and composition and colon cancer risk in women. *International Journal of Cancer, 118*, 1496–1500.

Martínez, M. E., Giovannucci, E., Spiegelman, D., et al. (1997). Leisure-time physical activity, body size, and colon cancer in women. *Journal of the National Cancer Institute, 89*, 948–955.

Matthews, C. E., Moore, S. C., Arem, H., et al. (2020). Amount and intensity of leisure-time physical activity and lower cancer risk. *Journal of Clinical Oncology, 38*, 686–697.

McTiernan, A. Mechanisms linking physical activity with cancer. *Nature Reviews Cancer, 8*, 205–211.

Meyerhardt, J. A., Heseltine, D., Niedzwiecki, D., et al. (2006). Impact of physical activity on cancer recurrence and survival in patients with stage III colon cancer: findings from CALGB 89803. *Journal of Clinical Oncology, 24*, 3535–3541

Mitsala. (2021). Artificial Intelligence in Colorectal Cancer Screening, Diagnosis and Treatment. *A New Era Curr Oncol, 3*, 1581–1607.

Muusses, L. D., van Weert, J. C. M., van Dulmen, S., et al. (2012). Chemotherapy and information-seeking behaviour: characteristics of patients using mass-media information sources. *Psychooncology, 21*(9), 993–1002.

National Health Service. (2021). Red meat and the risk of bowel cancer. https://www.nhs.uk/live-well/eat-well/food-guidelines-and-food-labels/red-meat-and-the-risk-of-bowel-cancer/ accessed 11 May 2022.

Norat, T., Lukanova, A., Ferrari, P., et al. (2002). Meat consumption and CRC risk: dose-response meta-analysis of epidemiological studies. *International Journal of Cancer, 98*, 241–256.

Othman, E. M., Leyh, A., & Stopper, H. (2013). Insulin mediated DNA damage in mammalian colon cells and human lymphocytes in vitro. *Mutation Research*, 745–746, 34–39.

Parkin, D. M., Boyd, L., & Walker, L. C. (2011). The fraction of cancer attributable to lifestyle and environmental factors in the UK in 2010. *British Journal of Cancer, 105* Suppl 2, S77–81.

Patel, V. R., Gereta, S., Blanton, C. J., et al. (2022). # ColonCancer: Social media discussions about CRC during the COVID-19 pandemic. *JCO Clinical Cancer Informatics, 6*, **e**2100180.

Pellino, G., Simillis, C., Qiu, S., et al. (2017). Social media and CRC: a systematic review of available resources. *PLoS One, 12*(8), e0183031. https://doi. org/10.1371/journal.pone.0183031.

Piraux., E, Reychler, G., Vancraeynest, D., et al. (2022). High-intensity aerobic interval training and resistance training are feasible in rectal cancer patients undergoing chemoradiotherapy: a feasibility randomized controlled study. *2*, 198–208 doi: 10.5603/RPOR. a2022.0036.

Realistic Medicine—Scottish Government (2021). What realistic medicine is and what it isn't. https://www.realisticmedicine.scot accessed 11 May 2022.

Rock, C. L., Thomson, C., Gansler, T., et al. (2020). American Cancer Society guideline for diet and physical activity for cancer prevention. *CA: A Cancer Journal for Clinicians, 70*, 245–271.

Rushton, M., Morash, R., Larocque, G., et al. (2015). Wellness Beyond Cancer Program: building an effective survivorship program. *Current Oncology, 22*(6), 419–434.

Sabesan et al. (2022). Implementation of the Australasian Teletrial Model: Translating ideas into action using implementation science frameworks. *J Telemed Telecare*, 8, 641-647. doi: 10.1177/1357633X211017805. Epub 2021 Jul 7.

Schmid, D., & Leitzmann, M. F. (2014). Association between physical activity and mortality among breast cancer and CRC survivors: a systematic review and meta-analysis. *Annals of Oncology, 25*, 1293–1311.

Segelov, E., & Garvey, G. (2020). Cancer and Indigenous populations: time to end the disparity. *JCO Global Oncology, 6*, 80–82.

Segelov, E., Underhill, C., Prenan, H., et al. (2020). Practical considerations for treating cancer patients in the COVID-19 pandemic. *JCO Oncol Pract.16*(8), 467–482.

Selva, A., Selva C,. Álvarez-Pérez Y., et al. (2021). Satisfaction and experience with CRC screening: a systematic review of validated patient reported outcome measures. *BMC Medical Research Methodology, 21*(1), 1–15.

Seivert, S., & Badowski, M. (2020). The rise of telemedicine: lessons from a global pandemic. *EMJ Innovations, 5*(1), 64–69.

Sharp, L., & Little, J. (2004). Polymorphisms in genes involved in folate metabolism and colorectal neoplasia: a HuGE review. *American Journal of Epidemiology, 159*, 423–443.

Shaw, E., Farris, M. S., Stone, C. R., et al. (2018). Effects of physical activity on CRC risk among family history and BMI subgroups: a systematic review and meta-analysis. *BMC Cancer, 18*, 71.

Simon, M. S., Thomson, C. A., Pettijohn, E., et al. (2011). Racial differences in CRC incidence and mortality in the Women's Health Initiative. *Cancer Epidemiology, Biomarkers & Prevention, 20*, 1368–1378.

Sjöström, L., Narbro, K., Sjströström, C. D., et al. (2007). Effects of bariatric surgery on mortality in Swedish obese subjects. *New England Journal of Medicine, 357*, 741–752.

Slawomirski, L., Auraaen, A., & Klazinga, N. S. (2017). The economics of patient safety: Strengthening a value-based approach to reducing patient harm at national level. OECD Health Working Papers No 96. https://doi.org/10.1787/5a9858cd-en.

Steins Bisschop, C. N., Courneya, K. S., Velthuis, M. J., et al. (2015). Control group design, contamination and drop-out in exercise oncology trials: a systematic review. *PLoS One, 10*, e0120996.

Sugimura, T., Wakabayashi, K., Nakagama, H., et al. (2004). Heterocyclic amines: mutagens/carcinogens produced during cooking of meat and fish. *Cancer Science, 95*, 290–299.

Sung, H., Ferlay, J., Siegel, R. L., et al. (2021). Global cancer statistics 2020: GLOBOCAN estimates of incidence and mortality worldwide for 36 cancers in 185 countries. *CA Cancer Journal for Clinicians, 71*, 209–249.

Szreter, S. The population health approach in historical perspective. (2003). *American Journal of Public Health, 93*(3), 421–431. https://doi.org/10.2105/AJPH.93.3.421.

Trock, B., Lanza, E., & Greenwald, P. (1990). Dietary fiber, vegetables, and colon cancer: critical review and meta-analyses of the epidemiologic evidence. *Journal of the National Cancer Institute, 82*, 650–661.

Tsugawa, Y., Jha, A. K., Newhouse, J. P., et al. (2017). Variation in physician spending and association with patient outcomes. *JAMA Internal Medicine, 177*(5), 675. https://doi.org/10.1001/jamainternmed.2017.0059.

Tual, S., Lemarchand, C., Giovannini, J., et al. (2022). Reliability of baseline self-reported information in the AGRICAN cohort. *Cancer Causes Control, 33*, 331–342.

Um, C. Y., Prizment, A., Hong, C.-P., et al. (2019). Associations of calcium, vitamin D, and dairy product intakes with CRC risk among older women: the Iowa Women's Health Study. *Nutrition and Cancer, 71*, 739–748.

Vallès, X., Alonso, M. H., López-Caleya, J. F., et al. (2018). CRC, sun exposure and dietary vitamin D and calcium intake in the MCC-Spain study. *Environment International, 121*, 428–434.

van Veen, M. R., Mols, F., Bours, M. J. L., et al. (2019). Adherence to the World Cancer Research Fund/American Institute for Cancer Research recommendations for cancer prevention is associated with better health-related quality of life among long-term CRC survivors: results of the PROFILES registry. *Support Care Cancer, 27*, 4565–4574.

Vaughan-Shaw, P. G., Buijs, L. F., Blackmur, J. P., et al. (2020). The effect of vitamin D supplementation on survival in patients with CRC: systematic review and meta-analysis of randomised controlled trials. *British Journal of Cancer, 123*, 1705–1712.

Vieira, A. R., Abar, L., Chan, D. S. M., et al. (2017). Foods and beverages and CRC risk: a systematic review and meta-analysis of cohort studies, an update of the evidence of the WCRF-AICR Continuous Update Project. *Annals of Oncology, 28*, 1788–1802.

Wang, Y., He, X., Nie, H., et al. (2020). Application of artificial intelligence to the diagnosis and therapy of colorectal cancer. *American Journal of Cancer Research, 10*, 3575–3598.

Wang, F., Cai, H., Gu, K., et al. (2020b). Adherence to dietary recommendations among long-term breast cancer survivors and cancer outcome associations. *Cancer Epidemiology, Biomarkers & Prevention, 29*, 386–395.

Wicks, P., & Chiauzzi, E. (2015). 'Trust but verify'—five approaches to ensure safe medical apps. *BMC Medicine, 2015;13*(1), 205. https://doi.org/10.1186/s12916-015-0451-z.

Wijler, L. A., Raats, D. A. E., Verheem, A., et al. (2022). Voluntary exercise influences metastatic organotropism in a murine CRC model. *JCSM Rapid Communications, 5*, 117–129.

Wolin, K. Y., Yan, Y., Colditz, G. A., et al. (2009). Physical activity and colon cancer prevention: a meta-analysis. *British Journal of Cancer, 100*, 611–616.

Women's Health Initiative Study. (1992). https://www.whi.org/ accessed 11 May 2022.

World Cancer Research Fund. (2018). Meat, fish, dairy and cancer risk. https://www.wcrf.org/diet-activity-and-cancer/risk-factors/meat-fish-dairy-and-cancer-risk/ accessed 11 May 2022.

World Health Organization. (1986). Ottawa Charter for Health Promotion. World Health Organization European Regional Office.

World Health Organization. (2015). Cancer: Carcinogenicity of the consumption of red meat and processed meat. https://www.who.int/news-room/questions-and-answers/item/cancer-carcinogenicity-of-the-consumption-of-red-meat-and-processed-meat accessed 11 May 2022.

World Health Organization. (2019). *Global status report on alcohol and health 2018*. World Health Organization.

World Health Organization. (2020). The Top 10 Causes of Death. https://www.who.int/news-room/fact-sheets/detail/the-top-10-causes-of-death accessed 12 March 2022.

Wu, F., Wang, B., Zhuang, P., et al. (2022). Association of preserved vegetable consumption and prevalence of colorectal polyps: results from the Lanxi Pre-CRC Cohort (LP3C). *European Journal of Nutrition, 61*, 1273–1284.

Yang, L., Morielli, A. R., Heer, E., et al. (2021). Effects of exercise on cancer treatment efficacy: a systematic review of preclinical and clinical studies. *Cancer Research, 81*, 4889–4895.

Zhang, X., Fang, Y.-J., Feng, X.-L., et al. (2020). Higher intakes of dietary vitamin D, calcium and dairy products are inversely associated with the risk of CRC: a case-control study in China. *British Journal of Nutrition, 123*, 699–711.

Ziegler, E., Hill, J., Lieske, B., et al. (2022). Empowerment in cancer patients: does peer support make a difference? A systematic review. *Psychooncology, 31*, 683–704.

Zoltick, E. S., Smith-Warner, S. A., Yuan, C., et al. (2021). Sugar-sweetened beverage, artificially sweetened beverage and sugar intake and CRC survival. *British Journal of Cancer, 125*, 1016–1024.

3

Molecular biology of sporadic colorectal cancer

Daniel Novelli and Marco Novelli

Introduction

In a seminal paper in 1954, Armitage and Doll postulated the multistage theory of carcinogenesis and inferred that six to seven specific, discrete, and stable events were required to turn a normal cell into a cancer (Armitage & Doll, 1954). It was not until some 34 years later that this theory was demonstrated in practice when Vogelstein described his adenoma–carcinoma sequence (Vogelstein et al., 1988). With genetic analysis in its infancy, researchers had been looking at families with the autosomal dominant inherited condition familial adenomatous polyposis. These patients develop thousands of adenomatous polyps in the large intestine and, if left untreated, these inevitably go on to develop colorectal adenocarcinoma. Vogelstein was able to map KRAS mutations, p53 mutations, and allelic deletions of chromosomes 5 and 18 onto various stages of adenoma and carcinoma development with production of his now eponymous Vogelgram in 1990 (Fig. 3.1) (Fearon & Vogelstein, 1990).

In the subsequent 30 years, Vogelstein's model has held up to investigation remarkably well. The main genetic players he described (APC, KRAS, and p53) remain the backbone of our current understanding of colorectal tumorigenesis (Fig. 3.2). What has changed is that it has since become apparent that this model, now known as the chromosomal instability (CIN) pathway of colorectal tumorigenesis, accounts for some 70–80% of sporadic colorectal cancers, leaving some 20–30% of tumours developing on other pathways. The combination of several different classification systems and varying nomenclature has led to this becoming a slightly confusing area but, seen simply, the vast majority of the remaining tumours develop via microsatellite instability (see also Chapter 1) with some overlap of these two main pathways.

Approximately 15% of colorectal cancers develop on a background of microsatellite instability (MSI). A small percentage of these (3% of total colorectal cancers) are hereditary colorectal cancers associated with Lynch syndrome, in which patients typically have a germline mutation in a mismatch repair gene. Most sporadic MSI tumours (approximately 12% of total CRCs) achieve microsatellite instability via the CpG island methylator phenotype (CIMP) pathway (Boland & Goel, 2010).

More recently, researchers have subdivided colorectal cancer into CIN tumours and 'hypermutated/ultramutated' tumours. This classification largely correlates with the CIN/MSI classification but has the added benefit that it incorporates non-MSI ultra-mutated tumours with mutations in other DNA repair genes (in particular POLE) and is also helpful when considering treatment options (e.g. immunotherapy) (Muzny et al., 2012). Lastly, there is also a classification based on consensus molecular subtypes which subdivides colorectal cancers into five categories, CMS1 to CMS4, with CMS1 representing the hyper/ultra-mutated tumours, CMS2 to CMS4 effectively subdividing the CIN tumours (CMS2 representing the classical canonical Wnt signalling pathway), leaving approximately 13% of tumours with mixed features unclassified (Guinney et al., 2015; Müller, Ibrahim, & Arends, 2016).

Adenoma–carcinoma sequence

Current models of the adenoma–carcinoma sequence (Fig. 3.2) retain loss/mutation in APC, KRAS, and p53, but in addition there has been progress in characterizing the 18q loss. 18q loss has been demonstrated in approximately 70% of colonic adenocarcinomas (Takayama et al., 2006). The deleted in colorectal cancer gene (DCC), now renamed 'Netrin receptor DCC', has been demonstrated to be mutated in only approximately 6% of colorectal cancers (Cho et al., 1994). DCC has since been implicated in the process of apoptosis (Mehlen et al., 1998) but the significance of DCC mutations in colorectal carcinogenesis remains uncertain. However, two established tumour suppressor genes, *SMAD2* and *SMAD4*, are also present at 18q. These genes function in transforming factor B (TF-b) signal transduction. *SMAD4* mutations have been demonstrated in up to 24% of colorectal carcinomas, with *SMAD2* mutations demonstrated at a level of 3.4% (Fleming et al., 2013).

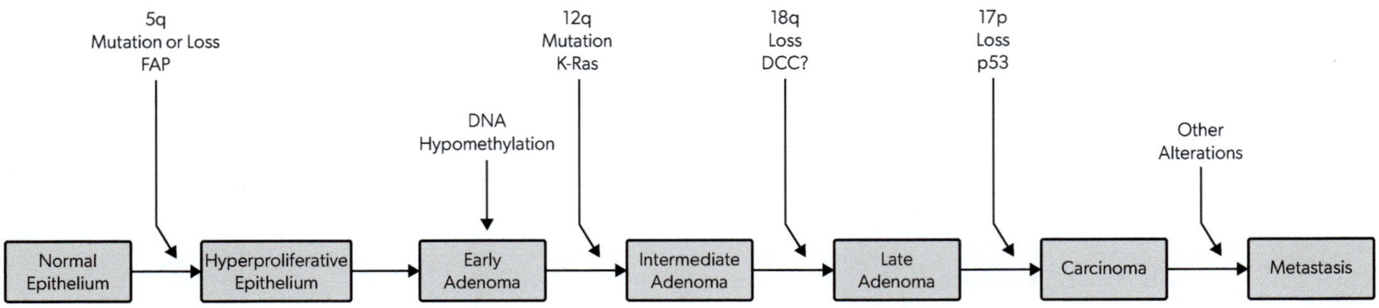

Figure 3.1 The Vogelgram (adapted from Fearon & Vogelstein, 1990).

APC—canonical pathway and Wnt signalling

In 1991, the tumour suppressor gene located at 5q21 was formally identified and named adenomatous polyposis coli (APC) (Kinzler et al., 1991). APC, often referred to as the gatekeeper gene, has been shown to be mutated in approximately 80% of sporadic colorectal carcinomas (Powell et al., 1992). APC appears to exert its main function via its interaction with B-catenin in the canonical pathway.

B-catenin is a key transcription protein expressed in a wide variety of tissues. It performs an essential role in promoting cellular proliferation within intestinal crypts. B-catenin acts by binding transcription factors, such as the TCF/LEF family, promoting downstream transcription of genes promoting proliferation (Schuijers et al., 2014). Intracellular levels of b-catenin are therefore carefully maintained through homeostatic Wnt signalling.

Extracellular Wnt binds cell surface receptors (e.g. frizzled), initiating a intracellular cascade of recruitment and phosphorylation events termed 'Wnt signalling'. Normal physiological Wnt signalling is controlled through a destruction complex ubiquitin ligase mechanism. When Wnt glycoprotein is absent, cytoplasmic b-catenin is held in a destruction complex composed of four core proteins: APC, Axin, GSK3, and CK1 (Clevers & Nusse, 2012b). Binding of the complex initiates a multistep phosphorylation sequence resulting in the recognition of b-catenin by an E3-ubiquitin ligase, named B-TrCP. The targeted recognition results in b-catenin polyubiquitination, and consequently proteasomal degradation. The degradation of b-catenin results in lower intracellular levels of b-catenin, downregulating the expression of pro-proliferative genes.

Active Wnt signalling inactivates the destruction complex preventing b-catenin degradation, causing an intracytoplasmic accumulation of b-catenin and enabling it to translocate to the nucleus where it activates TCF4-related gene transcription (Fig. 3.3).

Somatic mutation of genes coding for proteins in the b-catenin destruction complex results in ineffective b-catenin degradation leading to cellular proliferation (Fennell et al., 2020). APC is one of the most frequently mutated genes in colorectal tumorigenesis. Somatic mutations, primarily located within the mutation cluster region (MCR) between codons 1286 and 1513, result in an inactive/less efficient isoform of the APC protein (Smits et al., 2000). Most inactivating mutations reported are frameshift and nonsense mutations resulting in a truncated protein (Béroud & Soussi, 1996). Truncated APC proteins are unable to bind the b-catenin destruction complex resulting in a rise in cytoplasmic b-catenin levels, translocation of b-catenin to the nucleus, and subsequent activation and suppression of the expression of multiple genes resulting in tumour proliferation, survival, differentiation, migration/invasion, and stem cell markers (see Table 3.1).

Although mutations in the APC gene are the most common somatic mutations in the canonical pathway, mutations in genes coding for other proteins of the b-catenin destruction complex have also been shown to occur, including mutations in Axin and b-catenin

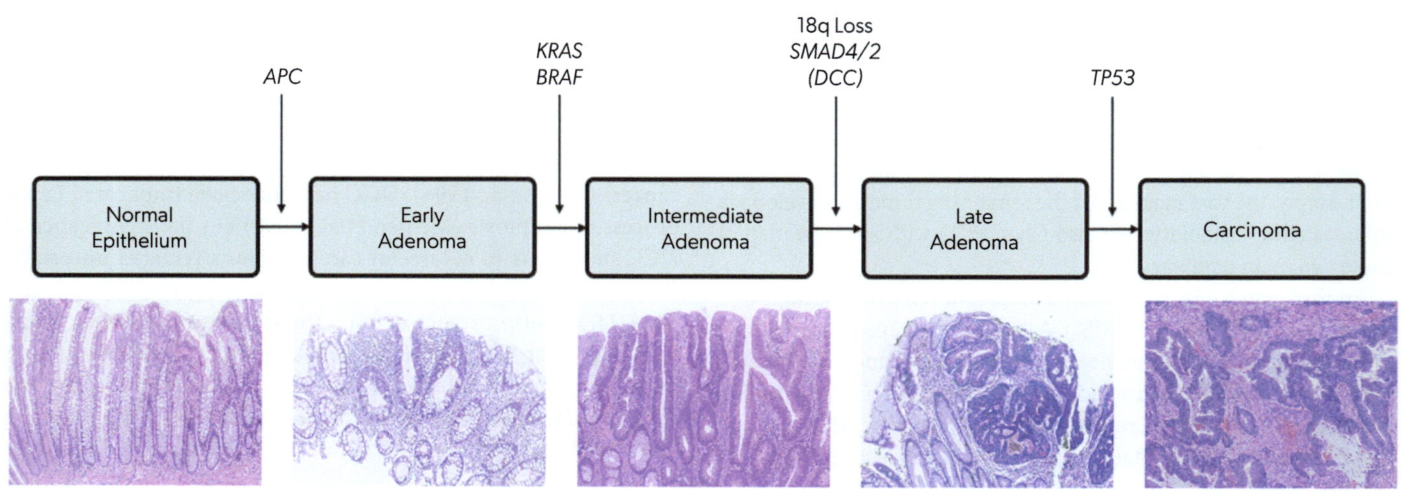

Figure 3.2 Current understanding of the adenoma carcinoma sequence.

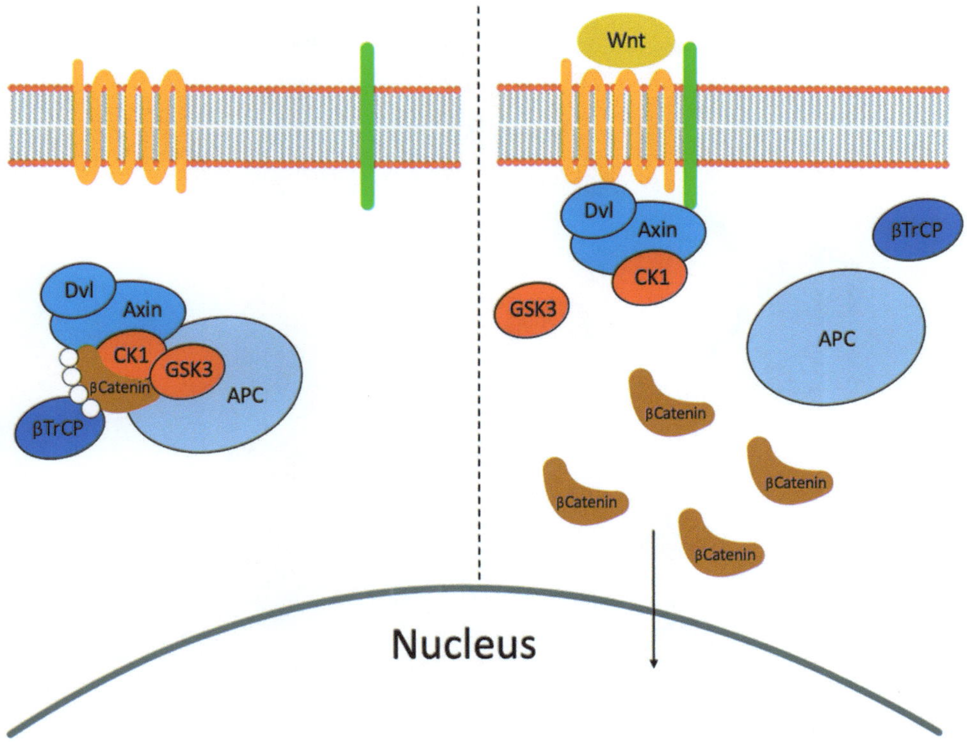

Figure 3.3 Model of Wnt signalling and the destruction complex (adapted from Clevers & Nusse, 2012).

itself. Such mutations and APC mutations are mutually exclusive but function in a similar fashion.

KRAS—MAPK/ERK pathway

A better understanding of the molecular pathways involved in colorectal tumorigenesis has widened the scope of potential targets for novel pharmaceutical therapies. The mitogen-activated protein kinase (MAPK/ERK) pathway is currently the most widely investigated and, arguably, most important pathway in colorectal cancer. The MAPK pathway is an evolutionary conserved and controlled physiological pathway involved in cellular proliferation, differentiation, survival, and death. The MAPK/ERK pathway (in particular the RAS/RAF/MEK/ERK kinase cascade) has been the subject of extensive research which has shown that it is one of the most frequently dysregulated pathways in human cancers. Such research has also led to the identification of a number of potential protein targets for therapeutic intervention and the development of multiple anti-cancer agents.

Table 3.1 B-catenin/TCF target genes (Adaped from Schneikert et al., 2007.)

PROLIFERATION	**c-Myc, Cyclin D, COX-2,** PGDH
SURVIVAL	**PPARR**, **COX-2**, PGDH, p62/SQSTM1
DIFFERENTIATION	E-cadherin
MIGRATION/INVASION	**MMP7**, **EphB**/Ephrin-B
STEM CELL MARKERS	**Lgr7**

Note: Upregulated genes are depicted in bold, downregulated are unbold.

Extracellular growth factors, such as epidermal growth factor (EGF), bind to and activate transmembrane receptor proteins known as receptor tyrosine kinases (e.g. EGFR). Activation of these transmembrane receptors initiates an intracellular cascade of kinases which activates RAS (see Fig. 3.4). Once activated, RAS activates RAF which in turn phosphorylates and activates MEK which then phosphorylates extracellular signal-regulated kinase (ERK). ERK then enters the nucleus initiating multiple transcription regulatory components through further phosphorylation, including those responsible for stimulating proliferation and cellular survival. In a similar fashion, receptor tyrosine kinase signalling can also activate the PI3K pathway.

RAS signalling pathways are some of the most well-studied and characterized signal transduction pathways in colorectal cancer progression. Highlighted in Vogelstein's initial description of the adenoma carcinoma sequence, RAS is a superfamily of genes encoding three ubiquitously expressed small GTPase transductor proteins (KRAS, HRAS, NRAS) (Hobbs, Der, & Rossman, 2016). RAS signalling enables external stimuli to alter and amplify nuclear expression of genes involved in cell proliferation and cellular survival. In colorectal carcinogenesis, KRAS is the most frequently mutated RAS protein (Dinu et al., 2014). Located on chromosome 12, the 21kDa protein, is made up of six beta strands and five alpha helices, and acts as a molecular switch through its intrinsic GTPase activity, driving cellular proliferation, survival, and ultimately metastasis. Mutations in the RAS superfamily have been reported in up to 30% of all human tumours. KRAS mutations account for up 85% of all RAS mutations and are present in 35–45% of all colorectal cancers. The most common KRAS mutations (90%) are located on codons 12 and 13 and result in constitutive activation of KRAS (Imamura et al., 2012). Such missense mutations typically function by either

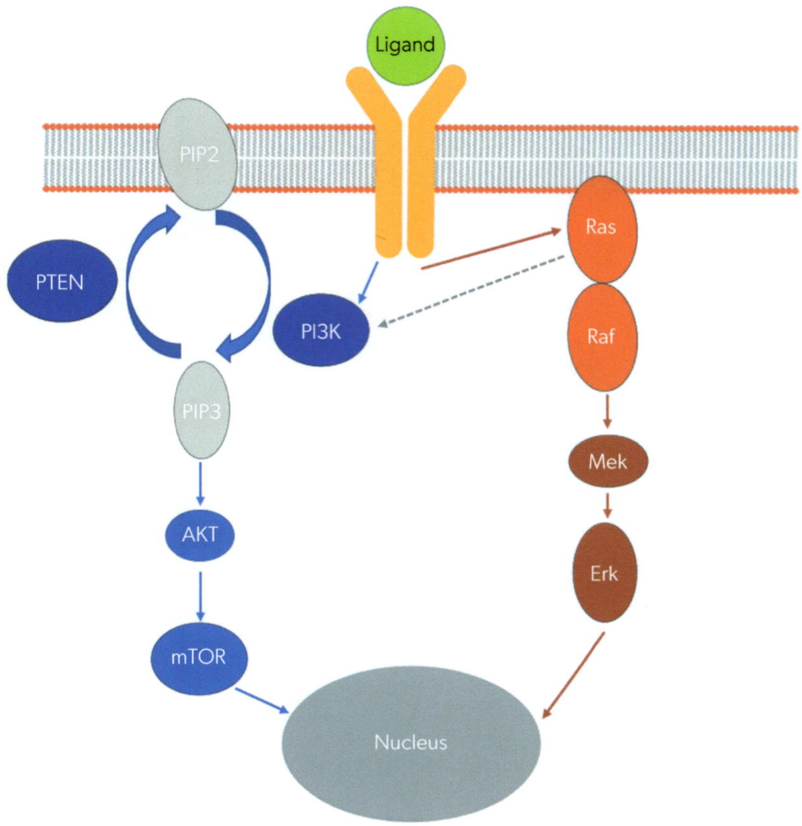

Figure 3.4 Receptor tyrosine kinase signalling pathways—MAPK and PI3K/pAKT pathways (adapted from (Loupakis et al., 2009).

disrupting GTP hydrolysis or enhancing nucleotide exchange resulting in the accumulation of constitutively activated KRAS (Cook et al., 2021).

RAF is a family of three serine/threonine-specific kinases (ARAF, BRAF, and CRAF) involved in the MAPK pathway. BRAF, located on gene 7, is the most frequently mutated RAF gene, with mutations demonstrated in 5–15% of colorectal cancers (Molina-Cerrillo et al., 2020). BRAF V600E is the most frequent BRAF mutation resulting in constitutively activated BRAF (Luu 2019).

Tumours with mutations in RAS or RAF genes typically demonstrate a poor response to anti- EGFR targeted therapies (e.g. cetuximab) in isolation or in combination with cytotoxics, as blocking EGFR-mediated signalling becomes ineffective when there is downstream activation of the MAPK pathway (Gong et al., 2016). KRAS and BRAF mutations act in a similar fashion so mutations in these genes are usually mutually exclusive.

SMAD2/4—transforming growth factor B (TGFB) pathway

The transforming growth factor B signalling pathway is a complex and crucial signalling pathway involved in a broad spectrum of cellular processes including embryogenesis, cell proliferation, cell differentiation, and cell death. Genetic aberrations involving this pathway have been demonstrated in both MSI-type colorectal cancers (primarily involving the TGFB receptor type 2) and MSS-type tumours (SMAD2+4). SMAD4 mutations have been associated with the CMS4: mesenchymal consensus molecular subtype (Müller, Ibrahim, & Arends, 2016) and are associated with a poor prognosis (Itatani, Kawada, & Sakai, 2019; Fang et al., 2021).

TP53

P53 has been dubbed the 'guardian of the genome'. This protein plays an important role as a controller of the cell cycle, ensuring that any DNA damage is identified and repaired before cell division. If DNA is badly damaged, p53 can also induce cell death via the process of apoptosis. P53 is widely regarded as the gene most frequently mutated during carcinogenesis in humans with p53 mutation demonstrated in 42% of twelve major human cancers and 59% of colorectal cancers (Kandoth et al., 2013). Dysregulation of p53 leads to chromosomal instability and ultimately aneuploidy. Given its importance in carcinogenesis, there has been a lot of research examining the potential for therapeutics targeting mutant p53 or its interaction with other proteins. Currently, no p53-based therapies are commercially available but this remains an area of ongoing investigation.

Hyperplastic polyp—sessile serrated lesion—carcinoma sequence

It had long been argued whether or not hyperplastic polyps are precursor lesions for colorectal malignancy. The demonstration of both BRAF mutations and CIMP in the microvesicular variant of hyperplastic polyps and KRAS mutations in the goblet cell variant of

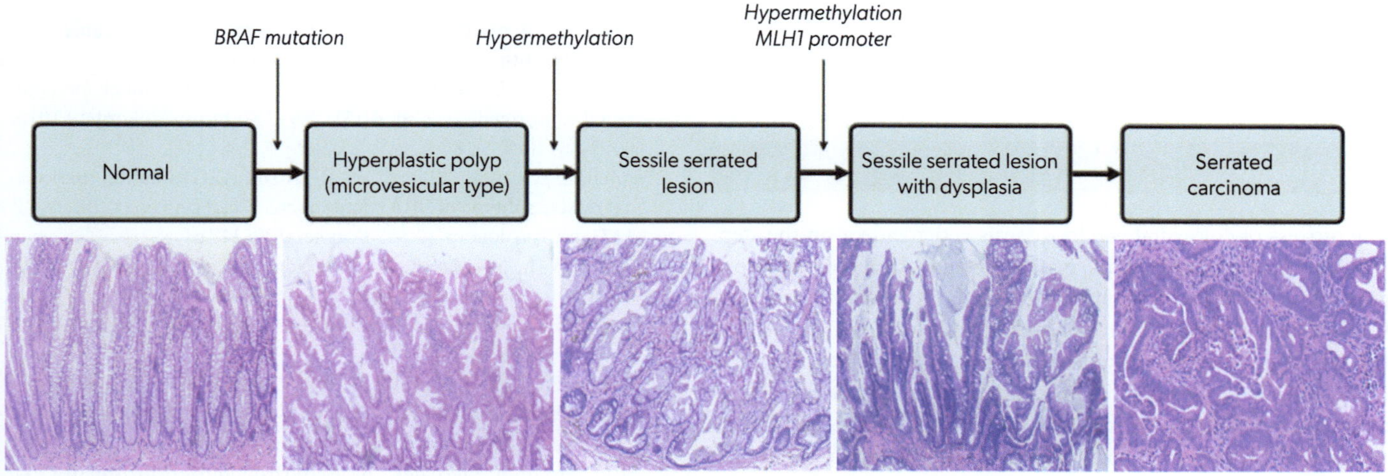

Figure 3.5 Current understanding of the hyperplastic polyp–sessile serrated lesion–carcinoma sequence.

hyperplastic polyps suggests that these lesions are almost certainly neoplastic and may well act as precursors lesions of colorectal cancer (Yang et al., 2004). The fact that BRAF mutations occur at a similar frequency in both hyperplastic polyps and sessile serrated lesions but that CIMP is much more frequent in sessile serrated lesions suggests there may well be progression from hyperplastic polyp, through sessile serrated lesion, to full-blown invasive carcinoma—the 'serrated carcinoma pathway' (Fig. 3.5).

Microsatellite instability

During DNA transcription there is a complex of seven proteins (MLH1, MLH3, MSH2, MSH3, MSH6, PMD1, and PMS2), known as the mismatch repair complex, which trails behind DNA polymerase. This complex proofreads the newly synthesized strand of DNA identifying and repairing mispaired bases. Microsatellites are repeat sequences of DNA which are scattered throughout the genome (in both coding and non-coding regions). DNA polymerase may experience 'slippage' when copying repeat sequences leading to DNA insertions and deletions. If there is a failure of mismatch repair this leads to frameshift mutations. PCR-based analysis is used to examine microsatellites to look for mismatch repair failure which, when demonstrated, is termed microsatellite instability. Screening for defective mismatch repair can also be performed using immunohistochemistry looking for loss of mismatch repair protein expression. When mismatch repair is deficient, frameshift mutations lead to changes in the resulting amino acid sequence and the generation of novel peptides. It has been postulated that these novel peptides can stimulate the immune system, which may explain the prominent lymphocytic infiltrate seen in many mismatch repair deficient tumours and their clinical response to immune checkpoint inhibitors.

In Lynch syndrome there is a germline mutation most commonly in one of four of the mismatch repair proteins: MLH1, MSH2, MSH6, and PMS2. In sporadic mismatch repair deficient colorectal adenocarcinomas mismatch repair is usually defective due to hypermethylation of the MLH1 promoter, an epigenetic phenomenon secondary to CIMP.

CpG methylator island phenotype (CIMP)

Methylation is a normal cellular process used to regulate gene expression without changing the DNA sequence. It is essential in normal cellular processes such as genomic imprinting and X-chromosome inactivation. Typically, around 4% of cytosine residues are methylated, mostly at CG dinucleotide sequences. Approximately 50% of CpG islands are located in gene promoter regions with methylation being utilized as a way of controlling gene expression. During carcinogenesis, cellular methylation can become aberrant, with hypermethylation causing silencing of tumour suppressor genes and hypomethylation upregulating oncogenes. Promoter CpG island methylation occurs across a wide range of human tumours. When this methylation occurs at multiple different loci it is referred to as CpG methylator island phenotype-high (CIMP-H). In CIMP, the MLH1 promoter is a frequent target leading to loss of MLH1 expression, failure of mismatch repair, and resulting microsatellite instability. In colorectal cancer CIMP is strongly associated with BRAF mutation (Weisenberger et al., 2006) and appears central to the serrated carcinoma pathway.

Somatic POLE mutation

POLE is the central catalytic subunit of DNA polymerase epsilon. The autosomal dominant inherited cancer syndrome polymerase proofreading-associated polyposis (PPAP) was described in 2014 with germline mutations demonstrated in both POLE and POLD1 (see Chapter 1). In a similar fashion to the mismatch repair proteins, POLE checks the transcription of DNA to ensure there are no errors in the newly generated DNA strand, but in the case of POLE this relates primarily to single base pair substitutions rather than insertions/deletions. Failure of POLE function leads to a very high burden of single nucleotide variants (SNVs). Since the discovery of PPAP it has become apparent that heterozygous somatic mutations in POLE are the driving mutations in a small percentage of sporadic colorectal adenocarcinomas (< 1%) (Domingo et al., 2016; Temko et al., 2018). Somatic mutation in POLE leads to early onset sporadic colorectal cancers with an ultra-mutated phenotype which tend to have a good prognosis and typically respond to immune checkpoint inhibitors (Domingo et al., 2016; Garmezy et al., 2022).

Discussion

The process of colorectal carcinogenesis is dependent on the stepwise accumulation of multiple genetic defects. An increased rate of genomic mutation accumulation seems to be central to this process. Colorectal cancers can be roughly divided into those that achieve this 'genomic instability' by deletions and gains in large pieces of DNA, so-called chromosomal instability, and those that have 'hyper and ultra-mutation'. The majority of sporadic colorectal cancers follow the chromosomal instability pathway (adenoma–carcinoma sequence). Novel targeted therapies for these tumours currently tend to focus on the MAPK/ERK pathway. The hypermutated tumours (MSI type) typically follow the serrated carcinoma pathway but the ultra-mutated tumours may well start as classical adenomas. For hyper and ultra-mutated tumours there are currently more potential treatment options, in particular, the use of immune checkpoint inhibitors. An understanding of the molecular biology of colorectal carcinogenesis is becoming increasingly important in the clinical management of colorectal cancer patients, providing information on patient prognosis, potentially directing surgery, and informing the use/choice of antitumour agents.

REFERENCES

Armitage, P., & Doll, R. (1954). The age distribution of cancer and a multi-stage theory of carcinogenesis. *British Journal of Cancer*, *8*(1),1–12. https://doi.org/10.1038/bjc.1954.1

Béroud, C., & Soussi, T. (1996). APC gene: database of germline and somatic mutations in human tumors and cell lines. *Nucleic Acids Research*, *24*(1), 121–124. https://doi.org/10.1093/nar/24.1.121

Boland, C. R., & Goel, A. (2010). Microsatellite instability in colorectal cancer. *Gastroenterology*, *138*(6), 2073–2087.e3. https://doi.org/10.1053/j.gastro.2009.12.064

Cancer Genome Atlas Network (2012). Comprehensive molecular characterization of human colon and rectal cancer. *Nature*, *487*(7407), 330–337. https://doi.org/10.1038/nature11252

Cho, K. R., Oliner, J. D., Simons, J. W., et al. (1994). The DCC gene: structural analysis and mutations in colorectal carcinomas. *Genomics*, *19*(3), 525–531. https://doi.org/10.1006/geno.1994.1102

Clevers, H., & Nusse, R. (2012). Wnt/β-catenin signaling and disease. *Cell*, *149*(6), 1192–1205. https://doi.org/10.1016/j.cell.2012.05.012

Cook, J. H., Melloni, G. E. M., Gulhan, D. C., et al. (2021). The origins and genetic interactions of KRAS mutations are allele- and tissue-specific. *Nature Communications*, *12*(1), 1808. https://doi.org/10.1038/s41467-021-22125-z

Dinu, D., Dobre, M., Panaitescu, E., et al. (2014). Prognostic significance of KRAS gene mutations in colorectal cancer—preliminary study. *Journal of Medicine and Life*, *7*(4), 581–587.

Domingo, E., Freeman-Mills, L., Rayner, E., et al. (2016). Somatic POLE proofreading domain mutation, immune response, and prognosis in colorectal cancer: a retrospective, pooled biomarker study. *Lancet Gastroenterology & Hepatology*, *1*(3), 207–216. https://doi.org/10.1016/S2468-1253(16)30014-0

Fang, T., Liang, T., Wang, Y., et al. (2021). Prognostic role and clinicopathological features of SMAD4 gene mutation in colorectal cancer: a systematic review and meta-analysis. *BMC Gastroenterology*, *21*(1), 297. https://doi.org/10.1186/s12876-021-01864-9

Fearon, E. R., & Vogelstein, B. (1990). A genetic model for colorectal tumorigenesis. *Cell*, *61*(5), 759–767. https://doi.org/10.1016/0092-8674(90)90186-i

Fennell, L. J., Kane, A., Liu, C., et al. (2020). APC mutation marks an aggressive subtype of BRAF mutant colorectal cancers. *Cancers*, *12*, 1171. https://doi.org/10.3390/cancers12051171

Fleming, N. I., Jorissen, R. N., Mouradov, D., et al. (2013). SMAD2, SMAD3 and SMAD4 mutations in colorectal cancer. *Cancer Research*, *73*(2), 725–735. https://doi.org/10.1158/0008-5472.CAN-12-2706

Garmezy, B., Gheeya, J., Lin, H. Y., et al. (2022). Clinical and molecular characterization of POLE mutations as predictive biomarkers of response to immune checkpoint inhibitors in advanced cancers. *JCO Precision Oncology*, *6*, e2100267. https://doi.org/10.1200/PO.21.00267

Gong, J, Cho, M, & Fakih, M. (2016). RAS and BRAF in metastatic colorectal cancer management. *Journal of Gastrointestinal Oncology*, *7*(5), 697–704. https://doi.org/10.21037/jgo.2016.06.12

Guinney, J., Dienstmann, R., Wang, X., et al. (2015). The consensus molecular subtypes of colorectal cancer. *Nature Medicine*, *21*(11), 1350–1356. https://doi.org/10.1038/nm.3967

Hobbs, G. A., Der, C. J., & Rossman, K. L. (2016). RAS isoforms and mutations in cancer at a glance. *Journal of Cell Science*, *129*(7), 1287–1292. https://doi.org/10.1242/jcs.182873

Imamura, Y., Morikawa, T., Liao, X., et al. (2012). Specific mutations in KRAS codons 12 and 13, and patient prognosis in 1075 BRAF wild-type colorectal cancers. *Clinical Cancer Research*, *18*(17), 4753–4763. https://doi.org/10.1158/1078-0432.CCR-11-3210

Itatani, Y., Kawada, K., & Sakai, Y. (2019). Transforming growth factor-β signaling pathway in colorectal cancer and its tumor microenvironment. *International Journal of Molecular Sciences*, *20*(23), 5822. https://doi.org/10.3390/ijms20235822

Kandoth, C., McLellan, M. D., Vandin, F., et al. (2013). Mutational landscape and significance across 12 major cancer types. *Nature*, *502*(7471), 333–339. https://doi.org/10.1038/nature12634

Kinzler, K. W., Nilbert, M. C., Vogelstein, B., et al. (1991). Identification of a gene located at chromosome 5q21 that is mutated in colorectal cancers. *Science*, *251*(4999), 1366–1370. https://doi.org/10.1126/science.1848370

Loupakis, F., Pollina, L., Stasi, I., et al. (2009). PTEN expression and KRAS mutations on primary tumors and metastases in the prediction of benefit from cetuximab plus irinotecan for patients with metastatic colorectal cancer. *Journal of Clinical Oncology*, *27*(16), 2622–2629. https://doi.org/10.1200/JCO.2008.20.2796

Luu, L.-J. (2019). BRAF mutation and its importance in colorectal cancer in TJPE-E Segelov (ed), Rijeka: (IntechOpen 2019) chapter 3.

Mehlen, P., Rabizadeh, S., Snipas, S. J., et al. (1998). The DCC gene product induces apoptosis by a mechanism requiring receptor proteolysis. *Nature*, *395*(6704), 801–804. https://doi.org/10.1038/27441

Molina-Cerrillo, J., San Román, M., Pozas, J., et al. (2020). BRAF mutated colorectal cancer: new treatment approaches. *Cancers*, *12*(6), 1571. https://doi.org/10.3390/cancers12061571

Müller, M. F., Ibrahim, A. E. K., & Arends, M. J. (2016) Molecular pathological classification of colorectal cancer. *Virchows Archiv*, *469*(2), 125–134. https://doi.org/10.1007/s00428-016-1956-3

Powell, S. M., Zilz, N., Beazer-Barclay, Y., et al. (1992). APC mutations occur early during colorectal tumorigenesis. *Nature*, *359*(6392), 235–237. https://doi.org/10.1038/359235a0

Schneikert, J., Grohmann, A., & Behrens, J. (2007). Truncated APC regulates the transcriptional activity of beta-catenin in a cell cycle dependent manner. *Human Molecular Genetics*, *16*(2), 199–209. https://doi.org/10.1093/hmg/ddl464

Schuijers, J., Mokry, M., Hatzis, P., et al. (2014). Wnt-induced transcriptional activation is exclusively mediated by TCF/LEF. *EMBO Journal*, *33*(2), 146–156. https://doi.org/10.1002/embj.201385358

Smits, R., Hofland, N., Edelmann, W., et al. (2000). Somatic Apc mutations are selected upon their capacity to inactivate the beta-catenin downregulating activity. *Genes, Chromosomes & Cancer*, *29*(3), 229–239. https://doi.org/10.1002/1098-2264(2000)9999:9999<::aid-gcc1033>3.0.co;2-r

Takayama, T., Miyanishi, K., Hayashi, T., et al. (2006). Colorectal cancer: genetics of development and metastasis. *Journal of Gastroenterology*, *41*(3), 185–192. https://doi.org/10.1007/s00535-006-1801-6

Temko, D., Van Gool, I. C., Rayner, E., et al. (2018). Somatic POLE exonuclease domain mutations are early events in sporadic endometrial and colorectal carcinogenesis, determining driver mutational landscape, clonal neoantigen burden and immune response. *Journal of Pathology*, *245*(3), 283–296. https://doi.org/10.1002/path.5081

Vogelstein, B., Fearon, E. R., Hamilton, S. R., et al. (1988). Genetic alterations during colorectal-tumor development. *New England Journal of Medicine*, *319*(9), 525–532. https://doi.org/10.1056/NEJM198809013190901

Weisenberger, D. J., Siegmund, K. D., Campan, M., et al. (2006). CpG island methylator phenotype underlies sporadic microsatellite instability and is tightly associated with BRAF mutation in colorectal cancer. *Nature Genetics*, *38*(7), 787–793. https://doi.org/10.1038/ng1834

Yang, S., Farraye, F. A., Mack, C., et al. (2004). BRAF and KRAS Mutations in hyperplastic polyps and serrated adenomas of the colorectum: relationship to histology and CpG island methylation status. *American Journal of Surgical Pathology*, *28*(11), 1452–1459. https://doi.org/10.1097/01.pas.0000141404.56839.6a

4

Impact of tumour microenvironment in governing invasion, growth, and metastasis

Faiz Jabbar and David N. Church

Introduction

As reviewed elsewhere in this text, colorectal cancer (CRC) initiation and local and metastatic spread are driven by genomic and epigenomic alterations intrinsic to malignant cells. However, similar to other solid tumours, there is a substantial and increasing awareness that these processes are also determined by the stromal and immune milieu in which these malignant cells reside; collectively referred to as the tumour microenvironment (TME) (Binnewies et al., 2018).

The importance of the TME was demonstrated more than a century ago by William Coley in one of the most cited of medical interventions. Coley injected a virulent strain of Streptococcus Pyogenes into the oesophageal cancer of patient suffering life-threatening symptoms. Following an acute, severe febrile illness, the tumour regressed and the patient made a complete recovery. Although not known at the time, this is now widely thought to be due to consequence of an immune-related cytokine-mediated tumoricidal reaction induced by the bacterium (Beutler & Cerami, 1986). The concept of the TME was birthed in 1889 by Stephen Paget. His seed and soil theory suggested that metastasis is not due to chance but rather that some tumour cells (seeds) grew preferentially in the microenvironment of select organs (soil). Consequently, metastases result only when the appropriate seed is implanted in its suitable soil. While his postulate was initially countered by the proponents of alternative, anatomical explanations based on tumour vascular and lymphatic drainage, it has since been validated by numerous studies that show tumour cells preferentially metastasize to specific organs (Paget, 1889; Fidler, 2008). While the mechanisms which determine local and distant tumour spread remain incompletely understood, it is now clear that the TME plays a critical role. Its importance in CRC is illustrated that the transcriptional profile of two of the four consensus molecular subtype (CMS) classes are driven by non-malignant cell types; that is immune-rich CMS1 tumours and stroma-rich CMS4 cases (Guinney et al., 2015).

The TME is dynamic. Its composition is established by bidirectional interactions between tumour cells and resident and infiltrating non-tumour cells. These communicate directly and indirectly to regulate cellular processes and exert selective pressures, thus shaping the other's phenotype. Such interactions are critical as to whether tumour cells lie dormant, are extinguished, or progress towards metastasis (Binnewies et al., 2018). Microenvironmental factors play opposing roles in tumour progression by either promoting or antagonising carcinogenesis; in fact, some can do either, depending upon which step in the disease process they are dysregulated. Interactions within the TME are mediated by cell-to-cell contact and soluble factors, such as cytokines, chemokines, and growth factors, derived both from the tumour and activated surrounding cells. These factors constantly remodel the TME and have local and systemic effects, which are not only crucial for generalized immunosuppression that enables the generation of pre-metastatic niches and successful metastatic establishment, but also closely affect patient prognosis and sensitivity to therapy (Binnewies et al., 2018).

As a disease arising in an immune-rich organ, CRC is notable for generating a strong immunosuppressive TME which hampers immunosurveillance and facilitates immune evasion and tumour dissemination. To escape eradication by the immune system, CRC recruits and polarizes immunosuppressive regulatory T cells (Tregs), tumour-associated macrophages (TAMs), and myeloid-derived suppressor cells (MDSCs). In addition, CRC inhibits or excludes immune cells with anti-tumour potential such as dendritic cells (DCs), natural killer (NK) cells, and effector T cells from the TME. The CRC TME consists of immune and stromal components such as the extracellular matrix (ECM), MAPs, blood vessels, and signalling molecules (**Fig. 4.1**). (Xiong, 2019).

In this chapter we detail the immune and stromal components of the CRC TME to understand its composition and diversity. We summarise the methods used to dissect the TME and the insights these have provided into its regulation of growth, invasion, and

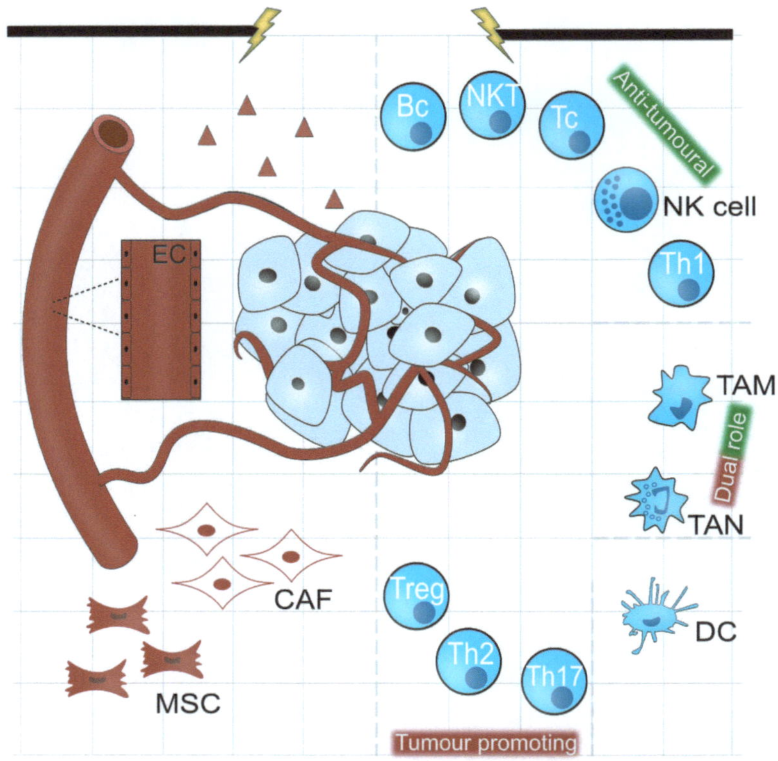

Figure 4.1 Overview of the tumour microenvironment (TME) in colorectal cancer.

Malignant epithelial cells are resident within and are infiltrated by non-malignant, yet dysregulated stromal and immune cells of the TME. Immune cell populations which typically exert an anti-tumour include cytotoxic T and B cells (CTL and Bc), Th1 cells and natural killer (NK) cells, and variant NK T cells (NKT). Other immune cell types such as regulatory T cells (Treg) Th2 and Th17 cells tend to promote tumour growth. A third group of immune cells including tumour-associated macrophages and neutrophils (TAMs and TANs) can have pro- or anti-tumour effect depending on their polarization. Dysregulated stromal cells include cancer-associated fibroblasts (CAFs) and mesenchymal stem cells (MSC). Tumour neovasculature populated by abnormal endothelial cells plays important roles in both transport of oxgen and nutrients but also signalling to both the epithelial component and other cells of the TME.

metastasis. Finally, we highlight the emerging interest in therapeutic targeting of the TME and the future perspectives in the field.

Composition of the TME in colorectal cancer

Immune component

Immune cells may comprise a substantial fraction of tumour bulk in CRC, with leucocyte proportion exceeding half of all tumour cells in some cases (Thorsson et al., 2018). In contrast, other CRCs display very low numbers of infiltrating immune cells. This variation in the extent to which tumours are infiltrated by immune cells is mirrored by substantial diversity in the type of immune cells within the CRC TME. To date, much research has focused on lymphocytes, and particularly T cells as a cell type capable of direct anticancer activity. B cells have also been studied as a cell type critical for humoural immunity via production of antibodies and cytokines, and one associated with tertiary lymphoid structures. Other important immune cell types include innate types such as tumour-associated macrophages (TAMs) and tumour-associated neutrophils (TANs), dendritic cells (DCs), and myeloid-derived suppressor cells (MDSCs). Nearly all of these have been shown to correlate with clinical outcome. As their levels are often strongly correlated or anticorrelated it is difficult to study associations in isolation; however the general picture is one in which CD8+ cytotoxic T cells (CTLs), memory T cells, CD4+ T Helper1 (Th1) cells, TFH cells, and B cells are associated with improved survival, while elevated densities of Treg cells, MDSCs, and neutrophils correlate with poor prognosis (discussed in detail below) (Schmitt & Greten, 2021).

T cells are perhaps the best characterized immune cell population within the TME. Clinically relevant T cell types include CTL, Th (of which many distinct subsets exist), Treg, and Natural Killer T cells (NKT). CTL cells recognize tumoral antigens via human leucocyte antigen (HLA) class I molecules and exert a killing function upon activation. Th cells are activated by interacting with MHC class II molecules on the surface of antigen presenting cells (APCs) and can differentiate into many subtypes (Th1, 2, 3, 17, TFH) which secrete different cytokines to promote diverse immune responses. Th1 responses produce IFN-γ, activate macrophages and CTLs, thus exerting an anti-tumour effect. In contrast Th2 responses typically promote tumour growth. The role of TH17 cells, beyond secretion of IL-17, is controversial. Treg cells are classically immunosuppressive, producing this effect through secretion of immunosuppressive molecules (IL-10, TGFb, IL-35), cell-mediated cytolysis, IL-2 mediated apoptosis, and DC and neutrophil suppression. NKT are pro-inflammatory lymphocytes of the innate immune system which produce IFN-γ and exert cytotoxic activity (Schmitt & Greten, 2021). The data linking T cell infiltrate with CRC outcome are abundant and discussed later in this chapter

As noted above, professional APCs are central to both the innate and adaptive immune responses. Arguably the most important of these are DCs, which exist as a heterogenous population within the TME. Upon stimulation by bacteria, viruses, or damaged tissues such as cancer, immature DCs (iDCs) begin a maturation process where costimulatory markers (CD40, CD80, CD83, CD86), HLA class I and II molecules, and inflammatory cytokines are produced, and cell fate is determined. The two major subsets arising from this process are plasmacytoid and conventional DC (pDC, cDC), but depending on the signals present in the TME, mature DCs can be further subdivided into stimulatory and regulatory DCs (sDCs and rDCs). Exposure to proinflammatory signals (i.e. pathogen-associated molecular patterns (PAMPs)) generates sDCs that express TNF-α, IL-6, IL-12, INF-α, and IFN-γ, stimulating T cell proliferation towards Th1, Th2, or Th17 phenotypes whilst impairing T-regulatory function, leading to an effective immune response. In contrast, tolerogenic signals (e.g. TGFβ, IL-10, and prostaglandins)—often arising from other cell types in the TME—generate DCs that express IL-10, TGFβ, indoleamine 2.3- dioxygenase (IDO), PD-1, and arginase that suppress Th/CTL activation and enable Treg cell differentiation and expansion, leading to tumour progression (Subtil et al., 2021). The density of tumour-infiltrating dendritic cells (TIDCs) in CRC has been suggested to predict reduced risk of metastasis and favourable outcome, although this finding is not universal. This discordance may reflect the heterogeneity of DC populations and their plasticity in reacting stimulatory or inhibitory signals from the TME, both of which require further investigation.

While much attention has focused on characterizing the adaptive immune response to CRC, exemplified by T cells as discussed above, innate immune cell types in the TME also play important roles. NK cells produce IFN-γ, proinflammatory cytokines, and have cytotoxic functions via granzyme B and perforin-mediated apoptosis. This helps to shape a proinflammatory anti-tumour microenvironment. Whilst NK cells typically exist at low density in the CRC TME, their presence is consistently associated with improved survival (Schmitt & Greten, 2021). Circulating monocytes recruited into the TME differentiate and polarise into TAMs which exist on wide spectrum between M1 and M2 subtypes. M1 TAMs secrete proinflammatory cytokines (IL-12, ROS) that prompt anti-tumour TH1 responses. M2 subtypes secrete anti-inflammatory IL-10 and TGFb cytokines, amongst others, that establish a tolerogenic TME and promote angiogenesis via vascular endothelial growth factor (VEGF) production. M2 TAMs also secrete matrix metalloproteinases (MMPs) and cathepsins to promote invasion. M1 and M2 TAM infiltration are typically associated with better and worse survival respectively in cancer, although in CRC the picture is clear as discussed below (Bruni et al., 2020). Like TAMs, neutrophils recruited to the TME differentiate into TANs with either tumour-suppressive (N1) or tumour-promoting (N2). N1 TANs express pro-inflammatory factors and have a greater ability to kill tumour cells *in vitro*, whereas N2 TANs have a reduced expression of immunoactive factors and produce large amounts of arginase, which suppresses T cell function. Tumour-suppressive N1-like subtypes are often found in the early stages of cancer but transform into a tumour-promoting N2-like subtype as tumours progress (Bruni et al., 2020). MDSCs are a heterogeneous population of immature myeloid cells (iMCS), which are generated when there is a pathological block in the differentiation process of iMCs. Their discovery and role in CRC has been recently characterised, with numerous studies showing MDSCs accumulate in CRC and may be an obstacle for cancer immunotherapy (Bruni et al., 2020).

Stromal and vascular component

Tumour stroma, consisting of acellular components such as the extracellular matrix (ECM), and specialized connective-tissue cells such as fibroblasts and mesenchymal stromal cells (MSCs), undergoes constant remodelling and provides both physical support and functional cues for malignant cells. Though relatively ignored compared to the epithelial component, it has emerged as a critical determinant of tumourigenesis, cancer progression, metastasis, and therapy resistance (Valkenburg et al., 2018).

Normal ECM is a highly organized structure of macromolecules with two major compartments; the basement membrane (BM) and interstitial ECM. Normal BM acts as a structural barrier and growth regulator, allowing immune cells but not fibroblasts through to the epithelial compartment. Interstitial ECM occupies the space between the epithelium and surrounding tissues and consists of macromolecules such as collagen, elastin, and fibronectin, and modulators like metalloproteinase (MMP) that cleave ECM components. ECM provides a reservoir of cytokines and growth factors and all components of the interstitial ECM contain binding domains for other macromolecules and cell-membrane receptors, which under normal conditions helps coordinate tissue structure and function (Valkenburg et al., 2018). Abnormal ECM in the CRC TME may contribute to immune exclusion and dysregulated signalling that promotes oncogenesis.

Fibroblasts are the most common stromal cell type in the CRC TME, and they sculpt the ECM in which they reside by synthesis, deposition, and turnover of macromolecules that build and degrade its components. Consequently, they influence mobility of other cells through the ECM and tissue integrity, among other processes. Cross-talk with malignant epithelium induces differentiation into cancer-associated fibroblasts (CAFs), which can release cytokines to influence tumour growth and invasion and promote angiogenesis, inflammation, and chemoresistance. This has led to CAFs being dubbed the architects of cancer pathogenesis in CRC (Valkenburg et al., 2018). MSCs are non-haematopoietic multipotent adult stromal cells that reside largely in bone marrow. MCSs support homeostasis in healthy tissue during regeneration and wound healing and are involved in regulation of intestinal inflammation, epithelial proliferation, stem cell maintenance, angiogenesis, and extracellular matrix remodelling and metastasis. MSCs have potent immunomodulatory capacity and are being investigated as a cellular therapy for use in a broad range of inflammatory diseases. Their ability to home to the sites of inflammation and injury and release growth factors or cytokines, to promote healing, dampen inflammation, and/or differentiate into various types of damaged tissues make them an attractive therapeutic target. The anti-inflammatory properties of MSCs are dependent on the ability of MSCs to respond to their environment and become 'activated'. Pro-inflammatory stimuli, including TNF-α, IL-1β, IL-6, or IFN-γ can enhance the immunosuppressive capabilities of MSCs (Wang et al., 2014). In the context of the tumour microenvironment, however, in the presence of a high level of pro-inflammatory signalling, these potent immunomodulatory properties can potentially influence the anti-tumour immune response and angiogenesis.

Endothelial cells (ECs) play critical roles in angiogenesis and regulating immune cell trafficking between blood and tissues. In a healthy state, ECs are typically found in a non-proliferating form.

However, they become activated upon environmental stressors, such as pro-angiogenic signals and hypoxia to initiate angiogenesis, or inflammatory triggers (TNF and interleukins) to enhance immune cell trafficking. Activated ECs are able to upregulate the expression of cell surface antigens (e.g. HLA molecules), adhesion molecules (selectins and integrins), and cytokines (e.g. IL-6 and IL-8) as well as to exhibit pro-thrombotic functions, ultimately resulting in a pro-immunogenic phenotype (Amersfoort et al., 2022). As a result they have potential to influence tumour growth, invasion, and metastasis

Summary of the TME

The above provides only a superficial summary of an extremely complex area, however it hopefully highlights the key players operative in the CRC TME (Fig. 4.1). The next section details the methods informative for its study, and the insights this has provided into the role of the TME in CRC development.

Methods used to study the tumour microenvironment

Quantification of immune cells in the TME can be done from a haematoxylin and eosin (H&E) stained sections from formalin-fixed paraffin-embedded (FFPE) samples generated in routine clinical practice. Systematic methods to do this, such as the Klintrup–Makinen score, have been developed and have prognostic significance. More detailed information on immune cell subsets within the TME is possible with immunohistochemistry (IHC), and more recently, multiplexed immunofluorescence which enables the identification of multiple protein markers and their spatial resolution. The emerging field of digital pathology combines these methods with rapid advances in machine learning and artificial intelligence to automate analysis, permitting resolution well beyond that possible to even expert pathologists (Bruni et al., 2020). Its use has already provided novel insights into the CRC TME and clinical outcome, and we anticipate further such results in the near term.

While lacking spatial resolution, flow cytometry permits measurement of dozens of markers at single cell level and has provided novel insights into the tumour-associated populations within the TME. For example, CRC tumours contain more of the highly immunosuppressive Treg cells compared to normal colon tissue or blood. There is a lower frequency of effector T cells (CD8+ CD69+) but a higher frequency of inflammatory Th cells (IL-17+) compared with normal bowel tissue. Another study showed that T cells in the TME produced more IL-17 and less IL-2 per cell than T cells from non-tumour-bearing tissue (Taylor et al., 2016).

In contrast to the protein-based methods above, which require prior knowledge of expected cell types under study to inform antibody selection, bulk and single cell RNAseq (scRNA-seq) provide an agnostic method of phenotyping TME-associated cells. Bulk RNAseq data provides a readout of infiltrating immune cells based on the level of their gene expression, codified in methods such as CIBERSORT and MCP-counter. The latter provides gene expression scores proportional to the amount of cells within the TME, allowing inter-sample comparisons, which have proved informative in the comparison of immune infiltrate between CRC consensus molecular subtypes (Guinney et al., 2015). scRNAseq permits unbiased analysis of rare cell types or cell states critical to tumourigenesis and holds great potential for study of the TME, however its use in this setting is in its relative infancy. Emerging methods for spatial transcriptomics permit combination of transcriptional profiles with spatial localization, potentially revealing genes that may be important in regulating cell–cell interactions and tumour growth or suppression (Ji et al., 2020). The high costs and low throughput of these technologies have limited their use, however the coming years are likely to see substantial advances in understanding in the TME as a result of these powerful technologies.

Past efforts to characterize the TME have provided a foundation for future efforts in which recent technological advances in techniques such as high-resolution single-cell RNA sequencing, flow cytometry, and imaging are expected to provide an unprecedented view of the composition, function, and location of immune cells within the TME.

The malignant epithelium in CRC

As noted earlier, molecular analysis of solid tumours has traditionally focused on the malignant epithelium. The genetic and epigenetic alterations that occur in its transformation from normal to cancer are well characterized and reviewed in detail in Chapters 2 and 3. Here we provide a brief recap to provide context to discussion of the interaction between malignant epithelium and the non-epithelial cells of the TME. The linear progression model developed by Vogelstein postulates that genetic alterations in CRC occur a tumour in a stepwise fashion leading to the acquisition of metastatic competency. Most follow the chromosomal instability (CIN) pathway, initiated by mutation in the *APC* tumour suppressor gene (TSG), followed by mutations in *KRAS*, *PIK3CA*, and *SMAD4*, loss of heterozygosity of chromosome 18 (LOH 18q), and *TP53* mutation. An alternative pathway enriched in right-sided CRCs is that of microsatellite instability (MSI) where dysfunction of DNA mismatch repair (MMR) causes genetic hypermutability. MSI often arises in association with a CpG island methylation phenotype (CIMP), though this association is not absolute, and CIMP may drive CRC development in the absence of MSI (Schmitt & Greten, 2021). Despite extensive characterization of these pathways and the tumoural mutational landscape they cause, there is a growing appreciation that interrogation of the epithelium in isolation is insufficient for prognostic and therapeutic purposes, and that valuable information is provided by its analysis within the context of its associated TME.

The TME as a regulator of CRC growth

Interactions between the TME and the malignant epithelium

Interactions between malignant epithelium and the TME shape all stages of CRC tumourigenesis. The plasticity of tumour and surrounding cells is driven by multiple factors, including direct cell–cell interaction, secreted factors, and other cues such as interstitial pressure. Activating mutations in oncogenes such as *KRAS* and *PIK3CA*, and loss of function of TSGs such as *APC* and *TP53* indirectly induces the production of pro-inflammatory cytokines, growth factors, and chemokines. These recruit pro-tumorigenic immune cells and establish an immunosuppressive TME in several ways. For example, *APC* mutation activates Wnt signalling resulting in a loss of intestinal barrier function allowing translocation of microbial products into the interstitial space and activates tissue resident IL-23 myeloid cells to release IL-17A, an interleukin that promotes early CRC (Grivennikov et al., 2012). Furthermore, as proliferating malignant epithelial cells exceed their blood supply, hypoxia-induced HIF1a expression activates CAFs to release TGFb amongst other chemokines, resulting in a tumour-promoting inflammatory response and further recruitment of immunosuppressive cell types to the TME (Ammirante et al., 2014). The mechanisms by which TGF-b achieves this are multiple, and include induction of Treg, inhibition of T cell proliferation and effector differentiation, attenuation of antigen presentation by DCs, inhibition of NK cells, and stimulation of B cells to class switch from IgM to immunosuppressive IgA phenotypes which secrete IL-10 to directly supress Tc. TGFβ in the TME also drives immune evasion via T cell exclusion (Astrid et al., 2017).

Roughly 5% of CRCs are thought to result in part as a consequence of chronic inflammation (CI), which has arisen due to environmental cues or inflammatory bowel disease among other causes. In addition to direct epigenetic effects on the epithelium, CI activates tissue-resident and recruited neutrophils and macrophages to produce reactive oxygen species which in turn induce mutations in epithelial cells. CI also results in the production of prostaglandins (PG) such as PGE2 which activate signalling pathways such as NOTCH, promoting neutrophil recruitment, tumour invasion, and NF-kB signalling, collectively inducing clonal expansion of cancer stem cells (CSCs). PGE2 also induces the differentiation of MDSCs and Treg cells, affects macrophage polarization, and inhibits the NK cell-dependent remodelling of the TME to enable immune evasion. Studies suggest that therapy-induced inflammation can also influence CRC growth by either promoting or suppressing carcinogenesis depending upon the mechanism of cell death they cause (Schmitt & Greten, 2021). Release of neoantigens from tumour cells that are undergoing apoptosis may improve immunosurveillance but the release of IL-1a from necrotic cells can promote angiogenesis, polarize fibroblasts towards tumour-promoting phenotypes, and induce malignant transformation and metastasis. Another important mechanism contributing to immunosuppression in CRC is the dysregulation of metabolic pathways to favour glycolysis, even in the presence of sufficient oxygen—referred to as the Warburg effect. The acidic, hypoxic ,and nutrient-poor environment this creates is hostile to T cells, leading to their exhaustion, among other effects (Schmitt & Greten, 2021).

TME-associated immune cells as regulators of tumour growth

A large and expanding body of literature documents the critical influence that immune cells within the TME exert on CRC growth. Th1, Tc cells, and their associated cytokines predict better prognosis in CRC, the association being strongest for Tc cells. IHC analysis of densities of CD45RO+ (later CD3+) and CD8+ cells in the centre of the tumour (CT) and invasive margin (IM) has been developed into the clinically approved Immunoscore®, which is now endorsed for prognostication by international guidelines (Bruni et al., 2020). NKT cells also correlate with improved outcome, likely through both direct (tumour cell lysis) and indirect (TH1 cell cytokine expression and modulation of immunosuppressive cells in the TME) mechanisms. The impact of Th2 and Th17 cells is less clear, although that of the latter may depend on whether they localize to the intraepithelial or intrastromal compartment (Schmitt & Greten, 2021).

Other types of immune cells exert pro-tumourigenic effects. Treg cells present in the CRC TME express immunosuppressive molecules (Tim-3, LAG-3, TGF-β, IL-10, CD25, and CTLA-4) at higher levels than those in the healthy colon. Their depletion in CRC caused CD4+ T cells to produce IFN-γ in a specific tumour antigen-shaped response and restored CD8+ T cell function in a preclinical model (Olguín et al., 2020). Interestingly, Treg have recently been shown to comprise two functionally distinct populations, with either high or low FOXP3 expression, the latter actually predicting better prognosis. Further complexity is illustrated by a recent study in rectal cancer which suggested that the spatial distance between Treg cells and CD8+ T cells in the epithelium and stroma correlated with differential survival. This highlights the growing clinical importance of including spatial information in understanding the true nature of the TME (Olguín et al., 2020). MDSCs cultivate an immunosuppressive TME via upregulation of iNOS and production of other immunosuppressive factors such as IDO1, IL-10, and TGFb. This suppresses T cell function, expands T-reg cells, and alters NK cell functionality. This effect is reflected by the finding that elevated levels of MDSCs within primary CRC and the circulation correlate with advanced TNM stages and lymph node metastasis and shorter overall survival (Bruni et al., 2020).

A third group of immune cells can exert pro-or anti-cancer effects depending on context. Promotion of T and NK cell cytotoxic activity by DCs is tumouricidal. However, the immunosuppressive CRC TME induces DC-mediated tolerance, contributing to immune escape and dampening of anti-tumour T cell responses. Clustering of TAMs, CAFs, and myeloid progenitor cells at the IM of the primary tumour interferes with DC differentiation and correlates with tumour progression, nodal and distant metastasis, and immunotherapy failure (Inagaki et al., 2021). The role of TAMs appears dependent on their location within the TME, possibly as a result of changes in plasticity and heterogeneity this correlates with. While most studies suggest a pro-tumorigenic role in most solid cancers, more studies are required to fully understand their biology and clinical correlates in CRC. B cells comprise an important component of the CRC TME. Occurrence of terminally differentiated B cells in tertiary lymphoid structures (TLSs)—ectopic lymphoid structures that develop within chronically inflamed areas like the TME—correlates with tumour suppression and improved outcome. TLSs are structurally and functionally similar to secondary lymphoid organs; their presence provides a location for antigen presentation, T and B cell differentiation in tumours, and may help T cell priming and shaping of an efficient antitumour response. While characterization of these structures and their associated cells is an area of intense study, TLSs in other cancer types such as hepatocellular carcinoma provide a niche for pro-tumoural mediators, complicating simplistic interpretation of their presence (Wang et al., 2021).

TME-associated stromal and vascular cells as regulators of tumour growth

As noted previously, CAFs are critical players in solid tumours. CAFs have diverse origins and can differentiate from several precursors in response to secretion of growth factors (TGFβ, PDGF, FGF) and interleukins from epithelial cells. This process appears to be driven by increased STAT3 signalling in CAFs and causes them to secrete growth factors (HGF, EGF IGF1, 2, FGF2,7, PGE-2, VEGF), C–X–C motif ligand 12 (CXCL-12), macrophage migration inhibitory factor (MIF), interleukins, and miRNAs, which promote tumour growth via inflammation, invasion, immune escape, and angiogenesis (Valkenburg et al., 2018). CAFs increase the number of tumour-initiating cells, a process augmented by TGFb signalling and promote CRC proliferation by secreting periostin and IL-6 to create a favourable environment for tumour cell proliferation that is modulated by various signalling pathways (PI3K-Akt, FGF-1/-3/FGFR4, and ERK5/PD-L1) and supported by reciprocal communication with CRC cells, via hydrogen sulphide, reinforcing proliferation. These findings have led to the hypothesis that non-genetic tissue changes in the stroma can also be a cause, rather than just a consequence, of the malignant process. CAFs are a vital source of immunosuppressive IL-6, which enhances VEGF production and angiogenesis. Recent findings suggest both IL-6-activated STAT3 and CAF-derived Wnt2 increase tumour angiogenesis in CRC. Therefore, it is tempting to speculate that the transcriptional reprogramming initiated by CAF-secreted IL-6 or Wnt2 could shift the balance toward proangiogenic signals in favour of tumour angiogenesis and proliferation (Deng, 2021). Due to their plasticity, MSCs are able both to promote and inhibit CRC growth, depending on TME context. MSCs can impede tumour initiation by dysregulating the Wnt and TGF-β-Smad signalling pathways, induce apoptosis, and inhibit proliferation through releasing exosomal miRNAs and inhibition proinflammatory cytokines. However, TGF-β signalling is capable of inducing differentiation of MSCs to CAFs, promoting tumour growth. MSCs and CRC cells can cooperate to drive CRC progression. MSCs help CRC resist senescence via posttranscriptional regulation of the P53/P21 pathway and promotes angiogenesis and tumour growth through paracrine proangiogenic factor IL-8 secretion. CRC cells induce morphological and functional changes on MSCs through secretion of exosomes, which is conducive to the growth and malignant progression (Li et al., 2020).

Tumour-associated endothelial cells (TECs) in the CRC TME can also promote carcinogenesis through secretion of VEGF and related angiogenic growth factors. VEGF and microvessel density are increased in pre-malignant colorectal lesions. This so-called angiogenic switch correlates with the transition of pre-malignant adenoma to carcinoma, and often occurs in response to hypoxia. Angiogenesis, a hallmark of cancer, is regulated by angiogenic factors (HIF, VEGFs, PDGFs) which recruit circulating ECs, endothelial and haematopoetic progenitors, and pericytes to the nascent TME. The high metabolism and Warburg effect in epithelial cells creates a hypoxic environment, stimulating the production of proangiogenic factors, resulting in aberrant vasculature. As a result, ECs provide nutrients for tumour growth, routes for metastatic dissemination, and drive therapeutic resistance. Tumour-associated ECs (TECs) have irregular morphology, express low levels of leukocyte adhesion molecules (ICAM1, VCAM1) and T cell-recruiting chemokines (Sparmann & Bar-Sagi, 2004). The resulting tumour blood vessels are tortuous, leaky, and have reduced pericyte coverage. This presents mechanical and chemical barriers to immune cell infiltration. However, if appropriate adhesion molecules are present in the tumour vasculature, immune cell infiltrate can promote the development of TLSs discussed earlier.

As with immune and stromal cells, the overall picture is of complex interplay with differential outcomes dependent on context and cues (Fig. 4.2).

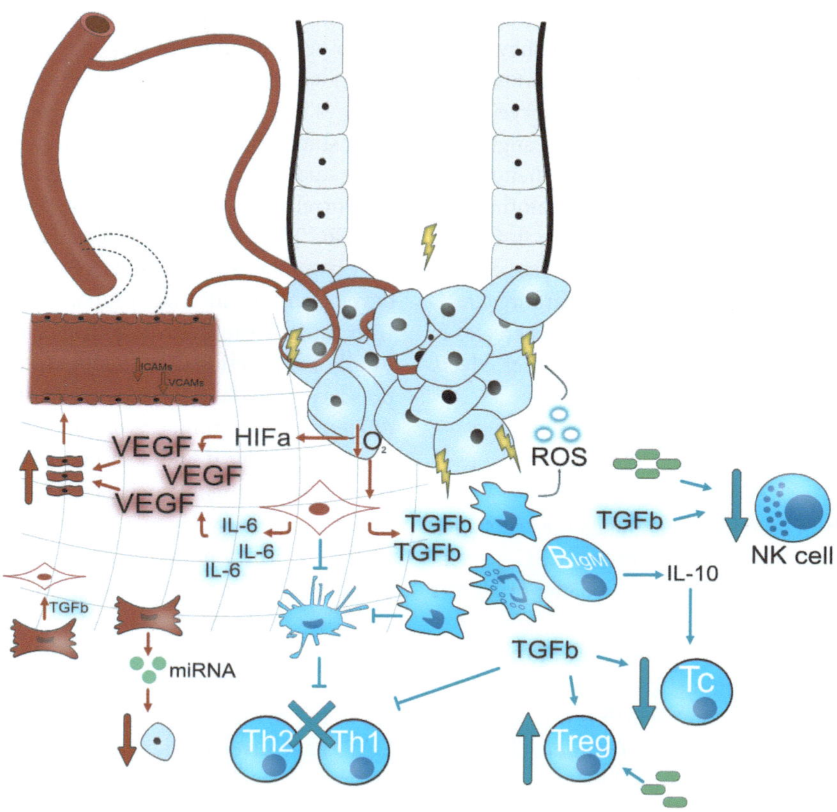

Figure 4.2 Interactions between malignant epithelium and the tumour microenvironment promote CRC growth.

The hypoxic microenvironment that results from the nascent tumour outgrowing its blood supply induces secretion of vascular endothelial growth factor (VEGF) by epithelial, stromal, and immune cells and promotes neovacularization, enabling tumour growth. Transforming growth factor beta (TGFb) produced by malignant epithelial cells acts on multiple cell types to induce an immunosuppressive microenvironment which favours tumour growth.

The TME governing invasion and metastasis of CRC

The metastatic cascade

While the processes that govern local CRC growth and invasion overlap with those that mediate distant dissemination, the key role of the TME in the latter merits specific focus.

The vast majority of CRC cells fail to metastasize, the process requiring the completion of a series of events termed the invasion–metastasis cascade. In this, epithelial cells in primary tumours (i) invade locally through surrounding ECM and stromal cell layers; (ii) intravasate into the lumina of blood vessels; (iii) survive transport through the host vasculature; (iv) arrest at distant organ sites; (v) extravasate into the parenchyma of distant tissues; (vi) become sufficiently immunologically quiescent to survive and form micrometastases, and (vii) re-initiate their proliferative programs to generate clinically detectable metastases (Hapach et al., 2019). The TME regulates each of these steps.

TME-associated immune cells, invasion, and metastasis

An important initiating event in primary tumour invasion is the transition of epithelial to an invasive mesenchymal phenotype: epithelial mesenchymal transition (EMT). Once metastatic colonization occurs, reversal of this process in a mesenchymal epithelial transition (MET), enables growth to occur. TGF-b mediates EMT by inducing transcription factors which suppress E-cadherin, an adhesion molecule dubbed the 'gatekeeper' of EMT. As discussed previously, multiple cells in the CRC TME, including immune cells, TAMs, platelets, and mesenchymal stem cells (MSCs) are all capable of TGFb secretion and thus can contribute this process (Zhang et al., 2021). CSCs are critical to this process, and their EMT has been suggested to play a critical role in CRC spread to distant organs. CSC number and fate is, in turn, determined by the TME, which provides pro/inhibitory-CRC cytokines that affect the CSCs pool and promote dissemination, for example CXCR4 appears to induce liver metastases. Thus, while CSCs have an intrinsic ability to invade and migrate, this process is regulated by the TME (Zhou et al., 2018).

The next steps in the cascade are also regulated by the TME. Once epithelial or stem cells have gained the ability to invade, their intravasation into the circulation is encouraged by TAMs which assist tumour cells to transverse blood vessel barriers. When in the circulation, platelets and components of the coagulation system protect tumour cells from cytotoxic immune cell recognition. Platelets escort tumour cells to the site of extravasation and bind to areas of vascular retraction helping tumour cells exit circulation into secondary organs. Fibroblasts at secondary sites upregulate fibronectin, which serves as a docking site for hematopoietic progenitor cells (HPCs) and subsequently tumour cells. Immunosuppressive TME-associated cells, such as MDSCs and NK cells, also populate premetastatic niches where they help to direct metastatic dissemination by creating a niche permissive to tumour colonization. Primary and secondary sites can communicate through exosomes, shed by primary tumour cells, NK cells, CAFs, and DCs. Factors contained in exosomes have the capacity to direct organ tropism, modulate immune evasion, support mesenchymal to epithelial transition (MET), and are predictive of metastasis and patient outcome. TANs migrate to metastatic sites, including liver and lung, to establish a pro-metastatic niche through CXCL1/CXCLR signalling. During migration TANs allow circulating tumour cells to adhere to them via Mac-1/ICAM-1 binding, forming a neutrophil extracellular trap (NET) to retain tumour cells at metastatic sites (Kaltenmeier et al., 2021).

The resulting micrometastases are triggered to proliferate and colonize their new environment by signals from cells within the metastatic TME. Malignant epithelial cells secrete CCL2 to recruit monocytes which differentiate into metastasis-associated macrophages (MAMs)—a subset of TAMs—in the liver, initiating CCL2/CCR2 signalling that encourages more MAM recruitment and tumour proliferation. MAMs secrete VEGFA, promoting extravasation via increasing vascular permeability and encouraging angiogenesis which facilitates persistent growth of migrating cancer cells. The final step before macrometastatic formation is the need to overcome immune destruction at their new metastatic site. In the liver, the most common metastatic site in CRC, liver sinusoidal endothelial cell lectin (LSECtin) actively inhibits T-cell immune responses and is a tropism promoting liver colonization. Nascent metastases accumulate myeloid cells and establish a pro-metastatic niche through IL-6-STAT3 signalling and exclusion of antitumour immune cells such as Tc and NK cells. They also recruit immune suppressor cells, including Treg and MDSCs, which further promote carcinogenesis (Quail & Joyce, 2013).

Therefore we can see how immune cells act to promote metastasis and established a complex TME that provides a suitable home for primary cancer cells to metastasize and grow in (Fig. 4.3).

TME-associated stromal cells, invasion, and metastasis

In addition to their central role in local invasion, CAFs are well recognized to promote metastasis in CRC. Metastasis-associated CAFs promote EMT, epithelial cell migration and lead to more aggressive phenotypes. The mechanisms underpinning this are not fully understood, although CAF-secreted factors are thought to establish a complex interaction network with malignant epithelial cells. For example, CAF-mediated secretion of STC1 and HGF induces PDGF signalling in epithelial cells which promotes metastasis. CAF-secreted HGF causes epithelial cells to adhere to ECs and induces EMT. EMT is also induced by Wnt2 and LOXL2 secretion that activate the focal adhesion kinase pathway, other growth factors including HGF, PDGF, FGF, and SDF-1, the latter of which promotes metastasis through activation of the CXCR4 axis. The ability of CAFs to undergo metabolic reprogramming can also promote dissemination. CAFs induced promotion of glutamine consumption by malignant epithelial cells, increased organ metastases in preclinical models (Tommelein et al., 2018) and lipidomic reprogramming, induces epithelial cell migration and invasion of CRC cells. The bidirectional cross-talk between CAFs and CRC and the immunosuppressive, pro-metastatic environment it induces illustrates the limitations of considering the tumour epithelium in isolation.

Other stromal cell types also play important roles in the metastatic cascade. Exosomal micro-RNAs released by MSCs inhibit epithelial cell invasion, EMT, and metastasis. One example is miR-3940-5p, which targets ITGA6 resulting in TGF-β1 inactivation. However, miRNAs within MSC-derived extracellular vesicles can also promote immune escape and metastasis. For example, miR-222

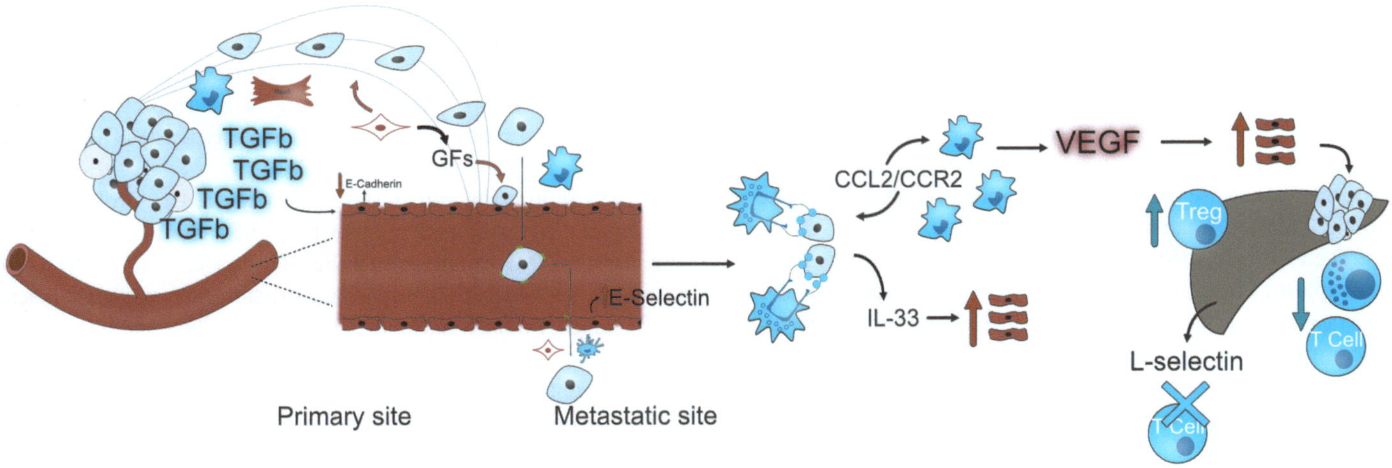

Figure 4.3 The tumour microenvironment as promoter of invasion and metastasis.
Secretion of TGFb and other growth factors by TME cells within the primary tumour promotes intravasation of malignant cells which can travel to distant sites. Extravasation is accompanied by establishment of a new TME at the distant site, enabling metastatic growth.

was shown to bind to and inhibit ATF3, resulting in the activation of the ATF3-regulated AKT pathway and a subsequent increase in CRC cell malignant phenotype and immune escape (Li et al., 2021). In addition to these indirect effects, MSCs can influence CRC metastasis via local interactions. Inflammation-activated MSCs secrete high levels of the pro-metastatic chemokine CCL5, which interacts with CCR1 on CRC cells, inducing the β-catenin/Slug pathway, EMT and a pro-metastatic programme (Chen et al., 2017).

Remodelling of the ECM is central to metastasis. Under homeostatic conditions, ECM components are isotropically arranged, with anisotropically arrangement a hallmark of a pathological TME. During tumourigenesis, ECM and BM degradation occurs through secretion of MMPs by CAFs, assisted by epithelial cells. Collagen deposition by CAFs, to replaces proteolytically degraded ECM proteins in an 'highway-style' linear arrangement that facilitates tumour cell invasion. Increased collagen density (desmoplasia) and enzymatic cross-linking of collagen during tumour progression can lead to matrix stiffening, with consequent activation of oncogenic signalling pathways such as the PI3 kinase (PI3K) in malignant cells. Desmoplasia also modulates the Snail transcription factor to downregulate E-cadherin resulting in promotion of EMT and metastasis in preclinical models (Wu, 2019).

In addition to its many effects discussed above, TGF-b also upregulates type XVI collagen formation, which is thought to induce anoikis resistance which enables cancer stem cells to initiate tumourigenesis and metastasis. Dysregulation of BM laminin proteins is also observed in the CRC TME. Upregulation of laminin-332, induces invasion and metastasis by binding integrins resulting in activation of EGFR and MAPK signalling and expression of matrix metalloproteinases such as MMP-2 (Giannelli et al., 1997).

Perhaps unsurprisingly given their function, TECs may play critical roles in metastasis of CRC. TECs in metastatic tumours express higher levels of vascular secretion factors than TECs in non-metastatic tumours and TEC apoptosis has been shown to inhibit liver metastasis. Metastatic liver tumours in CRC secrete IL-33 which induces TEC proliferation, migration, and differentiation resulting in neovascularization and subsequent CRC spreading. Blockage of IL-33 signalling could inhibit angiogenesis and reduce liver metastasis. TECs secrete Jagged-1, promoting the formation of CSCs which induce NOTCH signalling in tumour cells, an important factor in CRC metastasis. TECs also influence transendothelial migration of CRC cells by expressing E-selectin. Greater expression of E-selectin is associated with liver metastasis, possibly through E-selectin binding of death receptor-3 (DR-3) resulting in increased endothelial permeability, and trans-endothelial migration of cancer cells (Gout et al., 2006).

The data above demonstrate the CRC TME plays a critical role in determining metastasis through a highly complex network of interactions (Fig. 4.3). Thus the TME represents a rational target for therapy, and one that is the focus of much attention, as discussed in the following section.

Therapeutic targeting of the CRC TME

Strategies to manipulate the CRC TME are in their infancy when compared to those targeting the epithelial component in tumours such as chemotherapy and radiotherapy. However, the field has great potential with several lines of research being actively pursued (Fig. 4.4).

The development and application of therapeutics targeting immunosuppressive immune checkpoints such as PD1 and PDL1 represent a huge advance in the systemic therapy of cancer, as illustrated by their use across multiple cancer types. However, in CRC their activity is limited to the subset of tumours defined by DNA mismatch repair deficiency, comprising some 15% of early-stage disease but only 4% of metastatic disease. Furthermore, only half of patients with advanced metastatic disease respond to immune checkpoint inhibition. While some of the mechanisms of resistance are likely to be epithelial cell-intrinsic, emerging evidence points to an important contribution of the TME, particularly in the majority of MMR proficient cases. As discussed at length above, TGF-B can promote T cell exclusion, block the acquisition of a Th1 phenotype, inhibit antigen presentation by DCs, repress Tc-mediated cytolysis, and promote angiogenesis and EMT, encouraging metastasis. Inhibition of TGF-b results in preclinical models induces a potent and enduring CTL response against MSS CRC primary and

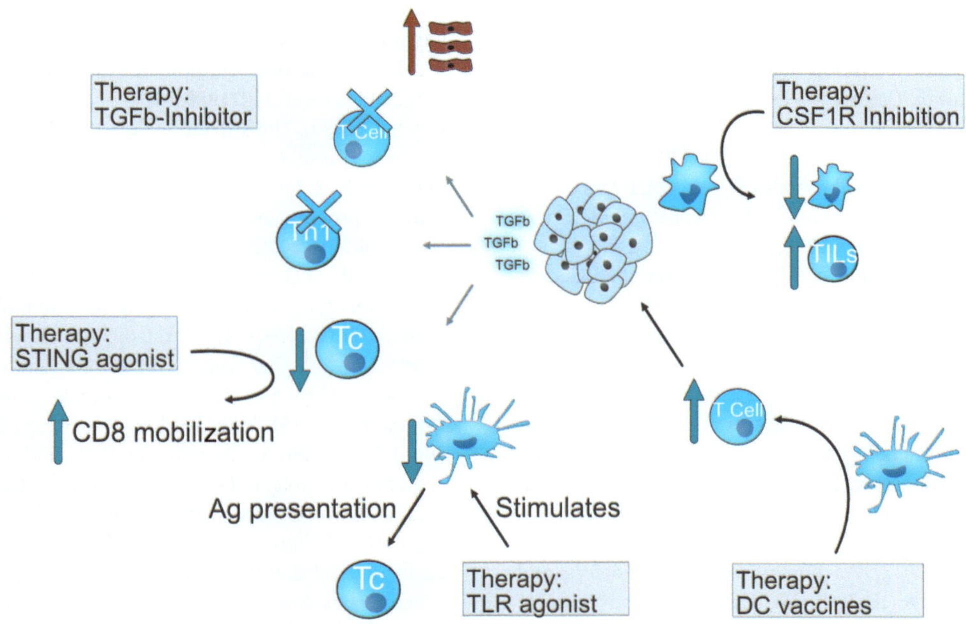

Figure 4.4 Therapies targeting the tumour microenvironment in CRC.

Multiple therapeutic approaches under investigation include immune checkpoint inhibition, and other immunotherapeutic approaches such as dendritic cell (DC) vaccination, toll-like receptor (TLR) agonists, and inhibition of immunosuppressive cytokines such as CSF1R. Reversal of the pro-tumour effects of TGFb by therapeutic targeting is in clinical trials.

metastatic tumours. Clinical trials using a bifunctional checkpoint inhibitor against PDL-1 and TGF-BR2 promotes CTL and NK cell activation, decreases tumour burden, and increases overall survival (Knudson et al., 2018). The importance of the immunosuppressive TME in CRC has been highlighted previously, and reversal of this is an important area of investigation. TLRs, when stimulated, lead to innate and adaptive immune responses such as increased antigen presentation to CTLs. TLR agonists are being trialled to overcome the immunosuppressive TME alongside agonists of the immune-modulating cell-intrinsic cGAS-STING pathway and macrophage manipulators. STING agonists promote CTL mobilization through stimulating production of interferons and pro-inflammatory cytokines. CSF1R regulates macrophage survival, differentiation and migration. Inhibition of this molecule reduces TAMs whilst simultaneously increasing TILs in CRC patients, re-engineering the TME to promote cancer destruction (Kamal et al., 2020).

Another promising area of TME-modulating therapy is use of dendritic cell vaccines to activate and expand tumour-directed cytotoxic T cells, thus improving their penetration of the TME and preventing their polarization into tolerogenic subtypes (Anguille et al., 2014).

While at present, most focus of TME modulation is directed at T cells, particularly CTLs, the strategies above and others illustrate the multiple mechanisms by which this make be examined. While inter- and intra-patient variation in the TME means that, as with epithelial targeting, a one-size-fits-all approach is likely to fall short of a personalized therapy directed to the key TME perturbations, this exciting area of research will hopefully result in improved therapies and patient outcomes.

Conclusions and future directions

This chapter has highlighted the increased awareness of the contribution that non-epithelial cells make to CRC tumourigenesis and clinical outcome, and summarized the complex interactions that underpin this. Rather than viewing CRC as a homogeneous population of malignant epithelial cells, it is now viewed as a complex ecosystem undergoing dynamic remodelling in response to intrinsic and extrinsic stressors. The lines of research we have outlined hold great promise to improve our understanding of this ecosystem, and to inform its rational therapeutic targeting for patient benefit.

REFERENCES

Amersfoort, J., et al. (2022). Immunomodulation by endothelial cells—partnering up with the immune system? *Nature Reviews Immunology*, *22*(9), 576–588. doi: 10.1038/s41577-022-00694-4. Epub 2022 Mar 14.

Ammirante, M., et al. (2014). Tissue injury and hypoxia promote malignant progression of prostate cancer by inducing CXCL13 expression in tumor myofibroblasts. *Proceedings of the National Academy of Sciences of the USA*, *111*(41), 14776–14781. doi: 10.1073/pnas.1416498111. Epub 2014 Sep 29.

Anguille, S. S., Lion, E., Tendeloo, V. F. V., & Berneman, Z. N. (2014). Clinical use of dendritic cells for cancer therapy. *Lancet Oncology*, *15*(7), e257–267. doi: 10.1016/S1470-2045(13)70585-0.

Westendorf, A. M., et al. (2017). Hypoxia enhances immunosuppression by inhibiting CD4+ effector T cell function and promoting Treg activity. *Cellular Physiology and Biochemistry*, *41*(4), 1271–1284. doi: 10.1159/000464429. Epub 2017 Mar 8.

Beutler, B., & Cerami, A. (1986). Cachectin and tumour necrosis factor as two sides of the same biological coin. *Nature*, *320*(6063), 584–588. doi: 10.1038/320584a0.

Binnewies, M., et al. (2018). Understanding the tumor immune microenvironment (TIME) for effective therapy. *Nature Medicine*, *24*(5), 541–550. doi: 10.1038/s41591-018-0014-x. Epub 2018 Apr 23.

Bruni, D., et al. (2020). The immune contexture and Immunoscore in cancer prognosis and therapeutic efficacy. *Nature Reviews Cancer*, *20*(11), 662–680. doi: 10.1038/s41568-020-0285-7. Epub 2020 Aug 4.

Chen, K., et al. (2017). Human MSCs promotes colorectal cancer epithelial–mesenchymal transition and progression via CCL5/β-catenin/Slug pathway. *Cell Death & Disease*, *8*(5), e2819. doi: 10.1038/cddis.2017.138.

Deng, L., Jiang, N., Zeng, J., Wang, Y., & Cui, H. (2021). The versatile roles of cancer-associated fibroblasts in colorectal cancer and therapeutic implications. *Frontiers in Cell Developmental Biology*, *9*, 733270. doi: 10.3389/fcell.2021.733270. eCollection 2021.

Fidler, I. J. (2008). The seed and soil hypothesis revisited. *Lancet Oncology*, *9*(8), 808. doi: 10.1016/S1470-2045(08)70201-8.

Gianni G. et al. (1997). Induction of cell migration by matrix metalloprotease-2 cleavage of laminin-5. *Science*, *277*(5323), 225–228. doi: 10.1126/science.277.5323.225.

Gout, S., et al. (2006). Death receptor-3, a new E-selectin counter-receptor that confers migration and survival advantages to colon carcinoma cells by triggering p38 and ERK MAPK activation. *Cancer Research*, *66*(18), 9117–9124. doi: 10.1158/0008-5472.CAN-05-4605.

Grivennikov, S. I., et al. (2012). Adenoma-linked barrier defects and microbial products drive IL-23/IL-17-mediated tumour growth. *Nature*, *491*(7423), 254–258. doi: 10.1038/nature11465.

Guinney, J., et al. (2015). The consensus molecular subtypes of colorectal cancer. *Nature Medicine*, *21*(11), 1350–1356. doi: 10.1038/nm.3967. Epub 2015 Oct 12.

Hapach, L. A., et al. (2019). Engineered models to parse apart the metastatic cascade. *NPJ Precision Oncology*, *3*(1), 20. doi: 10.1038/s41698-019-0092-3. eCollection 2019.

Inagaki, K., et al. (2021). Role of tumor-associated macrophages at the invasive front in human colorectal cancer progression. *Cancer Science*, *112*(7), 2692–2704. doi: 10.1111/cas.14940. Epub 2021 Jun 2.

Ji, A. L., et al. (2020). Multimodal analysis of composition and spatial architecture in human squamous cell carcinoma. *Cell*, *182*(2), 497–514.e422. doi: 10.1016/j.cell.2020.05.039. Epub 2020 Jun 23.

Kaltenmeier, C., et al. (2021). Neutrophil extracellular traps (NETs) in cancer metastasis. *Cancers (Basel)*, *13*(23), 6131. doi: 10.3390/cancers13236131.

Kamal, Y., et al. (2020). TME of CRC metastases. *Immunotherapy*, *12*(14), 1083–1100. doi: 10.2217/imt-2020-0026. Epub 2020 Aug 13.

Knudson, K. M., et al. (2018). M7824, a novel bifunctional anti-PD-L1/TGFβ Trap fusion protein, promotes anti-tumor efficacy as monotherapy and in combination with vaccine. *OncoImmunology*, *7*(5), e1426519. doi: 10.1080/2162402X.2018.1426519. eCollection 2018.

Li, G., et al. (2020). Human colorectal cancer derived-MSCs promote tumor cells escape from senescence via P53/P21 pathway. *Clinical and Translational Oncology*, *22*(4), 503–511. doi: 10.1007/s12094-019-02152-5. Epub 2019 Jun 19.

Li, S., et al. (2021). Extracellular vesicles-derived microRNA-222 promotes immune escape via interacting with ATF3 to regulate AKT1 transcription in colorectal cancer. *BMC Cancer*, *21*(1), 349. doi: 10.1186/s12885-021-08063-5.

Olguín, J. E., et al. (2020). Relevance of regulatory T cells during colorectal cancer Development. *Cancers (Basel)*, *12*(7), 1888. doi: 10.3390/cancers12071888.

Paget, S. (1889). The distribution of secondary growth in cancer of the breast. *Lancet*, *133*(3421), 571–573.

Quail, D. F., & Joyce, J. A. (2013). Microenvironmental regulation of tumor progression and metastasis. *Nature Medicine*, *19*(11), 1423–1437. doi: 10.1038/nm.3394.

Schmitt, M., & Greten, F. R. (2021). The inflammatory pathogenesis of colorectal cancer. *Nature Reviews Immunology*, *21*(10), 653–667. doi: 10.1038/s41577-021-00534-x. Epub 2021 Apr 28.

Sparmann, A., & Bar-Sagi, D. (2004). RAS-induced interleukin-8 expression plays a critical role in tumor growth and angiogenesis. *Cancer Cell*, *6*(5), 447–458. doi: 10.1016/j.ccr.2004.09.028.

Subtil, B., Cambi, A., Tauriello, D. V. F., & Vries, I. J. M. (2021). The therapeutic potential of tackling tumor-induced dendritic cell dysfunction in colorectal cancer. *Frontiers in Immunology*, *12*, 724883. doi: 10.3389/fimmu.2021.724883. eCollection 2021.

Taylor, E. S., et al. (2016). Functional impairment of infiltrating T cells in human colorectal cancer. *OncoImmunology*, *5*(11), e1234573. doi: 10.1080/2162402X.2016.1234573. eCollection 2016.

Thorsson, V., et al. (2018). The immune landscape of cancer. *Immunity*, *48*(4), 812–830.e814. doi: 10.1016/j.immuni.2018.03.023. Epub 2018 Apr 5.

Tommelein, J., Vlieghere, E. D., Verset, L., et al. (2018). Radiotherapy-activated cancer-associated fibroblasts promote tumor progression through paracrine IGF1R activation. *Cancer Research*, *78*(3), 659–670. doi: 10.1158/0008-5472.CAN-17-0524. Epub 2017 Dec 7.

Valkenburg, K. C., et al. (2018). Targeting the tumour stroma to improve cancer therapy. *Nature Reviews Clinical Oncology*, *15*(6), 366–381. doi: 10.1038/s41571-018-0007-1.

Wang, H., et al. (2021). Tumor-associated macrophages (TAMs) in colorectal cancer (CRC): from mechanism to therapy and prognosis. *International Journal of Molecular Sciences*, *22*(16), 8470. doi: 10.3390/ijms22168470.

Wang, Y., et al. (2014). Plasticity of mesenchymal stem cells in immunomodulation: pathological and therapeutic implications. *Nature Immunology*, *15*(11), 1009–1016. doi: 10.1038/ni.3002.

Wu, X. C., J; Zuo, Z., & Li, J (2019). Collagen facilitates the colorectal cancer stemness and metastasis through an integrin/PI3K/AKT/Snail signaling pathway. *Biomedicine & Pharmacotherapy*, *114*, 108708. doi: 10.1016/j.biopha.2019.108708. Epub 2019 Mar 24.

Xiong, Y. W. Y. T., K (2019). Tumor immune microenvironment and nano-immunotherapeutics in colorectal cancer. *Nanomedicine: Nanotechnology, Biology and Medicine*, *21*, 102034. doi: 10.1016/j.nano.2019.102034. Epub 2019 Jun 15.

Zhang, N., et al. (2021). Novel therapeutic strategies: targeting epithelial–mesenchymal transition in colorectal cancer. *Lancet Oncology*, *22*(8), e358–368. doi: 10.1016/S1470-2045(21)00343-0.

Zhou, Y., et al. (2018). Cancer stem cells in progression of colorectal cancer. *Oncotarget*, *9*(70), 33403–33415. doi: 10.18632/oncotarget.23607. eCollection 2018 Sep 7.

SECTION 2

Screening and staging

5

The importance of the gut microbiome in colorectal cancer risk and treatment

Jinlin Yang, Zijing Wang, Jin Wang, Tong Liu, Yuzhi Liu, Xian Zhang, Xiuhe Lv, and Li Yang

Introduction

The largest population of mammalian-associated microbiota resides in the gut. It includes bacteria, viruses, protozoa, and fungi, and comprises approximately 100 trillion cells (Temraz et al., 2019). Considered by some as a separate organ, the human gut microbiome is essential to health, playing key roles in food digestion, metabolism, host physiology, and immune system development (Britton & Young, 2014). This population of microorganisms, also known as the microbiota, regulates health, and alterations can contribute to disease. A growing body of evidence in recent years has demonstrated that the gut microbiota is an important environmental factor that influences multiple disorders including allergies (Prince et al., 2015), cardiovascular diseases (Tang et al., 2017), metabolic diseases (Bouter et al., 2017), inflammatory bowel disease (Ferreira et al., 2014), and many types of cancer, particularly colorectal cancer (CRC) (Gagnière et al., 2016; Omar Al-Hassi et al., 2018).

CRC poses a significant global health burden, which ranked third in incidence (over 1.8 million new cases) and second in mortality (over 860,000 deaths) in 2018 (Rawla et al., 2019). Depending on the mutation source, CRC is classified into inherited, inflammatory, or sporadic types, with the latter accounting for the majority (over 70%) of cases. The risk of developing CRC is associated with environmental factors as well as genetic factors (Mármol et al., 2017). Among the environmental factors, the importance of gut microbiota in CRC is increasingly being recognized. Since the gut microbiota was first reported by Weisburger et al. to correlate with colorectal neoplasia (Weisburger et al., 1975), its role in colorectal carcinogenesis has received increasing attention over the past few years, thus providing new ways to contemplate the prevention and treatment of CRC.

Gut microbiome association with CRC risk

As an important regulator of the intestinal microenvironment, the gut microbiota plays an indispensable role in colorectal carcinogenesis through various mechanisms, including energy harvesting, metabolism, and the immune response.

Metabolism and dietary components

The gut microbiota is a key regulator of the intestinal microenvironment, and it primarily comprises permanent residents and symbionts. However, the microbiota may become pathogenic through repeated exposure to environment and lifestyle factors (Pothuraju et al., 2021). The colorectal mucosa is continually exposed to dietary components, gut microbiota, and their secreted products, including toxin metabolites which directly interact with gut epithelial cells. Any changes in the gut metabolic environment can impair the intestinal mucosal barrier, allowing metabolites to diffuse into epithelial cells and blood vessels. Colitis induced by dextran sodium sulphate can increase the susceptibility to CRC by disrupting the intestinal mucosal barrier function. N-nitroso compounds and hydrogen sulphide generated from microbial metabolism have been reported to be pro-carcinogenic (Louis et al., 2014). Therefore, the toxin metabolites of the gut microbiota may be a critical risk factor for colorectal carcinogenesis.

Furthermore, the microbial metagenome encodes genes associated with the metabolism of many dietary nutrients, such as galacto-oligosaccharides and fructo-oligosaccharides, as well as host components such as bile acids (Adak & Khan, 2019). Short-chain fatty acids (SCFAs) are a major class of microbial metabolites produced from dietary components, such as indigestible fibre in the proximal colon. Several studies have identified that lower levels of SCFAs are associated with a higher risk of developing ulcerative colitis, advanced colorectal adenoma, and CRC (Abdulla et al., 2021). SCFAs, particularly butyrate, significantly decrease the pH in the colon, thus inhibiting pathogenic bacterial proliferation and preventing CRC cell proliferation (Sánchez-Alcoholado et al., 2020). In addition, butyrate promotes the anti-inflammatory properties of colonic macrophages and dendritic cells through interacting with G protein-coupled receptors, which further promoted the differentiation of Treg cells and IL-10-producing cells (Singh et al., 2014).

Bile acids are another class of metabolites processed by the microbiota in the intestines. Secondary bile acids significantly increase in the intestinal content after consumption of a high-fat diet (Wang et al., 2019). Mice fed a Western-style diet develop more colonic tumours than mice fed a control diet, because a high-fat diet impairs bile acid transport, dysregulates the activity of farnesoid X receptor, and eventually increases colon cell proliferation (Dermadi et al., 2017). Moreover, secondary bile acids have been identified to be genotoxic through generating reactive oxygen species (ROS) and causing oxidative DNA damage (Dvorak et al., 2007). Thus, the intermediate products of dietary metabolism can be metabolized by the microbiota, producing genotoxic or inflammatory regulators that guide colorectal carcinogenesis.

Inflammation and immune regulation

Chronic inflammation is an established risk factor for CRC. The gut microbiota plays an indispensable role in regulating the inflammatory response in the gastrointestinal tract by interacting with the host immune system and influencing the intestinal mucosal barrier (Brennan & Garrett, 2016). Recent metagenomics analyses have demonstrated that the numbers and communities of microbiota in CRC tissues differ from those in healthy host tissues, indicating the cancer-specific microbiota may contribute to the development of a pro-inflammatory microenvironment in CRC (Maghini et al., 2021). Host cells recognize pathogenic microbiota through various pattern recognition receptors, such as Toll-like receptors (TLRs), which mediate the inflammatory response to pathogens, such as lipopolysaccharides and bacterial flagella (Kawai & Akira, 2011). TLRs on tumour-infiltrating myeloid cells recognize and bind pathogenic bacteria and their components, and subsequently activate myeloid differentiation factor 88 (MyD88)-induced production of inflammatory cytokines (such as IL-6 and IL-23), which promote tumour cell proliferation by activating nuclear factor-κB (NF-κB) and the STAT3 signalling pathway (Vlantis et al., 2016).

Beyond generating a pro-inflammatory environment that promotes CRC progression through activation of the NF-κB pathway, *Fusobacterium nucleatum* recruits tumour-infiltrating immune cells in APC Min/+ mice (Kostic et al., 2013). Exosomes containing CXCL16 secreted by *F. nucleatum* also promote CRC metastasis *in vivo* (Guo et al., 2020). In APC Min/+ mice, inflammatory cytokines produced by *Peptostreptococcus anaerobius* sequentially recruit immunosuppressive myeloid-derived suppressor cells, tumour-associated macrophages, and tumour-associated neutrophils, thus promoting tumour immune evasion and contributing to CRC progression (Long et al., 2019). Regulation of inflammation and the immune response is another route through which the gut microbiota participates in colorectal carcinogenesis.

Genotoxins

DNA damage resulting from the microbiota is another carcinogenic mechanism in CRC. Some microorganisms, such as colibactin-producing *E. coli*, cause double-stranded DNA breaks in the host gut epithelial cells, thus resulting in genomic instability and increased mutation frequency (Cuevas-Ramos et al., 2010). *Enterococcus faecalis* is significantly higher in patients with CRC than in healthy individuals. *E. faecalis* infection induces excessive superoxide production, which caused DNA damage in epithelial cells (Huycke et al., 2002). Salmonella produces typhoid toxin, a genotoxin that induces DNA damage and genomic instability in APC-deficient CRC cells (Martin et al., 2019). The accumulation of mutations in epithelial cells results in uncontrolled proliferation and carcinogenesis.

As described, the gut microbiota, as a critical regulator of intestinal microenvironment homeostasis, plays an important role in colorectal carcinogenesis by producing toxic metabolites, reprocessing intermediate dietary products, regulating inflammation and the immune response, and causing DNA damage. These various functions of the gut microbiota suggest the possibility of modulating the microbiota for CRC screening, prevention, and treatment.

Roles of the gut microbiome in diagnosing and predicting CRC risk

Gut microbiome as CRC biomarkers

Population screening based on risk stratification can substantially decrease the incidence and mortality of colorectal cancer by detecting it at a curable stage; however, a universally feasible method for screening average-risk individuals remains a clinical challenge. Non-invasive stool-based tests usually have better patient adherence and compliance than endoscopic and blood-based tests. However, widely used faecal haemoglobin detection (gFOBT (guaiac faecal occult blood test) or FIT (faecal immunochemical testing)) and CRC genetic-targeted approaches (including multitarget stool DNA test) do not provide a good balance between accuracy and accessibility, particularly for the detection of precancerous adenoma, the precursor of most CRC cases (Quintero et al., 2012). The suboptimal sensitivity of the current methods justifies the exploration of accurate new biomarkers associated with CRC risk, presence, and severity.

Research on the associations between the gut microbiome and CRC risk and tumourigenesis has highlighted its potential CRC biomarkers. Accumulating evidence indicates prominent microbiome alterations in patients with CRC and adenoma, known as dysbiosis, compared with healthy individuals. Furthermore, several bacterial markers have been identified to be associated with CRC prognosis and therapeutic efficacy. These findings have highlighted the application of microbiome-related biomarkers in CRC monitoring, diagnosis, precise treatment, and prediction of clinical outcomes.

Microbiome biomarkers for CRC screening and detection

The potential of the gut microbiome to aid in CRC screening has been established on the basis of a significant divergence in its structure and composition between patients with CRC and healthy individuals. Using 16S rRNA gene or metagenomic shotgun sequencing, earlier investigations have observed differences in the diversity and richness of the gut microbiome in patients with CRC, although the results were not consistent among cohorts. Yu et al. reported reduction in gene richness and gene alpha diversity in the CRC patient microbiome, on the basis of metagenomic analysis (Yu et al., 2017), whereas another study described a stepwise increase in gene richness and diversity in the progression from normal epithelium to advanced adenoma to CRC (Feng et al., 2015). Therefore, more stable and definitive microbiome biomarkers for CRC are required.

Detailed analyses have detected alterations in the abundance of certain types of microbial species in patients with CRC or advanced colorectal adenoma. *F. nucleatum* has been shown to have tumourigenic effects in many studies in the past decade, and it is enriched in both faecal and mucosal samples from human colorectal adenomas and carcinomas (Brennan & Garrett, 2019). The efficacy of *F. nucleatum* screening for colorectal neoplasia has been validated in several populations across multiple ethnicities and geographical areas. A meta-analysis including 13 cohorts and seven colorectal adenoma cohorts reported an area under the receiver operating characteristic curve (AUROC) of 0.80 and 0.60 for predicting CRC and adenoma, respectively, with better efficacy than FIT alone (Zhang et al., 2019). However, the substantial heterogeneity among the included studies cannot be ignored. A combination of *F. nucleatum* abundance and FIT results has been found to significantly improve the neoplasia-detection performance for both CRC and advanced adenomas (Wong et al., 2017a). Furthermore, the *F. nucleatum* specific gene fadA has been suggested to promote colorectal carcinogenesis, and its copy levels might help define healthy, precancerous, and cancerous states (Rubinstein et al., 2013). Other microbial species enriched in colorectal neoplasia samples primarily cluster in the *Bacteroides*, *Campylobacter*, *Fusobacterium*, and *Parabacteroides*, whereas several species from *Faecalibacterium*, *Bifidobacterium*, and *Roseburia* are depleted in patients with CRC or advanced adenoma. Notably, oral taxa dislocation and colonization in the gut (including *F. nucleatum*, *Pavimonas micra*, and *Peptostreptococcus stomatis*) are prevalent features of the CRC-related microbiome, and the abundance of butyrate-producing species is often diminished in patients with CRC (Feng et al., 2015; Wang et al., 2012). However, discrepant findings associated with these species and genera in the CRC microbiome suggest that they are not valid enough as single biomarkers.

Approaches increasingly use multiple bacterial marker panels to screen and diagnose CRC or advanced adenoma, thus reflecting a more holistic view of the microbiome. Recent case-control studies have reported AUROCs of 0.85, 0.925, and 0.97 in distinguishing patients with CRC from healthy individuals by using 22, four, and five bacterial populations, respectively (Baxter et al., 2016; Osman et al., 2021; Rezasoltani et al., 2018). Metagenomic studies have also demonstrated reproducible panels of microbial biomarkers for CRC across cohorts, composed of microbial genes (Yu et al., 2017) or species abundance (Thomas et al., 2019), both of which achieved AUROCs above 0.80. However, few studies have validated the value of microbiota in CRC risk stratification from a translational viewpoint. Moreover, the complexity of the gut microbiota far exceeds that of bacteria, and a recent study integrating eight cohorts has highlighted 16 multi-kingdom markers, including 11 bacterial, four fungal, and one archaeal features, providing robust and improved predictability in CRC diagnosis (average AUROC of 0.83) compared with single-kingdom markers (Liu et al., 2022). Given the emerging understanding of the contributions of fungi and viruses to the pathogenesis of colitis and CRC, the signatures of these non-bacterial communities may be highly valuable in CRC risk evaluation and diagnosis.

Microbiome biomarkers for CRC prognosis and treatment efficacy

Beyond the diagnostic values of the microbiota in detecting colorectal neoplasia, accumulating data have illustrated the relationships between gut microbiome markers and clinical outcomes of CRC, including survival, relapse, and response to treatments.

Associations between CRC survival and tumour-related bacterial abundance have been identified, and the most compelling evidence has been found for *F. nucleatum*. Mima et al. reported that the amount of *F. nucleatum* DNA in CRC tissue is positively associated with pT stage and CRC-specific mortality, independently of clinical, pathological, and major tumour molecular features (Mima et al., 2016). Two meta-analyses published in 2020 also suggested that F. *nucleatum* positivity in CRC tumour tissue is associated with poorer overall survival and disease-free survival, and higher levels of *F. nucleatum* are associated with poorer CRC prognosis even after curative surgery, thus suggesting the practicality of bacteria-focused interventions during the peri-operative period (Colov et al., 2020; Gethings-Behncke et al., 2020). *Bacteroides fragilis* has also been described as an indicator of advanced tumour stage, poor survival, and unfavourable immune infiltration in CRC, whereas *Faecalibacterium prausnitzii* has been found to be more abundant in patients with earlier tumour stages and prolonged survival (Colov et al., 2020; Wei et al., 2016). Enterotoxigenic *B. fragilis*, along with *P. stomatis* and *Parvimonas micra*, comprise a faecal bacterial signature defining the existence and malignancy of laterally spreading tumours, which are primary precursor lesions in CRC (Shen et al., 2021). Approaches to detecting microbial translocation and microbiota-related markers in the blood of patients with CRC have also shown prognostic value (Raza et al., 2022). A study has measured the presence of gene fragments from *B. fragilis*, *Escherichia coli*, and *Candida albicans*, and observed more disease metastasis and significantly shorter survival in patients with detectable bacterial DNA in the blood (Messaritakis et al., 2020). Currently, prognostic bacterial markers are retrieved primarily from tumour tissue or blood samples, whereas few data on non-invasive methods have been reported, thus hindering promptness and compliance with prognostication. Robust signatures of multiple microbiome markers and the combination of microbial features with other clinical parameters may also offer better solutions for CRC prognostication.

From a translational perspective, numerous investigations have clarified the value of gut microbiome biomarkers in predicting patient responses to chemo-, radio- and immunotherapy in CRC, as well as the occurrence of adverse effects after treatments. These discoveries have shed new light on optimal personalized treatment selection and adjustment, and have resulted in intense interest in manipulating microbial composition in patients with CRC to improve clinical outcomes. Details are described and discussed in the next section.

Role of the gut microbiome response to CRC treatments

In recent years, the role of gut microbiota in CRC has received increasing attention. The gut microbiota and its metabolites promote carcinogenesis by inducing inflammatory signalling pathways, gene mutations, epigenetic disorders, and other mechanisms (Peters et al., 2016), and can also affect metabolism, immune regulation, bacterial translocation, enzymatic degradation, and the diversity of flora. The gut microbiota affects the efficiency of chemotherapeutic drugs and regulates the host's response to the drug, thereby is expected to become a new means of improving outcomes of anticancer treatment.

Gut microbiota in CRC chemotherapy

Recent chemotherapy studies suggest that the gut microbiota mediates the response to chemotherapy, including that with 5-fluorouracil (5-FU), platinum, and irinotecan, through a variety of mechanisms including microbial translocation, immune regulation, and metabolic enzyme degradation (García-González et al., 2017; Iida et al., 2013). Treatment with 5-FU inhibits thymidine nucleotide synthase and blocks the conversion of deoxyuracil nucleotides to deoxythymidine pyrimidine nucleotides, thereby inhibiting DNA biosynthesis. In addition, it inhibits the synthesis of RNA by preventing the incorporation of uracil and orotic acid into RNA, thereby affecting protein biosynthesis. The gut microbiota represented by *E. coli*, *Bifidobacterium*, and *Lactobacillus* has been found to be involved in the regulation of 5-FU mediated by vitamins B6 and B12 (Scott et al., 2017). In addition, the gut microbiota improves therapeutic efficacy through 5-FU-induced host cell autophagy and cell death (Scott et al., 2017). Thus, the gut microbiota affects the metabolic conversion of 5-FU, thereby affecting the therapeutic effect of this compound.

Platinum chemotherapy drugs including oxaliplatin, cisplatin, carboplatin, and lobaplatin, by acting on cell DNA and forming Pt-DNA compounds, result in apoptosis of tumour cells. The gut microbiota, such as *Lactobacillus acidophilus*, stimulates immune cells to secrete ROS, which enhances DNA damage and blocks DNA repair and transcription in tumour cells, thus enhancing the efficacy of platinum (Firwana et al., 2018; Iida et al., 2013).

Irinotecan, a prodrug of SN-38, is commonly used to treat CRC. Irinotecan and SN-38 have anti-tumour effects by inhibiting topoisomerase I, which is necessary for DNA replication in human cells, thus inducing DNA single-strand damage and blocking DNA replication. Pharmacologically, SN-38 is glucuronidated to form an inactive conjugate (SN-38G) and secreted to the gut via biliary excretion, then the inactive conjugate is hydrolysed back to active SN-38 by gut bacterial β-glucuronidase enzymes. However, because of its low water solubility, this drug can easily cause severe diarrhoea. Selective inhibition of bacterial β-glucuronidases has recently been demonstrated to alleviate gastrointestinal toxicity caused by irinotecan in mice (Wallace et al., 2015). Furthermore, oral administration of probiotics has been found to ameliorate intestinal mucositis caused by 5-FU in a mouse model (Kato et al., 2017; Yeung et al., 2015), suggesting the ability to decrease chemotherapy's adverse effects by altering the gut microbiota in patients with CRC in the future.

Gut microbiota in CRC immunotherapy

Immunotherapy is now widely used in the treatment of many malignant tumours and has revolutionized the treatment of cancer. In addition to the expression of programmed cell death ligand 1 (PD-L1), the tumour mutation load, oncogenic mutations, and the presence of tumour-infiltrating lymphocyte, the gut microbiota can also influence the efficacy of immunotherapy (Santarpia & Karachaliou, 2015; Topalian et al., 2016). On the one hand, the gut microbiota stimulates immune activation by recruiting immune cells to the mucosa, promoting maturation of the intestinal-associated lymphoid tissue and stimulating protective epithelial cells, enhancing the infiltration of T cells in the tumour microenvironment, thus improving the efficacy of immunotherapy (Sivan et al., 2015). On the other hand, anti-CTLA-4 drugs activate local lymphocytes, promote the deterioration of the epithelial barrier, and thus propel translocation of *Bacteroides*, which may play a role in activating antigen-presenting cells (including dendritic cells), and consequently enhancing the response of anti-tumour T cells (Vétizou et al., 2015). Anti-PD-L1 drugs appear to have a synergistic effect with the gut microbiota, thereby enhancing the antigen presentation function of dendritic cells and the T cell response (Rescigno, 2015).

Some immunotherapy drugs including anti-PD-1 and anti-CTLA-4 checkpoint inhibitors might only play a therapeutic role in metastatic CRC patients with microsatellite instability-high or DNA mismatch repair-deficient CRC, as these types of CRC exhibit higher mutational loads, tumour neoantigen epitope, and tumour-infiltrating lymphocytes (Brahmer et al., 2010; Topalian et al., 2012). It seems that the gut microbiota plays an important role in improving treatment response and minimizing possible adverse effects.

Faecal microbiota transplantation in CRC therapy

Faecal microbiota transplantation (FMT) was first described in 1958, when it was used to treat *Clostridium difficile* infection (Eiseman et al., 1958). Increasing evidence has indicated that FMT plays a promising therapeutic role in other disorders involving gut dysbiosis (Filip et al., 2018).

To date, no conclusive data from clinical trials have been reported about FMT therapy for CRC in humans. However, two recent studies using mouse models showed its potential. One study indicated that laboratory mice reconstituted with natural microbiota improved resistance against mutagen/inflammation-induced colorectal tumorigenesis (Rosshart et al., 2017). Another study has shown that the faecal microbiota from patients with CRC promotes tumour formation in germ-free and conventional mice (Wong et al., 2017b). Overall, FMT is a promising strategy for the treatment of patients with CRC, although several questions and potential risks remain to be assessed. However, it is controversial in various aspects regarding the use of FMT, such as the optimal storage conditions for faeces, the standardization of procedures, the selection of donors and recipients, and the establishment of appropriate cycles for FMT administration, dosage, and frequency. The potential risks of FMT include the transmission of pathogens to recipients, particularly immunocompromised patients, and the transmission of silent recessive elements in healthy donors (Sbahi & Di Palma, 2016). Therefore, future studies should focus on identifying the gut microbiota, determining its function, and developing defined microbial communities as alternatives to the whole FMT.

Role of the gut microbiome in response to CRC prevention strategies

As many as 29% of incident CRC cases in the United Kingdom and 42% of incident CRC cases in the United States have been suggested to be preventable via lifestyle modifications, thus highlighting the importance of risk factor management in CRC prevention (Choi et al., 2021; Islami et al., 2018). Symbiotic microorganisms directly influence the risk of CRC development and mediate the effects of other risk factors including diet patterns, obesity, physical activity, and smoking. Gut microbiota interventions, either directly or through lifestyle modification, therefore have great potential for decreasing CRC incidence and mortality.

Dietary modification

Epidemiological studies and randomized control trials have extensively described the association between CRC incidence and dietary patterns, specifically the consumption of red and processed meat, fibre, and alcohol. The diet is also a principal determinant of the gut microbiome, governing its dynamic composition and metabolism and resulting in a divergence in microbiota-related CRC risk (David et al., 2014). The role of the microbiota in diet-oriented CRC prevention is increasingly being appreciated. In several diet interventional or observational studies, populations with different CRC rates and similar genetic backgrounds have been characterized with different microbial structures and composition, mostly because of dietary differences (O'Keefe et al., 2015; Rothschild et al., 2018). A two-week reciprocal diet switching in two African populations has been found to significantly perturb mucosal biomarkers, the abundance of deleterious taxa, and the metabolome known to affect cancer risk. Alterations in the gut community towards a pro-CRC signature have been found to occur with high-fat and low-fibre diets, thus indicating that a short-term intervention of diet may have remarkable beneficial effects on CRC prevention through reshaping the gut microbiota (O'Keefe et al., 2015). In precancerous lesions, high-fibre dietary patterns have also been found to decrease the risk of advanced colorectal adenoma in a dose-dependent and microbiota-mediated manner (Nucci et al., 2021). However, high-fibre and low-fat dietary intake (either alone or together) has failed to prevent recurrent colorectal adenomas in patients with an adenoma history (Lanza et al., 2007; Schatzkin et al., 2000), thereby suggesting a limited protective effect.

A modest association of alcohol consumption (wine, beer, or spirits) with increased CRC rates has also been observed in a dose-dependent manner (McNabb et al., 2020). This effect might be partially due to gut dysbiosis, because chronic ethanol exposure diminishes butyrate-producing taxa, compromises barrier integrity, and induces bacterial dislocation in the gut (Leclercq et al., 2014). Whether abstinence from alcohol has a protective value in CRC requires further clarification, and the duration of abstinence remains to be determined. Several studies have evaluated the negative association of circulating vitamin D (McCullough et al., 2019) and omega-3 fatty acids (Yang et al., 2014) with CRC risk. Genome-wide association analysis has identified the vitamin D receptor as a microbiota-associated regulator, whereas the mechanisms through which vitamin D intake inhibits CRC development through the gut microbiota remain unclear (Wang et al., 2016). Extensive results have revealed that regular omega-3 fatty acid supplementation reshapes the gut microbiome by increasing *Lactobacillus* and *Bifidobacterium* and suppressing *Fusobacterium nucleatum*, LPS-producing bacteria (Shen et al., 2014). The protective value of dietary supplementation may be considered in clinical practice, although modification of whole dietary habits cannot be replaced. Clinicians and nutritionists should also be cautious regarding the toxicity caused by excessive supplement intake.

Weight reduction and physical activity

The positive association between adiposity in adulthood and the risk of CRC has been repeatedly illustrated in epidemiologic studies. Excessive body weight is associated with increased CRC risk in a non-linear manner in populations with a BMI exceeding 27 kg/m^2, and has been found to contribute to approximately 5% of incident CRC cases in the United States (Islami et al., 2018). Weight control through bariatric surgery (Bailly et al., 2020) and physical activity (Friedenreich et al., 2021) significantly decreases the risk of CRC, particularly in men (Keum et al., 2015). The mechanisms underlying the obesity–CRC relationship have been extensively researched and found to include systemic inflammation, dysregulated insulin/insulin-like growth factor 1 metabolism, adipokines, and sex hormones. Increasing evidence suggests the role of the gut microbiome in this interplay. Diet-induced obesity remodels the transcriptomic landscape of colonic epithelium towards cancer progression, in a microbiota-dependent but diet type-independent manner (Li et al., 2014; Qin et al., 2018). Bariatric surgery, an effective weight reduction method, induces rapid and persistent changes in gut microbiota diversity and composition. However, whether these changes promote a shift towards a lean microbiome phenotype remains unclear (Palleja et al., 2016). Notably, the gut microbiota after bariatric surgery may be improved but still impaired with respect to a population with normal body weight, thus suggesting that its effects should not be over-exaggerated (Aron-Wisnewsky et al., 2019). In both animal models and human studies in athletes, exercise has been found to alter the composition of the butyrate-producing gut microorganisms and increase the intestinal concentrations of SCFAs, both of which are perturbed in CRC (Barton et al., 2018; Evans et al., 2014).

Smoking cessation

Tobacco smoking has been demonstrated to be associated with increased CRC risk in a manner dependent on intensity and duration. Although the latent hazardous effect of smoking may be prolonged up to 25 years after cessation, smoking cessation remains recommended to decrease the risk of CRC (Botteri et al., 2020). Causes of smoking-associated colorectal neoplasia development remain to be elucidated, but perturbation of the gut microbiota may be partially responsible. Smoking-induced modification of the microbiome has been observed in the oral cavity, airway, faeces, and intestinal mucosa (Huang & Shi, 2019). In patients with Crohn's disease, smoking exerts detrimental effects on the mucosal barrier, decreases the microbiome gene richness and diversity, and is associated with higher *Bacteroides–Prevotella* abundance, which has a pro-inflammatory effect on mucosa (Huang & Shi, 2019). The results of depleted butyrate-producing microorganisms and increased pro-inflammatory factors in smokers are associated with features of gut microbiome disturbance in patients with CRC. However, the diversity and composition of microorganisms in the gut recover after smoking cessation, alongside the restoration of an intact intestinal mucosal barrier (Biedermann et al., 2014), thus further suggesting the importance and benefits of smoking cessation in CRC prevention.

Probiotics and prebiotics

Probiotics are live microorganisms that confer health benefits, and prebiotics are chemicals inducing the growth or activity of health-promoting microorganisms in the gut. Studies have indicated the anti-tumour properties and mechanisms of several probiotics and prebiotics in CRC, including *Bifidobacterium*, *Lactobacillus* spp., and non-digestible polysaccharides metabolized by bacteria into beneficial SCFAs (Zitvogel et al., 2017). Preclinical and clinical trials have also evaluated the efficacy of oral administration of probiotics, mostly from the genera *Lactobacillus* and *Bifidobacterium* (Sivamaruthi et al., 2020). In high-risk patients with a history of colonic polyps, epithelial barrier function has been found to improve, and cell proliferation has been found to decrease, after oral administration of prebiotic inulin combined with the probiotics *Lactobacillus rhamnosus GG* and *Bifidobacterium lactis* Bb12 (Rafter et al., 2007). However, more clinical data are required to define the potential preventive roles of probiotics and prebiotics in CRC, given the current inconsistent results. Metformin, an anti-diabetic drug with recently discovered cancer-preventive effects, also modifies the composition of the gut microbiota via prebiotic routes (Al Kattar et al., 2020).

Conclusion

The gut microbiota, a critical regulator of intestinal microenvironment homeostasis, regulates health and alterations contributing to CRC initiation, possibly because the microbiome produces toxic metabolites, reprocesses intermediate dietary products, modulates immune and inflammatory responses, and causes DNA damage. Furthermore, the gut microbiome is currently being investigated as a potential biomarker for CRC early detection, monitoring, and prognosis. Thus, the gut microbiome might be modified in CRC treatment or preventive strategies, providing an promising approach to decreasing the risk of CRC development. However, the mechanisms through which the gut microbiota influences CRC development, and the clinical effects and applications remain to be elucidated. In the near future, integrated prospective studies and high-quality mechanistic experimental studies might open new avenues for studying the roles of gut microbiota in CRC risk, screening, treatment, and prevention.

REFERENCES

Abdulla, M.-H., Agarwal, D., Singh, J. K., et al. (2021). Association of the microbiome with colorectal cancer development (review). *International Journal of Oncology*, *58*, 17.

Adak, A., & Khan, M. R. (2019). An insight into gut microbiota and its functionalities. *Cellular and Molecular Life Sciences*, *76*, 473–493.

Al Kattar, S., Jurjus, R., Pinon, A., et al. (2020). Metformin and probiotics in the crosstalk between colitis-associated colorectal cancer and diabetes in mice. *Cancers*, *12*, 1857.

Aron-Wisnewsky, J., Prifti, E., Belda, E., et al. (2019). Major microbiota dysbiosis in severe obesity: fate after bariatric surgery. *Gut*, *68*, 70–82.

Bailly, L., Fabre, R., Pradier, C., et al. (2020). Colorectal cancer risk following bariatric surgery in a nationwide study of French individuals with obesity. *JAMA Surgery*, *155*, 395–402.

Barton, W., Penney, N. C., Cronin, O., et al. (2018). The microbiome of professional athletes differs from that of more sedentary subjects in composition and particularly at the functional metabolic level. *Gut*, *67*, 625–633.

Baxter, N. T., Ruffin, M. T., Rogers, M. A. M., et al. (2016). Microbiota-based model improves the sensitivity of fecal immunochemical test for detecting colonic lesions. *Genome Medicine*, *8*, 37.

Biedermann, L., Brülisauer, K., Zeitz, J., et al. (2014). Smoking cessation alters intestinal microbiota: insights from quantitative investigations on human fecal samples using FISH. *Inflammatory Bowel Disease*, *20*, 1496–1501.

Botteri, E., Borroni, E., Sloan, E. K., et al. (2020). Smoking and colorectal cancer risk, overall and by molecular subtypes: a meta-analysis. *American Journal of Gastroenterology*, *115*, 1940–1949.

Bouter, K. E., van Raalte, D. H., Groen, A. K., et al. (2017). Role of the gut microbiome in the pathogenesis of obesity and obesity-related metabolic dysfunction. *Gastroenterology*, *152*, 1671–1678.

Brahmer, J. R., Drake, C. G., Wollner, I., et al. (2010). Phase I study of single-agent anti-programmed death-1 (MDX-1106) in refractory solid tumors: safety, clinical activity, pharmacodynamics, and immunologic correlates. *Journal of Clinical Oncology*, *28*, 3167–3175.

Brennan, C. A., & Garrett, W. S., (2016). Gut microbiota, inflammation, and colorectal cancer. *Annual Review of Microbiology*, *70*, 395–411.

Brennan, C. A., & Garrett, W. S. (2019). Fusobacterium nucleatum — symbiont, opportunist and oncobacterium. *Nature Reviews Microbiology*, *17*, 156–166.

Britton, R. A., & Young, V. B. (2014). Role of the intestinal microbiota in resistance to colonization by Clostridium difficile. *Gastroenterology*, *146*, 1547–1553.

Choi, J., Jia, G., Wen, W., et al. (2021). Healthy lifestyles, genetic modifiers, and colorectal cancer risk: a prospective cohort study in the UK Biobank. *American Journal of Clinical Nutrition*, *113*, 810–820.

Colov, E. P., Degett, T. H., Raskov, H., et al. (2020). The impact of the gut microbiota on prognosis after surgery for colorectal cancer—a systematic review and meta-analysis. *Acta Pathologica, Microbiologica, et Immunologica Scandinavica*, *128*, 162–176.

Cuevas-Ramos, G., Petit, C. R., Marcq, I., et al. (2010). Escherichia coli induces DNA damage in vivo and triggers genomic instability in mammalian cells. *Proceedings of the National Academy of Sciences of the USA*, *107*, 11537–11542.

David, L. A., Maurice, C. F., Carmody, R. N., et al. (2014). Diet rapidly and reproducibly alters the human gut microbiome. *Nature*, *505*, 559–563.

Dermadi, D., Valo, S., Ollila, S., et al. (2017). Western diet deregulates bile acid homeostasis, cell proliferation, and tumorigenesis in colon. *Cancer Research*, *77*, 3352–3363.

Dvorak, K., Payne, C. M., Chavarria, M., et al. (2007). Bile acids in combination with low pH induce oxidative stress and oxidative DNA damage: relevance to the pathogenesis of Barrett's oesophagus. *Gut*, *56*, 763–771.

Eiseman, B., Silen, W., Bascom, G. S., et al. (1958). Fecal enema as an adjunct in the treatment of pseudomembranous enterocolitis. *Surgery*, *44*, 854–859.

Evans, C. C., LePard, K. J., Kwak, J. W., et al. (2014). Exercise prevents weight gain and alters the gut microbiota in a mouse model of high fat diet-induced obesity. *PLoS One*, *9*, e92193.

Feng, Q., Liang, S., Jia, H., et al. (2015). Gut microbiome development along the colorectal adenoma–carcinoma sequence. *Nature Communication*, *6*, 6528.

Ferreira, C. M., Vieira, A. T., Vinolo, M. A. R., et al. (2014). The central role of the gut microbiota in chronic inflammatory diseases. *Journal of Immunological Research*, *2014*, 689492.

Filip, M., Tzaneva, V., & Dumitrascu, D. L. (2018). Fecal transplantation: digestive and extradigestive clinical applications. *Clujul Medical Journal*, *91*, 259–265.

Firwana, B., Avaritt, N., Shields, B., et al. (2018). Do checkpoint inhibitors rely on gut microbiota to fight cancer? *Journal of Oncology Pharmacology Practice*, *24*, 468–472.

Friedenreich, C. M., Ryder-Burbidge, C., & McNeil, J. (2021). Physical activity, obesity and sedentary behavior in cancer etiology: epidemiologic evidence and biologic mechanisms. *Molecular Oncology, 15*, 790–800.

Gagnière, J., Raisch, J., Veziant, J., et al. (2016). Gut microbiota imbalance and colorectal cancer. *World Journal of Gastroenterology, 22*, 501–518.

García-González, A. P., Ritter, A. D., Shrestha, S., et al. (2017). Bacterial metabolism affects the C. elegans response to cancer chemotherapeutics. *Cell, 169*, 431–441.e8.

Gethings-Behncke, C., Coleman, H. G., Jordao, H. W. T., et al. (2020). Fusobacterium nucleatum in the colorectum and its association with cancer risk and survival: a systematic review and meta-analysis. *Cancer Epidemiology, Biomarkers & Prevention, 29*, 539–548.

Guo, S., Chen, J., Chen, F., et al. (2022). Exosomes derived from Fusobacterium nucleatum-infected colorectal cancer cells facilitate tumour metastasis by selectively carrying miR-1246/92b-3p/27a-3p and CXCL16. *Gut, 71*, e1–3.

Huang, C., & Shi, G. (2019. Smoking and microbiome in oral, airway, gut and some systemic diseases. *Journal of Translational Medicine, 17*, 225.

Huycke, M. M., Abrams, V., & Moore, D. R. (2002). Enterococcus faecalis produces extracellular superoxide and hydrogen peroxide that damages colonic epithelial cell DNA. *Carcinogenesis 23*, 529–536.

Iida, N., Dzutsev, A., Stewart, C. A., et al. (2013). Commensal bacteria control cancer response to therapy by modulating the tumor microenvironment. *Science, 342*, 967–970.

Islami, F., Goding Sauer, A., Miller, K. D., et al. (2018). Proportion and number of cancer cases and deaths attributable to potentially modifiable risk factors in the United States: potentially preventable cancers in US. *CA, Cancer Journal for Clinicians, 68*, 31–54.

Kato, S., Hamouda, N., Kano, Y., et al. (2017). Probiotic Bifidobacterium bifidum G9-1 attenuates 5-fluorouracil-induced intestinal mucositis in mice via suppression of dysbiosis-related secondary inflammatory responses. *Clinical and Experimental Pharmacology and Physiology, 44*, 1017–1025.

Kawai, T., & Akira, S. (2011). Toll-like receptors and their crosstalk with other innate receptors in infection and immunity. *Immunity 34*, 637–650.

Keum, N., Greenwood, D. C., Lee, D. H., et al. (2015). Adult weight gain and adiposity-related cancers: a dose-response meta-analysis of prospective observational studies. *Journal of the National Cancer Institute, 107*, djv088.

Kostic, A. D., Chun, E., Robertson, L., et al. (2013). Fusobacterium nucleatum potentiates intestinal tumorigenesis and modulates the tumor-immune microenvironment. *Cell Host & Microbe, 14*, 207–215.

Lanza, E., Yu, B., Murphy, G., et al. (2007). The polyp prevention trial continued follow-up study: no effect of a low-fat, high-fiber, high-fruit, and -vegetable diet on adenoma recurrence eight years after randomization. *Cancer Epidemiology, Biomarkers & Prevention, 16*, 1745–1752.

Leclercq, S., Matamoros, S., Cani, P. D., et al. (2014). Intestinal permeability, gut-bacterial dysbiosis, and behavioral markers of alcohol-dependence severity. *Proceedings of the National Academy of Science of the USA, 111*, E4485–4493.

Li, R., Grimm, S. A., Chrysovergis, K., et al. (2014). Obesity, rather than diet, drives epigenomic alterations in colonic epithelium resembling cancer progression. *Cell Metabolism, 19*, 702–711.

Liu, N.-N., Jiao, N., Tan, J.-C., et al. (2022). Multi-kingdom microbiota analyses identify bacterial–fungal interactions and biomarkers of colorectal cancer across cohorts. *Nature Microbiology, 7*, 238–250.

Long, X., Wong, C. C., Tong, L., et al. (2019). Peptostreptococcus anaerobius promotes colorectal carcinogenesis and modulates tumour immunity. *Nature Reviews Microbiology, 4*, 2319–2330.

Louis, P., Hold, G. L., & Flint, H. J. (2014). The gut microbiota, bacterial metabolites and colorectal cancer. *Nature Reviews Microbiology, 12*, 661–672.

Maghini, D. G., Moss, E. L., Vance, S. E., et al. (2021). Improved high-molecular-weight DNA extraction, nanopore sequencing and metagenomic assembly from the human gut microbiome. *Nature Protocols, 16*, 458–471.

Mármol, I., Sánchez-de-Diego, C., Pradilla Dieste, A., et al. (2017). Colorectal carcinoma: a general overview and future perspectives in colorectal cancer. *International Journal of Molecular Science, 18*, E197.

Martin, O. C. B., Bergonzini, A., D'Amico, F., et al. (2019). Infection with genotoxin-producing Salmonella enterica synergises with loss of the tumour suppressor APC in promoting genomic instability via the PI3K pathway in colonic epithelial cells. *Cell Microbiology, 21*, e13099.

McCullough, M. L., Zoltick, E. S., Weinstein, S. J., et al. (2019). Circulating vitamin D and colorectal cancer risk: an international pooling project of 17 cohorts. *Journal of the National Cancer Institute, 111*, 158–169.

McNabb, S., Harrison, T.A., Albanes, D., et al. (2020). Meta-analysis of 16 studies of the association of alcohol with colorectal cancer. *International Journal of Cancer, 146*, 861–873.

Messaritakis, I., Vogiatzoglou, K., Tsantaki, K., et al. (2020). The prognostic value of the detection of microbial translocation in the blood of colorectal cancer patients. *Cancers, 12*, 1058.

Mima, K., Nishihara, R., Qian, Z. R., et al. (2016). Fusobacterium nucleatum in colorectal carcinoma tissue and patient prognosis. *Gut, 65*, 1973–1980.

Nucci, D., Fatigoni, C., Salvatori, T., et al. (2021). Association between dietary fibre intake and colorectal adenoma: a systematic review and meta-analysis. *International Journal of Environmental Research and Public Health, 18*, 4168.

O'Keefe, S. J. D., Li, J. V., Lahti, L., et al. (2015). Fat, fibre and cancer risk in African Americans and rural Africans. *Nature Communication, 6*, 6342.

Omar Al-Hassi, H., Ng, O., & Brookes, M. (2018). Tumour-associated and non-tumour-associated microbiota in colorectal cancer. *Gut, 67*, 395.

Osman, M. A., Neoh, H., Ab Mutalib, N.-S., et al. (2021. Parvimonas micra, Peptostreptococcus stomatis, Fusobacterium nucleatum and Akkermansia muciniphila as a four-bacteria biomarker panel of colorectal cancer. *Scientific Reports, 11*, 2925.

Palleja, A., Kashani, A., Allin, K. H., et al. (2016). Roux-en-Y gastric bypass surgery of morbidly obese patients induces swift and persistent changes of the individual gut microbiota. *Genome Medicine, 8*, 67.

Peters, B. A., Dominianni, C., Shapiro, J. A., et al. (2016). The gut microbiota in conventional and serrated precursors of colorectal cancer. *Microbiome, 4*, 69.

Pothuraju, R., Chaudhary, S., Rachagani, S., et al. (2021). Mucins, gut microbiota, and postbiotics role in colorectal cancer. *Gut Microbes, 13*, 1974795.

Prince, B. T., Mandel, M. J., Nadeau, K., et al. (2015). Gut microbiome and the development of food allergy and allergic disease. *Pediatric Clinics of North America, 62*, 1479–1492.

Qin, Y., Roberts, J. D., Grimm, S. A., et al. (2018). An obesity-associated gut microbiome reprograms the intestinal epigenome and leads to altered colonic gene expression. *Genome Biology*, *19*, 7.

Quintero, E., Castells, A., Bujanda, L., et al. (2012). Colonoscopy versus fecal immunochemical testing in colorectal-cancer screening. *New England Journal of Medicine*, *366*, 697–706.

Rafter, J., Bennett, M., Caderni, G., et al. (2007). Dietary synbiotics reduce cancer risk factors in polypectomized and colon cancer patients. *American Journal of Clinical Nutrition*, *85*, 488–496.

Rawla, P., Sunkara, T., & Barsouk, A. (2019). Epidemiology of colorectal cancer: incidence, mortality, survival, and risk factors. *Polish Journal of Gastroenterology*, *14*, 89–103.

Raza, A., Khan, A. Q., Inchakalody, V. P., et al. (2022). Dynamic liquid biopsy components as predictive and prognostic biomarkers in colorectal cancer. *Journal of Experimental Clinical Cancer Research*, *41*, 99.

Rescigno, M. (2015. A 'fit' microbiota to potentiate cancer immunotherapy. *Genome Medicine*, *7*, 131.

Rezasoltani, S., Sharafkhah, M., Asadzadeh Aghdaei, H., et al. (2018). Applying simple linear combination, multiple logistic and factor analysis methods for candidate fecal bacteria as novel biomarkers for early detection of adenomatous polyps and colon cancer. *Journal of Microbiological Methods*, *155*, 82–88.

Rosshart, S. P., Vassallo, B. G., Angeletti, D., et al. (2017). Wild mouse gut microbiota promotes host fitness and improves disease resistance. *Cell*, *171*, 1015–1028.e13.

Rothschild, D., Weissbrod, O., Barkan, E., et al. (2018). Environment dominates over host genetics in shaping human gut microbiota. *Nature*, *555*, 210–215.

Rubinstein, M. R., Wang, X., Liu, W., et al. (2013). Fusobacterium nucleatum promotes colorectal carcinogenesis by modulating E-cadherin/β-catenin signaling via its FadA adhesin. *Cell Host & Microbe*, *14*, 195–206.

Sánchez-Alcoholado, L., Ramos-Molina, B., Otero, A., et al. (2020). The role of the gut microbiome in colorectal cancer development and therapy response. *Cancers (Basel)*, *12*, E1406.

Santarpia, M., & Karachaliou, N. (2015). Tumor immune microenvironment characterization and response to anti-PD-1 therapy. *Cancer Biology and Medicine*, *12*, 74–78.

Sbahi, H., & Di Palma, J. A. (2016). Faecal microbiota transplantation: applications and limitations in treating gastrointestinal disorders. *BMJ Open Gastroenterology*, *3*, e000087.

Schatzkin, A., Lanza, E., Corle, D., et al. (2000). Lack of effect of a low-fat, high-fiber diet on the recurrence of colorectal adenomas. *New England Journal of Medicine*, *342*, 1149–1155.

Scott, T. A., Quintaneiro, L. M., Norvaisas, P., et al. (2017). Host-microbe co-metabolism dictates cancer drug efficacy in *C.* elegans. *Cell*, *169*, 442–456.e18.

Shen, W., Gaskins, H. R., & McIntosh, M.K. (2014). Influence of dietary fat on intestinal microbes, inflammation, barrier function and metabolic outcomes. *Journal of Nutritional Biochemistry*, *25*, 270–280.

Shen, X., Li, J., Li, J., et al. (2021). Fecal enterotoxigenic bacteroides fragilis–peptostreptococcus stomatis–parvimonas micra biomarker for noninvasive diagnosis and prognosis of colorectal laterally spreading tumor. *Frontiers in Oncology*, *11*, 661048.

Singh, N., Gurav, A., Sivaprakasam, S., et al. (2014). Activation of Gpr109a, receptor for niacin and the commensal metabolite butyrate, suppresses colonic inflammation and carcinogenesis. *Immunity*, *40*, 128–139.

Sivamaruthi, B. S., Kesika, P., & Chaiyasut, C. (2020). The role of probiotics in colorectal cancer management. *Evidence-Based Complementary and Alternative Medicine*, *2020*, 3535982.

Sivan, A., Corrales, L., Hubert, N., Williams, J. B., et al. (2015). Commensal bifidobacterium promotes antitumor immunity and facilitates anti-PD-L1 efficacy. *Science*, *350*, 1084–1089.

Tang, W. H. W., Kitai, T., & Hazen, S. L. (2017). Gut microbiota in cardiovascular health and disease. *Circulation Research*, *120*, 1183–1196.

Temraz, S., Nassar, F., Nasr, R., et al. (2019). Gut microbiome: a promising biomarker for immunotherapy in colorectal cancer. *International Journal of Molecular Science*, *20*, E4155.

Thomas, A. M., Manghi, P., Asnicar, F., et al. (2019). Metagenomic analysis of colorectal cancer datasets identifies cross-cohort microbial diagnostic signatures and a link with choline degradation. *Nature Medicine*, *25*, 667–678.

Tilg, H., Adolph, T. E., Gerner, R. R., et al. (2018). The intestinal microbiota in colorectal cancer. *Cancer Cell*, *33*, 954–964.

Topalian, S. L., Hodi, F. S., Brahmer, J. R., et al. (2012). Safety, activity, and immune correlates of anti-PD-1 antibody in cancer. *New England Journal of Medicine*, *366*, 2443–2454.

Topalian, S. L., Taube, J. M., Anders, R. A., et al. (2016). Mechanism-driven biomarkers to guide immune checkpoint blockade in cancer therapy. *Nature Reviews Cancer*, *16*, 275–287.

Vétizou, M., Pitt, J. M., Daillère, R., et al. (2015). Anticancer immunotherapy by CTLA-4 blockade relies on the gut microbiota. *Science*, *350*, 1079–1084.

Vlantis, K., Polykratis, A., Welz, P.-S., et al. (2016). TLR-independent anti-inflammatory function of intestinal epithelial TRAF6 signalling prevents DSS-induced colitis in mice. *Gut*, *65*, 935–943.

Wallace, B. D., Roberts, A. B., Pollet, R. M., et al. (2015). Structure and inhibition of microbiome β-glucuronidases essential to the alleviation of cancer drug toxicity. *Chemistry & Biology*, *22*, 1238–1249.

Wang, J., Thingholm, L. B., Skiecevičienė, J., et al. (2016). Genome-wide association analysis identifies variation in vitamin D receptor and other host factors influencing the gut microbiota. *Nature Genetics*, *48*, 1396–1406.

Wang, K., Liao, M., Zhou, N., et al. (2019). Parabacteroides distasonis alleviates obesity and metabolic dysfunctions via production of succinate and secondary bile acids. *Cell Reports*, *26*, 222–235.e5.

Wang, T., Cai, G., Qiu, Y., et al. (2012). Structural segregation of gut microbiota between colorectal cancer patients and healthy volunteers. *ISME Journal*, *6*, 320–329.

Wei, Z., Cao, S., Liu, S., et al. (2016). Could gut microbiota serve as prognostic biomarker associated with colorectal cancer patients' survival? A pilot study on relevant mechanism. *Oncotarget*, *7*, 46158–46172.

Weisburger, J. H., Reddy, B. S., Narisawa, T., et al. (1975). Germ-free status and colon tumor induction by N-methyl-N'-nitro-N-nitrosoguanidine. *Proceedings of the Society of Experimental Biology & Medicine*, *148*, 1119–1121.

Wong, S. H., Kwong, T. N. Y., Chow, T.-C., et al. (2017a). Quantitation of faecal fusobacterium improves faecal immunochemical test in detecting advanced colorectal neoplasia. *Gut*, *66*, 1441–1448.

Wong, S. H., Zhao, L., Zhang, X., Nakatsu, G., Han, J., et al. (2017b). Gavage of fecal samples from patients with colorectal cancer promotes intestinal carcinogenesis in germ-free and conventional mice. *Gastroenterology*, *153*, 1621–1633.e6.

Yang, B., Wang, F.-L., Ren, X.-L., et al. (2014). Biospecimen long-chain N-3 PUFA and risk of colorectal cancer: a meta-analysis of data from 60,627 individuals. *PLoS One*, *9*, e110574.

Yeung, C.-Y., Chan, W.-T., Jiang, C.-B., et al. (2015). Amelioration of chemotherapy-induced intestinal mucositis by orally administered probiotics in a mouse model. *PLoS One*, *10*, e0138746.

Yu, J., Feng, Q., Wong, S. H., et al. (2017). Metagenomic analysis of faecal microbiome as a tool towards targeted non-invasive biomarkers for colorectal cancer. *Gut*, *66*, 70–78.

Zhang, X., Zhu, X., Cao, Y., et al. (2019). Fecal Fusobacterium nucleatum for the diagnosis of colorectal tumor: A systematic review and meta-analysis. *Cancer Medicine*, *8*, 480–491.

Zitvogel, L., Daillère, R., Roberti, M. P., et al. (2017). Anticancer effects of the microbiome and its products. *Nature Reviews Microbiology*, *15*, 465–478.

6

Innovations in population screening

Anoop Kozhippatu Varghese and James E. East

Introduction

Despite being the third highest cause of cancer-related death worldwide, colorectal cancer is a preventable disease. Many countries have therefore implemented screening programmes for colorectal cancer that can be opportunistic or organized at a regional or national level. Screening for colorectal cancer has consistently been shown to be cost effective and to reduce colorectal cancer-related mortality, although an effect on overall mortality has not been demonstrated.

In 2017 the US Multi-Society Task Force (USMSTF) on Colorectal Cancer recommended screening should start at the age of 50 years. USMSTF ranked CRC screening tests into a 'menu' with three tiers based on performance features, cost, and practical considerations. First-tier tests were colonoscopy every 10 years and annual faecal immunochemical test (FIT). Second-tier tests include CT colonography every five years, flexible sigmoidoscopy every five to ten years, and FIT with multi-target stool DNA every three years. Third-tier tests include capsule colonoscopy every five years (Rex et al., 2017); however, in 2018 the American Cancer Society (ACS) recommended a reduction in the age at which screening should be started from 50 to 45 years of age in those at average risk, driven by data that showed that colorectal cancer was increasing in incidence in younger patients in many higher income countries.

In 2006, the National Health Service (NHS) introduced the Bowel Cancer Screening Programme (BCSP) in England and Wales with an aim to detect colorectal carcinomas early and thereby improve the outcomes and mortality of CRC. The BCSP initially targeted a population of 60 to 69 years of age in whom a guaiac faecal occult blood test (gFOBt) was done biennially (Logan et al., 2012). A positive faecal occult blood test was then followed up with a whole colon test, most commonly colonoscopy. In 2013 the 'Bowelscope' programme was also launched in England in which a flexible sigmoidoscopy was offered to the population at the age of 55 years and a colonoscopy followed, for those with significant findings at flexible sigmoidoscopy (see below). In 2019 the NHS BCSP switched from gFOBt to FIT testing due to modelling suggesting improved test performance and cost effectiveness, with subsequent abandonment of Bowelscope in 2021.

This series of changes, while relatively slow, show that screening programmes evolve over time to include new concepts and technologies, and that this is likely to continue, with some of the technologies described below becoming part of the opportunistic or organized screening programme armamentarium. Current options internationally are summarized in Table 6.1.

Colonoscopy

Colonoscopy remains the criterion standard for bowel cancer screening and is the final common pathway after other screening tests. It is effective both for early detection of even small colorectal cancers and also for therapy of precancerous polyps which can stop their progression to cancer. The National Polyp Study in 1980s in the United States led to widespread adoption of colonoscopy as the preferred screening tests in that country, on the basis of an approximate 50% reduction in colorectal cancer and CRC-related death compared to SEER data. The fact that prevention of CRC is not 100% suggests that there is room for improvement in the procedure to prevent post-colonoscopy colorectal cancer which accounts for 7–9% of all colorectal cancers detected (Fig. 6.1).

Historically colonoscopy has focussed on adenomas as the primary target and by disrupting the adenoma–carcinoma sequence by polypectomy, there is now strong evidence that this reduces future colorectal cancer risk, however the risk reduction is not evenly distributed throughout the colon, with much greater reductions in the left colon and rectum than in the right colon. The reasons for this are multiple and include that polyps in the right colon often have a flatter shape, can be hidden behind deep haustral folds, but are also more frequently serrated lesions. Serrated lesions were not previously considered as colorectal cancer precursors, however in the last decade or so it has become increasingly clear that they account for up to one-third of colorectal cancers, especially post-colonoscopy colorectal cancers in the right colon (East et al., 2017).

Serrated lesions are almost universally flat in shape and are often pale or transparent (Fig. 6.2). This makes them both difficult to detect, and even when detected difficult to resect comprehensively, with one large study suggesting that the rate of residual polyp was four-fold higher after resection of serrated polyps compared to adenomatous lesion. Appreciation of the importance of serrated

Table 6.1 International Recommendations on methods for colorectal cancer screening

Method	USPSTF	USMSTF/ACS/ACR	ACG	Asia Pacific	European
Colonoscopy every 10 y	+	+	+	+	+
High-sensitivity gFOBT every 1 y	+	No comment	+	+	+
FIT every 1 y	+	+	+	+	+
MTsDNA every 1–3 y	+	+	+	No comment	Not recommended
CT colonography every 5 y	+	+	+	Not recommended	Not recommended
Flexible sigmoidoscopy every 5–10 y	+	+	+	+	+
Capsule colonoscopy every 5 y	+	+	+	No comment	Not recommended
Septin 9	No comment	Not recommended	Not recommended	No comment	No comment
Double Contrast Barium Enema	Not recommended	+	Not recommended	Not recommended	No comment

Adapted from AGA clinical practice update on approach to the use of noninvasive colorectal cancer screening options: commentary (Burke et al., 2022).

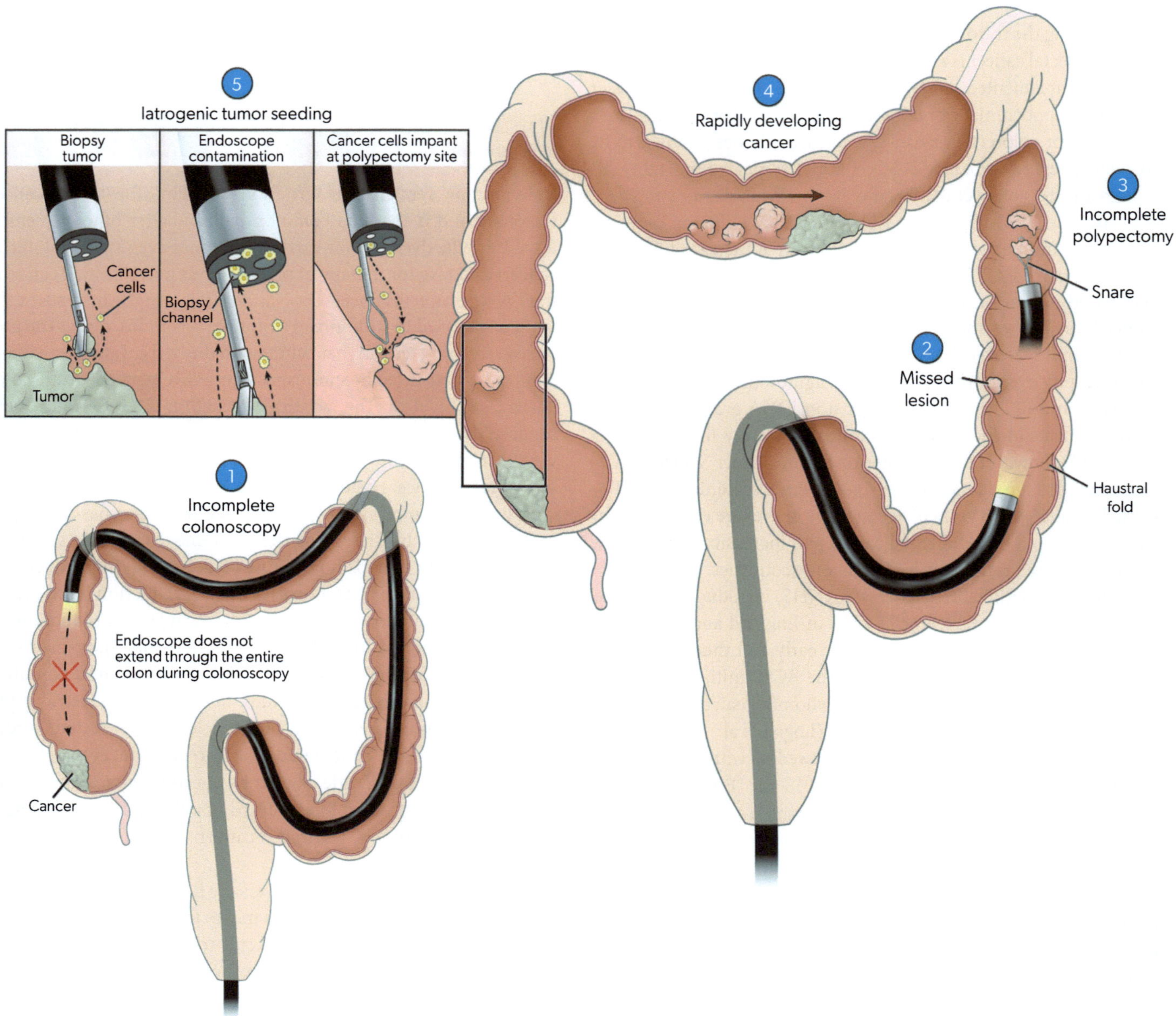

Figure 6.1 Mechanisms of post-colonoscopy colorectal cancer development (reproduced from East, J. E. (2019). Can colonoscopy sow the seeds of colorectal cancer? *Gastroenterology*, *157*(5), 1192–1195. doi:10.1053/j.gastro.2019.09.004. Copyright 2019 by the AGA Institute (Elsevier)).

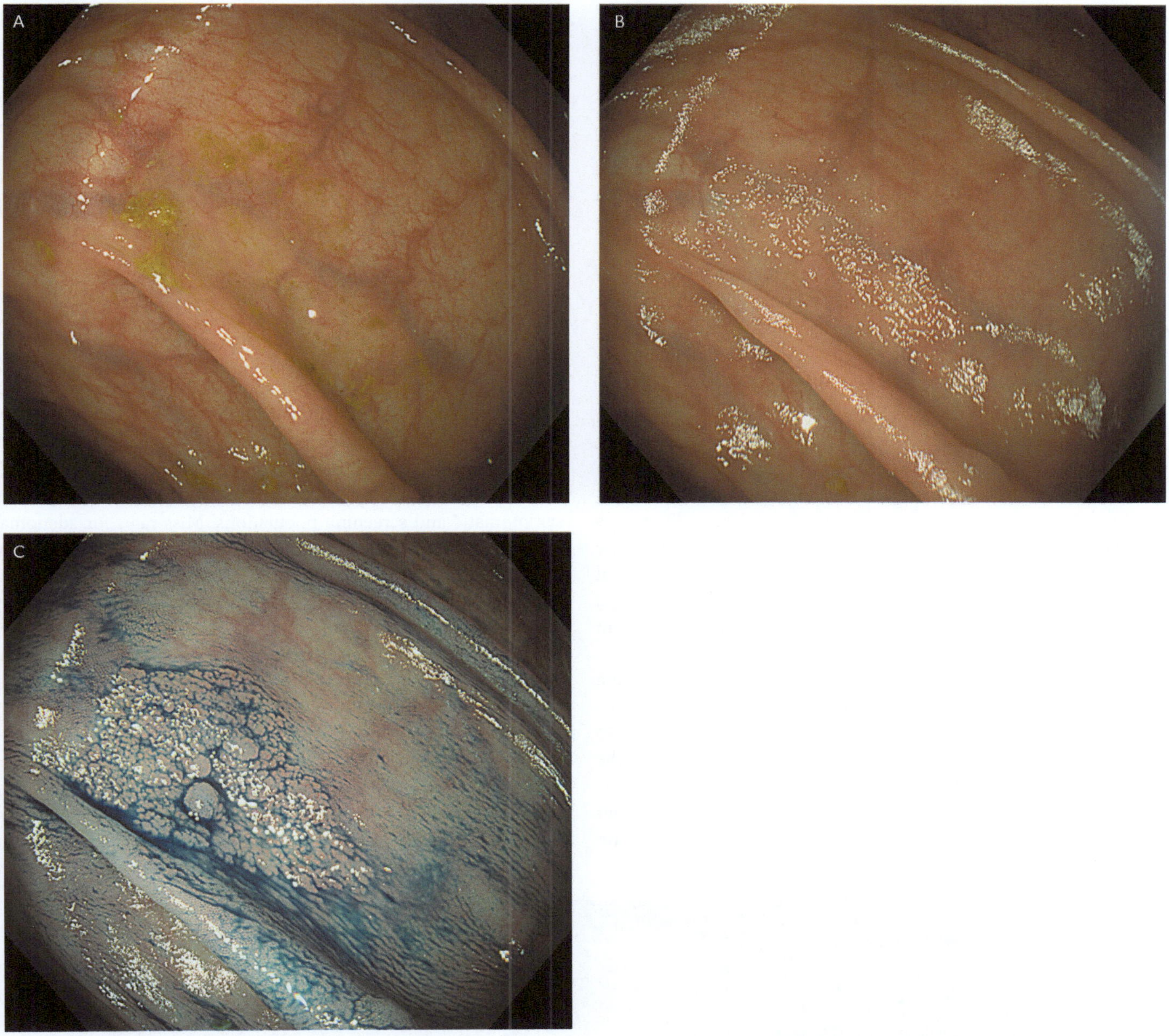

Figure 6.2 **A.** 20 mm sessile serrated lesion ascending colon; note subtle blurring of blood vessel pattern and adherent bile stained mucus. **B.** After washing the polyp becomes almost invisible. **C.** After application of blue dye (chromoendoscopy) to the bowel lining the serrated lesion is much clearer (reproduced from East, J. E. (2019). Endoscopic polypectomy. *WGO handbook on early diagnosis and treatment of GI cancer* <https://wdhd.worldgastroenterology.org/UserFiles/file/WGOF/WDHD2019/WDHD2019Handbook.pdf>).

lesions by the screening community is expected to lead to an improvement in the cancer prevention effectiveness of colonoscopy in the right colon.

Imaging

The move to video colonoscopes in the 1980 and 1990s was a huge step forward in image quality and operator comfort. However the advent of high-definition colonoscopy that become widely available after 2005 has had less of an impact on screening performance with modest increases in adenoma detection rates. Therefore endoscopists have sought other imaging enhancements to try to optimize polyp detection and therefore colorectal cancer prevention. Chromoendoscopy (dye-spray) involves spraying blue dye on the colonic mucosa to highlight subtle abnormalities and it can increase adenoma detection rates by approximately 20%; however, it is time-consuming and cumbersome, adds cost (dye-spray catheters), and has not been adopted at a population level (Fig. 6.2).

Optical or digital mucosal enhancement offered the potential for better detection without these disadvantages, at the press of a button. Techniques included narrowed spectrum endoscopy (NBI, FICE, i-SCAN) which use shorter wavelengths to highlight superficial microvessels, and autofluorescence endoscopy which relies on differing tissue properties (NADPH, flavins) to build up a false colour image. Despite being more convenient than dye-spray, the benefits were limited and there has not been widespread adoption in screening programmes, despite widespread clinical availability.

Devices

While efforts have been made to improve detection in the visual field, the risk remains that polyps can be hidden in areas that can be more difficult to visualize despite a skilled endoscopist such as behind haustral folds or at colonic flexures. Devices have therefore been developed that try to reveal more mucosa, either by the use of attachments that press down on mucosal folds (e.g. Endocuff, Endorings, G-EYE) or devices that provide a different angle of view (e.g. Third eye retroscope, FUSE). While these provide a modest increase in adenoma detection, they can make the intubation phase of colonoscopy more challenging. Despite support for the use of, for example, Endocuff by the UK National Institute for Health and Care Excellence (NICE) as part of the NHS bowel cancer screening programme, their use has not become widespread in screening.

Quality

Colonoscopy is an operator-dependant technique with large variation in the ability of endoscopists to detect adenomas and serrated polyps in screening populations reported. These differences in adenoma detection rate correlate strongly with post-colonoscopy colorectal cancer rates and death from post-colonoscopy colorectal cancer, with endoscopists in the lowest detection quintile having a three-fold higher post-colonoscopy CRC death rate than those in the highest detecting quintile (Corley et al., 2014).

Therefore monitoring of adenoma detection rates has become a key performance indicator (KPI) at colonoscopy in screening programmes at both an individual and unit level, with feedback given to endoscopists every six months in the United Kingdom as part of the requirement for Endoscopy units to remain accredited. Interventions to support adenoma detection, for example evidence bundles and feedback, can lead to long-term improvements in adenoma detection for poorer performing operators. In those where intervention leads to improvements in adenoma detection, the post-colonoscopy colorectal cancer (PCCRC) rate falls. There has therefore been considerable effort to implement quality assurance programmes within bowel cancer screening internationally, with a reduction in PCCRC seen in symptomatic practice over time. Polyp detection rates and other KPIs are already captured by endoscopy reporting software tools, and it is likely this will become increasing automated and sophisticated with support by artificial intelligence (AI).

Artificial intelligence

The use of AI (deep convolutional neural networks) in endoscopy has proceeded rapidly as image analysis tools have evolved from existing work on facial recognition technologies. Polyp detection algorithms have rapidly advanced and are now available commercially as computer-aided detection (CADe) (e.g. GI Genius (Medtronic), CAD-EYE (Fujinon)), and have demonstrated effectiveness in both symptomatic and screening populations. Miss rates for adenomas can be reduced by 50% and absolute overall detection increased from 19.3% to 29.6%, relative risk 1.52 (1.31–1.77) in a recent meta-analysis (Barua et al., 2021). Improvements are seen in both poorer performers and experts (Fig. 6.3). The technology is very user-friendly and can be added to existing systems without the need for different colonoscopes or video towers. It is likely that these systems will become widespread in both symptomatic and screening practice in the next few years.

Artificial intelligence is likely to have further impact in providing real-time evaluation of the quality of bowel cleaning (e.g. Endoangel), which also correlates with adenoma detection rates, and to assess the proportion of mucosa visualized, encouraging the

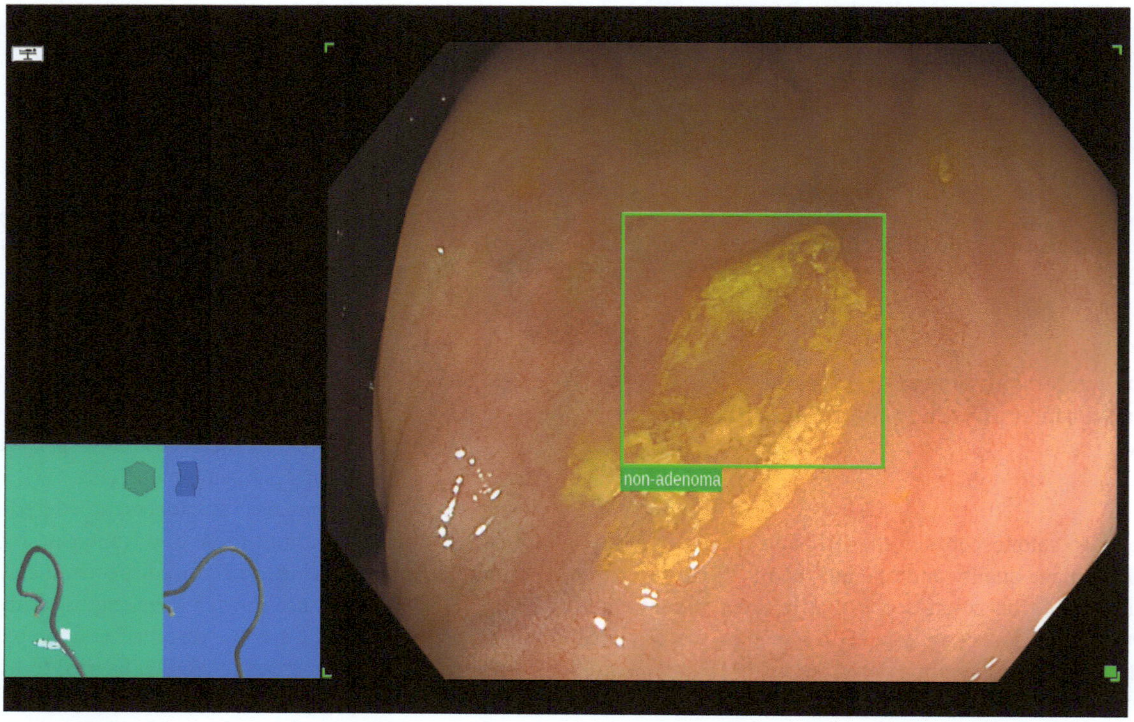

Figure 6.3 A serrated lesion highlighted (green bounding box) by the GI Genius endoscopy AI system (Medtronic) with histological characterisation (non-adenoma as text below bounding box).

endoscopist to explore behind folds and flexures meticulously, and providing real-time quality assurance feedback. In combination, such algorithms are likely to enhance the full screening colonoscopy workflow, including automated report writing and recommending surveillance intervals, which may reduce variability. However, these are likely to be clinician support tools rather than fully autonomous algorithms. Data are still lacking that AI-supported colonoscopy will have lower post-colonoscopy CRC rates, but large-scale trials are planned. AI-supported adenoma detection is cost effective in modelling studies in the long term but may increase short-terms costs (Ariea et al., 2022). Currently AI-supported colonoscopy is not reimbursed but other medical AI technology has achieved this, and reimbursement is likely to accelerate adoption (Mori et al., 2023)

FIT and FIT+

Faecal immunochemical testing (FIT) is an antibody-based test for human globin in stool. It has largely replaced guaiac testing as it is automated, quantitative, and reproducible in population-based screening programmes. It is recommended as a screening test option by all international guideline groups. FIT is straightforward to administer at scale and is effective at detecting early cancer; however, it is much less effective at detecting colorectal cancer precursors, for example advanced adenomas which are an important target in screening programmes which aim to prevent the development of colorectal cancer rather than detect it at an earlier and curable stage. There has therefore been considerable interest in developing 'FIT plus' tests where FIT is combined with an additional biomarker to try to improve performance, especially for colorectal cancer precursor lesions.

FIT+ multitarget stool DNA

Colonic cells are continuously shed into the faecal stream from both healthy and diseased mucosa. Cancers and precancerous lesions have typical genetic aberrations which can be detected with sequencing techniques from DNA extracted from stool samples. Cologuard® is a combination of a FIT test and stool DNA analysis available commercially in the United States. This detects aberrantly methylated BMP3 and NDRG4 promoter regions, and mutant KRAS with an improvement in test performance compared to FIT alone for colorectal cancer from 0.89 to 0.94 (area under ROC curve), and for advanced colorectal neoplasia from 0.67 to 0.73. Of particular note, the sensitivity for serrated lesion 10 mm or larger increased from 5% to 42% (Imperiale, 2014). However, in order to perform the analysis a whole stool is required which makes it far less easy for patients to perform the test and makes for more challenging transport logistics compared to FIT.

FIT+ microbiome

The role of the microbiome has become much better appreciated in recent years with the development of new genomic methods (Shotgun metagenomic sequencing and 16S RNA sequencing) which has enabled the detection of a much wide range of microbes than traditional culture techniques. As FIT testing collects a sample of stool, this might also be available for microbiome as well as blood in stool analysis. Colorectal cancer patients have changes in the stool microbiome that may be both carcinogenic themselves and also reflect microbiome changes due to the presence of the cancer, or cancer precursors. Analysis of these changes, including the virome and mycobiome, can improve the diagnostic performance of FIT both for cancer and precursors.

A study in a Chinese population used metagenomic analysis to demonstrate that a faecal bacterial marker *m3* (*Lachnoclostridium sp.*) can improve the detection of even non-advanced adenomas, sensitivity 48.3%, and in combination with FIT had a sensitivity for advanced adenomas of 56.8% compared to 16.1% for FIT alone. A wider combination of four faecal bacterial markers plus FIT had a sensitivity of 93.8% and specificity of 81.2% for CRC (Liang et al., 2020),

FIT+ polygenic risk

Polygenic risk describes the small heritable changes in colorectal risk that patients acquire through the actions of multiple genes, rather than the action of a single mendelian driver mutation in, for example, familial adenomatous polyposis. Polygenic risk is thought to account for up to about 10% of colorectal cancer risk. Whole genome sequencing or SnP chip-based approaches have developed rapidly recently, meaning that the costs have fallen, which might make this approach viable in a screening setting, perhaps as a saliva/buccal swab combined with FIT. The results might be used to individualize FIT cut-off values, or for those at highest polygenic risk to select an alternative screening methodology (e.g. colonoscopy), or be combined with other environmental risk factors in a compound risk score

Initial analysis using combinations of tens to hundreds of SnPs known to be associated with colorectal cancer from genome-wide association studies did not support enhanced discrimination, nor have AI-supported approaches helped. Using a Bayesian approach and all of the dataset, however, some improvement in discrimination is possible that is equivalent to knowing a patient's family history. As nuclear families become smaller, and therefore less family history data are available to clinicians, this may be of value, although the effect size is small. The datasets that these models are drawn from are predominantly from patients of European ancestry, and so may not be applicable to populations worldwide (Chapter 1).

Polygenic risk can also be combined with environmental risk factors to enhance the effectiveness of future cancer prediction. One large-scale model using QCancer-10, based on UK primary care datasets and UK biobank data, was able to show an improvement in model prediction, but the overall net gains were small, and it is not clear that the benefits would be cost effective (Briggs et al., 2022).

Flexible sigmoidoscopy

Flexible sigmoidoscopy examines the rectum and left colon, and can detect cancer, but it can also detect and remove adenomas, potentially preventing colorectal cancer developing. It does not require sedation and preparation is usually with an enema. It is suggested that most adenomas in the distal colon will have developed by age 60 and so a one-off flexible sigmoidoscopy might be effective for CRC prevention, although US guidelines recommend screening with this every five years.

In the FlexiScope trial which was conducted in United Kingdom which randomized 170,000 screenees, offering once-only flexible sigmoidoscopy reduced the colorectal cancer incidence by 23% and colorectal cancer mortality by 31% (Atkin et al., 2010). The rate of distal colorectal cancer prevention (i.e. in the area that had been examined and cleared of precursors lesion) was 50% during 11 years of follow-up, and the effect continued in an extension study that reviewed outcomes at 17 years. The proximal colon was only examined in a subsequent colonoscopy if there was identification of a CRC, an advanced adenoma, ≥ 3 adenomas, or ≥ 20 hyperplastic polyps above the rectum. Perhaps because of this, there was no effect on proximal cancer prevention. Three other large trials of flexible sigmoidoscopy screening, the US Prostate, Lung, Colorectal and Ovarian cancer screening trial (PLCO), the Italian Screening for Colon and Rectum trial (SCORE), and the Norwegian Colorectal Cancer Prevention trial (NORCCAP), and a combined analysis all showed a similar level of reduction in colorectal cancer incidence and mortality, with a greater effect in men than in women, perhaps because of the CRC sidedness divergence between the sexes.

In 2013, the UK government initiated an NHS programme of one-off flexible sigmoidoscopy at age 55 on the basis of these data, the 'Bowelscope' programme, with biannual FIT for patients aged 60–74. However the logistics were formidable, especially the requirement to train sufficient endoscopists to perform the procedures. This screening programme has now been abandoned, with the FIT starting age reduced to 50 to compensate. Attempts to improve patient experience with underwater intubation, or adenoma detection with the Endocuff devices (WASH and BADENOMA studies, respectively) were not effective.

Therefore, despite high-quality randomized data from multiple studies, flexible sigmoidoscopy is not widely used as a broad screening tool, and it is currently difficult to see how it might be optimized further to be a core part of general screening programmes.

CT colonography

CT colonography (CTC) is a high-resolution CT examination used for detecting colorectal carcinomas and advanced colonic polyps, requiring pre-procedure colonic preparation and peri-procedure colonic insufflation. The Radiology Clinical and Professional Group for the NHS Bowel Cancer Screening Programme (BCSP) has developed guidelines to define standards for the delivery of high-quality colonic imaging and recommends CTC as an alternative, when colonoscopy is incomplete or when the patient is medically unfit for the procedure. A recent meta-analysis of CT colonography with bowel prep from the US Preventative Services Taskforce, showed a sensitivity 0.89 and a specificity of 0.94 in detecting adenomas ≥ 10 mm in a screening population (Lin et al., 2021).

CTC is a safe and better tolerated procedure when compared to other modalities for imaging the large bowel without sedation. CT colonography has two main safety issues, in the form of risk of colonic perforation and pneumoperitoneum, which is an extremely rare event, < 1:10,000, and the exposure to ionizing radiation. CT colonography is contraindicated in patients with active colitis, diverticulitis, recent colorectal surgery, colonic perforation, and small bowel obstruction. Misinterpretation of CT colonography can result in false negative (missed) or false positive results, and quality assurance and training programmes are being developed as in colonoscopy. Missed lesions on CTC depends on many factors including lesion characteristics, anatomic location of the lesion, and study technique. In general, flat lesions are more commonly missed than sessile or pedunculated lesions, which means CTC is less effective for detecting sessile serrated lesions, now recognized as an important CRC precursor. Also, CTC is less accurate in detecting diminutive polyps < 5 mm where sensitivity may be only 50%.

Although there remain the positives described above, CTC has not become a major part of screening programmes, despite being an option in US guidelines, and despite possible advantages in detecting extra luminal pathology that may also be relevant to wider screening (e.g. abdominal aortic aneurysm), although harm through over investigation of incidental findings is also possible. In part, this reticence may relate to the need for follow-up colonoscopy in one-third of cases due to a polyp being detected. As lower radiation dose, lower toxicity protocols are developed, particularly combined with AI-supported interpretation, the role of CTC may become more prominent, potentially combining with CT-based lung cancer screening which might increase engagement.

Colon capsule endoscopy

Colon capsule endoscopy (CCE) can provide views of the entire colon, and the sensitivity for detection of smaller polyps has increased significantly from first-generation (CCE I) colon capsules to second-generation (CCE II) colon capsules (Fig. 6.4). The European Society of Gastrointestinal Endoscopy has recommended CCE II in the case of a positive faecal occult blood test (FOBT) or FIT with incomplete or unfeasible colonoscopy, within organized population screening programmes. The US Food and Drug Administration (FDA) has approved CCE II for patients with a previous incomplete colonoscopy and for evaluation of lower gastrointestinal bleeding. Colon capsule endoscopy carries minimal risks since it is a non-invasive test which requires no sedation and can be carried out at home. CCE II has various advantages over CCE I, which include a nearly 360° field of view and the ability to vary the number of recorded images (i.e. the adaptive frame rate), which saves battery life

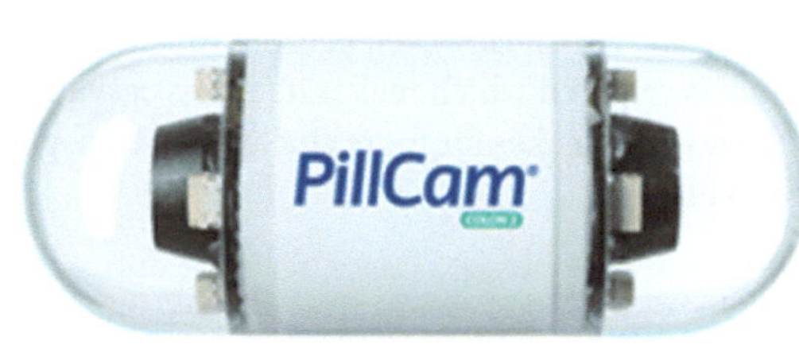

Figure 6.4 Colon capsule endoscope showing double ended configuration (reproduced from I. Papalia et al. (2021). Colon capsule endoscopy in the assessment of mucosal healing in Crohn's disease. *Inflammatory Bowel Diseases*, *27* (Suppl_2), S25–32. <https://doi.org/10.1093/ibd/izab180>.

and increases the time available for the procedure. In this way, the colon and rectum can be examined completely.

CCE II has a new type of data recorder that communicates bidirectionally with the capsule. The capsule can be monitored and any delay can be managed using prokinetic agents. The disadvantages of CCE that have been mentioned are the extended period of time for results and future requirement of a colonoscopy when significant lesions are found. Also, the patient requires a higher degree of colonic cleansing since air insufflation, cleaning, and suctioning are not possible as they are in a colonoscopy. The patient may require booster medications to propel the capsule across the small bowel and colon for a complete visualization of the colon. A meta-analyses looking at studies of CCE in screening populations showed a sensitivity for polyps ≥ 6 mm of 88% (95% CI: 0.84–0.91), and specificity 94% (95% CI: 0.92–0.95), although incomplete examinations occurred in 11.6% of cases and preparation was adequate in only 54–92% of cases. (Sulbaran et al., 2022)

Artificial intelligence can perform automated reviewing of the CCE images, which leads to time saving for the clinicians. Early AI models have reported high sensitivity 79.0% and specificity 87.0% for detection of polyps and colorectal malignancies (Yamada et al., 2021).

This potentially opens up a new model for screening based on home-delivered CCE, avoiding the inconvenience of attending a hospital appointment, combined with predominantly AI reading of the result, reducing costs, especially time needed for reading which can be tenfold less than a standard human read. Amazon and Medtronic are currently exploring a partnership to offer this and it is likely that others could offer a similarly disruptive model.

Check cap

The need for a patient-friendly colorectal cancer screening test led to the development of Check Cap which requires no bowel preparation or sedation. Check Cap is an imaging capsule which consists of an X-ray emitter, a short-lived radioisotope, which is collimated and rotated to form three beams which scans when it moves through the colon. The capsule transmits data to an externally worn recorder and transmits electromagnetic signals which allows the recorder to identify the three-dimensional position and orientation of the capsule. A small amount of radiopaque contrast may be required to increase the contrast in the colon walls and differentiate stool from polyps.

Early data from 45 patients suggests the technique is safe. Sensitivity for polyp detection was 78% and specificity of 90% in those where colon imaging was more than 50%, and the radiation dose is low, 0.05 mSv (approximately one chest X-ray) (Gluck et al., 2019).

Liquid biopsy

Liquid biopsy has been defined as the analysis of bodily fluids, primarily blood, to detect both genomic as well as proteomic assessment of a wide array of tumour-derived targets such as circulating tumour cells (CTCs), circulating tumour DNA (ctDNA), tumour-derived extracellular vesicles, and circulating cell-free RNA (cfRNA), composed of small RNAs/miRNAs. These can detect a range of tumours including early CRC and is increasingly sensitive for early tumours, however the role of liquid biopsy in detecting premalignant lesions for prevention is less clear. Liquid biopsy analysis can include DNA mutations, copy number alterations (CNAs), transcriptome and proteome profiling, epigenetic changes, and metabolite profiling.

SEPT9 is a promising non-invasive and convenient biomarker in detection of colorectal carcinomas, with varying diagnostic sensitivities documented in different published literatures. SEPT9 DNA is released into the circulation from necrotic and apoptotic cancer cells during CRC carcinogenesis, and the risk of CRC can be determined by identifying the degree of DNA methylation of specific promoter regions of SEPT9 in blood. SEPT9 has higher sensitivity for diagnosing cancer in the colon than in the rectum, the right colon than left colon, and metastatic disease than cancers in early stage. The PRESEPT which was a multicentre study conducted in the United States and Germany and revealed a sensitivity of 48.2–68% and specificity of 80–91.5% in diagnosing CRCs (Church et al., 2014). The exact interval screening interval has not been established and it is not recommended by any guideline groups.

Colorectal cancer is a target of multi-cancer early detection (MCED) blood test panels that seek to use liquid biopsy methods to detect cancer at an early stage. CancerSEEK is perhaps the best known exemplar of this approach which combines immunoassays for proteins (e.g. carcinoma embryonic antigen (CEA)) with multiplex PCR analysis of cell-free tumour DNA to detect and localize a range of cancers including CRC using a supervised machine learning-based approach to the dataset. This has shown a sensitivity for surgically resectable stage I–III colorectal cancer of 69% (Cohen et al., 2018). Combined with PET-CT imaging, this approach doubled the rate of cancer detection compared to standard of care screening in the DETCECT-A study of 10,006 women with no prior history of cancer.

It is likely that the performance of MCED approaches will improve both with advances in analytics for specific targets (e.g. BEAMing) as well as combining multiple targets (e.g. proteins, exosomes, and cfDNA). While not currently effective in detecting colorectal cancer precursor lesions, it is likely that such tests will become widespread due to their ability to screen for multiple cancers, and that patients may be more willing to have a blood test rather than a stool test or other invasive test, however colorectal cancer prevention by removing precursor lesion may be compromised.

Volatile organic compounds, metabolomics and Smart toilets

Detection of volatile organic compounds in urine, breath, and other body fluids has shown promise in detecting colorectal cancer via an 'electronic nose' in which an array of diverse chemical sensors are used to sense odours rather than individual analyses. These can be portable and is easy to use, compared with more formal gas chromatography–mass spectrometry. Colorectal BReath Analysis (COBRA) study is an ongoing prospective cohort study analysing the possibility of breath volatile organic compounds (VOCs) for detecting CRC and adenomatous polyps.

PolypDx is a urine-based metabolomic test which can detect adenomatous polyps. In a validation study of 1,000 Chinese patients,

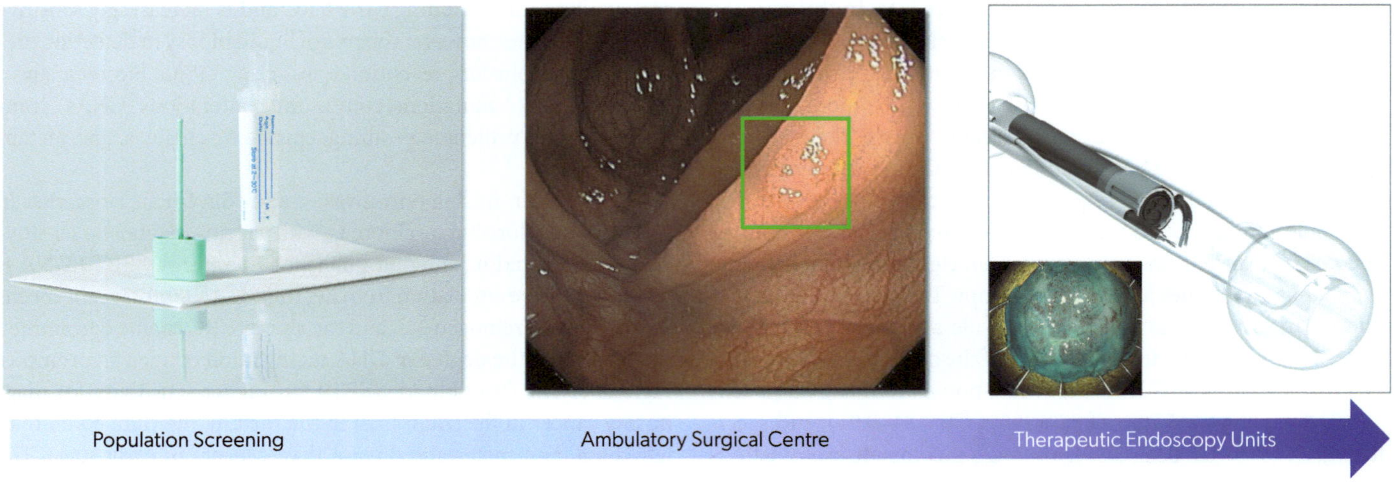

High-performance biomarkers
- FIT + methylation (Cologuard)
- FIT + Microbiome
- FIT + polygenetic risk score
- Liquid biopsy (cfDNA)

AI-enhanced colonoscopy
- 40% increase in adenoma detection
- Improved serrated lesion detection
- Differentiate cancer from non-invasive

Organ-preserving endotherapy
- New endoluminal platforms
- Full thickness endoscopic resection
- Endoscopic submucosal dissection

Figure 6.5 Proposed future screening strategy combining high performance biomarkers, AI supported colonoscopy and advanced endoluminal resection techniques.

sensitivity of 82.6% and a specificity of 42.4% was reported, similar to that of the original Canadian study (Deng et al., 2017).

The 'Smart toilet' concept is a monitoring device which can be attached to any toilet or integrated into the toilet or toilet seat and can regularly scan the human waste using optical and additional sensors. Once scanned, the information is analysed using machine learning algorithm-based analysis and can detect a range of markers seen in colorectal cancers, that might include changes in stool form, frequency, blood, or urine (see above) or other biomarkers (Park, 2020).

Conclusion

The initial promise of colorectal cancer population-based screening using guaiac faecal occult blood tests and colonoscopy that developed in the 1990s has made major steps forward, with the change to FIT-based testing and the focus on quality in bowel cancer screening colonoscopy. However, these advances have not eliminated PCCRC, nor have they focused our ongoing limited resources in a way that optimizes value for both those paying for colorectal cancer screening programmes, and the populations that they serve. One of the greatest challenges may be changing clinical behaviour where fee-per-service models of colonoscopy-based screening exist which drive business revenue.

It seems inevitable that improvements in biomarker performance, be these stool or blood based, will occur in the next decade, although it remains unclear which technologies will become dominant and scalable across all populations, and widely acceptable to patients (Chan et al., 2023). Technologies which can identify cancer precursors more effectively, including both adenomas and serrated lesions, are likely to offer immediate benefit, and this is already being seen commercially with, for example, Cologuard. Using high-performance biomarkers which are widely acceptable to the population being screened should help identify those who need colonoscopy, getting closer to the goal that 'every colonoscopy should be a therapeutic colonoscopy'. Nevertheless, even enriching the population coming for colonoscopy, there is still a miss rate for subtle premalignant lesions and endoscopist variability. AI-supported colonoscopy is straightforward to implement and commercially available to enhance detection and in theory will reduce PCCRC, and is likely to be widely available at scale in the next few years.

The combination of a new generation of high-performance biomarkers with AI-supported colonoscopy has the potential to lead to a step change in the clinical and cost effectiveness of colorectal cancer screening programmes. Screening is already leading to higher levels of detection of advanced, large premalignant lesions that with new endoscopic resection devices can be resected endoscopically with organ-preserving techniques, avoiding surgery which is expensive, invasive, and has higher complication rates.

There is therefore an opportunity to see a new model of screening in the next decade where linking hubs which deliver population-based high-performance biomarker analysis with local quality-assured, AI-supported colonoscopy screening centres, and regional centres for advanced endoscopic resection may become a reality (Fig. 6.5). However, it is equally possible that we will move to a model of repeated blood tests using liquid biopsy followed by PET for tumour localization as part of a wider MCED cancer detection strategy.

REFERENCES

Areia, M., Mori, Y., Correale, L., et al. (2022). Cost-effectiveness of artificial intelligence for screening colonoscopy: a modelling study. *Lancet Digital Health*, *4*(6), e436–444. doi: 10.1016/S2589-7500(22)00042-5

Atkin, W. S., Edwards, R., Kralj-Hans, I., et al. (2010). UK Flexible Sigmoidoscopy Trial Investigators. Once-only flexible sigmoidoscopy screening in prevention of colorectal cancer: a multicentre randomised controlled trial. *Lancet*, *375*(9726), 1624–1633. doi: 10.1016/S0140-6736(10)60551-X

Barua, I., Vinsard, D. G., Jodal, H. C., et al. (2021). Artificial intelligence for polyp detection during colonoscopy: a systematic review and meta-analysis. *Endoscopy*, *53*(3), 277–284. doi: 10.1055/a-1201-7165

Briggs, S. E. W., Law, P., East, J. E., et al. (2022). Integrating genome-wide polygenic risk scores and non-genetic risk to predict colorectal cancer diagnosis using UK Biobank data: population based cohort study. *British Medical Journal*, *379*, e071707. doi: 10.1136/bmj-2022-071707

Burke, C. A., Lieberman, D., & Feuerstein, J. D. (2022). AGA clinical practice update on approach to the use of noninvasive colorectal cancer screening options: commentary. *Gastroenterology*, *162*(3), 952–956. doi: 10.1053/j.gastro.2021.09.075

Chan, F. K. L., Wong, M. C. S., Chan, A. T., et al. (2023). Joint Asian Pacific Association of Gastroenterology (APAGE)-Asian Pacific Society of Digestive Endoscopy (APSDE) clinical practice guidelines on the use of non-invasive biomarkers for diagnosis of colorectal neoplasia. *Gut, 72*(7), 1240–1254. https://doi.org/10.1136/gutjnl-2023-329429

Church, T. R., Wandell, M., Lofton-Day, C., et al. (2014). Prospective evaluation of methylated SEPT9 in plasma for detection of asymptomatic colorectal cancer. *Gut*, *63*(2), 317–325. doi: 10.1136/gutjnl-2012-304149

Cohen, J. D., Li, L., Wang, Y., et al. (2018). Detection and localization of surgically resectable cancers with a multi-analyte blood test. *Science*, *359*(6378), 926–930. doi: 10.1126/science.aar3247

Corley, D. A., Jensen, C. D., Marks, A. R., et al. (2014). Adenoma detection rate and risk of colorectal cancer and death. *New England Journal of Medicine* , *370*(14), 1298–1306. doi: 10.1056/NEJMoa1309086

Deng, L., Fang, H., Tso, V. K., et al. (2017). Clinical validation of a novel urine-based metabolomic test for the detection of colonic polyps on Chinese population. *International Journal of Colorectal Disease*, *32*(5), 741–743. doi: 10.1007/s00384-016-2729-9

East, J. E., Atkin, W. S., Bateman, A. C., et al. (2017). British Society of Gastroenterology position statement on serrated polyps in the colon and rectum. *Gut*, *66*(7), 1181–1196. doi: 10.1136/gutjnl-2017-314005

Gluck, N., Half, E. E., Bieber, V., et al. (2019). Novel prep-less X-ray imaging capsule for colon cancer screening: a feasibility study. *Gut*, *68*(5), 774–775. doi: 10.1136/gutjnl-2018-316127

Imperiale, T. F., Ransohoff, D. F., Itzkowitz, S. H., et al. (2014). Multitarget stool DNA testing for colorectal-cancer screening. *New England Journal of Medicine*, *370*(14), 1287–1297. doi: 10.1056/NEJMoa1311194

Liang, J. Q., Li, T., Nakatsu, G., et al. (2020). A novel faecal Lachnoclostridium marker for the non-invasive diagnosis of colorectal adenoma and cancer. *Gut*, *69*(7), 1248–1257. doi: 10.1136/gutjnl-2019-318532

Lin, J. S., Perdue, L. A., Henrikson, N. B., et al. (2021). Screening for colorectal cancer: updated evidence report and systematic review for the US Preventive Services Task Force. *Journal of the American Medical Association*, *325*(19), 1978–1998. doi: 10.1001/jama.2021.4417

Logan, R. F., Patnick, J., Nickerson, C., et al. (2012). Outcomes of the Bowel Cancer Screening Programme (BCSP) in England after the first 1 million tests. *Gut*, *61*(10), 1439–1446. doi: 10.1136/gutjnl-2011-300843

Mori, Y., East, J. E., Hassan, C., et al. (2023). Benefits and challenges in implementation of artificial intelligence in colonoscopy: World Endoscopy Organization position statement. *Digestive endoscopy: official journal of the Japan Gastroenterological Endoscopy Society*, *35*(4), 422–429. https://doi.org/10.1111/den.14531

Park, S. M., Won, D. D., Lee, B. J., et al. (2020). A mountable toilet system for personalized health monitoring via the analysis of excreta. *Nature Biomedical Engineering*, *4*(6), 624–635. doi: 10.1038/s41551-020-0534-9

Rex, D. K., Boland, C. R., Dominitz, J. A., et al. (2017). Colorectal cancer screening: recommendations for physicians and patients from the U.S. Multi-Society Task Force on Colorectal Cancer. *Gastroenterology*, *153*(1), 307–323. doi: 10.1053/j.gastro.2017.05.013

Sulbaran, M., Bustamante-Lopez, L., Bernardo, W., et al. (2022). Systematic review and meta-analysis of colon capsule endoscopy accuracy for colorectal cancer screening. An alternative during the Covid-19 pandemic? *Journal of Medical Screening*, *29*(3), 148–155. doi: 10.1177/09691413221074803

Yamada, A., Niikura, R., Otani, K., et al. (2021). Automatic detection of colorectal neoplasia in wireless colon capsule endoscopic images using a deep convolutional neural network. *Endoscopy*, *53*(8), 832–836. doi: 10.1055/a-1266-1066

7

Pathology, tumour staging, and prognostic and predictive biomarkers

Dan Jiang, Xian Zhang, and Zijian Lu

Introduction

Documentation of the pathology of disease stretches back at least 3,500 years, with Ancient Egyptian medicine being described in the Edwin Smith Papyrus and Papyrus of Ebers. However, for centuries, the only pathological documentation was in the form of gross pathology that could be seen with the naked eye. A couple of millennia later, Hippocrates (approximately 400 BC) described the humoural theory of the nature of the disease, with extensive descriptions of inflammation, tumours, and tuberculosis. Galen (*c.* 150 AD) carried out extensive dissections of pigs and monkeys and described the 'crab-like' growth of tumours. The Italian Renaissance brought a renewed interest in human dissection of cadavers and a greater understanding of macroscopic anatomy with Vesalius and others. Anatomy became a discipline in its own right but the real revolution started with William Harvey (*c.* 1600) who, through his dissection work, described the circulatory system and diseases of the heart. About 100 years later, Morgagni, a medical student in Bologna, started to correlate the symptoms of patients with the findings on autopsy after their deaths, really consolidating that disease had a very anatomical 'organic' basis. John Hunter (*c.* 1750) described experimental pathology and used primitive microscopes. The Hunterian Museum in the Royal College of Surgeons, London, is a testament to his extensive work. By the early 1800s, microscopes were being developed and starting to be used, in particular, Virchow was routinely using the microscope to correlate with his findings from 'gross pathology' from autopsies. Virchow was the father of cellular pathology, showing at a deeper and more granular level that disease was not just 'organ based' but rather 'cell based'. By 1850, the specialty of 'pathology' rather than just anatomy was born. Fixing and embedding of tissue became routine by the end of the nineteenth century, and the discovery of monoclonal antibodies for staining in the first half of the twentieth century, followed by the discovery of DNA and the polymerase chain reaction, have completely revolutionized anatomy and pathology again. All these techniques are used in the routine assessment of pathological specimens that are removed from the body, either as biopsies or as a full resection, to dictate the next course of action in a patient's treatment pathway.

Full removal of a colorectal lesion at endoscopy

Sometimes the whole of a lesion visualized at endoscopy is removed in a single diagnostic/therapeutic step. pTis colorectal cancer (CRC) refers to carcinoma with invasion of the lamina propria and/or muscularis mucosa, and pT1 refers to a lesion with tumour invasion of submucosa but not extending into the muscularis propria (Amin et al., 2017), which may be removed by endoscopic mucosal resection (EMR) or endoscopic submucosal dissection (ESD). High-quality specimen handling and detailed histological evaluation are needed, as these determine subsequent treatment strategies.

Specimen handling

It is important for colorectal pathologists to have an excellent understanding of and a careful approach to dealing with these small lesions so that very accurate staging can be achieved.

Pinning, fixation

The sampled tissue is flattened with the mucosal surface up and pinned out on a styrofoam block along its borders in the fresh state (Fig. 7.1A). However, overextension should be avoided. For a flat lesion, the oral and anal orientation should be marked. For malignant polyps, a pin into the stalk can prevent stalk shrinkage and curling. The samples should be immersed in 10% neutral buffered formalin as soon as possible to avoid tissue degeneration, and less than 1 hour is acceptable when the sample is stored in physiological saline, which can allow the tissue to remain moist but does not avoid tissue autolysis (Kumarasinghe et al., 2020). The fixation time should be no less than 6 hours in total, and a shorter fixation time may lead to contracted and curling tissue, which hinders the subsequent correct orientation and sectioning by the pathologist (Kumarasinghe et al., 2020).

Sectioning

The practical aspects of sectioning somewhat depend on anatomical shape of the resected tissue, as below

For malignant flat/elevated lesions, it is important to cut along or against the marked orientation if the negative margin is obvious. If the lesion is close to one point of the resection margin, the tangent of the nearest margin is taken as the reference and then cut perpendicular to the reference (Nagata & Shimizu, 2012). It is optimal to use two-colour inking in the base of the specimen to help ascertain the orientation of each tissue strip (Fig. 7.1B). Serial sectioning of the whole specimen is performed every 2–3 mm, and all tissue strips are numbered, photographed, and embedded in order.

For malignant pedunculated lesions, en bloc resection with the stalk is crucial for accurate pathological staging and invasion depth measurement. The burned margin (or marked with ink) could be used as a marker to identify the resection margin. If the diameter of the stalk is more than 2 mm, the sections should be cut perpendicular to the resection margin at approximately 1 mm from the centre of the stalk and then cut parallel at an interval of 2–3 mm (Kumarasinghe et al., 2020). If the diameter of the stalk is less than 2 mm, the specimen should be sectioned perpendicular to the resection margin at the equivalent interval, but the stalk should be kept as a whole (Kumarasinghe et al., 2020). All tissue sections should be embedded in the same direction.

Histological assessment

Invasion depth measurement

The distance between the inferior edge of the muscularis mucosae and the deepest invasion is measured and recorded as the invasion depth for pT1 lesions (Fig. 7.1C). Superficial submucosal invasion is referred to as an invasion depth of < 1 mm, and deep submucosal invasion is defined as the invasion depth ≧ 1 mm but not extending to the muscularis propria (Hashiguchi et al., 2020). An alternative way to record the invasion depth is to apply the Kikuchi classification, which divides the submucosa into three parts (one-third, two-thirds, or three-thirds) and corresponds to SM1, SM2, or SM3 (Kikuchi et al., 1995).

In cases with unrecognizable muscularis mucosae, presenting as disappearance, disarray, or desmoplastic reaction around the muscularis mucosae, the muscularis mucosae is not appropriate as the reference line and may underestimate the depth of submucosal invasion (Hashiguchi et al., 2020). The invasion depth can be measured from the surface of the lesion to the deepest invasion point (Hashiguchi et al., 2020). However, there is controversy over the latter measurement; note that the measurement method in the pathological report is necessary.

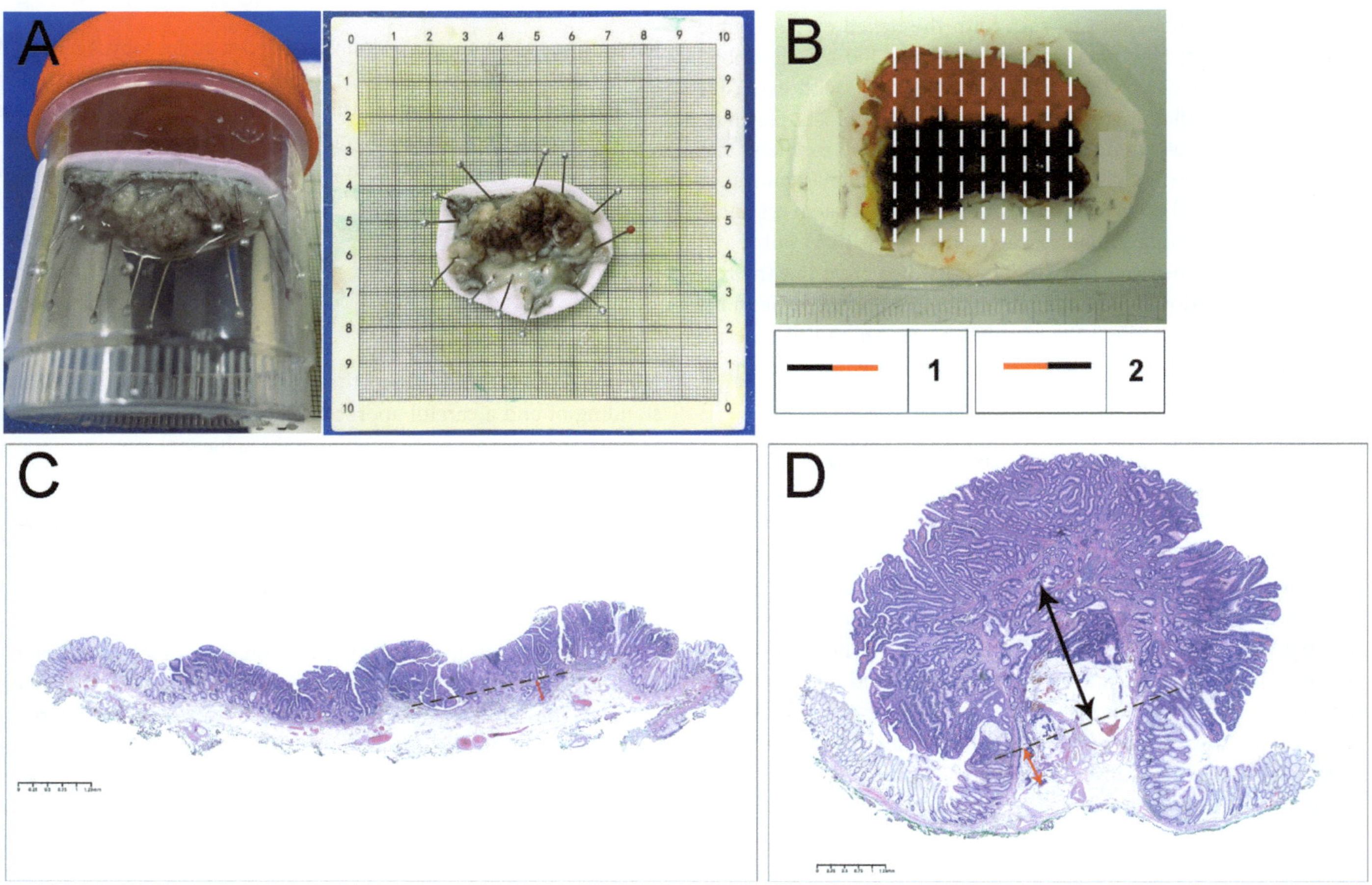

Figure 7.1 Endoscopically removed specimen.

A Sampling tissue is flattened and pinned to a styrofoam block along its borders in the fresh state. **B** Two-colour inks marking the base of the specimen to help identify the orientation of each tissue strip. **C** Flat lesion (H&E staining), the submucosal invasion depth is measured from the lower edge of the muscularis mucosa (dotted line) to the deepest part of the tumour invasion (red arrow). **D** Pedunculated lesion (H&E staining), there is an imaginary line between the tumour and nontumour junction from both sides (dotted line). The invasion above the line is regarded as head invasion (black arrow), and the invasion below is regarded as stalk invasion (red arrow).

There is a concept of head/stalk invasion in malignant pedunculated lesions. It is important to make an imaginary line between the tumour and non-tumour junction from both sides. The invasion above this reference line is regarded as head invasion (within the polyp head), and the invasion below the line is regarded as stalk invasion (Fig. 7.1D) (Hashiguchi et al., 2020). Reporting head or stalk invasion is required when the muscularis mucosae is tangled or unidentifiable. It is important to report both the invasion pattern (head or stalk) and the depth of invasion when the muscular mucosa can be identified, considering that the prognosis may differ between head and stalk invasion even with the same submucosal invasion depth (Shaukat et al., 2020).

Margin evaluation

Horizontal margins (HM, lateral/mucosal margin) and vertical margins (VM, deep/intramural margin) should be evaluated and reported separately (Hashiguchi et al., 2020). The nearest distance from the tumour front to the margin and the number of positive margins should be recorded. In HM, using 180-degree level sections to estimate the other side is necessary if the lesion is present on the first or last tissue strip. It could help determine the embedding direction and accurately assess the HM. Histological type (intraepithelial neoplasia/invasive cancer) of the lesion involving HM should be reported.

Histological subtypes, grading, lymphovascular invasion assessment, and tumour budding assessment are all described below as per radical operation specimen.

Radical operation specimen

The radical operation allows accurate staging and potential cure of early CRC. Pathological evaluation offers critical information for subsequent management of the patient and prognosis prediction. A comprehensive pathological report includes at least pT and pN staging evaluation and other essential histopathological features.

Gross examination

Macroscopic appearance

Colorectal carcinoma grows in different morphological patterns, including polypoid, ulcerative, diffusely infiltrating, and other types (Figs. 7.2A and 7.2B) (Bosman et al., 2019). These must be recorded as they impact on behaviour of the tumour, and their classification may be useful for research purposes.

Tumour perforation

Perforation is a macroscopically visible, full-thickness defect through the tumour. Tumour perforation *in situ* within the abdominal cavity is considered likely to increase the risk of tumour seeding within the peritoneal cavity and therefore predict future relapse within the abdominal cavity, hence such cases are best regarded as pT4a disease (Loughrey et al., 2022). It is important to note that cases in which the proximal bowel is perforated as a result of a distal obstructing tumour, and cases where there is an iatrogenic defect occurring on the specimen once it is outside the abdominal cavity are *not* counted as tumour perforation as they do not have the deleterious effect on prognosis. The presence or absence of tumour perforation should be recorded in the pathological report.

Specimen handling for radial/circumferential margin evaluation

The radial/circumferential resection margin (CRM) refers to any aspect of the resection specimen that is not covered by the peritoneum (Amin et al., 2017). The fresh specimen is opened anteriorly to the upper border of the mesorectum (at least 2 cm away from the tumour) to aid the fixation buffer permeation (Loughrey et al., 2022). The CRM of the fresh specimen could be marked with a clip

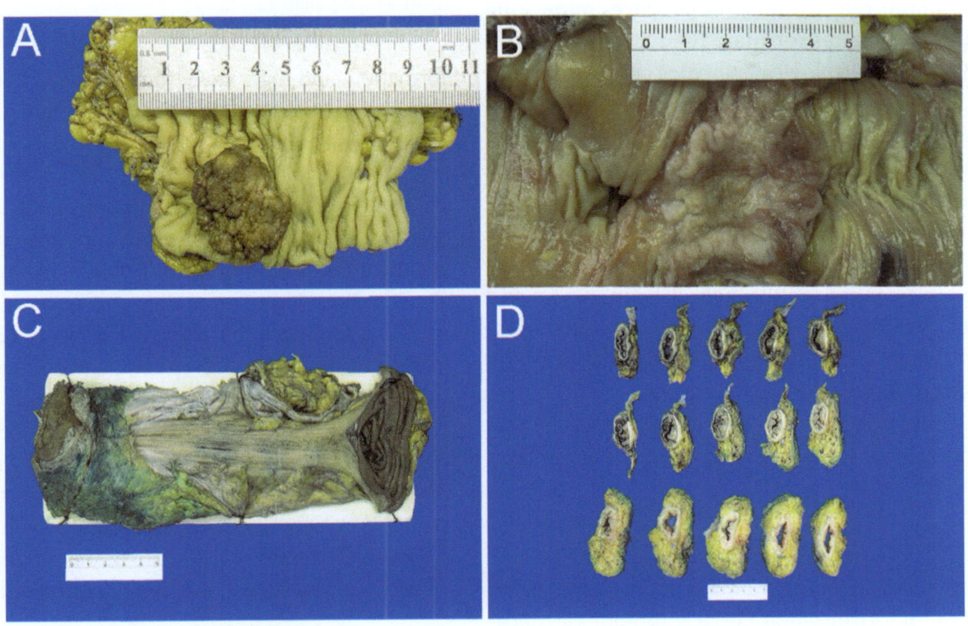

Figure 7.2 Gross examination of operative specimens.

A Polypoid lesion in gross appearance. **B** Ulcerative lesion in gross appearance. **C** The circumferential resection margin (CRM) is shown in green, and the specimen is pinned to a foam board for subsequent histopathological analysis. **D** Transverse dissection at 5 mm intervals perpendicular to the long axis of the mesorectum for a CRM specimen. All sections are numbered and photographed.

or suture by the surgeons and then pinned to a foam board and sent for pathological analysis (Fig. 7.2C) (Loughrey et al., 2022). The specimens are fixed with 10% neutral buffered formalin. The recommended fixation time is 48–72 hours (Van Cutsem et al., 2016).

The CRM is inked before specimen dissection to assist in identifying the margin and measuring the distance between the margin and the invasion front. A section at 5 mm intervals is transversely perpendicular to the long axis of the mesorectum (Loughrey et al., 2022). All slices are numbered and photographed (Fig. 7.2D).

Gross lymph node examination

Lymph node sampling should be documented and grouped according to the direction of lymphatic drainage by surgeons (Amin et al., 2017). The total number of nodes examined from the radical resection specimen should be at least 12 nodes. If < 12 lymph nodes are found at first examination, then resubmission for more potential lymph nodes and re-examination is recommended (Amin et al., 2017).

Microscopic examination

Histological assessment and staging

Histological subtypes

The majority (90%) of all cancers in the colon and rectum are adenocarcinomas (Bosman et al., 2019). Most cases are diagnosed as adenocarcinoma NOS (Fig. 7.3A), but several distinct histological subtypes can be identified (Bosman et al., 2019).

Signet-ring cell carcinoma (Fig. 7.3B) consists of at least 50% of the tumour being signet-ring cells (Bosman et al., 2019). Mucinous adenocarcinoma (Fig. 7.3C) is diagnosed when more than 50% of the lesion is composed of extracellular mucin, with cancerous epithelium strips or clumps (including signet-ring cells) (Bosman et al., 2019). Micropapillary adenocarcinoma (Fig. 7.3D) is characterized by a small cluster of tumour cells within stromal spaces mimicking vascular channels, which accounts for more than 5% of the lesion (Bosman et al., 2019). These histological subtypes appear more aggressive biological behaviour than adenocarcinoma NOS (Kuhn et al., 2018). Reporting each component's histological sub-type and proportion is recommended if the proportion does not meet the diagnostic cut-off value.

The medullary carcinoma (Fig. 7.3E) is characterized by sheets of malignant cells with vesicular nuclei, prominent nucleoli, and abundant eosinophilic cytoplasm, with infiltration of lymphocytes and neutrophilic granulocytes (Bosman et al., 2019). It is frequently associated with microsatellite instability-high (MSI-H) status, which indicates a favourable prognosis (Kuhn et al., 2018).

Other histological subtypes occur less frequently, including serrated adenocarcinoma and adenoma-like adenocarcinoma (Bosman et al., 2019).

Histological grading

A two-tier grading system for adenocarcinoma NOS is recommended by the 2019 World Health Organization (WHO) tumour classification (Bosman et al., 2019). Low-grade tumours (equivalent to well to moderately differentiated) are characterized by glandular differentiation similar to normal colorectal glands with more than 50% gland formation, and high-grade tumours (equivalent to poorly differentiated) are characterized by poor and atypical glandular formation.

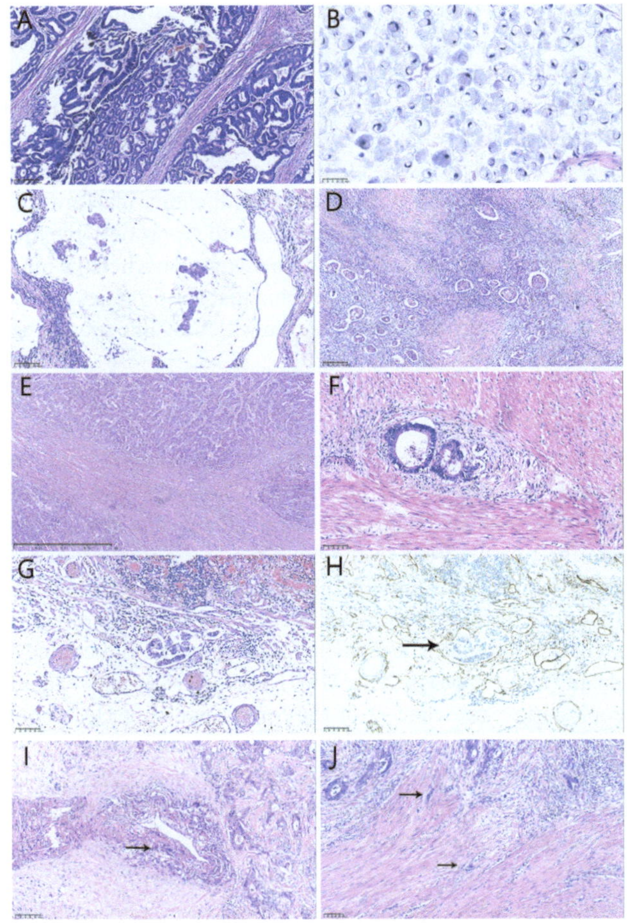

Figure 7.3 Histopathological assessment of colorectal adenocarcinoma (H&E staining).

A Adenocarcinoma none of specific. **B** Signet-ring cell carcinoma. **C** Mucinous adenocarcinoma. **D** Micropapillary adenocarcinoma. **E** Medullary carcinoma (this is an MMR deficiency; case confirmed by immunohistochemistry (IHC)). **F** Perineural invasion. **G** Lymphovascular invasion (black arrow). **H** D2-40 IHC indicating lymphatic vessel invasion (black arrow); both G and H show the same case. **I** Venous wall invasion (black arrow). **J** Tumour budding (black arrow).

Invasion depth (pT staging) evaluation

pT stages refer to the local invasion depth of CRC and they are among the most important prognostic factors, necessitating very accurate assessment and documentation. Using the criteria in the 8th edition of the American Joint Committee on Cancer's (AJCC) *Staging manual*, invasion depth is recorded as pT1, pT2, pT3 when the tumour extends into the submucosa (pT1), penetrating through the submucosa into but not through the muscularis propria (pT2), and penetrating through the muscularis propria (pT3), respectively (Amin et al., 2017). pT4 refers to tumour involvement of the serosal surface (pT4a) or direct invasion of a surrounding organ and structure (pT4b) (Amin et al., 2017). Note that in perforation cases with tumour cells being continuous with the serosal surface through inflammation, they are also considered T4a, as described above (Amin et al., 2017).

Perineural invasion

Perineural invasion (PNI) is defined as the growth of tumour cells along nerves, in which tumour cells surround at least one-third of the nerve circumference and can be present in any layer of the nerve (Fig. 7.3F) (Hashiguchi et al., 2020). The conventional approach is to use haematoxylin and eosin (H&E) slides to identify PNI, and S100 immunohistochemical (IHC) staining could be considered for identifying PNI.

Lymphovascular invasion

Lymphovascular invasion (LVI) is the invasion of cancer cells into the lymphatic or blood vessels (Amin et al., 2017). The histological diagnosis of lymphovascular invasion on H&E staining slides includes the presence of tumour cells within an endothelium-lined space and hyaline thrombus or erythrocytes surrounding the tumour cells (Fig. 7.3G). CD34 and D2-40 IHC staining can help identify the vascular or lymphatic endothelium (Fig. 7.3H). Pathologists should definitely report positive or negative lymphovascular invasion, but reporting is not mandatory for subtyping microlymphatic vessel or microvessel invasion (Hashiguchi et al., 2020) because it is difficult to distinguish them on H&E-stained slides and cross-reactivity exists between the different IHC markers (Hashiguchi et al., 2020).

Intramural and extramural vascular invasion

Venous invasion in H&E sections refers to cancer cells present within an endothelium-lined space that is either surrounded by a rim of muscle or contains red blood cells (Fig. 7.3I). Victoria blue staining or Elastica van Gieson staining can be applied to identify venous vessels (Vass et al., 2004). The anatomic sites of the involved veins are classified as extramural (veins extend beyond the muscularis propria) and intramural venous invasion (identified within the submucosa or muscularis propria) (Loughrey et al., 2022).

Tumour budding

Tumour budding is defined as a single cancer cell or a small cluster consisting of less than four or five cancer cells at the invasive front of the tumour (Fig. 7.3J) (Lugli et al., 2017). All tissue slides are scanned at a low power to identify the area with the highest number of tumour buds and then counted under the microscopic field of a 20-objective lens (Lugli et al., 2017). Tumours with 0 to 4, 5 to 9, and ≥ 10 tumour buds in an area of 0.785 mm^2 a (20–objective lens) are classified as low (G1), medium (G2), and high (G3) grade, respectively (Lugli et al., 2017).

Response to neoadjuvant therapy

Four-tier tumour regression grade (TRG) is used to evaluate the pathological response to neoadjuvant therapy, which is based on the residual tumour cells and the degree of fibrosis (Amin et al., 2017). TRG 0 (complete response) denotes no viable tumour cells observed (Fig. 7.4A). TRG 1 (near-complete response) denotes that single tumour cells or rare small groups of tumour cells remained (Fig. 7.4B). TRG 2 (minimal response) denotes residual cancer with a desmoplastic response (Fig. 7.4C). TRG 3 (poor response) denotes extensive residual tumour with minimal or no evidence of tumour cell death (Fig. 7.4D). Residual tumour cells indicate viable cells without necrosis. A mucinous lake without cellular component is designated a complete response. According to the AJCC *Staging manual*, tumour regression should be thoroughly assessed and recorded at the primary tumour sites, in regional nodes, and in any other tumour deposits (Amin et al., 2017).

Radial (circumferential) margin evaluation

The distance is measured from the tumour front, metastatic lymph nodes, or tumour deposit to the CRM (Amin et al., 2017). A distance ≤ 1 mm is recorded as a positive margin, otherwise it is recorded as negative (Amin et al., 2017). The distance to the margin should be recorded wherever possible as well as the R0 versus R1 status.

Histological assessment of lymph nodes

Metastatic lesions in lymph nodes can be evaluated in H&E tissue slides and sometimes confirmed by applying IHC (using cytokeratin antibody, etc.). It is important to count the number of metastatic lymph nodes and report pN staging following the newest edition of TNM staging.

Micrometastases are defined by a cluster of 10–20 tumour cells or clumps of tumour cells. ≥ 0.2 mm but ≤ 2 mm in diameter and

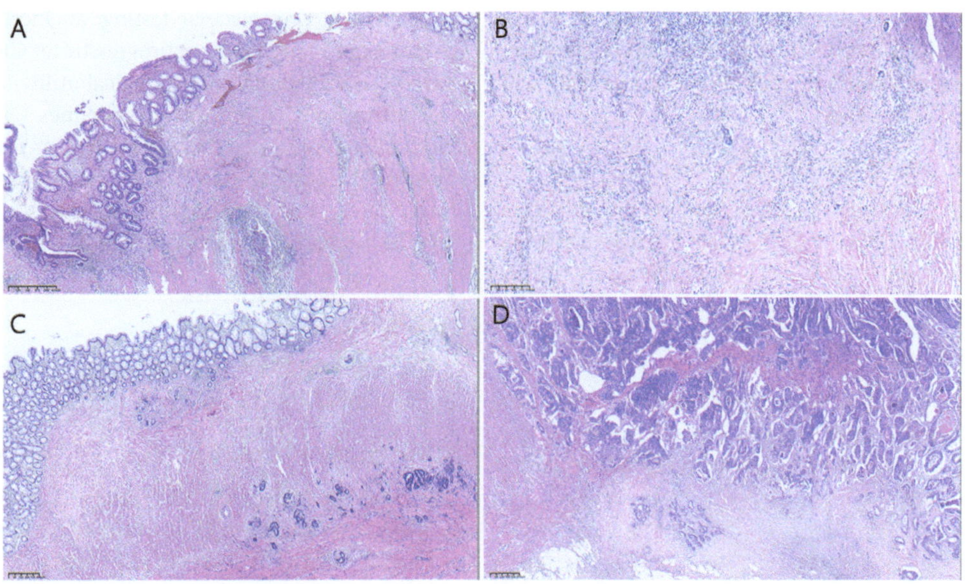

Figure 7.4 Representative images of tumour regression grade (TRG) (H&E staining).

A TRG 0 No residual tumour cells. **B** TRG 1 Single cells or rare small groups of tumour cells remained. **C** TRG 2 Residual cancer with desmoplastic response. **D** TRG3 Extensive residual tumour with minimal or no evidence of tumour response.

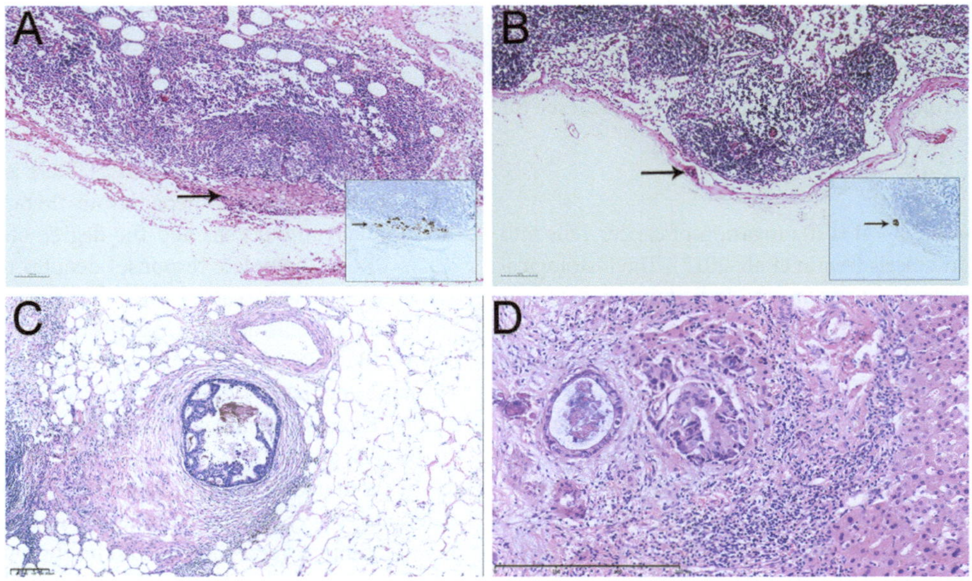

Figure 7.5 Metastasis of colorectal adenocarcinoma (H&E staining).
A Micrometastases in the lymph node (black arrow). **B** Isolated tumour cells in the lymph node (black arrow). **C** Tumour deposits; **D** Histologically confirmed distant metastasis.

should be recorded as positive lymph nodes (pN+) (Fig. 7.5A) (Benson et al., 2021). Cancerous cells < 0.2 mm are considered isolated tumour cells and recorded as pN0 (i+) ('i' is isolated tumour cell) (Fig. 7.5B) (Benson et al., 2021).

Tumour deposits

Tumour deposits are characterized as discrete tumor nodules within the lymphatic drainage of the primary carcinoma without recognizable lymph nodes, blood vessels, or nerve structures (Fig. 7.5C) (Amin et al., 2017). When tumour deposits are found within the vessel wall or around the neural structure, they should be categorized as venous or perineural invasion (Amin et al., 2017). If there is no regional lymph node metastases, the tumour deposit is designated N1c, regardless of its number, size, and shape (Amin et al., 2017). Instead, if there is regional lymph node metastasis, the number of tumour deposits should be counted and reported but not counted into the number of positive lymph nodes (Amin et al., 2017). However, this remains controversial and should be staged in accordance with the most recent version of the TNM.

Histological assessment for distant metastasis

The designation of M0 is not usually the responsibility of the pathologist unless a questionable lesion outside of the colorectum has been biopsied and histologically confirmed. If there has been histological confirmation of distant metastasis, then this can be recorded as pM1 (Fig. 7.5D).

Additional abnormalities

Any pathological abnormalities of the surrounding bowel segments, including polyps, adenomas, inflammatory bowel diseases, or special infections, should be recorded for completeness and because it can direct future treatment.

The pathological report

A thorough pathological report is needed for CRC, including pathological tumour staging, histological features mentioned above, and any established biomarkers that have been introduced as per below. All required parameters should be listed in a formatted report and displayed in the order mandated by the local multidisciplinary team (MDT). Communication of pathology information to the MDT is essential, and the report temple should be regularly updated by adding any newly established items in light of recent new knowledge. MDT discussion can suggest the inclusion of some non-core pathological information. Included here is an example of pathological report template used in the radical resection of rectal cancer specimens (Fig. 7.6).

Biomarkers standardly used for prognosis and prediction

With the advanced knowledge of the pathogenesis of CRC and the improvement of molecular testing, an increasing number of biomarkers can be predictive or prognostic for CRC. Several biomarkers have been validated for their clinical utility in the appropriate clinical setting for CRC by existing guidelines. On the other hand, many biomarkers are partly established and/or under development. All biomarker testing should be performed only in accredited laboratories by utilizing the accredited methods/kits. Table 7.1 summarizes the biomarkers in CRC.

Established prognostic/ predictive biomarkers

Below is an outline of the established prognostic and predictive biomarkers for colorectal cancer.

Microsatellite instability/mismatch repair

Microsatellite instability (MSI) refers to simple repeated nucleotide sequences arising from DNA mismatch repair (MMR) protein deficiency (dMMR) (Boland et al., 1998). MSI/MMR status defines therapeutic opportunities and gives prognostic information as well as providing screening information for possible Lynch syndrome (Benson et al., 2021). For example, patients with stage II tumours of MSI-H or MMR deficiency (dMMR) may have a better prognosis

Rectal Cancer Histopathology Report

Gross Description

Tumour Size: __cm × __cm × __cm

Gross type: ☐Ulcerative, ☐Polypoid, ☐Infiltrative, ☐Cannot be determined.

Tumour Site: ☐Anterior, ☐Left side, ☐Right side, ☐Posterior, ☐Circumferential, ☐Cannot be assessed.

Tumour Perforation: ☐Not identified, ☐Present, ☐Cannot be determined.

Mesentery Integrity: ☐3, ☐2, ☐1, ☐Cannot be determined.

Miles Assessment: ☐D, ☐C, ☐B, ☐A, ☐Cannot be determined.

Microscopy Description

Histological Type: ____________________ **Histological Grade:** ☐Low grade, ☐High grade.

Invasion Depth (pT stage): ☐No evidence of primary tumour pT0, ☐Intraepithial or lamina propria pTis, ☐Submucosa pT1, ☐Muscularis propria pT2, ☐Pericolorectal tissues pT3, ☐Peritoneum pT4a, ☐Other organs or structures pT4b, ☐Cannot be assessed.
Distance of tumour exceeds muscularis propria ___ mm.

Perineural Invasion(PNI): ☐Not identified, ☐Present, ☐Cannot be determined.

Lymphovascular Invasion(LVI): ☐Not identified, ☐Present, ☐Cannot be determined.

Extramural Veins Invasion: ☐Not identified, ☐Present, ☐Cannot be determined.

Tumor Budding: ☐G1(<5), ☐G2 (5-9), ☐G3(≥10).

Neoadjuvant treatment Effect: Neoadjuvant radiochemotherapy (nCRT) ☐Yes, ☐No, ☐Not clear.
nCRT case: ☐Complete response (TRG0), ☐Near-complete response (TRG1), ☐Minimal response(TRG2), ☐Poor response (TRG3).

Circumferential Margin: Distance of tumour to nearest margin __mm. ☐Positive≤1mm, Negative >1mm.

Mesentery Involvement: ☐Cannot be identified, ☐Involved (☐≤1/3, ☐1/3~2/3, ☐≥2/3), ☐Cannot be determined.

Cut ends Margin: Proximal Margin ☐Negative, ☐Positive, ☐Cannot be determined.
Distal Margin ☐Negative, ☐Positive, ☐Cannot be determined.

Resection Integrity: ☐R0, Complete, ☐R1, Residual tumour can be identified under microscope, ☐R2, Residual tumour can be identified by gross examination, ☐Cannot be determined.

Lymph Nodes: Evaluated Number:___ ; Positive Number:___ ☐Cannot be determined.

pN Stage: ☐pNx, ☐pN0: 0, ☐pN1a: 1, ☐pN1b: 2~3, ☐pN1c: Tumor Deposits (LN negative), ☐pN2a: 4~6, ☐pN2b: ≥7 LN.
Detailed description:______________________________

pM Stage: (can be ignored if there is no specimen) ☐pM1 (☐pM1a: metastasis confined to one organ, ☐pM1b: metastasis in more than one organ, ☐pM1c: metastasis to peritoneum with or without other organ involvement). Detailed description:______________________________

AJCC 8th pTNM Stage: pT__pN___pM___(ypT__pN___pM___), ☐Cannot be determined.

Abnormal of Surrounding Mucosa: ☐Not identified, ☐Present,______________________

Additional Pathological Findings:______________________________

Immunohistochemistry: MLH1( ), PMS2( ), MSH2( ), MSH6( ), Her2( ), BRAF V600E( ).

Comments:______________________________

Signature:______________ Date:__________

Figure 7.6 Example of a pathological report (essential features for a standard assessment).

Table 7.1 Prognostic/predictive biomarkers in colorectal carcinoma

Biomarkers	Type of abnormality	Type of recommended specimen	Type of testing	Predictive applicability
Established prognostic/predictive biomarkers				
Microsatellite instability/ mismatch repair	Instability of microsatellites	Tissue and blood	IHC PCR NGS	Stage II MSI-H patients may have a good prognosis and do not benefit from 5-fluorouracil adjuvant therapy; Predictive response to immune checkpoint inhibitor therapy; Screening for Lynch syndrome;
RAS genes	KRAS exons 2, 3 and 4 (codons 12, 13, 59, 61, 117 and 146); NRAS exons 2, 3 and 4 (codons 12, 13, 59, 61 and 117);	Tissue and blood	PCR Sanger NGS	Anti-EGFR therapy is ineffective in colorectal cancers with these mutations;
BRAF	BRAF V600E	Tissue and blood	IHC PCR Sanger NGS	Negative predictive response to anti-EGFR therapy with chemotherapy; Predictor of response to anti-EGFR therapy with encorafenib; Predictive poor response to neoadjuvant chemoradiation therapy in locally advanced rectal cancer; Presence of BRAF V600E mutation is consistent with sporadic dMMR colorectal cancer;
Biomarkers partly established and/or under development				
HER2	HER2 amplification/ over-expression	Tissue	IHC FISH NGS	Predictive resistance to anti-EGFR therapy and shorter progression disease survival; Anti-HER2 therapy is only indicated in HER2-amplified tumours that are also RAS and BRAF wild type;
NTRK fusions	NTRK fusions	Tissue	IHC FISH RT-PCR NGS	NTRK inhibitions have been shown to have activity only in cases with NTRK fusion;
POLE	Mutations within the proofreading (exonuclease) domain	Tissue	Sanger NGS	Predictive response to immune checkpoint inhibitors; Predictive in prognosis;
TMB	Total amount of somatic coding mutations within the average 1 MB range of coding proteins	Tissue	NGS	Predictive response to immune checkpoint inhibitors
DPYD	DPYD deficiency mainly results from genetic variants due to genetic polymorphisms in DPYD gene locus	Blood	PCR Sanger NGS	Predictive biomarker for exaggerated fluorouracil toxicity
PIK3CA	Exon 9 (E542K, E545K) and exon 20 (H1047R)	Tissue	PCR Sanger NGS	Predictive poor response rate to anti-EGFR therapy and shorter progression-free survival; Aspirin improves colorectal cancer-specific survival in patients with mutated-PIK3CA colorectal cancers;
c-Met	MET over-expression or gene amplification	Tissue	NGS	Predictive in prognosis; Possibly predictive response to anti-EGFR therapy;
Oncotype DX	12-gene expression assay	Tissue	NGS	Tumour recurrence score; Predictive in prognosis;
ColDx	634-probes based multigene assay	Tissue	NGS	Prognostic marker for recurrence in patients with stage II colon cancer;
ctDNA	Circulating tumour DNA	Blood	PCR NGS	ctDNA to detect minimal residual disease, response to adjuvant therapy, and identify patients at high risk of recurrence;
TME	Tumour microenvironment	Tissue	IHC, *et al*	Predictive markers of immunotherapy efficacy and prognosis;

IHC, immunohistochemistry; PCR, polymerase chain reaction; NGS, next-generation sequencing; MSI-H, microsatellite instability-high; EGFR, epidermal growth factor receptor; HER2, human epidermal growth factor receptor 2; FISH, fluorescence *in situ* hybridization; NTRK, neurotrophic tyrosine receptor kinase; RT-PCR, reverse transcription PCR; POLE, polymerase epsilon; TMB, tumour mutational burden; DPYD, dihydropyrimidine dehydrogenase; c-MET, proto-oncogene mesenchymal-epithelial transition factor; ctDNA, circulating tumour DNA; TME, tumour microenvironment.

but some authors believe they do not benefit so much from 5-fluorouracil (5-FU) adjuvant therapy (Bertagnolli et al., 2009); advanced CRCs with MSI-H/dMMR are candidates for immune checkpoint inhibitor therapy (Luchini et al., 2019). Approximately 15% of CRCs present MSI-H/dMMR (Burgart et al., 2021).

MMR IHC testing (Figs. 7.7A and 7.7B) is a cost-effective method using antibodies against four MMR proteins: MLH1, MSH2, MSH6, and PMS2. Tumours in which all four MMR proteins are expressed are termed MMR proficient (pMMR). At least one MMR protein absent in tumour cell nuclei is characterized as MMR-deficient (dMMR). Internal positive control (positive lymphocytes, fibroblasts in the background) should be present if designating a dMMR result, otherwise repeat the IHC staining to confirm the results. Additionally, *BRAF* V600E mutation or *MLH1* promoter methylation testing should be performed if only an absent *MLH1* (+/– *PMS2*) protein is found, which is associated with sporadic dMMR cancers (Benson et al., 2021). The MMR IHC result is now standardly recommended to be integrated into all routine pathological report forms.

As well as IHC definition of pMMR versus dMMR, MSI status can be assessed by multiplex fluorescence polymerase chain reaction (PCR) with capillary electrophoresis (Boland et al., 1998). MSI-H is defined as loss of stability in more than 30–40% of microsatellite markers; otherwise it is MSS/MSI-L (Boland et al., 1998). Next-generation sequencing represents an alternative molecular test to assess MSI.

RAS genes

GTPase proteins encoded by *RAS* family genes are regulated by the upstream epidermal growth factor receptor (EGFR) signal and participate in regulating cell growth, differentiation, proliferation, and survival (De Roock et al., 2010). Forty to 50 per cent of CRCs harbour *KRAS* mutations, and approximately 3.8% have *NRAS* mutations (Van Cutsem et al., 2016). *RAS* (*KRAS* and *NRAS*) mutation status has been confirmed as a negative predictive marker of treatment response for anti-EGFR therapy in patients with metastatic CRC (mCRC) (De Roock et al., 2010), so in the setting of non-resectable or metastatic CRC, it is absolutely necessary to assess CRC tumours for *RAS* mutation in order to open as many avenues for therapeutic intervention as possible.

The *RAS* testing recommended includes *KRAS* exons 2, 3, and 4 (specifically codons 12, 13, 59, 61, 117, and 146) and *NRAS* exons 2, 3, and 4 (codons 12, 13, 59, 61, 117, and 146) (Burgart et al., 2021). Testing for *RAS* can be accomplished by Sanger sequencing, PCR, and next-generation sequencing (NGS) (Benson et al., 2021).

A neoplastic cell content in the sequenced sample is recommended to be greater than 20% in order to give the best chance of accurate mutational status assessment. Where the proportion of tumour cells is insufficient, pathologists may enrich the tumour cell content by macrodissection (Van Cutsem et al., 2016).

BRAF

BRAF is a molecule of the *RAS/RAF/MAPK/ERK* signalling pathway (Tol et al., 2009). A number of mutations in the *BRAF* gene can occur and these are now classified as Class 1, Class 2, and Class 3 mutations. *BRAF* V600E accounts for more than 90% of the *BRAF* mutations observed and is called the Class 1 mutation. It is considered the most important as it causes continuous activation and signal transduction, regardless of external stimulus. The presence of the *BRAF* V600E mutation is an unfavourable prognostic marker for patients with metastatic CRC and a negative predictive biomarker for response to EGFR antibody therapy, unless they are used in combination with *BRAF* inhibitors such as encorafenib (Tol et al., 2009). *BRAF* V600E is also a predictor for poor response to neoadjuvant chemoradiation therapy in locally advanced rectal cancer (Jiang et al., 2019). *BRAF* V600E mutation is found in 8–12% of patients with mCRC (Van Cutsem et al., 2016) and is associated with sporadic (non-Lynch) dMMR status, so the two should always be done together. Testing for *BRAF* V600E can be accomplished via IHC, Sanger sequencing, PCR, and NGS (Fig. 7.7C). Class 2 and Class 3 mutations are the subject of many ongoing studies to define their prognostic relevance and to assess their impact upon the efficacy of various therapeutic interventions.

Biomarkers partly established and/or under development

There is much ongoing research looking at a huge spectrum of markers that may be important, not only in terms of predicting

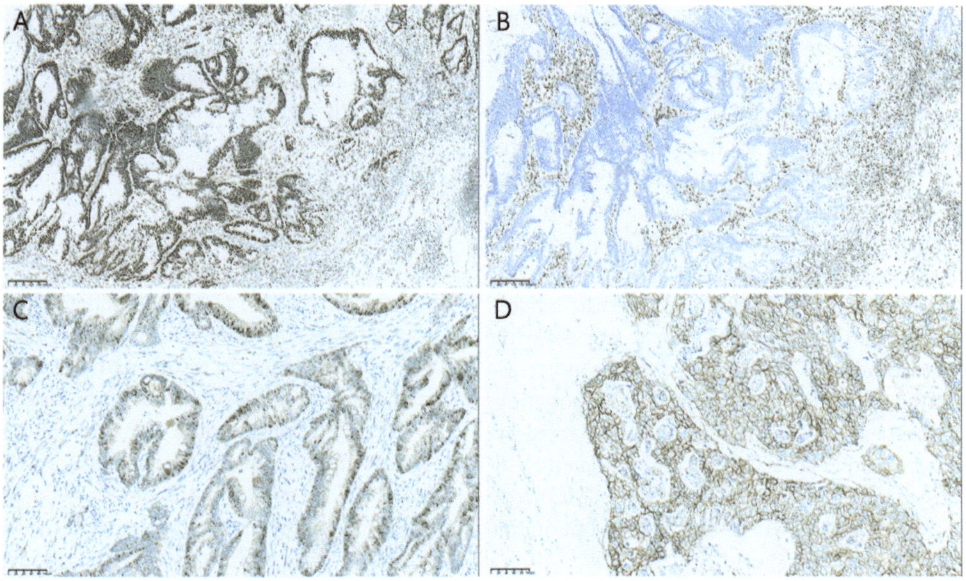

Figure 7.7 Immunohistochemistry.

A Positive mismatch repair (MMR) protein expression (MMR proficiency) is characterized as positive expression in the nuclei of tumour cells. **B** MMR absent (MMR deficiency) refers to negative expression in tumour cell nuclei when compared to positive expression in background lymphocytes and fibroblasts. **C** *BRAF V600E* positivity shows expression in the cytoplasm of tumour cells (case result confirmed by genetic sequencing). **D** HER2 expression is recorded as 3 + staining showing strong staining of the cellular membrane in more than 50% of tumour cells (case result confirmed by fluorescence *in situ* hybridization).

prognosis and response to various classes of therapeutic agents but also in predicting toxicity from various drugs. Both categories will be explored below.

Putative Markers of Prognosis and Therapeutic Prediction

HER2

Human epidermal growth factor receptor 2 (HER2) is a member of the same family of signalling kinase receptors as EGFR (Burgart et al., 2021). Overall, only 3% of CRC tumours display HER2 amplification/over-expression, but the prevalence of such over-expression is higher in *RAS/BRAF*-wild type tumours, where it is observed in 5–14% (Van Cutsem et al., 2016). Increasing evidence indicates that HER2 over-expression can predict resistance to anti-EGFR therapy and shorter progression-free survival (Sartore-Bianchi et al., 2019). Experts agree that *HER2* gene amplification should be evaluated for patients with metastatic CRC, but this is not done routinely. There is certainly an argument for such testing in cases where a patient displays resistance to standard chemotherapy plus anti-EGFR to enrich the population being tested. Anti-HER2 therapy is not currently recommended for mCRC outside of a clinical trial (Benson et al., 2021).

Diagnostic testing includes IHC, fluorescence *in situ* hybridization (FISH), or NGS. In IHC, HER2 3+ is recorded as positive, showing strong staining of the cellular membrane in more than 50% of tumour cells (Fig. 7.7D) (Valtorta et al., 2015). A score of 2+ requires further FISH evaluation (Valtorta et al., 2015). A HER2:CEP17 ratio ≥ 2 in more than 50% of tumour cells is recorded as HER2 amplification. However, the optimal cut-off for screening candidates to receive HER2-targeted therapies needs further investigation. A future direction for establishing a new HER2 scoring system, instead of the traditional positive/negative system, may be considered with the emergence of antibody-dependent cellular cytotoxicity drugs (Oh & Bang, 2020).

NTRK fusions

Oncogenic neurotrophic tyrosine receptor kinase (*NTRK*, including *NTRK1*, *NTRK2*, and *NTRK3*) gene fusions lead to the structural activation of its encoding tropomyosin receptor kinase (TRK) proteins, thus activating various cancer-related downstream signalling pathways (Gatalica et al., 2019). TRK inhibitors have been approved as a valid treatment for *NTRK* fusion positive solid tumours (Okamura et al., 2018). *NTRK* fusion is reported with a frequency of < 1% in CRC, especially in pan wild-type *RAS* and *BRAF* (Okamura et al., 2018). The international expert consensus recommends that *NTRK* fusions testing could be considered in patients with advanced CRC in order to avoid missing the opportunity for treatment with a TRK inhibitor (Benson et al., 2021). However, this is not currently the standard of care and its testing and therapeutic targeting is largely limited to clinical trials. *NTRK* fusions can be detected by IHC, FISH, reverse transcription PCR (RT-PCR) and validated NGS methods. The European Society for Medical Oncology (ESMO) recommendation has taken RNA-based NGS as the optimal option for the detection of *NTRK* fusions (Marchiò et al., 2019).

POLE

Proofreading by DNA polymerase is another cellular check that facilitates high-fidelity DNA replication in human cells, in addition to the function of the MMR system (Valle et al., 2014). Mutations in the exonuclease domain in DNA polymerase epsilon (*POLE*) cause impaired proofreading function, resulting in massively increased tumour mutational burden (TMB) (Mo et al., 2020). POLE-mutant CRCs have been reported to have an excellent prognosis (Mo et al., 2020). Somatic mutations within the domain of *POLE* are found in 1–2% of CRCs (Valle et al., 2014). Pathogenic *POLE* hotspot mutations in the exonuclease domain (exons 9, 11, 13, and 14) are being evaluated by Sanger sequencing or NGS in ongoing clinical trials (Palles et al., 2013).

Tumour mutational burden (TMB)

TMB is defined as the total amount of somatic coding mutations within the average 1 MB range of coding regions, including gene coding errors, base substitution, gene insertion or deletion, and other forms of genetic changes (Domingo et al., 2018). The US Food and Drug Administration (FDA) has approved immune checkpoint inhibitor treatment for patients with unresectable or metastatic solid tumours with a high tumour mutation load (TMB-high defined by ≥ 10 mutations/megabase) (Schrock et al., 2019). It could be quantified using NGS techniques. At present, routine TMB detection is not carried out or recommended in CRC, although there is likely to be increasing pressure for it to be assessed in the future to allow more patients access to immune checkpoint inhibitors.

PIK3CA

Phosphatidylinositol-3 kinase (PI3K) is the downstream pathway of EGFR parallel to the *RAS* pathway, the subunits of which are *PIK3CA/PIK3CB* (De Roock et al., 2010). *PIK3CA* mutations occur in approximately 10–18% of CRCs, mainly in exon 9 (E542K, E545K) and exon 20 (H1047R), and lead to increased PI3K activity and high oncogenic transformation ability (Burgart et al., 2021). Several studies indicate that *PIK3CA* mutation is associated with a poorer response rate to anti-EGFR therapy and shorter progression-free survival (PFS) in advanced CRC patients (Mao et al., 2012). Additionally, it has been reported that aspirin can improve CRC-specific survival in patients harbouring *PIK3CA* mutation (Liao et al., 2012). To date, *PIK3CA* mutational analysis of CRC tissue outside a clinical trial is not routinely performed, although it is being assessed in adjuvant trials with the use of aspirin.

c-MET

The proto-oncogene mesenchymal epithelial transition factor (c-MET) is a tyrosine kinase cell surface receptor for its ligand, hepatocyte growth factor (HGF), which activates downstream effector pathways and is involved in CRC carcinogenesis (Pietrantonio et al., 2016). Targeted therapy of this pathway in CRC is under active research (Pietrantonio et al., 2016). Additionally, recent data have also suggested that tumours with *MET* alterations (over-expression or gene amplification) showed a reduced disease control rate and shorter PFS in mCRC patients with wild-type *KRAS* treated with anti-EGFR inhibitors suggesting c-MET over-expression as a novel mechanism of resistance to EGFR-antibody therapy (Pietrantonio et al., 2016). It also opens up potential therapeutic avenues for combining anti-EGFR antibodies with c-MET inhibitors to counteract or prevent resistance. No recommendation data are currently available for routine testing for c-MET.

Oncotype DX

One of the criticisms of single gene testing in terms of evaluating prognosis is that each individual gene only tells one part of the story and does not set the whole scene for that specific tumour. In contradistinction to this approach, the Oncotype DX colon cancer assay is a 12-gene expression assay of seven known cancer recurrence-related genes and five reference genes, which provides a recurrence score (RS, 0 to 100) using RNA extracted from formalin-fixed paraffin-embedded (FFPE) tissue (Venook et al., 2013). According to the calculated tumour RS, patients are divided into one of three levels, low (< 18), intermediate (18–30), and high (31–100). The three different categories have possibilities of distant recurrence at three years of 12%, 18%, and 22%, respectively, in stage II and III colon cancer (Venook et al., 2013; Yamanaka et al., 2016). Moreover, evidence also indicates that the score is prognostic for disease-free survival (DFS) and overall survival (OS), and patients with a higher RS may derive more absolute benefit from oxaliplatin (Yothers et al., 2013).

ColDx

ColDx is a 634-probe-based multi-gene assay used as a prognostic marker for recurrence in patients with stage II colon cancer (Kennedy et al., 2011). Clinical validation indicated that patients identified as high risk by ColDx in stage II colon cancer had a shorter recurrence-free interval (Niedzwiecki et al., 2016).

ctDNA

Circulating tumour DNA (ctDNA) is free DNA released into blood by apoptotic tumour cells, a kind of circulating free DNA (Reinert et al., 2019). Post-surgical ctDNA has potential utility for monitoring tumour recurrence in patients with stage I–III colon cancer (Tie et al., 2019). Considering that the content of ctDNA in peripheral blood is low, ctDNA testing is necessarily based on more sensitive methods, consisting of quantitative real-time PCR (qPCR), RT-PCR, droplet digital PCR (ddPCR), and NGS. ctDNA liquid biopsies are emerging as a new tool to guide treatment decisions but they are currently largely being investigated in clinical trials rather than being a standard part of routine practice.

Tumour micro-environment (TME)

The TME plays a crucial role in tumour biobehaviour in CRC either via direct intercellular communication or through chemokine/cytokine signallings (Liu et al., 2022). The role of distinct immune cell types in modulating cancer progression and response to immunotherapy is increasingly emerging. The Immunoscore, which quantifies and qualifies the infiltrating T lymphocytes within the tumour microenvironment, is proposed to complement TNM classification for CRC (Guinney et al., 2015).

Other researchers, however, feel that it is not only individual immune effectors that are important as much as the whole environment and the supporting cells around the tumour cells. The combination of DNA ploidy and stroma fraction is able to stratify patients with stage II CRC into three risk groups which correlate with five-year cancer-specific survival (Danielsen et al., 2018). A combination biomarker consisting of intratumoural CD8+ T-lymphocytes and stroma fraction is reported as a prognostic marker for early CRC (Jiang et al., 2021). In summary, evidence of the importance of the form and content of the TME as a predictive and prognostic biomarker is building.

Markers of therapeutic toxicity

As well as predicting effectiveness of oncological interventions, it is important to ensure that patients are not put at excessive risk. In the same way that patients are considered carefully in terms of their cardiovascular and respiratory well-being before having a general anaesthetic, it is imperative to screen for potential harm to any patients who may be at specific increased risk of an anticancer agent. Such increased risk can be dictated by Pharmacogenomics, the presence of mutations in the genes important in drug metabolism.

DPYD

Dihydropyrimidine dehydrogenase (DPYD), coded by the *DPYD* gene, is the initial and rate-limiting enzyme in the catabolism of 5-FU metabolism in vivo (Rosmarin et al., 2014). Variants or polymorphisms in the *DPYD* gene are known to affect enzymatic activity, leading to impaired fluoropyrimidine catabolism and therefore to increased systemic toxicity, particularly in terms of the risk of neutropenia (Rosmarin et al., 2014). DPYD deficiency occurs at a frequency of 0–3% with some geographical variation (Van Cutsem et al., 2016). The European Medicines Agency recommends *DPYD* genotyping or detecting the uracil blood level for all patients receiving fluoropyrimidine-based treatment to improve its safety (Hodroj et al., 2021). Four variants are currently commonly screened and associated with 5-FU toxicity (*DPYD*∗2A or rs3918290, *DPYD*∗13 or rs55886062, c.2846A>T or D949V or rs67376798, HapB3 or rs75017182 or rs56038477) (Rosmarin et al., 2014). However, other single nucleotide polymorphisms do exist, and it is a subject of ongoing research to define the best routine testing for a specific geographical population. Universal testing for *DPYD* genotyping is not yet performed (Benson et al., 2021).

Conclusions

The role of the pathologist in preparing and analysing the pathology of colorectal cancer is growing all the time. It now includes preparing tumour tissue to undergo IHC or sequencing to elucidate prognostic and predictive markers. In the, it is likely also to encompass collating data from novel methods such as ctDNA testing. Research and novel technologies have radically altered our approach, particularly over the last 20 to 30 years.

REFERENCES

Amin, M. B., Edge, S. B., Greene, F. L., et al. (2017). *AJCC cancer staging manual* 8th Ed. Springer.

Benson, A. B., Venook, A. P., Al-Hawary, M. M., et al. (2021). Colon cancer, Version 2.2021, NCCN clinical practice guidelines in oncology. *Journal of the National Comprehensive Cancer Network 19*, 329–359.

Bertagnolli, M. M., Niedzwiecki, D., Compton, C. C., et al. (2009). Microsatellite instability predicts improved response to adjuvant therapy with irinotecan, fluorouracil, and leucovorin in stage III colon cancer: Cancer and Leukemia Group B Protocol 89803. *Journal of Clinical Oncology*, *27*, 1814–1821.

Boland, C. R., Thibodeau, S. N., Hamilton, S. R., et al. (1998). A National Cancer Institute Workshop on microsatellite instability for cancer detection and familial predisposition: development of international criteria for the determination of microsatellite instability in colorectal cancer. *Cancer Research*, *58*, 5248–5257.

Burgart, L. J., Chopp, W. V., Jain, D., et al. (2021). Template for reporting results of biomarker testing of specimens from patients with carcinoma of the colon and rectum. <https://www.cap.org/protocols-and-guidelines/cancer-reporting-tools/cancer-protocol-templates> accessed 17 June 2025.

Danielsen, H. E., Hveem, T. S., Domingo, E., et al. (2018). Prognostic markers for colorectal cancer: estimating ploidy and stroma. *Annals of Oncology*, *29*, 616–623.

De Roock, W., Claes, B., Bernasconi, D., et al. (2010). Effects of KRAS, BRAF, NRAS, and PIK3CA mutations on the efficacy of cetuximab plus chemotherapy in chemotherapy-refractory metastatic colorectal cancer: a retrospective consortium analysis. *Lancet Oncology* *11*, 753–762.

Domingo, E., Camps, C., Kaisaki, P. J., et al. (2018). Mutation burden and other molecular markers of prognosis in colorectal cancer treated with curative intent: results from the QUASAR 2 clinical trial and an Australian community-based series. *Lancet Gastroenterology & Hepatology*, *3*, 635–643.

Gatalica, Z., Xiu, J., Swensen, J., et al. (2019). Molecular characterization of cancers with NTRK gene fusions. *Modern Pathology*, *32*, 147–153.

Guinney, J., Dienstmann, R., Wang, X., et al. (2015). The consensus molecular subtypes of colorectal cancer. *Nature Medicine*, *21*, 1350–6.

Hashiguchi, Y., Muro, K., Saito, Y., et al. (2020). Japanese Society for Cancer of the Colon and Rectum (JSCCR) guidelines 2019 for the treatment of colorectal cancer. *International Journal of Clinical Oncology*, *25*, 1–42.

Hodroj, K., Barthelemy, D., Lega, J. C., et al. (2021). Issues and limitations of available biomarkers for fluoropyrimidine-based chemotherapy toxicity, a narrative review of the literature. *ESMO Open*, *6*, 100125.

Jiang, D., Wang, X., Wang, Y., et al. (2019). Mutation in BRAF and SMAD4 associated with resistance to neoadjuvant chemoradiation therapy in locally advanced rectal cancer. *Virchows Archiv* *475*, 39–47.

Jiang, D., Hveem, T. S., Glaire, M., et al. (2021). Automated assessment of CD8(+) T-lymphocytes and stroma fractions complement conventional staging of colorectal cancer. *EBioMedicine*, *71*, 103547.

Kennedy, R. D., Bylesjo, M., Kerr, P., et al. (2011). Development and independent validation of a prognostic assay for stage II colon cancer using formalin-fixed paraffin-embedded tissue. *Journal of Clinical Oncology*, *29*, 4620–4626.

Kikuchi, R., Takano, M., Takagi, K., et al. (1995). Management of early invasive colorectal cancer. Risk of recurrence and clinical guidelines. *Diseases of the Colon & Rectum*, *38*, 1286–1295.

Kuhn, E., Morbini, P., Cancellieri, A., et al. (2018). Adenocarcinoma classification: patterns and prognosis. *Pathologica*, *110*, 5–11.

Kumarasinghe, M. P., Bourke, M. J., Brown, I., et al. (2020). Pathological assessment of endoscopic resections of the gastrointestinal tract: a comprehensive clinicopathologic review. *Modern Pathology*, *33*, 986–1006.

Liao, X., Lochhead, P., Nishihara, R., et al. (2012). Aspirin use, tumor PIK3CA mutation, and colorectal-cancer survival. *New England Journal of Medicine*, *367*, 1596–1606.

Liu, Y., Zhang, Q., Xing, B., et al. (2022). Immune phenotypic linkage between colorectal cancer and liver metastasis. *Cancer Cell*, *40*, 424–437.e5.

Loughrey, M. B., Webster, F., Arends, M. J., et al. (2022). Dataset for pathology reporting of colorectal cancer: recommendations from the International Collaboration on Cancer Reporting (ICCR). *Annals of Surgery*, *275*, e549–561.

Luchini, C., Bibeau, F., Ligtenberg, M. J. L., et al. (2019). ESMO recommendations on microsatellite instability testing for immunotherapy in cancer, and its relationship with PD-1/PD-L1 expression and tumour mutational burden: a systematic review-based approach. *Annals of Oncology*, *30*, 1232–1243.

Lugli, A., Kirsch, R., Ajioka, Y., et al. (2017). Recommendations for reporting tumor budding in colorectal cancer based on the International Tumor Budding Consensus Conference (ITBCC) 2016. *Modern Pathology*, *30*, 1299–1311.

Mao, C., Yang, Z. Y., Hu, X. F., et al. (2012). PIK3CA exon 20 mutations as a potential biomarker for resistance to anti-EGFR monoclonal antibodies in KRAS wild-type metastatic colorectal cancer: a systematic review and meta-analysis. *Annals of Oncology*, *23*, 1518–1525.

Marchiò, C., Scaltriti, M., Ladanyi, M., et al. (2019). ESMO recommendations on the standard methods to detect NTRK fusions in daily practice and clinical research. *Annals of Oncology*, *30*, 1417–1427.

Mo, S., Ma, X., Li, Y., et al. (2020). Somatic POLE exonuclease domain mutations elicit enhanced intratumoral immune responses in stage II colorectal cancer. *Journal of Immunotherapy Cancer*, *8*, e000881

Nagata, K., & Shimizu, M. (2012). Pathological evaluation of gastrointestinal endoscopic submucosal dissection materials based on Japanese guidelines. *World Journal of Gastrointestinal Endoscopy*, *4*, 489–499.

Nagtegaal, I. D., Odze, R. D., Klimstra, D., et al. (2020). The 2019 WHO classification of tumours of the digestive system. *Histopathology*, *76*, 182–188.

Niedzwiecki, D., Frankel, W. L., Venook, A. P., et al. (2016). Association between results of a gene expression signature assay and recurrence-free interval in patients with stage II colon cancer in Cancer and Leukemia Group B 9581 (Alliance). *Journal of Clinical Oncology*, *34*, 3047–3053.

Oh, D. Y., & Bang, Y. J. (2020). HER2-targeted therapies—a role beyond breast cancer. *Nature Reviews Clinical Oncology*, *17*, 33–48.

Okamura, R., Boichard, A., Kato, S., et al. (2018). Analysis of NTRK alterations in pan-cancer adult and pediatric malignancies: implications for NTRK-targeted therapeutics. *JCO Precision Oncology*, *2018*, PO.18.00183.

Palles, C., Cazier, J. B., Howarth, K. M., et al. (2013). Germline mutations affecting the proofreading domains of POLE and POLD1 predispose to colorectal adenomas and carcinomas. *Nature Genetics*, *45*, 136–144.

Pietrantonio, F., Oddo, D., Gloghini, A., et al. (2016). MET-driven resistance to dual EGFR and BRAF blockade may be overcome by switching from EGFR to MET inhibition in BRAF-mutated colorectal cancer. *Cancer Discovery*, *6*, 963–971.

Reinert, T., Henriksen, T. V., Christensen, E., et al. (2019). Analysis of plasma cell-free DNA by ultradeep sequencing in patients with stages I to III colorectal cancer. *JAMA Oncology*, *5*, 1124–1131.

Rosmarin, D., Palles, C., Church, D., et al. (2014). Genetic markers of toxicity from capecitabine and other fluorouracil-based regimens: investigation in the QUASAR2 study, systematic review, and meta-analysis. *Journal of Clinical Oncology*, *32*, 1031–1039.

Sartore-Bianchi, A., Amatu, A., Porcu, L., et al. (2019). HER2 positivity predicts unresponsiveness to EGFR-targeted treatment in metastatic colorectal cancer. *Oncologist*, *24*, 1395–1402.

Schrock, A. B., Ouyang, C., Sandhu, J., et al. (2019). Tumor mutational burden is predictive of response to immune checkpoint inhibitors in MSI-high metastatic colorectal cancer. *Annals of Oncology*, *30*, 1096–1103.

Shaukat, A., Kaltenbach, T., Dominitz, J. A., et al. (2020). Endoscopic recognition and management strategies for malignant colorectal polyps: recommendations of the US Multi-Society Task Force on Colorectal Cancer. *Gastroenterology, 159*, 1916–1934.e2.

Tie, J., Cohen, J. D., Wang, Y., et al. (2019). Circulating tumor DNA analyses as markers of recurrence risk and benefit of adjuvant therapy for stage III colon cancer. *JAMA Oncology, 5*, 1710–1717.

Tol, J., Nagtegaal, I. D., & Punt, C. J. (2009). BRAF mutation in metastatic colorectal cancer. *New England Journal of Medicine, 361*, 98–99.

Valle, L., Hernández-Illán, E., Bellido, F., et al. (2014). New insights into POLE and POLD1 germline mutations in familial colorectal cancer and polyposis. *Human Molecular Genetics, 23*, 3506–3512.

Valtorta, E., Martino, C., Sartore-Bianchi, A., et al. (2015). Assessment of a HER2 scoring system for colorectal cancer: results from a validation study. *Modern Pathology, 28*, 1481–1491.

Van Cutsem, E., Cervantes, A., Adam, R., et al. (2016). ESMO consensus guidelines for the management of patients with metastatic colorectal cancer. *Annals of Oncology, 27*, 1386–1422.

Vass, D. G., Ainsworth, R., Anderson, J. H., et al. (2004). The value of an elastic tissue stain in detecting venous invasion in colorectal cancer. *Journal of Clinical Pathology, 57*, 769–72.

Venook, A. P., Niedzwiecki, D., Lopatin, M., et al. (2013). Biologic determinants of tumor recurrence in stage II colon cancer: validation study of the 12-gene recurrence score in cancer and leukemia group B (CALGB) 9581. *Journal of Clinical Oncology, 31*, 1775–1781.

Yamanaka, T., Oki, E., Yamazaki, K., et al. (2016). 12-gene recurrence score assay stratifies the recurrence risk in stage II/III colon cancer with surgery alone: The SUNRISE Study. *Journal of Clinical Oncology, 34*, 2906–2913.

Yothers, G., O'Connell, M. J., Lee, M., et al. (2013). Validation of the 12-gene colon cancer recurrence score in NSABP C-07 as a predictor of recurrence in patients with stage II and III colon cancer treated with fluorouracil and leucovorin (FU/LV) and FU/LV plus oxaliplatin. *Journal of Clinical Oncology, 31*, 4512–4519.

8

Artificial intelligence and digital pathology

Andreas Kleppe, Tarjei S. Hveem, Knut Liestøl, and Håvard Danielsen

Introduction

With enough data and proper design, modern artificial intelligence (AI) systems show high proficiency in recognizing patterns in complex data, such as images. Since the field of pathology relies heavily on the interpretation of information in image form, these AI systems have the potential to transform current clinical practice by easing repetitious diagnostic tasks and improving precision (Bera et al., 2019). By now, AI systems have been constructed for identifying areas of interest within slides, efficient classification of cancers into sub-types, detection of mutational status from images, and survival prediction for various cancer types (**Fig. 8.1**), together confirming the potential for AI to alter the workflow in pathology markedly.

Artificial intelligence is a broad term referring to machine-based approaches typically used to make different kinds of classifications or predictions. Natural intelligent systems inspire the field's name, and modern AI approaches apply artificial neural networks, which share some similarities with the processing found in the mammalian visual system from the retina to the visual cortex. To develop AI systems, the computer can be instructed to learn from data in some specific but autonomous manner. This process is known as machine learning (ML), and the focus of this chapter will be on systems trained in such a manner. Traditionally, these systems used handcrafted features calculated from the input data to predict the output. However, modern AI systems applying neural networks typically leverage the data also to learn the features through learning many simple transformations that create successively more abstract representations of the input data before ending up with the predicted output. These so-called deep learning (DL) models, and convolutional neural network (CNN) models, in particular, prospered the advances in digital image analysis and the use of AI in pathology because they often outperformed more traditional approaches and also removed the need for intelligently predefining features (van der Laak et al., 2021).

The history of artificial neural networks dates back to the 1940s, with a surge in activities from the 1980s and onwards. The superiority of DL models in terms of performance was established around 2010 when the advancements in methodological techniques, computer hardware, and curated data allowed efficient training of sufficiently large and deep neural networks to outperform more traditional approaches in competitions on various pattern recognition tasks. DL soon became utterly dominant in pattern recognition tasks related to images and natural language processing. This paved the way for medical applications, for instance, demonstrated by DL models showing supremacy in detecting mitotic figures.

The utilization of AI in pathology depends on the ongoing digitalization of the pathological workflow. One vital step was the development of fluorescent and bright-field slide scanners enabling the production of high-quality whole slide images (WSI). The availability of WSIs, accompanied by the large output of images in radiology, has led to profound growth in publications on the use of AI for image-based medical diagnostics. We searched PubMed on the 13 September 2022 for DL studies in cancer diagnostics using the same user query described previously (Kleppe et al., 2021) and found 241 search results published in 2016, 451 in 2017, 945 in 2018, 1945 in 2019, 3237 in 2020, and 4778 in 2021. The number of scientific publications and the yearly increase of 50–100% clearly show that DL is a very active and rapidly growing field of research in cancer diagnostics.

A key factor for DL models is good generalizability properties so that the models perform equally well on patient samples from other hospitals with differences in laboratory handling. Good generalizability properties partly depend on good design choices in terms of neural network and training techniques to avoid learning details only found in the training data, a common issue encountered in ML that is usually referred to as overfitting. Secondly, good generalizability partly depends on having sufficient amounts of training data as well as training data that is representative of the kind of data later seen when evaluating new cases. Usually, one tries to reach the desired level of size and variation partly through using representative and varied real-life data and partly by utilizing artificially created data. The artificial data is typically obtained by so-called augmentation, where new information is generated by transforming real-life data. For image data, common transformations are simple rotations, mirror reversals, and changes in brightness, hue, and contrast (Shorten & Koshgoftaar, 2019).

The inherent high complexity of DL models and the challenges of obtaining sufficient and representative training data makes good generalization ability uncertain until testing and validation on external datasets are verified. In recent years, it has become more common to report external tests in DL studies in cancer diagnostics, in particular for publications in leading scientific journals. However, validation in clinic-near settings is still lacking in many studies,

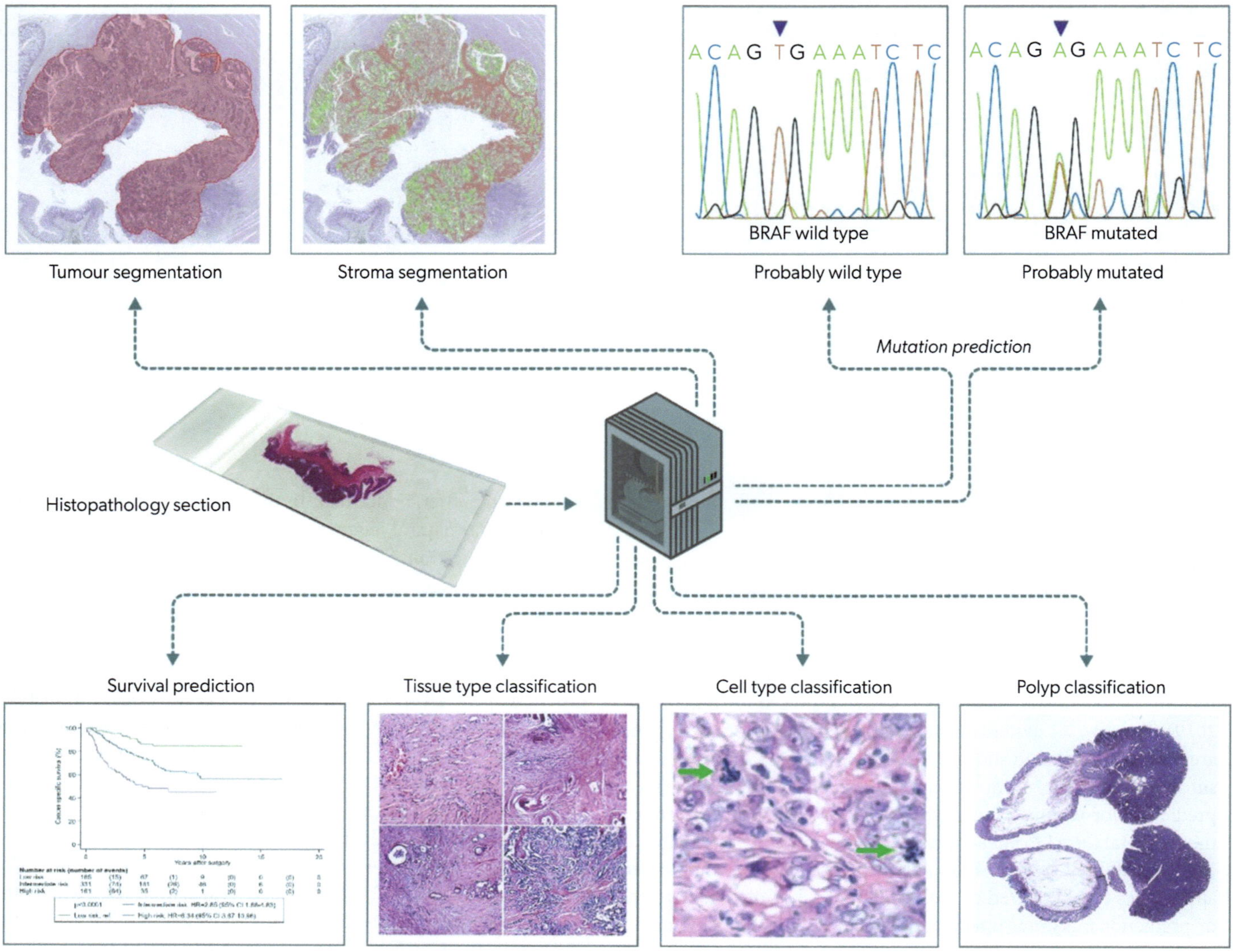

Figure 8.1 Prediction tasks using conventional histopathology section images.

Examples of information that can be automatically extracted with machine learning from a whole slide image (WSI) of a routine haematoxylin and eosin-stained tissue section from colorectal cancer. Some information can also be manually assessed by pathologists, while other information is not visible to the human eye or not adequately described and tested to be assessed by pathologists in clinical practice. Tumour segmentation allows the delineation of the epithelial tumour component in the tissue section. This annotation is required for many subsequent analyses. The stroma component of the epithelial tumour can also be segmented, resulting in an estimate of the stroma-tumour fraction, which is shown to be prognostic in several studies. Also DNA mutation status can be estimated for specific genes, for example *BRAF*, which can be used to select samples for conventional molecular testing. Deep learning models have been trained to predict survival directly from the WSI, using patient outcome to label samples in the training phase. Several studies have shown the ability of machine learning to detect tissue types and relate the tissue type composition to clinical parameters. Cell types are another entity for quantification, where, for example, mitotic figures can be identified and counted. Examination of bowel polyps represents a massive workload for pathologists when screening programmes are implemented. Machine learning models can aid the histopathological examination by, for example, identifying a fraction of the low-risk polyps that do not require examination by a pathologist.

making reliable validation an essential factor to consider when evaluating AI systems (Kleppe et al., 2021; Homeyer et al., 2022).

In the following, we will attempt to describe the status of AI research in digital pathology for colorectal cancer (CRC), focusing on the kind of systems being developed, on the level on testing and validation, and finally on the prospects of getting more understandable AI systems.

AI in polyp classification

Organized bowel screening to detect premalignant polyps and CRCs is now implemented in several countries and is shown to reduce both incidence and mortality rates significantly (Levin et al., 2018). Implementing bowel cancer screening programmes requires substantial endoscopy and pathology resources to perform the bowel examinations and analyse the resected polyps. The histopathological characterization of the resected polyps is the foundation for the current risk assessment and follow-up recommendations, where high-risk polyps are distinguished from low-risk polyps based on histology, size, and numbers (Rutter et al., 2020).

Automating the histopathological characterization and corresponding risk classification may significantly streamline the implementation of bowel screening programmes, where low-risk polyps constitute the majority. ML has been used for the classification of polyp histology in a few studies (Korbar et al., 2017; Wei et al., 2020), where DL models have been trained to distinguish hyperplastic polyps, sessile serrated adenoma, traditional serrated adenoma, tubular adenoma, and tubulovillous or villous adenomas. CNN's were used for the classification, where the input to the network in the study by Korbar et al. was image crops from 697 WSIs scanned at 20× magnification from one institution for training and 239 WSIs from the same institution for testing (Korbar et al., 2017). In contrast, Wei et al. three years later used image crops from 508 WSIs scanned at 40× magnification from one institution for training and an external dataset consisting of 238 slides from 24 different institutions in 13 US states for testing (Wei et al., 2020). Both studies predicted histology class for each image crop; Korbar et al. (2017) used the most common histology class to represent the WSI, whereas Wei et al. (2020) used histology-type classification rules with thresholds established in the training dataset to predict the histology class for the WSI. The published studies indicate the approach's feasibility, although confirmatory validation studies are warranted before applying these systems in clinical practice.

Nasir-Moin et al. (2021) used the AI system developed by Wei et al. (2020) to aid pathologists in their classification of polyps. The AI system predicted histology classes for overlapping image crops as well as an expected histology class for the entire WSI. The area quantifications and overall histology class prediction were visualized to the pathologists during their review. In total, 15 pathologists participated in the study to evaluate the effect of being aided by the AI system on time and accuracy. The polyp classes predicted by the pathologists aided by the AI system were compared to the traditional microscope-based polyp examinations carried out by the same pathologists. The classification accuracy improved from 73.9% to 80.8%, but the mean examination time per slide increased from 13.0 seconds to 21.7 seconds overall. However, the increase in examination time was nearly half for the last 20% of slides, indicating that the increase could be relatively small when pathologists become familiar and experienced with being aided by the AI system.

With the increasing use of bowel screening, the incidence of diagnosed T1 CRCs will increase. There is a need for markers that can inform the selection of treatment of CRC patients with submucosal invasion (T1) tumours, in particular, to distinguish the patients that are cured after the endoscopic resection from those with a higher chance of lymph node metastasis and therefore where formal intestinal resection with lymph node dissection is needed. With current guidelines for deciding on surgical resection, only about 10% of the patients with T1 CRC undergoing surgical resection have lymph node metastasis (Ichimasa et al., 2021). Studies have indicated the ability of DL models to predict lymph node status based on WSIs of biopsy sections stained with haematoxylin and eosin (HE) (Iizkua et al., 2020; Song et al., 2022; Takamatsu et al., 2022). The proposed system by Takamatsu et al. (2022) was developed in a stepwise manner using ground truth from pathologists, where the first model separated cancer from non-cancer tiles, the second model classified tiles according to histological type and risk for lymph node metastasis. In contrast, the last model was a random forest classifier that combined cancer and lymph node metastasis predictions with tumour location into a sample level lymph node metastasis prediction. In total, 551 patients from one hospital were used for training and 236 patients from the same hospital were used to test the system's ability to predict lymph node metastasis, achieving an area under the receiver operating characteristic curve (AUC) of 0.971 in the training set and 0.760 in the test set. Better test performance has been observed by combining only clinical and pathological markers using AI (Kudo et al., 2021). However, the results are not consistent across studies, as Song et al. similarly observed an AUC of 0.764 in a test subset consisting of 80 patients for a model trained using DL and WSIs of HE-stained sections from 320 patients, but worse test performance when combining only clinical and pathological markers using AI and no improvement by incorporating clinical features with the DL model (Song et al., 2022).

The prediction of lymph node status is important to tailor treatment after surgery for patients with T-stage higher than T1. Kwak et al. trained a DL model for detection of tissue types and identified the peri-tumoural stroma fraction (Kwak et al., 2021). The peri-tumoural stroma fraction was compared in primary tumours from colon cancer patients with lymph node metastasis (specifically stage III) from those without (specifically stage I and II) in the Cancer Genome Atlas (TCGA). It was found to be higher in the former group. Liu et al. developed a DL system for the prediction of lymph node metastasis where features from HE-stained WSIs were extracted and combined with a DL representation of molecular analyses in blood samples from the patients (Liu et al., 2022). The authors compared the results with preoperative radiology-imaging diagnosis in the development cohort. They found that the DL approach performed better, particularly by correctly classifying more patients without lymph node metastasis.

Tumour tissue detection and delineation

Discrimination between tumour and non-tumour tissue is fundamental in cancer pathology and is an appropriate first step for many AI-based digital pathology tasks. To obtain ground truth, data for training DL models to segment the tumour region can be marked with a digital delineation, or sub-images of the WSI can be classified as tumour or non-tumour according to their tumour content. Due to the large memory usage, the gigapixel WSIs pose a technical challenge for ML models that provide predictions on the entire WSI. Commonly used strategies to overcome the challenge are to reduce the image size by down-sampling or to use image crops. Down-sampling the WSI reduces the image's size and information content. Image crops, on the other hand, maintain the high-resolution information in relatively small image tiles but removes their spatial context. Skrede et al. developed a DL model for tumour segmentation in WSIs from CRC using images resized to fit in a frame of 1600 × 1600 pixels while keeping the aspect ratio (Skrede et al., 2020). Other studies have used image crops (Fu et al., 2020; Xu et al., 2020; Ben Hamida et al., 2021). To evaluate the results, a predicted tumour segmentation can be compared with the ground truth using established metrics for segmentation accuracy, such as the Dice coefficient (Dice, 1945) and Jaccard index (Jaccard, 1912), or using metrics more common for classification tasks, in particular if the prediction and ground truth only concern whether or not a tile contains tumour. Although high accuracies are reported for most models, typically with more than 90% of pixels or tiles correctly classified according to the ground truth, most studies use internal test sets, whereas examples of external validations are less common.

Tissue type classification

The importance of the tumour microenvironment (TME) for the understanding and predicting carcinogenesis and its outcome is now largely recognized (Anderson & Simon, 2020). The interplay between cancer cells and their local environment is important for cancer progression. Quantifying cell and tissue type composition is therefore a sensible approach for TME characterization and for automation of existing pathology examinations. ML has been used to develop models for the automatic identification of cell and tissue type in WSIs of HE-stained sections, collectively providing a detailed TME characterization on multiple levels of resolution.

Competitions have facilitated the development of DL models in digital pathology, primarily by providing curated and well annotated datasets and benchmarks for comparing different approaches. The objective of the GlaS@MICCAI2015 colon gland segmentation challenge was to automatically segment glands in WSIs of HE-stained sections (Sirinukunwattana et al., 2017). In total, 13 solutions were submitted, and conventional metrics for evaluation of segmentation accuracy were used to rank the solutions based on the performance in independent test samples. The best-performing solutions used CNNs to segment glands in the input WSIs.

Tissue patterns within the tumour region have been quantified using different AI systems to estimate the stroma–tumour ratio and degree of tumour differentiation, and tumour budding (Awan et al., 2017; Danielsen et al., 2018; Kather et al., 2019; Geesink et al., 2019; Pai et al., 2021). These are all well-known prognostic markers that may benefit from the consistent assessment provided by AI systems. These histopathological properties have traditionally been assessed manually by pathologists, but AI systems for automatic assessment have been developed, first using traditional image analysis and, more recently, using DL.

The stroma–tumour ratio can be assessed in HE-stained sections, and a higher stroma content relative to the epithelial tumour content is a marker of poor prognosis (Mesker et al., 2007; van Pelt et al., 2018). Danielsen et al. developed an AI system for the automatic segmentation of stroma in HE-stained WSIs using traditional image analysis and used the system to estimate the stroma-tumour ratio (Danielsen et al., 2018). In a study of 1,029 patients with stage II CRC from three different cohorts, a risk classification combining stroma–tumour ratio and DNA ploidy status was a significant predictor of cancer-specific survival (Danielsen et al., 2018). After adjusting for age, adjuvant treatment, and pathological T-stage, the patients with high stroma content (more than 50%) and non-diploid ploidy status had a hazard ratio (HR) of 2.95 (95% CI 1.73–5.03, $p < 0.001$) compared to patients with low stroma content (50% or less) and diploid ploidy status. Kather et al. trained a DL model to classify image crops from HE-stained WSIs as one of nine tissue types and combined the output from this model into a 'deep stroma score' comprising information from different types of non-tumour components of the tumour (Kather et al., 2019). The 'deep stroma score' was categorized into 'low' and 'high' using the median score for 500 patients in the CRC datasets from TCGA (TCGA-COAD and TCGA-READ) as threshold. The resulting 'deep stroma classification' was shown to provide supplemental prognostic information in an external test using 409 stage I–IV CRC patients recruited between 2003 and 2007 at multiple institutions in Germany; the hazard ration (HR) in the multivariable analysis was 1.63 (95% CI 1.14–2.33, $p = 0.008$) in the analysis of overall survival and 2.29 (95% CI 1.5–3.48, $p = 0.0004$) in the analysis of cancer-specific survival. Zhao et al. (2020) followed a similar approach as Kather et al. (2019) to develop a fully automated AI system for stroma quantification in CRC and observed an HR of 2.08 (95% CI 1.26–3.42; $p = 0.004$) in multivariable analysis of overall survival using 315 patients from a different Chinese hospital than the one used for training. Jiang et al. developed a DL system for the automatic quantification of different morphological properties in stage III CRC, including stroma (Jiang et al., 2020). Based on the different properties, they defined a classifier that was observed to predict disease-free survival and overall survival in a small external dataset consisting of 47 TCGA-COAD patients with more than 36 months of follow-up. Li et al. developed another DL model to identify tissue types in CRC and used it to define a DL system outputting three risk groups (Li et al., 2022). In analysis of an external dataset consisting of 246 TCGA patients with stage II or III CRC, they observed that adjuvant chemotherapy was significantly associated with improved overall survival in the patients identified as high risk by their DL system (HR 0.2, 95% CI 0.05–0.65, $p = 0.009$), but not in the patients identified as low or medium risk by their DL system (Li et al., 2022).

The assessments of tumour budding have used pan-cytokeratin or HE staining and involve the identification of single tumour cells or small tumour cell clusters at the invasion front of the tumour. The presence and level of this pattern are associated with an adverse patient outcome (Lugli et al., 2021). Weis et al. used a combination of traditional image analysis and ML to automatically segment and quantify tumour buds in sections immunohistochemically (IHC) stained with pan-cytokeratin (Weis et al., 2018). They found a good correlation with ground truth annotations and nodal status when using the number of budding hotspots. Pai et al. developed a DL system for automatically segmenting histological features including tumour buds and poorly differentiated clusters using HE-stained tissue micromicroarrayss) with manual annotation of different cells and tissue types (Pai et al., 2021). CNNs were trained to separate types of cells and tissue layer-wise (Pai et al., 2021). The automatically segmented tumour buds and poorly differentiated clusters correlated well with manual assessments and significantly associated with lymph nodes and distant metastasis. Awan et al. developed a DL system for objective assessment of tumour differentiation and observed accuracy of 97% when classifying normal versus cancer and 91% when classifying normal versus low-grade cancer versus high-grade cancer in threefold cross-validation (Awan et al., 2017).

While human experts can perform these and many other visual assessments, the subjective nature of the quantification process results in a suboptimal agreement between observers and between multiple assessments by a single human observer. AI systems can aid or even replace an observer if accurate enough in routine clinical settings. If a system is being applied in clinical practice, its robustness and accuracy should be monitored to ensure that changes in, for example, sample preparation or imaging techniques do not bias the system.

Cell type classification

Cells have been automatically identified and classified according to cell type using HE-stained WSIs, and the resulting composition of cell types is associated with clinical and pathological features (Sirinukunwattana et al. 2016; Sirinukunwattana et al. 2018; Shapcott et al., 2019). Sirinukunwattana et al. (2016) trained a DL model to detect and classify cell nuclei as epithelial, inflammatory, fibroblast, or miscellaneous, and later (2018) extended their AI system also to characterize tissue regions and showed that the identified features were predictive for distant metastasis of CRC in an analysis of 72 patients from one institution and 30 patients from another institution. The best performing feature was the inflammation ratio, achieving an HR of 0.389 (95% CI 0.189–0.803, p = 0.004) in multivariable analysis in the dataset comprising 72 patients, but the AI system was not tested in an external dataset. Shapcott et al. used similar training data to develop a DL model which was tested in an external dataset of 142 HE-stained WSIs of colon cancer from TCGA, where they observed an association between the estimated cellular composition and clinical and pathological features such as metastasis, vascular invasion, and mucinous carcinoma (Shapcott et al., 2019).

Several recent studies have focused on tumour-infiltrating lymphocytes (TILs), which are white blood cells (immune effectors) that have moved from the blood into the tumour. The host immune response is important in carcinogenesis, and the type, density, and site of TILs are prognostic markers in CRC (Idos et al., 2020). The presence of TILs in tumours is associated with better clinical outcomes and could be relevant information for tailoring treatment. T-cell density has been quantified by AI systems using WSIs of sections immunohistochemically (IHC) stained for specific types, such as CD8 for cytotoxic T-cells that promote apoptosis of cancer cells and CD3 for T-cells that activate cytotoxic T-cells and T helper cells. Glaire et al. developed an AI system to quantify CD8 expression and observed that decreased CD8 expression predicted poor patient outcome in stage II and III CRC (Glaire et al., 2019). Jiang et al. combined the CD8 expression and stroma–tumour fraction into a prognostic marker and indicated its clinical usability for low- and high-risk stage II and III CRC patients (Jiang et al., 2021). Xu et al. used HE-stained WSIs with manually assessed TIL categories in one dataset to develop a DL system for automatic TIL quantification (Xu et al., 2022). Higher TIL density was observed to be associated with improved progression-free survival in the multivariable analysis of an external dataset from TCGA consisting of 268 CRC patients (Xu et al., 2022). Also, Abousamra et al. trained a DL system to predict TIL status and analysed CRC patients from TCGA but they reported results for CRC only when analysed together with other cancer types (Abousamra et al., 2022).

DNA ploidy and chromatin analysis

DNA ploidy analysis by image cytometry is another type of digital pathology method where the tumour sample is prepared into a cell suspension that is spun onto a glass slide and stained with the DNA-specific Feulgen stain (Fig. 8.2). The Feulgen stain is stoichiometric, and the transmitted light through a cell nucleus is, therefore, proportional to its DNA content. The DNA content in cell nuclei is calculated for all cell nuclei in a tumour specimen to yield a histogram of the distribution of DNA content in the measured sample. A normal DNA content distribution where most cells are in interphase with two copies of each chromosome is called a diploid state. In contrast, deviations from the normal DNA content distribution are referred to as a non-diploid state. Non-diploid ploidy status is related to large-scale genomic instability and is associated with an adverse prognosis in most cancer types, including in patients with CRC and patients with initially resectable CRC liver metastasis (Hveem et al., 2014; Danielsen et al., 2016; Peng et al., 2021; Li et al., 2022).

Another analysis that can be performed after the same sample preparation used for DNA ploidy measurement is chromatin analysis, where the DNA organisation in cell nuclei is automatically quantified using texture analysis (Fig. 8.2). An ML system has been developed to classify each sample as chromatin homogeneous or chromatin heterogeneous. External validations have shown that patients with chromatin heterogeneous tumours have a worse outcome than patients with chromatin homogeneous tumours in several cancer types (Kleppe et al., 2018). In CRC, the HR in analysis of cancer-specific survival was observed to be 2.6 (95% CI 1.2–5.6, p = 0.016) in an external trial-based dataset with 391 stage II CRC patients and 1.9 (95% CI 1.1–3.2, p = 0.026) in an external community-based dataset with 442 stage I or II CRC patients after adjusting for established prognostic patient characteristics in multivariable analyses (Kleppe et al., 2018). The findings have been validated by independent research teams using new external datasets. These studies also indicate that chromatin analysis can be combined with markers of DNA ploidy and stroma–tumour fraction to enhance risk stratification in stage II CRC further (Yang et al., 2020; Zhao et al., 2021). Yang et al. found that both DNA ploidy and chromatin heterogeneity were significant in multivariable analysis of disease-free survival, resulting in an HR of 2.6 (95% CI 1.2–5.5, p = 0.015) for DNA ploidy alone, 3.3 (95% CI 1.7–6.6, p = 0.001) for chromatin heterogeneity alone, and 4.4 (95% CI 1.9–10.3) for high versus low risk of the three-grouped marker combining DNA ploidy and chromatin heterogeneity (Yang et al., 2020). Zhao et al. investigated the prognostic impact of DNA ploidy, chromatin heterogeneity, and stroma–tumour fraction in stage I, II, and IV CRC and confirmed the prognostic value of all three markers in stage II CRC, also after adjusting for T-stage, microsatellite instability (MSI) status, and adjuvant treatment in multivariable analysis of disease-free survival and overall survival (Zhao et al., 2021). They observed that patients where at least one of the three markers indicated worse clinical outcome had better disease-free survival and overall survival when receiving adjuvant treatment than when not receiving adjuvant therapy and concluded that the combination of the three markers was an accurate prognostic tool that could guide treatment decisions in stage II CRC. It has been indicated that assessments of DNA ploidy and chromatin heterogeneity are resilient against deviations in sample preparation and imaging (Danielsen et al., 2016; Kleppe et al., 2018), providing consistent measurements across multiple imaging devices (Kleppe & Danielsen, 2018), and can thus be expected to handle the diversity of routine clinical practice well.

Molecular characterization

Automatically detecting tumours and characterizing the tumour microenvironment can assist pathologists, relieving them from tedious assessments and allowing them to handle specimens more efficiently, in addition to providing more objective and consistent pathological assessments. However, it is also anticipated that DL can be used to perform tasks currently not done by pathologists using

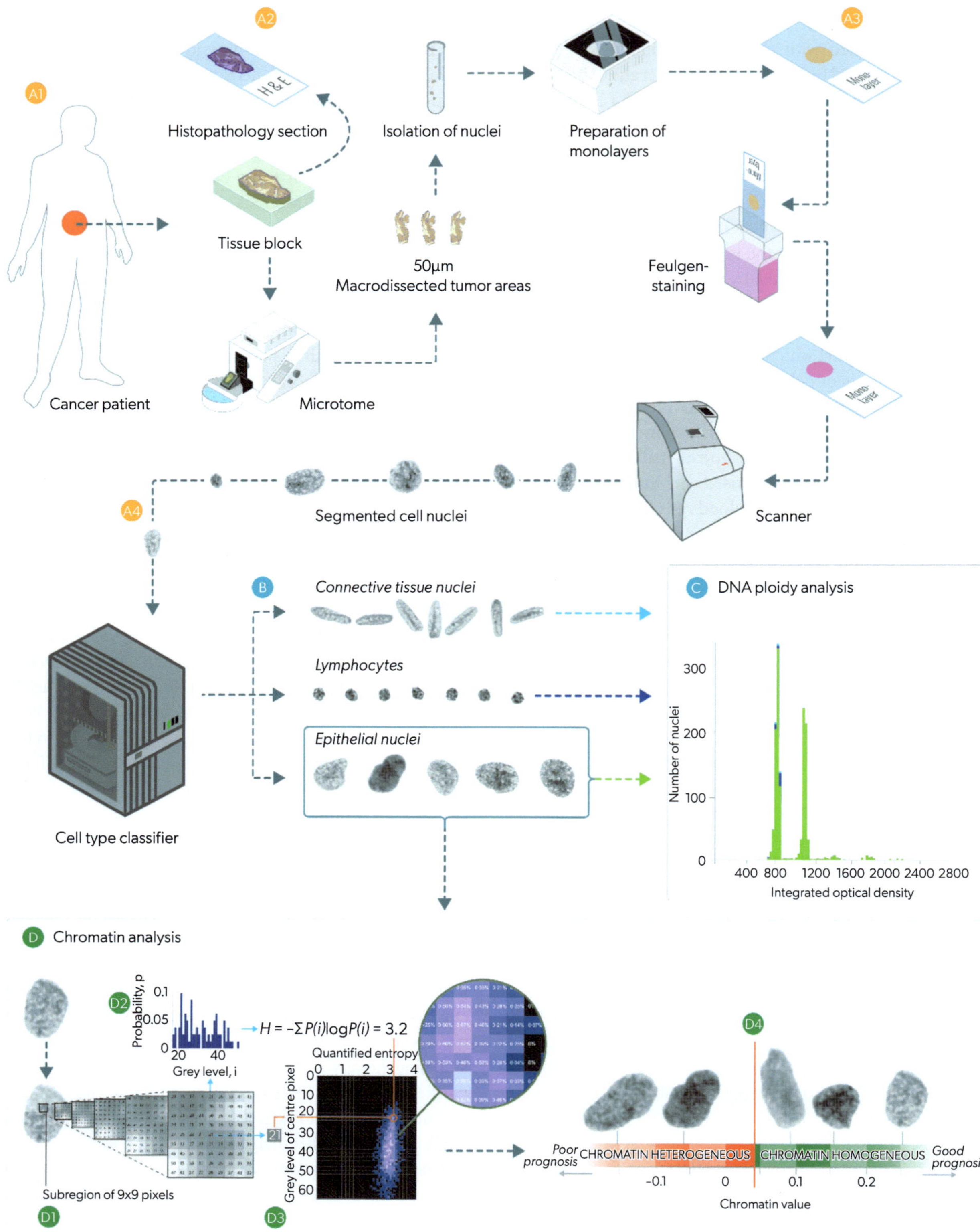

Figure 8.2 Pipeline for assessment of DNA ploidy and chromatin heterogeneity.

A1: An individual cancer patient. A2: The surgical specimen is partitioned, and each piece is formalin-fixated and paraffin-embedded. Tumour is macrodissected from a 50 μm section cut from a tumour tissue block and used to make a cell suspension. Intact cell nuclei are isolated and spun onto a monolayer (A3) glass slide. The monolayer specimen is stained with a DNA-specific Feulgen stain and imaged on a scanner. Cell nuclei are automatically segmented from the digital image (A4) and sorted according to cell type using a machine learning system (B). C: Optical density in Feulgen-stained cell nuclei is proportional to DNA content. A histogram of the optical density of each epithelial nucleus in a cell population represents the DNA content distribution and, thus, the DNA ploidy of that cell population. In a normal diploid DNA content distribution, most nuclei have two copies of each chromosome. A minority are undergoing division, seen as one major peak termed 2c in the DNA ploidy histogram and a small peak with twice the amount of DNA, termed 4c. Deviations from this pattern are called a non-diploid DNA ploidy state and are associated with an inferior patient outcome. The optical density of other cell types, such as fibroblasts or lymphocytes, may be included to support the analysis by providing a reference for the diploid population's DNA content. D: For chromatin analysis, subregions of the cell nucleus image (D1) are analysed by extracting two quantities: the grey level of the centre pixel (here 21) and the Shannon entropy of the grey levels in the subregion (here 3.2) (D2). The two quantities extracted from the subregion will identify a position in a matrix (D3). The occurrence is counted by incrementing the value in the matrix at that position (initially, all matrix values are 0), and the computation of the two quantities and incrementation of the corresponding matrix value is performed for every subregion of the nuclear image. The resulting matrix describes the frequency of each pair of centre grey levels and surrounding entropy for a cell nucleus image. It is normalised by its total count to provide the bivariate probability mass function called the grey level entropy matrix (GLEM). The GLEM is a representation of the chromatin organisation in a cell nucleus and can be aggregated to a patient-level representation by averaging the GLEMs for all cell nuclei for a patient. This patient-level GLEM can then be converted to a chromatin value using a weighting function learned from a training dataset. D4: Depiction of five nuclear images and their chromatin value. The threshold applied to dichotomise the chromatin value was 0.044.

histopathology sections, typically because it would have been too time-consuming, considered not possible with sufficient accuracy, or the relevant morphological patterns have not yet been described sufficiently well. One example of this is the prediction of mutations using HE-stained histopathology sections.

Several studies have applied DL to develop models for predicting MSI or mismatch repair deficiency (dMMR) from images of histopathology sections of CRC tissue (Kather et al., 2019; Cao et al., 2020; Echle et al., 2020; Kather et al., 2020; Ke et al., 2020; Schmauch et al., 2020; Bilal et al., 2021; Lee et al., 2021a; Lee et al., 2021b; Yamashita et al., 2021a; Yamashita et al., 2021b; Schrammen et al., 2022; Echle et al., 2022). A recent study applied more than 8,000 patients to train and validate the performance of models classifying tumours as either MSI/dMMR or microsatellite stable (MSS)/proficient mismatch repair (pMMR) across different countries and ethnicities (Echle et al., 2022). The results indicate that it will be possible to detect nearly 50% of CRC patients where MSI is very unlikely, thus substantially reducing the workload required to test for MSI/dMMR (Fig. 8.3). However, current models are still not adequately robust to allow reliable usage in routine clinical practice (Kleepe, 2022). The possibility of using DL to enable such prediction could have been anticipated because earlier observations indicated that pathological assessments such as tumour-infiltrating lymphocytes, Crohn's-like inflammatory reaction, and tumour differentiation are independent predictors of MSI (Greenson et al., 2003), and that the combination of such assessments and clinical parameters such as age and tumour location can predict MSI quite accurately (Jenkins et al., 2007; Greenson et al., 2009). After being made sufficiently robust and accurate, DL models allowing automatic prediction of MSI/dMMR status from HE-stained WSIs could facilitate more extensive and cost-effective usage of MSI/dMMR status to guide treatment decisions in CRC.

Several pan-cancer studies have explored the possibility of predicting molecular characteristics in multiple cancer types, including CRC. Kather et al. indicated that DL models can be trained to predict genetic mutation of *BRAF*, *KMT2B*, *KMT2D*, *KRAS*, *PIK3CA*, *RNF43*, and *TP53* using only HE-stained WSIs (Kather et al., 2020). Similarly, Fu et al. observed many significant associations between genomic alterations and features extracted from WSIs using a DL model (Fu et al., 2020). Komura et al. also used a DL model to extract features from HE-stained WSIs (Komura et al., 2022). They indicated that the same features could be utilized to retrieve tiles looking histologically similar to a query tile and to predict 19 mutations in colon cancer, including *BRAF*, *KMT2D*, *KRAS*, *RNF43*, and *TP53*, and four mutations in rectal cancer, specifically *ATM*, *NRAS*, *SCR*, and *FLT3*. While these studies indicate that DL models can be trained to predict some genetic mutations in CRC, they all apply the same public data from TCGA for training and testing. Schrammen et al. used a different dataset to train DL systems for prediction of *BRAF* and *KRAS* status and observed an AUC of 0.821 for *BRAF* status prediction and 0.609 for *KRAS* status prediction, suggesting that at least *BRAF* status could be predictable from

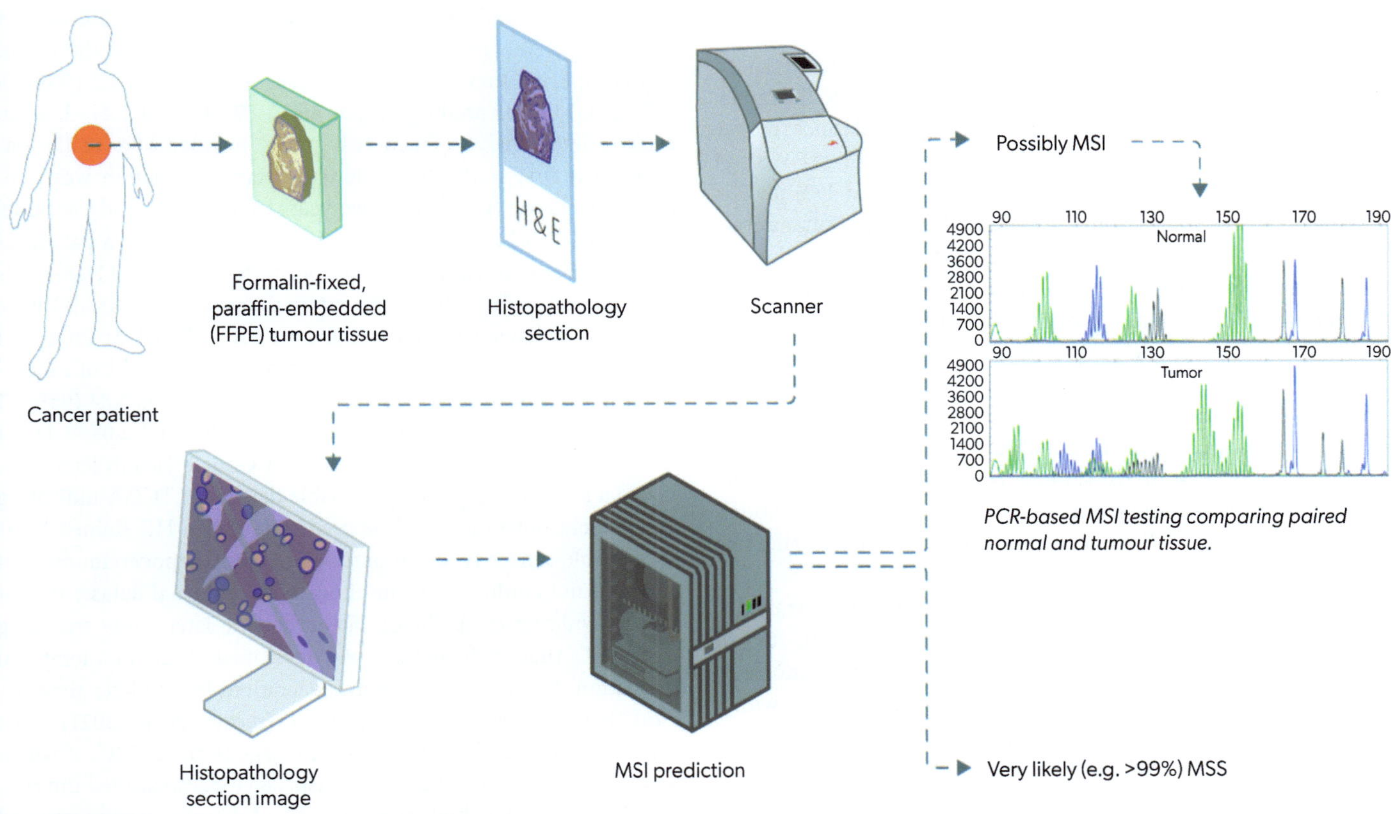

Figure 8.3 Microsatellite instability (MSI) prediction and possible usage.

A practical example of how a machine learning system can streamline the assessment of MSI status is using a whole slide image of a tissue section stained with haematoxylin and eosin (H&E). After surgery, the resected tumour is stored as formalin-fixed and paraffin-embedded tissue blocks. A thin section is cut from a tumour block, mounted on a glass slide, and stained with H&E. The slide is imaged using a pathology scanner to provide a digital image of the histopathology section. A deep learning model analyses the image to predict MSI status with corresponding confidence. Microsatellite stable (MSS) tumours constitute the majority, and samples predicted MSS with high confidence can be reasonably regarded as MSS. In contrast, the remaining samples can be tested for MSI using polymerase chain reaction (PCR).

HE-stained WSIs (Schrammen et al., 2022). More recently, studies analysing external datasets have confirmed these findings (Saldanha et al., 2023; Niehues et al., 2023).

Since the same genetic mutation can be predicted in multiple cancer types, it might be hypothesized that the patterns found through DL to predict the mutation are the same for multiple cancer types. In line with this hypothesis, Noorbakhsh et al. trained DL models to predict *TP53* mutation status using HE-stained WSIs from one cancer type and tested the model on a different cancer type using TCGA data (Noorbakhsh et al., 2020). While it appeared to be possible to predict *TP53* mutation status across cancer types, the observed performance was best when trained on the same cancer type, in particular for colon cancer.

Kather et al. (2020) and Fu et al. (2020) also found that HE-stained WSIs can be used to predict gene expression and gene expression signatures in CRC using DL. Similarly, Schmauch et al. determined the spatial localization of T cells by predicting expression of *CD3D*, *CD3E*, *CD3G*, and *CD247* and the spatial localization of B cells by predicting expression of *CD19* and *CD20* using HE-stained WSIs of colon cancer (Schmauch et al., 2020). While promising, these findings were based solely on TCGA data and need to be confirmed in external validations.

Kather et al. additionally predicted consensus molecular subtype using TCGA data (Kather et al., 2020). Prediction of molecular subtypes from HE-stained WSIs using CNNs was reported by Popovici et al. (2017) in 2017 using data from the PETACC-3 trial on stage III colon cancer (Van Cutsem et al., 2009). While these studies lacked external validation, the more recent study by Sirinukunwattana et al. (2021) developed a DL model to predict consensus molecular subtype using 510 HE-stained WSIs from 278 patients with advanced CRC in the FOCUS trial (Seymour et al., 2007) and tested the model performance on external data from TCGA and a rectal cancer biopsy dataset. They observed an average accuracy of 60% for 431 WSIs of resection specimens from 430 patients in TCGA and 49% for 265 WSIs of biopsy specimens from 144 patients (Sirinukunwattana et al., 2021). Adaptations to parts of the external datasets, using domain adversarial learning and a random forest to determine better thresholds for biopsy specimens, increased the average accuracy to 64% for the TCGA dataset and 72% for the biopsy dataset. Considering that an average accuracy of 25% could be expected from a random classifier because there are four consensus molecular subtypes, these findings suggest that it may be possible to determine the consensus molecular subtype from HE-stained WSIs with a rather good accuracy, but improvements should be considered to make the models more accurate and resilient against technical differences affecting the resulting WSIs.

Collectively, these studies suggest that it is possible to train DL models to predict some molecular characteristics from HE-stained WSIs. Characteristics that correlate with visually apparent morphological or cellular features are more likely to be identifiable with a high accuracy using AI systems. The best example seems to be prediction of MSI/dMMR status, which is approaching a state where an AI system could be considered for clinical implementation. While it seems to be possible to predict consensus molecular subtype and at least *BRAF* status substantially better than random guessing, it is unclear whether such AI systems have clinical utility if not made more accurate. For other molecular characteristics, the current results are more suggestive than assertive and need verification in external datasets.

Direct prediction of patient outcome

An aim of many of the studies that characterize different aspects or entities in the tumour is to predict how aggressive the disease is and whether the patient is likely to die of the cancer. More accurate estimation of the patient's prognosis enables more personalized treatment. For adjuvant chemotherapy, which is currently the most relevant treatment option for the majority of CRC patients, the treatment appears to reduce the risk of recurrence and death proportionally similar in different patient subgroups defined by conventional clinical and pathological characteristics (Gray et al., 2007; André et al., 2009). This implies that for patient groups with high survival probability, adjuvant chemotherapy will save few lives compared to patient groups with low survival probability. Consequently, the identification of patients with excellent cancer-specific survival can directly indicate patients that should not be given adjuvant chemotherapy and thereby be spared from the associated side effects. Better stratification into high- and low-risk groups will also increase the survival difference between these groups and make the risk stratification more useful for clinical decisions and communication with patients.

While patient outcome can be indicated by tumour characterizations that AI models can identify, DL can also be used to train models that predict patient outcome directly from a WSI (Fig. 8.4A). An early study on this was published in 2018, where Bychkov et al. presented a DL model for prediction of five-year disease-specific outcome (Bychkov et al., 2018). The model was trained, tuned, and tested using cross-validation in a CRC dataset containing 420 patients with Dukes' stage A to D, and the HR of disease-specific survival for high versus low risk was 2.3 (95% CI 1.79–3.03) in univariable analysis and 1.89 (95% CI 1.41–2.53) in multivariable analysis. Each risk group included 50% of the patients. The first study that included external validation was published by Skrede et al. (2020) two years later. In that study, a model was trained and tuned using 2,473 patients to classify a patient as having either good, uncertain, or poor prognosis. Of 1,110 patients with stage II or III CRC in the external dataset, 704 (63.4%) were classified as having a good prognosis, 136 (12.3%) as uncertain prognosis, and 270 (24.3%) as poor prognosis. The HR of cancer-specific survival for poor versus good prognosis was 3.84 (95% CI 2.72–5.43) in univariable analysis and 3.04 (95% CI 2.07–4.47) in multivariable analysis. Wulczyn et al. at Google Health later published a study using publicly available data from TCGA indicating that patient outcome could be predictable from HE-stained WSIs in multiple cancer types, in particular colon adenocarcinoma, but they did not confirm their findings in any external dataset in that study (Wulczyn et al., 2020). However, in a later study analysing only CRC, they evaluated a newly developed model in a temporal validation dataset; that is, a dataset acquired from a later time period than the development dataset (Wulczyn et al., 2021). That dataset consisted of 738 patients with stage II or III CRC, of which 281 (38.1%) were classified as low risk, 283 (38.3%) as medium risk, and 174 (23.6%) as high risk. The HR of disease-specific survival for high versus low risk was 3.55 (95% CI 2.58–4.89) in univariable analysis. Recently, Chen et al. proposed a new DL network based on vision transformers that was observed to increase the performance compared to previous approaches, but the evaluation was performed using cross-validation in TCGA datasets and not using any

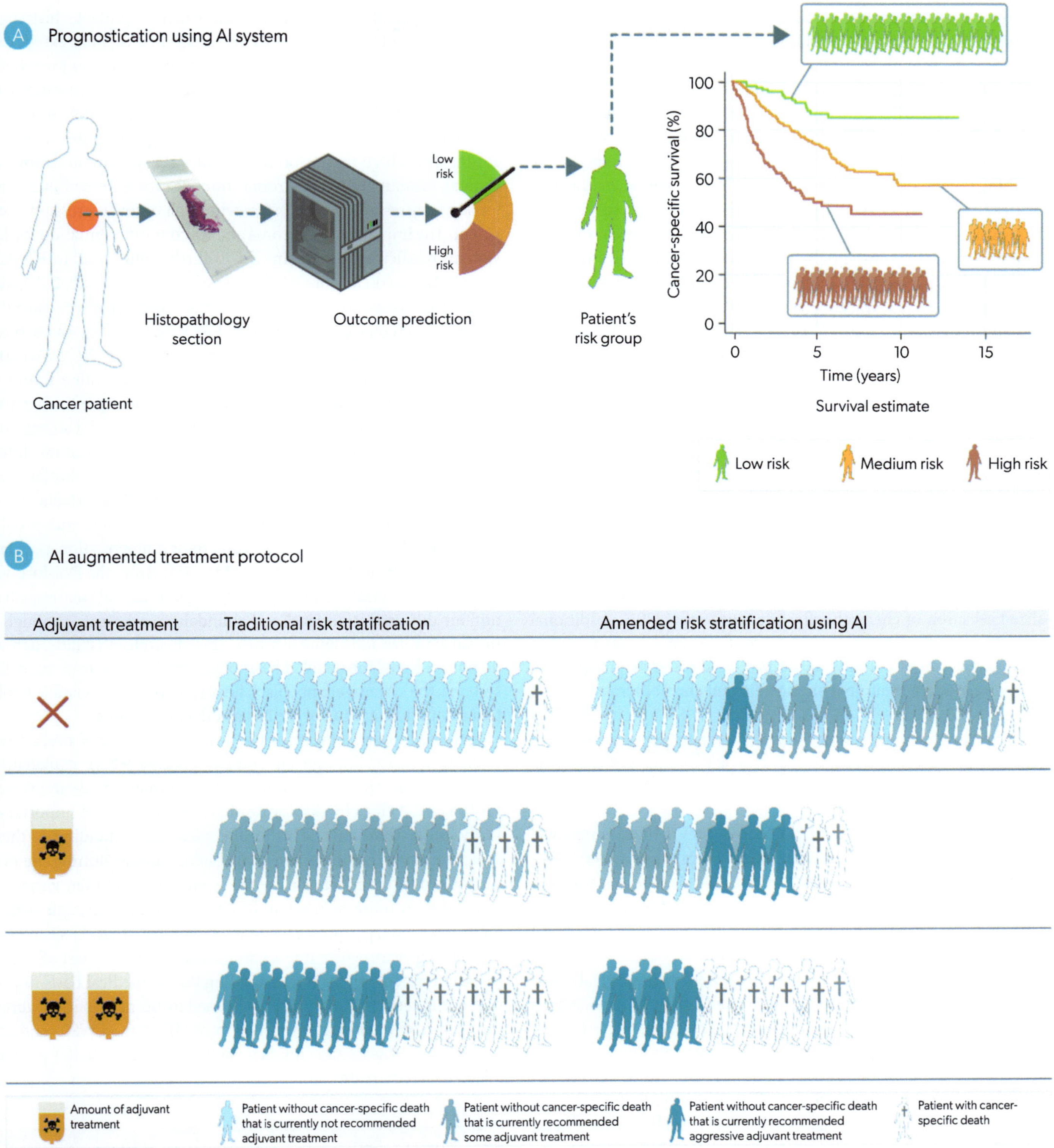

Figure 8.4 Direct prediction of patient outcome and integration with treatment protocol.

A: A whole slide image of an H&E stained tissue section from a patient's resected tumour is analysed using a deep learning model to predict the patient's survival. The prediction is usually a continuous value but can be categorised into, for example, three risk categories representing a low, intermediate, and high risk for recurrence and cancer death following surgery. **B:** Treatment protocols based on pathological and clinical parameters are used to identify patients that should be offered adjuvant chemotherapy. A challenge with the current protocols is the limited ability to separate patients likely to benefit from adjuvant therapy from those better left without, especially in high-risk stage II and stage III cancers. The integration of an AI system's risk prediction has the potential to substantially improve patient stratification for adjuvant treatment. Offering more adjuvant therapy to patients at very high risk of recurrence and no adjuvant treatment to those at very low risk may result in improved survival and quality of life for cancer patients and cost savings.

external dataset (Chen et al., 2022). Another alternative that might improve the accuracy is to include genomic data as input to a DL system that also analyse an HE-stained WSI (Boehm et al., 2022). A few studies have found this to improve the prediction of patient outcome (Mobadersany et al., 2018; Chen et al., 2021), but it has not yet been confirmed in external datasets nor explored in CRC.

While DL models appear capable of predicting patient outcome directly from an HE-stained WSI and providing prognostic information supplemental to clinical, pathological, and molecular markers used in current clinical practice, the models are currently not accurate enough to replace all other markers. The additional prognostic value of a DL model should therefore be leveraged by integrating its prediction with the markers currently in clinical use (Fig. 8.4B). Kleppe et al. learned such an integration from 997 patients with stage II or III CRC, resulting in a scheme that can be used to classify an individual patient as low, intermediate, or high risk (Kleppe et al., 2022). The HR of cancer-specific survival for high versus low risk was 10.71 (95% CI 6.39–17.93) in an external dataset, which was substantially higher than for a risk stratification system reflecting current guidelines (HR 6.12, 95% CI 3.09–12.10). The proposed risk stratification system included three times as many patients in the low-risk group. These low-risk patients had excellent cancer-specific survival, similar to the patients currently not recommended adjuvant chemotherapy because the net survival benefit is expected to be minuscule or even negative and the entailed side effects are often substantial. When also considering that all patients in this external dataset received the same adjuvant chemotherapy and that adjuvant chemotherapy causes a proportionally similar reduction in risk of recurrence and death, it appears that not treating patients in the low-risk group of the proposed risk stratification with adjuvant chemotherapy will reduce morbidity and treatment costs. Thus, utilizing the prognostic value of a DL marker allowed better risk stratification and could translate into better and more individualized selection of chemotherapy after surgery of CRC. Additional validation studies are warranted to confirm the excellent cancer-specific survival of patients in the proposed low-risk group when receiving modern treatment but no adjuvant chemotherapy.

Towards understandable deep learning systems

Predictions are and should be easier to accept if their biomedical basis is understood. Thus, revealing the basis of an AI system's predictions is key for the widespread clinical use of such systems. For certain systems, like those estimating mitotic index, this is less of a problem because the biological rationale is well established and manual inspection can reveal whether the AI system made any errors. For many other systems, like those predicting survival based on HE-stained WSIs, it is much more challenging to explain why the AI system ended up with a specific prediction. Since limited explainability is a general concern with DL systems, this is a highly active research area. Several methods for explaining AI predictions have been developed. Some of these methods, for instance Layer-wise Relevance Propagation (LRP) (Bach et al., 2015)[88] and Integrated Gradients (IG) (Sundararajan et al., 2017) generate so-called attribution maps that highlight which regions of an image contribute the most to the predictions. Such methods are expected to provide insight into what DL systems utilize to make their predictions, but it can be difficult to integrate the explanation of each image in a large dataset into an overarching and concise explanation of the DL system, in particular when there is limited knowledge about what the system should utilize. Understanding the biomedical basis may also be beneficial for improving the DL systems.

More traditional approaches may also hint at features used by an AI system to make predictions. For instance, Wulczyn et al. derived clusters of similarly looking and human-interpretable histologic sub-images of HE-stained WSIs and examined to what extent different clusters explained the score from their DL system for prediction of survival (Wulczyn et al., 2021). Highest regression coefficient was seen for a cluster characterized by small, moderately to poorly differentiated tumour areas adjacent to adipose tissue. Another cluster with a high regression coefficient was abundant in stroma. In general, tumour grade and stroma–tumour ratio emerged as characteristic features of several clusters with high or low regression coefficient. The importance of stroma and tumour differentiation for DL systems predicting survival in CRC is further illustrated in Fig. 8.5. The CNN-based DoMore-v1-CRC marker (Skrede et al., 2020) can be used to create heatmaps indicating areas the marker associates with poor outcome (shown in red in Fig. 8.5A). In some cases, these areas largely align to stromal areas (shown in red in Fig. 8.5B). The patterns most clearly signifying poor outcome are often found in the stroma, but the model prediction is also clearly influenced by features in the epithelial areas. Skrede et al. described a strong correlation between the DoMore-v1-CRC class and the tumour differentiation level as classified by a specialist pathologist (Skrede et al., 2020). This is confirmed by directly examining the epithelial areas, where well differentiation clearly tends to be associated with predictions of good outcome (Fig. 8.5C) and poor differentiation associate with predictions of poor outcome (Fig. 8.5D). Thus, the DoMore-v1-CRC marker is clearly quantifying known biomedical factors such as tumour differentiation level and abundance of stroma, although it may also utilize additional features. This illustrates that although we do not yet know the detailed basis of the predictions from many DL systems, the systems are not black boxes where it is impossible to obtain any understanding of the basis of the predictions.

Increased understanding of the basis of DL systems' predictions is likely to arise through an iterative process where explanation techniques like those generating attribution maps guide the search for biological clues by displaying structures of specific importance to the prediction task. Gains in biological understanding of these structures may then help reveal the biology underpinning the predictions, paving the way for better predictions and then visualizations of even more focused and important areas. Through similar cross-disciplinary processes, one may anticipate that AI systems in the coming years evolve into a natural and integrated part of cancer researchers' toolbox for understanding the biomedical basis of predictions in tasks currently not performed by humans, such as direct prediction of mutations or survival from HE-stained WSIs, and as a tool for pathologists and clinicians in their search for better patient-adapted cancer treatment.

Conclusions and future directions

The rapid development of new DL systems in medicine and beyond is facilitated by an exceptionally important informal convention in the DL community, namely that the source codes used to develop the systems are made publicly available with few or no restrictions. Large technology companies have contributed by developing comprehensive ML frameworks that greatly simplify the development of new DL systems, for instance PyTorch by Facebook Artificial Intelligence Research (now Meta AI) and TensorFlow by the Google Brain team. These frameworks are free and open source, and most

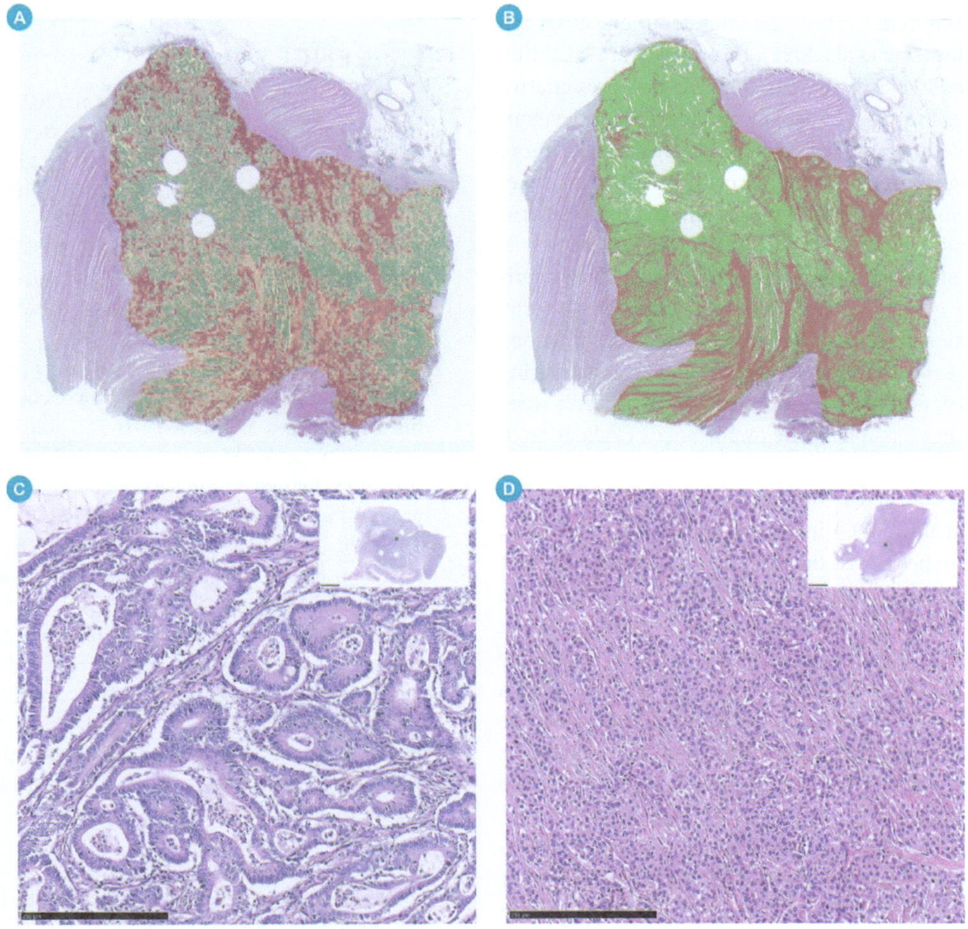

Figure 8.5 DoMore-v1-CRC's relation to stroma and tumour differentiation.

A: The DoMore-v1-CRC marker can be used to provide a score for small sub-images indicating the likelihood of cancer-specific death. Sub-images indicating poor outcomes are shown in red, while sub-images indicating good outcomes are shown in green. **B:** Assessment of areas with predominantly epithelial cells (shown in green) and stroma (shown in red). For details on the assessment method, see Danielsen et al., 2018. **C:** An example of a well-differentiated epithelial region with a DoMore-v1-CRC score indicating a good outcome. **D:** An example of a poorly differentiated epithelial region with a DoMore-v1-CRC score indicating poor outcome. C-D: The scale bar in the extracted region is 250 μm. The region extracted from the whole slide image (WSI) is indicated by a black square in the inserted WSI. Scale bar in the inserted WSI is 5 mm.

source codes for training DL systems use such frameworks. Thus, there exist a wide range of open-source codes for training DL systems that anyone can download, use, and relatively easily modify to fit their application and hypotheses. One example of an important advancement prospering on the openness of the DL community is the neural networks called transformers. Originally designed for use in natural language processing (Vaswani et al., 2017), the twin advantage of excelling in handling of long-range dependencies in sequences (like sentences) and efficient use of parallel processing hardware has made these systems completely dominant on language translation and similar tasks. Re-using open-source code available from language applications, Dosovitskiy et al. demonstrated that the same type of network architecture attains excellent results compared to state-of-the-art CNNs for image tasks while requiring substantially less computational resources to train (Dosovitskiy et al., 2021). Such re-use of source code speeds up developmental processes greatly and facilitates the use of new advancements in other applications. Thus, a continued inflow of new and improved techniques is expected to enable the development of gradually better DL systems for histopathology.

A critical step currently largely lacking in AI-based digital pathology is the transformation of promising DL systems into clinically useful and accepted systems. In addition to being able to explain the basis of the predictions, rigorous evaluation is necessary to be able to trust the AI systems. Failure to evaluate new AI systems properly may have far-reaching consequences, including reduced credibility of findings in AI research more generally and systems of limited value or even harmful to patients if used for decisions on treatment. The challenges arise both from scarcity of suitable data and a lack of routines on how to validate the system performance and test the clinical utility.

The data challenge is partly a straightforward consequence of the demands for data in the development of AI systems and DL systems in particular. Large and representative sets are needed for training an accurate and robust model, and external and representative sets are needed to evaluate its performance reliably in the intended medical setting (Kleppe et al., 2021; Homeyer et al., 2022). Thus, the future development of AI systems is not only a matter of methodological and technical inventions but also of advances in terms of access to well curated data. Such data, from different sources, are not only important to achieve the necessary quantities but also to provide access to heterogeneous data. Representing the diversity naturally occurring in the intended medical setting is seemingly at least as important as size to develop robust DL systems and to evaluate their performance in different parts of the intended medical setting (Kleppe et al., 2021; Homeyer et al., 2022). Positively, the availability of open datasets is growing. Still, increased access to representative data will remain among the most critical factors for further development and clinical implementation of medical AI. This calls for more efforts to solve limiting factors like privacy concerns and legal issues as well as to ensure well-deserved academic credit to those who provide high-quality data.

Reliable validation of AI systems is challenging. It includes verifying that the system generalizes well and performs satisfactorily when evaluated on external cohorts representative of the intended medical setting as well as when input data are obtained using differing laboratory procedures or alternative equipment. This has been a weak point of many studies, but fortunately the importance of validation in external datasets now seems largely adopted by the community and the majority of studies published in high-impact journals now include external tests (Kleppe et al., 2021). What is still often lacking, however, is testing of the performance across the range of differences in patient and sample characteristics as well as predefined protocols identifying both the validation datasets to be used, including what they represent in terms of medical setting and target population, and the primary and secondary analyses to be conducted (Kleppe et al., 2021). Such protocols are essential both for facilitating thorough pre-planning the evaluation process and to prevent repeated or multiple evaluations, which are well known as important contributors to biased inference and irreproducible results.

Compared to drug clinical trials, studies of AI systems for diagnostic purposes may to a larger extent, utilize retrospective data, for example, from earlier clinical trials. However, retrospective studies tend to overlook practical issues and irregularities and may give over-optimistic results. Thus, to bring AI systems into the clinic, we expect in the coming years to see studies specifically designed to evaluate the clinical utility of a specific AI system, including randomized studies designed similarly to pharmaceutical phase 3 trials by using the AI system to intervene directly with the current standard of care. Such studies require time but may be needed to ensure the real-life efficacy of the systems and then also to generate the necessary trust in the AI systems.

Declaration of interests

TSH, KL, and HED report filing of a patent application entitled 'Histological image analysis' with International Patent Application Number PCT/EP2018/080828. AK, TSH, KL, and HED report filing of a patent application entitled 'Histological image analysis' with International Patent Application Number PCT/EP2020/076090.

Acknowledgements

The authors thank Marian Seiergren for their help with creating the figures and Ole-Johan Skrede for comments.

Håvard Emil Danielsen passed away far too soon, before the publication of this work. Håvard's dedication and expertise greatly enriched our work and will continue to inspire us. His wide-ranging contributions to digital pathology, medical diagnostics and cancer biomedicine will have a lasting impact on the field and play a vital role in advancing personalized treatments for the benefit of cancer patients. Rest in peace, dear colleague and friend.

REFERENCES

Abousamra, S., Gupta, R., Hou, L., et al. (2022). Deep learning-based mapping of tumor infiltrating lymphocytes in whole slide images of 23 types of cancer. *Frontiers in Oncology*, *11*, 806603.

Anderson, N. M., & Simon, M.C. (2020). The tumor microenvironment. *Current Biology*, *30*(16), R921–R5.

André, T., Boni, C., Navarro, M., et al. (2009). Improved overall survival with oxaliplatin, fluorouracil, and leucovorin as adjuvant treatment in stage II or III colon cancer in the MOSAIC Trial. *Journal of Clinical Oncology*, *27*(19), 3109–3116.

Awan, R., Sirinukunwattana, K., Epstein, D., et al. (2017). Glandular morphometrics for objective grading of colorectal adenocarcinoma histology images. *Science Reports*, *7*(1), 16852.

Bach, S., Binder, A., Montavon, G., et al. (2015). On pixel-wise explanations for non-linear classifier decisions by layer-wise relevance propagation. *PLoS One*, *10*(7), e0130140.

Ben Hamida, A., Devanne, M., Weber, J., et al. (2021). Deep learning for colon cancer histopathological images analysis. *Computers in Biology and Medicine*, *136*: 104730.

Bera, K., Schalper, K. A., Rimm, D. L., et al. (2019). Artificial intelligence in digital pathology—new tools for diagnosis and precision oncology. *Nature Reviews Clinical Oncology*, *16*(11), 703–715.

Bilal, M., Raza, S. E. A., Azam, A., et al. (2021). Development and validation of a weakly supervised deep learning framework to predict the status of molecular pathways and key mutations in colorectal cancer from routine histology images: a retrospective study. *Lancet Digital Health*, *3*(12), e763–772.

Boehm, K. M., Khosravi, P., Vanguri, R., et al. (2022). Harnessing multimodal data integration to advance precision oncology. *Nature Reviews Cancer*, *22*(2), 114–26.

Bychkov D., Linder N., Turkki R., et al. (2018). Deep learning based tissue analysis predicts outcome in colorectal cancer. *Science Reports*, *8*(1), 3395.

Cao, R., Yang, F., Ma, S.-C., et al. (2020). Development and interpretation of a pathomics-based model for the prediction of microsatellite instability in colorectal cancer. *Theranostics* *10*(24), 11080–11091.

Chen, R. J., Chen, C., Li, Y., et al. (2022). Scaling vision transformers to gigapixel images via hierarchical self-supervised learning. *Proceedings of the IEEE Conference on Computer Vision and Pattern Recognition*, 16144–16155.

Chen, R. J., Lu, M. Y., Weng, W. H., et al. (2021). Multimodal co-attention transformer for survival prediction in gigapixel whole slide images. *Proceedings of the IEEE Conference on Computer Vision and Pattern Recognition*, 3995–4005.

Danielsen, H. E., Pradhan, M., & Novelli, M. (2016). Revisiting tumour aneuploidy–the place of ploidy assessment in the molecular era. *Nature Reviews Clinical Oncology*, *13*(5), 291–304.

Danielsen, H. E., Hveem, T. S., Domingo, E., et al. (2018). Prognostic markers for colorectal cancer: estimating ploidy and stroma. *Annals of Oncology*, *29*(3), 616–623.

Dice, L. R. (1945). Measures of the amount of ecologic association between species. *Ecology*, *26*(3), 297–302.

Dosovitskiy, A., Beyer, L., Kolesnikov, A., et al. (2021). An image is worth 16×16 words: transformers for image recognition at scale. *Proceedings of the International Conference on Learning Representation.*

Echle, A,. Ghaffari Laleh, N., Quirke, P., et al. (2022). Artificial intelligence for detection of microsatellite instability in colorectal cancer—a multicentric analysis of a pre-screening tool for clinical application. *ESMO Open*, *7*(2)

Echle, A., Grabsch, H. I., Quirke, P., et al. (2020). Clinical-grade detection of microsatellite instability in colorectal tumors by deep learning. *Gastroenterology*, *159*(4), 1406–1416.e11.

Fu, Y., Jung, A. W., Torne, R. V., et al. (2020). Pan-cancer computational histopathology reveals mutations, tumor composition and prognosis. *Nature Cancer*, *1*(8), 800–810.

Geessink, O. G. F., Baidoshvili, A., Klaase, J. M., et al. (2019). Computer aided quantification of intratumoral stroma yields an independent prognosticator in rectal cancer. *Cell Oncology*, *42*(3), 331–341.

Glaire, M. A., Domingo, E., Sveen, A., et al. (2019). Tumour-infiltrating CD8+ lymphocytes and colorectal cancer recurrence by tumour and nodal stage. *British Journal of Cancer*, *121*(6), 474–482.

Gray, R., Barnwell, J., McConkey, C., et al. (2007). Adjuvant chemotherapy versus observation in patients with colorectal cancer: a randomised study. *Lancet*, *370*(9604), 2020–2029.

Greenson, J. K., Bonner, J. D., Ben-Yzhak, O., et al. (2003). Phenotype of microsatellite unstable colorectal carcinomas: well-differentiated and focally mucinous tumors and the absence of dirty necrosis correlate with microsatellite instability. *American Journal of Surgical Pathology*, *27*(5), 563–570.

Greenson, J. K., Huang, S.-C., Herron, C., et al. (2009). Pathologic predictors of microsatellite instability in colorectal cancer. *American Journal of Surgical Pathology*, *33*(1), 126–133.

Homeyer, A., Geißler, C., Schwen, L. O., et al. (2022). Recommendations on compiling test datasets for evaluating artificial intelligence solutions in pathology. *Modern Pathology*.

Hveem, T. S., Merok, M. A., Pretorius, M. E., et al. (2014). Prognostic impact of genomic instability in colorectal cancer. *British Journal of Cancer*, *110*(8), 2159–2164.

Ichimasa, K., Kudo, S.-E., Miyachi, H., et al. (2021). Risk stratification of T1 colorectal cancer metastasis to lymph nodes: current status and perspective. *Gut Liver*, *15*(6), 818–826.

Idos, G.E., Kwok, J., Bonthala, N., et al. (2020). The prognostic implications of tumor infiltrating lymphocytes in colorectal cancer: a systematic review and meta-analysis. *Science Reports*, *10*(1), 3360.

Iizuka, O., Kanavati, F., Kato, K., et al. (2020). Deep learning models for histopathological classification of gastric and colonic epithelial tumours. *Science Reports*, *10*(1), 1504.

Jaccard, P. The distribution of the flora in the alpine zone. (1912). *New Phytologist*, *11*(2), 37–50.

Jenkins, M. A., Hayashi, S., O'Shea, A.-M., et al. (2007). Pathology features in Bethesda Guidelines predict colorectal cancer microsatellite instability: a population-based study. *Gastroenterology*, *133*(1), 48–56.

Jiang, D., Hveem, T. S., Glaire, M., et al. (2021). Automated assessment of CD8+ T-lymphocytes and stroma fractions complement conventional staging of colorectal cancer. *EBioMedicine*, *71*.

Jiang, D., Liao, J., Duan, H., et al. (2020). A machine learning-based prognostic predictor for stage III colon cancer. *Science Reports*, *10*(1), 10333.

Kather, J. N., Heij, L. R., Grabsch, H. I., et al. (2020). Pan-cancer image-based detection of clinically actionable genetic alterations. *Nature Cancer*, *1*(8), 789–799.

Kather, J. N., Krisam, J., Charoentong, P., et al. (2019). Predicting survival from colorectal cancer histology slides using deep learning: A retrospective multicenter study. *PLoS Medicine*, *16*(1), e1002730.

Kather, J. N., Pearson, A. T., Halama, N., et al. (2019). Deep learning can predict microsatellite instability directly from histology in gastrointestinal cancer. *Nature Medicine*, *25*(7), 1054–1056.

Ke, J., Shen, Y., Wright, J. D., et al. (2020). Identifying patch-level MSI from histological images of colorectal cancer by a knowledge distillation model. *Proceedings of the IEEE International Conference on Bioinformatics and Biomedicine*, 1043–1046.

Kim, H., Yoon, H., Thakur, N., et al. (2021). Deep learning-based histopathological segmentation for whole slide images of colorectal cancer in a compressed domain. *Science Reports*, *11*(1), 22520.

Kleppe, A. (2022). Area under the curve may hide poor generalisation to external datasets. *ESMO Open*, *7*(2).

Kleppe, A., & Danielsen, H. E. (2018). Clinical utility of chromatin analysis. *Oncotarget*, *9*(65), 32406–32407.

Kleppe, A., Albregtsen, F., Vlatkovic, L., et al. (2018). Chromatin organisation and cancer prognosis: a pan-cancer study. *Lancet Oncology*, *19*(3), 356–369.

Kleppe, A., Skrede, O.-J., De Raedt, S., et al. (2021). Designing deep learning studies in cancer diagnostics. *Nature Reviews Cancer*, *21*(3), 199–211.

Kleppe, A., Skrede, O.-J., De Raedt, S., et al. (2022). A clinical decision support system optimising adjuvant chemotherapy for colorectal cancers by integrating deep learning and pathological staging markers: a development and validation study. *Lancet Oncology*, *23*(9), 1221–1232.

Komura, D., Kawabe, A., Fukuta, K., et al. (2022). Universal encoding of pan-cancer histology by deep texture representations. *Cell Reports*, *38*(9).

Korbar, B., Olofson, A., Miraflor, A., et al. (2017). Deep learning for classification of colorectal polyps on whole-slide images. *Journal of Pathology Informatics*, *8*(1), 30.

Kudo, S.-E., Ichimasa, K., Villard, B., et al. (2021). Artificial intelligence system to determine risk of T1 colorectal cancer metastasis to lymph node. *Gastroenterology*, *160*(4), 1075–1084.e2.

Kwak, M. S., Lee, H. H., Yang, J. M., et al. (2021). Deep convolutional neural network-based lymph node metastasis prediction for colon cancer using histopathological images. *Frontiers in Oncology*, *10*.

Lee, H., Seo, J., Lee, G., et al. (2021a) Two-stage classification method for MSI status prediction based on deep learning approach. *Applied Science*, *11*(1), 254.

Lee, S. H., Song, I. H., & Jang, H.-J. (2021b) Feasibility of deep learning-based fully automated classification of microsatellite instability in tissue slides of colorectal cancer. *International Journal of Cancer*, *149*(3), 728–740.

Levin, T. R., Corley, D. A., Jensen, C. D., et al. (2018). Effects of organized colorectal cancer screening on cancer incidence and mortality in a large community-based population. *Gastroenterology*, *155*(5), 1383–1391.e5.

Li, X., Jonnagaddala, J., Yang, S., et al. (2023). A retrospective analysis using deep-learning models for predicting survival outcome and benefit of adjuvant I chemotherapy in stage II/III colorectal cancer. *Journal of Cancer Research and Clinical Oncology*.

Li, Y., Liao, L., Kong, L., et al. (2022). DNA ploidy and stroma predicted the risk of recurrence in low-risk stage III colorectal cancer. *Clinical and Translational Oncology*, *25*, 218–225.

Liu, H., Zhao, Y., Yang, F., et al. (2022). Preoperative prediction of lymph node metastasis in colorectal cancer with deep learning. *BME Frontiers*, *2022*: 9860179.

Lugli, A., Zlobec, I., Berger, M. D., et al. (2021). Tumour budding in solid cancers. *Nature Reviews Clinical Oncology*, *18*(2), 101–115.

Mesker, W. E., Junggeburt, J. M. C., Szuhai, K., et al. (2007). The carcinoma–stromal ratio of colon carcinoma is an independent factor for survival compared to lymph node status and tumor stage. *Cell Oncology*, *29*: 387–398.

Mobadersany, P., Yousefi, S., Amgad, M., et al. (2018). Predicting cancer outcomes from histology and genomics using convolutional networks. *Proceedings of the National Academy of Sciences USA, 115*(13), E2970.

Nasir-Moin, M., Suriawinata, A. A., Ren, B., et al. (2021). Evaluation of an artificial intelligence–augmented digital system for histologic classification of colorectal polyps. *JAMA Network Open, 4*(11), e2135271.

Noorbakhsh, J., Farahmand, S., Foroughi Pour, A., et al. (2020). Deep learning-based cross-classifications reveal conserved spatial behaviors within tumor histological images. *Nature Communication, 11*(1), 6367.

Pai, R. K., Hartman, D., Schaeffer, D. F., et al. (2021). Development and initial validation of a deep learning algorithm to quantify histological features in colorectal carcinoma including tumour budding/poorly differentiated clusters. *Histopathology, 79*(3), 391–405.

Peng, J., Li, W., Fan, W., et al. (2021). Prognostic value of a novel biomarker combining DNA ploidy and tumor burden score for initially resectable liver metastases from patients with colorectal cancer. *Cancer Cell International, 21*(1), 554.

Popovici, V., Budinská, E., Dušek, L., et al. (2017). Image-based surrogate biomarkers for molecular subtypes of colorectal cancer. *Bioinformatics, 33*(13), 2002–2009.

Rutter, M. D., East, J., Rees, C. J., et al. (2020). British Society of Gastroenterology/Association of Coloproctology of Great Britain and Ireland/Public Health England post-polypectomy and post-colorectal cancer resection surveillance guidelines. *Gut, 69*(2), 201–223.

Schmauch, B., Romagnoni, A., Pronier, E., et al. (2020). A deep learning model to predict RNA-Seq expression of tumours from whole slide images. *Nature Communication, 11*(1), 3877.

Schrammen, P. L., Ghaffari Laleh, N., Echle, A., et al. (2022). Weakly supervised annotation-free cancer detection and prediction of genotype in routine histopathology. *Journal of Pathology, 256*(1), 50–60.

Seymour, M. T., Maughan, T. S., Ledermann, J. A., et al. (2007). Different strategies of sequential and combination chemotherapy for patients with poor prognosis advanced colorectal cancer (MRC FOCUS): a randomised controlled trial. *Lancet, 370*(9582), 143–152.

Shapcott, M., Hewitt, K. J., & Rajpoot, N. (2019). Deep learning with sampling in colon cancer histology. *Frontiers in Bioengineering and Biotechnology, 7*: 52.

Shorten, C., & Khoshgoftaar, T. M. (2019). A survey on image data augmentation for deep learning. *Journal of Big Data, 6*(1), 60.

Sirinukunwattana, K., Domingo, E., Richman, S. D., et al. (2021). Image-based consensus molecular subtype (imCMS) classification of colorectal cancer using deep learning. *Gut, 70*(3), 544–554.

Sirinukunwattana, K., Pluim, J. P. W., Chen, H., et al. (2017). Gland segmentation in colon histology images: the GlaS challenge contest. *Medical Image Analysis, 35*: 489–502.

Sirinukunwattana, K., Raza, S. E. A., Tsang, Y. W., et al. (2016). Locality sensitive deep learning for detection and classification of nuclei in routine colon cancer histology images. *IEEE Transactions on Medical Imaging, 35*(5), 1196–1206.

Sirinukunwattana, K., Snead, D., Epstein, D., et al. (2018). Novel digital signatures of tissue phenotypes for predicting distant metastasis in colorectal cancer. *Science Reports, 8*(1), 13692.

Skrede, O.-J., De Raedt, S., Kleppe, A., et al. (2020). Deep learning for prediction of colorectal cancer outcome: a discovery and validation study. *Lancet, 395*(10221), 350–360.

Song, J. H., Hong, Y., Kim, E. R., et al. (2022). Utility of artificial intelligence with deep learning of hematoxylin and eosin-stained whole slide images to predict lymph node metastasis in T1 colorectal cancer using endoscopically resected specimens; prediction of lymph node metastasis in T1 colorectal cancer. *Journal of Gastroenterology, 57*(9), 654–666.

Sundararajan, M., Taly, A., & Yan, Q. (2017). Axiomatic attribution for deep networks. *Proceedings of the 34th International Conference on Machine Learning, 70*: 3319–3328.

Takamatsu, M., Yamamoto, N., Kawachi, H., et al. (2022). Prediction of lymph node metastasis in early colorectal cancer based on histologic images by artificial intelligence. *Science Reports, 12*(1), 2963.

Van Cutsem, E., Labianca, R., Bodoky, G., et al. (2009). Randomized phase III trial comparing biweekly infusional fluorouracil/leucovorin alone or with irinotecan in the adjuvant treatment of stage III colon cancer: PETACC-3. *Journal of Clinical Oncology, 27*(19), 3117–3125.

van der Laak, J., Litjens, G., & Ciompi, F. (2021). Deep learning in histopathology: the path to the clinic. *Nature Medicine, 27*(5), 775–784.

van Pelt, G. W., Sandberg, T. P., Morreau, H., et al. (2018). The tumour–stroma ratio in colon cancer: the biological role and its prognostic impact. *Histopathology, 73*(2), 197–206.

Vaswani, A., Shazeer, N., Parmar, N., et al. (2017). Attention is all you need. *Advances in Neural Information Processing Systems, 30*: 1–11.

Wei, J. W., Suriawinata, A. A., Vaickus, L. J., et al. (2020). Evaluation of a deep neural network for automated classification of colorectal polyps on histopathologic slides. *JAMA Network Open, 3*(4), e203398.

Weis, C.-A., Kather, J. N., Melchers, S., et al. (2018). Automatic evaluation of tumour budding in immunohistochemically stained colorectal carcinomas and correlation to clinical outcome. *Diagnostic Pathology, 13*(1), 64.

Wulczyn, E., Steiner, D. F., Xu, Z., et al. (2020). Deep learning-based survival prediction for multiple cancer types using histopathology images. *PLoS One, 15*(6), e0233678.

Wulczyn, E., Steiner, D. F., Moran, M., et al. (2021). Interpretable survival prediction for colorectal cancer using deep learning. *NPJ Digital Medicine, 4*(1), 71.

Xu, H., Cha, Y. J., Clemenceau, J. R., et al. (2022). Spatial analysis of tumour-infiltrating lymphocytes in histological sections using deep learning techniques predicts survival in colorectal carcinoma. *Journal of Pathology: Clinical Research, 8*(4), 327–339.

Xu, L., Walker, B., Liang, P.-I., et al. (2020). Colorectal cancer detection based on deep learning. *Journal of Pathology Informatics, 11*(1), 28.

Yamashita, R., Long, J., Banda, S., et al. (2021a). Learning domain-agnostic visual representation for computational pathology using medically-irrelevant style transfer augmentation. *IEEE Transactions on Medical Imaging, 40*(12), 3945–3954.

Yamashita, R., Long, J., Longacre, T., et al. (2021b). Deep learning model for the prediction of microsatellite instability in colorectal cancer: a diagnostic study. *Lancet Oncology, 22*(1), 132–141.

Yang, L., Chen, P., Zhang, L., et al. (2020). Prognostic value of nucleotyping, DNA ploidy and stroma in high-risk stage II colon cancer. *British Journal of Cancer, 123*(6), 973–981.

Zhao, K., Li, Z., Yao, S., et al. (2020). Artificial intelligence quantified tumour-stroma ratio is an independent predictor for overall survival in resectable colorectal cancer. *eBioMedicine, 61*.

Zhao, Z., Zhang, X., Li, Z., et al. (2021). Automated assessment of DNA ploidy, chromatin organization, and stroma fraction to predict prognosis and adjuvant therapy response in patients with stage II colorectal carcinoma. *American Journal of Cancer Research, 11*(12), 6119–6132.

9

Artificial intelligence and radiomics

Meng Dou, Zhebin Chen, Xianhong Xu, Xiaojing Gu, Xuejiao Li, and Xin Wang

Introduction

Medical imaging began in 1895 when German physicist Wilhelm Konrad Rontgen discovered X-rays. There was a relative lull in development until, in 1978, G. N. Hounsfield published computed tomography (CT) technology, which is considered to be one of the greatest achievements of science and technology in the twentieth century. Since then, medical imaging has developed rapidly, and various new medical imaging devices and technologies have been continuously presented. Medical imaging has played a vital role in cancer screening, diagnosis, and treatment of patients. On the other hand, the rise of modern artificial intelligence in recent years has led to breakthroughs in computer vision and pattern recognition, and the growth of medical big data provides an excellent opportunity for artificial intelligence applications to medical imaging analysis and correlation with the multiple molecular events that are associated with diseases initiation and progression. In this context, radiomics emerges as a new research area that integrates artificial intelligence and machine learning to extract pathophysiological information from region of interests (ROIs), thus enabling cancer diagnosis, tumour staging, therapeutic evaluation, and prognosis assessment.

In recent years, due to advances in storage and information technology, the medical image information has been well preserved digitally. Compared with previous research based on small samples, the ever-growing number of medical images brings new research opportunities: (i) based on a large amount of imaging data, a more accurate machine learning model can be established to improve the level of diagnosis and detection of computer-aided diagnosis systems so that its accuracy is comparable to human-level diagnosis; (ii) more complex and expressive machine learning methods can play a better role with big data, thus mining more potential models and information from massive imaging data. The accumulation of medical image big data and the rapid development of artificial intelligence technology directly promote a novel comprehensive method of analysis in medicine.

Radiomics is an emerging medical image analysis method proposed by (Lambin et al., 2012), which refers to the high-throughput extraction of a large number of image features from radiological images. In the same year, Kumar et al. supplemented the definition of radiomics to high-throughput extraction and analysis of a large number of advanced quantitative image features from CT, positron emission tomography (PET), and magnetic resonance imaging (MRI) (Kumar et al., 2012), expanding the imaging modality and adding quantification analysis. In 2014, Aerts et al. published a breakthrough application in *Nature Communications*, pointing out the prognostic ability of radiomics (Aerts et al., 2014). In general, radiomics refers to the extraction and analysis of highly representative quantitative image features from clinically large-scale imaging data—that is, using a large number of automated data feature description algorithms, the imaging data were transformed into high-dimensional extensible feature space, and the disease diagnosis and prediction of the case data were completed by comparing and analysing the imaging data with clinical information. Furthermore, the radiomics analysis is based on the assumption that the quantitative image-based parameters have a certain correlation with the molecular phenotype or genotype of the tumour. Radiomics post-processes the medical images that need to be collected in clinical diagnosis and treatment, extracts information that is impossible to see with the naked eye, and combines with other genomic, metabolic, and protein data to improve the treatment response prediction and prognosis of the tumour. Thus, personalized treatment of the patient can be achieved.

Radiomics generally refers to the use of CT, PET, MRI, or ultrasound imaging as input data, extracting expressive features from massive image-based databanks, and then using machine learning or statistical models for quantitative analysis. Compared with the traditional practice of using only manual viewing, radiomics analysis can extract high-dimensional features that are difficult to describe quantitatively in human visuals and correlate them with clinical and pathological information to achieve the prediction of certain diseases or genes. Using advanced bioinformatics tools and machine learning methods, researchers are able to develop potential models that improve the prediction accuracy of diagnostic and prognostic approaches (Gillies et al., 2016).

Due to the pathological characteristics of different tumour types, they can have different imaging appearances. Different tumour image features also can suggest completely different treatment methods, which can then directly affect the prognosis. At present, based on the subjective clinical experience of the clinician, prejudgement of the tumour is achieved through medical images. Based on the existing medical image feature analysis, some multidimensional texture features can accurately reflect the pathological information of the diseased tissue, which has important research value for the realization of individualized medical treatment. Therefore, a complete feature database can filter the subsequent key features and provide more comprehensive data support. The use of radiomics methods to assist in the predictive analysis of tumours and to give credible recommendations has the potential to be of great practical significance.

Radiomics analysis mainly extracts and quantifies the features associated with a diagnosis from images. For example, in the CT images of tumours, there are differences in the shape, size, and texture and these can be associated with different pathological grades. These features are often used by clinicians as a basis for manual diagnosis, but the diagnostic results are subjective and relevant to the radiologists' experience, which makes it difficult to realize objective and repeatable diagnosis results. However, in the analysis of radiomics, the features of these clinicians' qualitative descriptions can be quantitatively described by mathematical expressions from the perspective of images, thus providing an objective and repeatable diagnosis. Radiomics attempts to extract image features associated with diagnostic results through a large number of medical images, and directly analyses results via the images, rather than just simple image processing, thereby allowing a much more objective assessment. For example, researchers extracted high-dimensional image features of primary cancer by radiomics and found that these features were highly correlated with the staging of colorectal cancer, and a radiomics signature was generated using these features to discriminate stage I–II and stage III–IV colorectal cancer (Liang et al., 2016).

In traditional genetic analysis, whether a gene is mutated is determined by gene sequencing of tumour tissue sampled from a certain location of the tumour. However, due to the heterogeneity of the tumour, genetic mutations may occur in other parts of the tumour that are not sampled. Therefore, traditional genetic analysis may have sampling errors. The mutated gene affects the growth of the tumour and is thus expressed in the imaging data (Gillies et al., 2016). Radiomic features can be extracted from the overall tumour image, which contains more complete topological information. The genetic analysis in radiomics can complement the traditional genetic analysis to improve diagnostic accuracy. At present, the clinical application of radiomics mainly includes auxiliary diagnosis, treatment evaluation, and prognosis prediction. With the development of medical image big data, more abundant image data will further enable the application of artificial intelligence methods. At the same time, excellent clinical manifestations obtained by various advanced pattern recognition methods also enable the application of radiomics in auxiliary diagnosis, treatment evaluation, and prognosis prediction (Parmar et al., 2015).

Methodology of radiomics

The key technologies of radiomics include the ROIs segmentation, feature extraction, feature selection, radiomics model construction, and model evaluation. In order to measure the performance of the radiomics model, a unified quality assessment system is also needed to measure the clinical value of the developed model. In radiomics research, it is necessary to use artificial or automatic algorithms for tumour segmentation (detection), then massive radiomics feature extraction for the tumour ROI region. Since the extracted features contain high-latitude irrelevant information, feature dimensionality reduction of radiomic features is needed to identify key radiomic features. Finally, a small number of key radiomic features are used for the modelling analysis to provide clinically available radiomics models (Fig. 9.1).

Image acquisition and ROI segmentation

Due to the different reconstruction methods and slice thickness of different scanners, the parameters (such as resolution) of images are also greatly different. In order to reduce the differences, on the one hand it is possible to reduce the difference in parameters as much as possible by formulating a series of clinical medical image acquisition specifications. On the other hand, it is possible to select features that have high reproducibility between different patients, sufficient dynamics range (Balagurunathan et al., 2014), and which are insensitive to image acquisition protocols and reconstruction algorithms in the analysis process.

Radiomics analysis extracts features from the ROIs, including tumours, normal tissues, and other anatomical structures. The accurate segmentation of the ROIs is very important for feature quantification, feature extraction, and statistical analysis. The manual segmentation results of experienced radiologists are often used as the gold standard, but this method is very time-consuming and has very large subjectivity. Therefore, it is not suitable for radiomics analysis based on large data volume medical images. The research of robust automatic or semi-automatic segmentation methods is a very important part of radiomics analysis, such as pulmonary nodules segmentation, pulmonary nodules segmentation based on the central pooling convolutional neural network (Wang et al., 2017) (CF-CNN), and tumour segmentation based on full convolution. Tumour segmentation determines the region of interest that will be analysed in subsequent steps of radiomics.

Feature extraction

Radiomic feature extraction is a crucial step in radiomics that captures quantitative characteristics of ROIs. This process can be performed after the tumour area is segmented. There are various methods available for extracting rich tumour information with clinical value from medical imaging. Radiomics features can be divided into two categories: artificial design features and deep learning features.

Artificial design features are classical method that describe image information. These features include low-level visual features and high-dimensional non-linear features, which can reflect tumour information from multiple scales. Artificial design features can be divided into three categories: intensity features, shape features, and texture features. Although these features have a clear calculation formula and strong interpretability, they are difficult to design and lack adaptability for different investigations. For example, the definition formula is required to design new features, which leads to inflexibility, dependence on expert knowledge, and weak scalability. Additionally, it is difficult to take different clinical labels into account for different clinical research. In the design of artificially designed features, research generally focuses on depicting tumour information from multiple perspectives, but designing features consistent

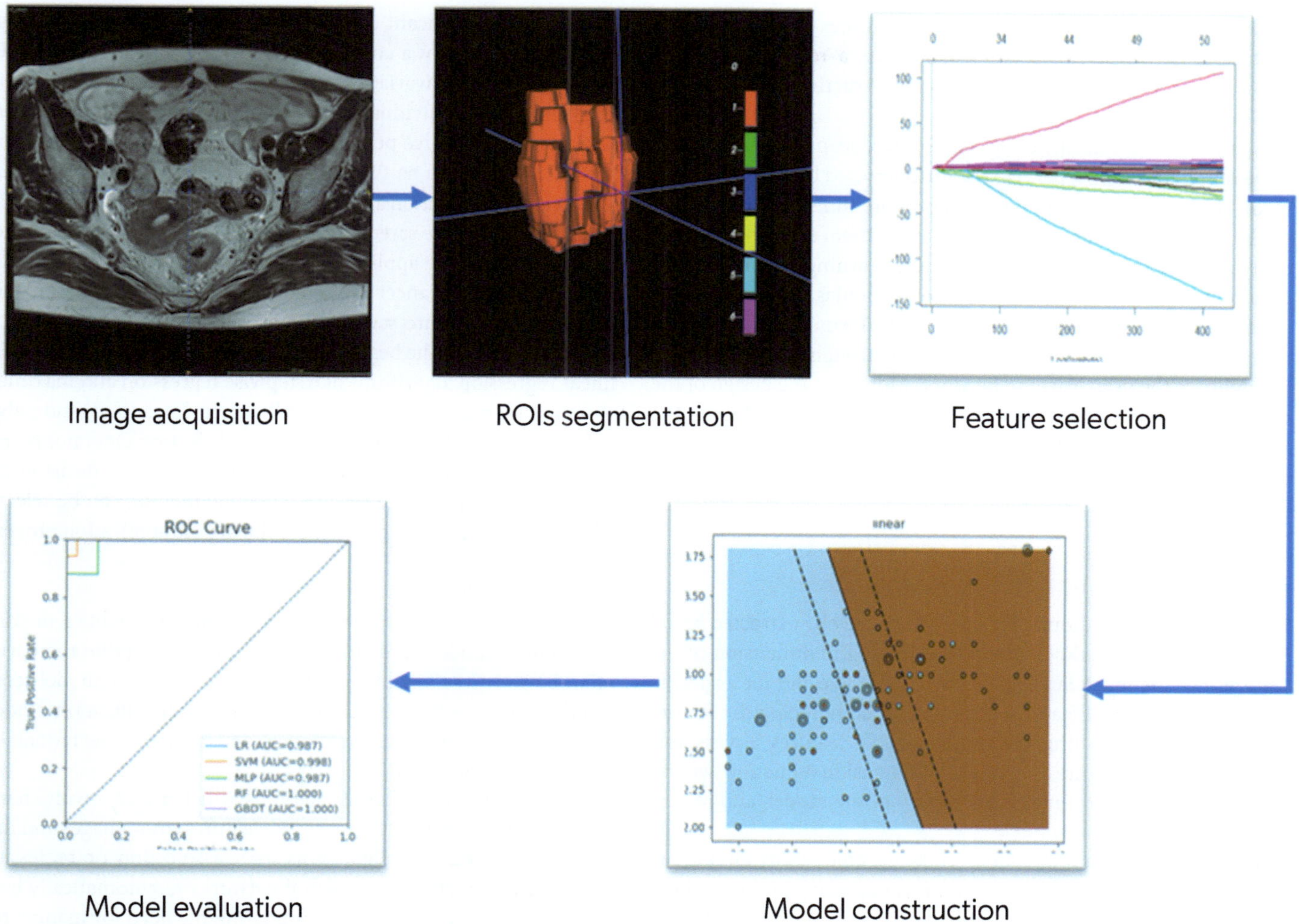

Figure 9.1 An MRI-based radiomics analysis workflow.

with clinical labels or designing different features for different topics is sometimes unfeasible (Table 9.1).

In contrast, deep learning has the ability to learn features automatically from data through its powerful self-learning feature rather than relying on manual feature design. Deep learning algorithms use a stacked neural network structure, and feature extraction can be achieved in two ways: (i) by training a deep model such as convolutional neural networks or transformer-based networks then regarding the output of its fully connected layer as a deep learning feature; (ii) by training an auto-encoder with unlabelled data and regarding the output of the encoder as a deep learning feature. When there are labelled data available to train the supervised learning model, researchers usually train a small network and apply the first method to extract the deep learning feature, collecting the output of its fully connected layer as the deep learning feature. In the study by Yu et al. (2017), researchers constructed a three-layer CNN to predict epidermal growth factor receptor (EGFR) gene mutations in lung cancer. After the CNN is trained, the author extracted 30-dimensional deep learning features of the fully connected layer and trained the SVM classifier separately. In the test set, the deep learning feature reached 0.668 area under receiver operating characteristic (ROC) curve (AUC). When the set of labelled data is extremely small to train the supervised CNN, the auto-encoder help to learn the features of deep learning automatically by unsupervised learning. In another study (Wang et al., 2018), a typical model of auto-encoder is constructed to extract deep learning features.

The training of the auto-encoder only requires the medical image, without the need for clinical labels. In contrast to supervised learning, the auto-encoder utilizes an encoder network to extract deep learning features. These features are then used by the decoder network to reconstruct the original images, allowing for the evaluation of the amount of information contained within the deep learning features. When the deep learning features successfully

Table 9.1 Details of different radiomics settings

Filters	Features
Laplacian of Gaussian	First-order Statistics
Wavelet	Shape-based (2D and 3D)
Square	Grey Level Co-occurrence Matrix
Square Root	Grey Level Run Length Matrix
Logarithm	Grey Level Size Zone Matrix
Exponential	Grey Level Dependence Matrix
Gradient	Neighbouring Grey Tone Difference Matrix
Local Binary Pattern (2D /3D)	

reconstruct the original input images, it indicates that they already capture most of the image information. As a result, these deep learning features play a crucial role in constructing the model for clinical prediction.

Compared to artificially designed features, deep learning features are acquired through supervised or unsupervised learning from the medical image. As a result, these features are inherently connected to clinical labels or tumour images, making them superior to artificially defined features. Additionally, deep learning features do not require manual definition of calculation formulas. This means that certain features, which may be difficult to formulate but are still meaningful, can be automatically obtained through the self-learning capability of the deep learning network. Moreover, the design of the deep learning network structure is flexible. By simply altering the network structure or training mode, different deep learning features can be achieved. However, it should be noted that features learned through deep learning on small-scale data are not as robust as features designed artificially.

Feature selection and dimension reduction

A large number of radiomic features can usually be extracted based on the extraction methods described above. The dimension of the features may be much larger than the sample size, but for a specific analysis target not all features are valuable, so reducing the feature dimension, and selecting the most valuable features is very important. Through feature selection and dimension reduction, we will reduce overfitting, promote the accuracy of the model, and reduce the training time of the model.

Since there is often redundancy or strong collinearity among the extracted high-dimensional features, it is necessary to screen these features and identify the best combination to enhance the prediction accuracy of the model. In situations where there are numerous features, a three-step feature screening process is typically employed. This process involves eliminating features with significant differences between observers, conducting univariate feature screening, and finally performing multivariable feature screening. The steps are as follows: (i) eliminate features with large intra-observer and inter-observer differences: to reduce the impact of human factors on feature calculation, compare the differences in features between observers and within observers. The robustness of features can be reflected by calculating the inter-group consistency coefficient, and features with significant differences can be eliminated by setting a threshold. Generally, a consistency coefficient threshold of 0.7~0.8 can be used. (ii) Univariate feature screening: analyse the predictive performance of individual features one by one to identify features with higher predictive performance. This method includes various statistical tests such as two independent samples t-test, rank sum test, Pearson correlation analysis, and recursive elimination method. Additionally, feature screening methods based on the double difference method can be applied to evaluate the efficacy of neoadjuvant therapy for rectal cancer and obtain key feature information. (iii) Multi-variable feature screening: find the optimal combination of features to achieve the best prediction effect. This can be done using linear regression algorithms like stepwise regression and maximum R-square increment method, as well as non-linear regression algorithms like Least Absolute Shrinkage and Selection Operator regression (LASSO regression), elastic-net regression, and decision tree analysis. The appropriate feature screening method can be selected based on the specific circumstances during the application process.

Model construction and evaluation

After the completed feature selection and dimensionality reduction, a radiomics model needs to be established to describe the correlation between the feature and the predicted tag. The models commonly used in radiomics include basic linear classification models, tree models, linear regression models, and deep learning models developed in recent years.

Unlike traditional radiomic methods, which usually involve hand-designed feature extractors to extract features from images and then use machine learning algorithms for classification or regression, deep learning methods use neural networks to automatically learn features from images, thereby eliminating the need for manual feature extractors. Deep learning methods typically require more data and computing resources, but often achieve better performance. CNN is a feed-forward neural network and treats each pixel in the image and the points around it as a whole by convolution, so that small images can be learned as features instead of learning from each pixel (Fig. 9.2). This allows the classifier to learn the features and methods from the picture itself, rather than providing features to the classifier by humans. On the one hand, it breaks through the limitations of human design features, and on the other hand, it completes an end-to-end work-flow that can automatically study the problem.

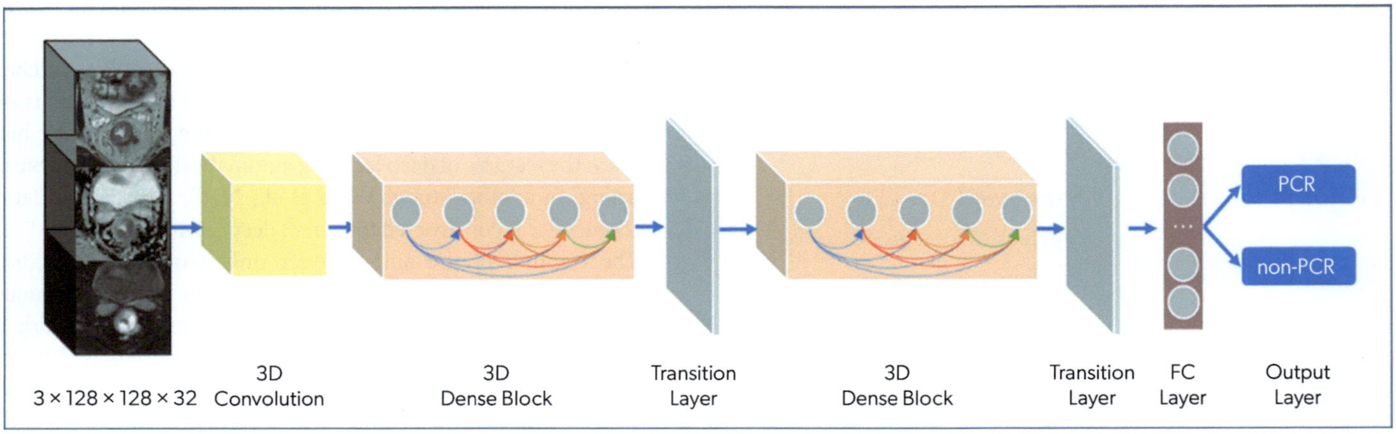

Figure 9.2 CNN network to predict outcome in rectal cancer using multi-parametric MRI images.

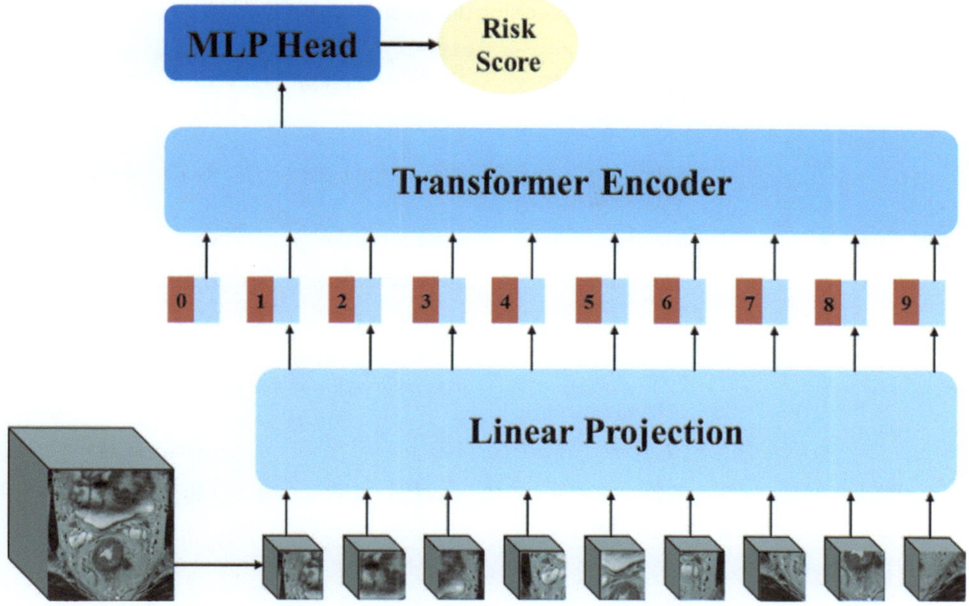

Figure 9.3 Vision transformer network to predict outcome in rectal cancer. MLP = multilayer perceptron.

The Vision Transformer (VIT) is a transformer specifically designed for computer vision. Originally intended for natural language processing, the transformer was adapted to computer vision in 2020, resulting in VIT. The basic structure of VIT involves decomposing the input image into patches, tokenizing it, and then applying the tokens to the standard transformer architecture (Fig. 9.3). The attention mechanism in VIT repeatedly transforms the representation vector of image patches to incorporate more semantic relationships in the image. Compared to CNN, VIT uses a self-attention mechanism to capture global relationships in images, enabling it to handle global information better. As a result, VITs are increasingly used in the field of medical image analysis.

The model's performance can be assessed using indicators such as accuracy, sensitivity, and specificity. The area under the curve (AUC) is also a commonly used indicator for evaluating model performance. All the evaluation indicators have values between 0 and 1. The closer the value is to 1, the better the model's prediction performance. Additionally, the calibration curve can be used to assess the consistency between the model's predicted efficacy and the true efficacy. The decision analysis curve can evaluate the potential clinical benefits that the model may offer to patients. To facilitate clinical application, the model can also be visualized by creating a nomogram.

Application of radiomics

Precision diagnosis of colorectal cancer

Assisted diagnosis is one of the main clinical applications of radiomics and can be considered as the development of traditional computer-aided diagnosis (CAD) methods based on medical images. The application of radiomics in assisted diagnosis focuses on specific clinical needs, mining a large number of high-throughput features from standardized medical images, and ultimately establishing a generalized quantitative model with high diagnostic efficiency (Lambin et al., 2012). Compared with traditional CAD, the radiomics method is more targeted at the enrolled population and clinical problems, and therefore has more practical value (Gillies et al., 2016). Based on routinely used medical images, radiomics can be widely used in cancer diagnosis, such as screening and staging (Table 9.2).

Colorectal cancer screening

Early screening and diagnosis can greatly help improve patient outcomes, especially those with poor survival rates. Available modalities for CRC screening include invasive (colonoscopy and flexible sigmoidoscopy) and minimally invasive (capsule endoscopy) techniques, imaging tests (computed tomography colonography (CTC)), blood and stool tests, and more. Radiomics can be used as a non-invasive and cost-effective method to screen large populations for colorectal cancer risk using personal health data. In recent years, there have been many radiomics studies on colorectal cancer screening.

Colonoscopy is the most commonly used and widely accepted technique for screening colon cancer, serving as the gold standard. In particular, the identification of polyps in colonoscopy images is crucial for early detection and prevention of cancer. It is also the preferred technology for early diagnosis and prevention of colon cancer. Gessert et al. (2019) utilized two powerful deep learning architectures to detect colon cancer in confocal laser microscopy (CLM) images. These models were pre-trained on the ImageNet dataset, enabling transfer learning due to the limited size of their dataset. These cases illustrate the potential of deep learning architectures in classifying and detecting colon cancer in CLM images.

CTC is a modified CT examination. To improve colorectal polyp detection and classification, artificial intelligence-based algorithms can provide computer-assisted solutions to achieve optimal diagnostic performance and image quality in CTCs. Grosu et al. (2021) developed a machine learning method to differentiate between benign and precancerous CTC-detected colorectal polyps

Table 9.2 Description of studies in the radiomics analysis in precision diagnosis of colorectal cancer

Author, year	Modality	Study population	Outcome	Method	AUC/ACC/C-index
Gessert et al. (2019)	Confocal laser microscopy (CLM)	1,577 images	Cancer detection	CNN	ACC:0.891
Grosu et al. (2021)	CT	63 (training) 59 (validation)	Benign or premalignant	Random Forest	AUC:0.91
Godkhindi and Gowda (2017)	CT	825 cases	polyp detection	CNN	ACC:0.87
Liang et al., (2016)	CT	286 (training) 208 (validation)	preoperative staging	LASSO	AUC:0.79
Sun et al., (2018)	T2 MRI	119 cases	T stage	LASSO	AUC:0.852
Huang et al. (2018)	CT	222 (training) 144 (validation)	high-grade vs low-grade	LASSO	AUC:0.735
Dou et al. (2022)	CT	32 cases	T stage	Decision Tree	-
Huang et al. (2016)	CT	326 cases	Lymph Node Metastasis	Logistic Regression	C-index:0.778

in average-risk asymptomatic CRC screening samples. The current classification algorithm showed promising results with a sensitivity of 82%, a specificity of 85%, and an AUC of 0.91. Godkhindi and Gowda (2017) used CNN after applying some image processing techniques to fully automated cancer diagnosis in CT colonography. This practice divides the colon into types 1, 2, and 3, which can aid in the diagnosis of cancer. Their results showed that CNN with pre-processed CT colonography images is suitable for detecting CRC.

Colorectal cancer staging

Accurate cancer staging determines decisions about cancer treatment strategies, and there are significant differences in the effectiveness of cancer treatment and palliative care at different stages. The tumour lymph node metastasis (TNM) staging system proposed by the American Joint Committee on Cancer (AJCC) is one of the main cancer staging methods (Amin et al., 2017). Based on accurate TNM staging, patients can avoid over-treatment in the early stage and receive timely and effective treatment in the late stage, which helps to formulate individualized treatment strategies and achieve reasonable allocation of medical resources (Glastonbury et al., 2016).

In T staging, radiomic features of CT and MRI have been studied in previous studies and have been shown to be useful (Liang et al., 2016; Sun et al., 2018). In a study by Huang et al. (2018), radiomic signatures were identified from CT images and used to preoperatively differentiate high-grade CRC from low-grade CRC. Their results showed the effectiveness of radiomics signatures with larger areas under the curve. In their study, only portal venous phase CT images were used to identify radiomic features without involving any dynamic contrast enhancement (DCE) parameters. Dou et al. (2022) studied the value of functional and radiomic parameters of CT in T-stage assessment of patients with CRC. The CT image functional and radiomic parameters and clinical information of 32 CRC patients were analysed using decision trees, and six rules were determined, and it was found that the shape elongation rate of nodules, blood flow extraction, and blood volume in the tumour area are of great significance. This study shows that the combination of CT functional parameters and radiomics parameters is helpful for the diagnosis and T staging of CRC.

Accurate prediction of lymph node metastasis (LNM) status is of great significance for prognostic monitoring and treatment planning of colorectal cancer patients. Several histopathological findings (i.e. tumour differentiation and lymph vascular invasion) are known as indicators of LNM; however, they are only available after surgery (Smith et al., 2010). Pre-operative prediction of LNM status provides valuable information and support for treatment decisions before adjuvant therapy and surgical resection. Huang et al. (2016) attempted to construct and validate a radiomics nomogram involving clinicopathological risk factors and radiomics features for preoperative prediction of LNM in colorectal cancer. The LASSO regression method was used to select 24 potential features and construct a radiomics score. The model showed good discrimination, with a C-index of 0.736 (C-index, 0.759 and 0.766 through internal validation), and good calibration.

Treatment evaluation and prognosis analysis

Currently, the evaluation of treatment and prediction of prognosis for colorectal cancer using medical imaging relies on the experience of clinicians and requires pathological testing. However, radiologic assessment is subjective and influenced by the observations of the radiologist. Radiomics can extract high-throughput quantitative features to capture the histopathological changes of lesions preoperatively. This enables the detection of subtle changes in radiology that correlate with post-operative prognosis and aid in personalized medicine. The quantification of medical imaging using radiomics has the potential to improve the accuracy of treatment assessment and prognostic prediction of cancer (Table 9.3).

Treatment evaluation of colorectal cancer

For locally advanced rectal cancer (LARC), guidelines recommend neoadjuvant chemoradiotherapy followed by tumour resection and removal of the mesorectal envelope with lymph nodes, followed by adjuvant chemotherapy. Approximately 20% of patients can achieve a pathological complete response (pCR) with

Table 9.3 Description of studies in the radiomics analysis in treatment evaluation and prognosis analysis of colorectal cancer

Author, year	Modality	Study population	Outcome	Method	AUC/ACC/C-index
Shaish et al. (2020)	CT	132 cases	PCR/TRG/NAR	Logistic Regression	AUC:0.80/0.80/0.66
Zhang et al. (2020)	MRI	308 cases/ 104 cases	PCR/TRG/T downstaging	CNN	AUC:0.99/0.70/0.79
Giannini et al. (2020)	CT	141 lesions	Response to HER2-targeted therapy	Naïve Bayesian	-
Dercle et al. (2020)	CT	667 cases	Tumour response	Random Forest	AUC:0.80
Liu et al. (2019)	T2 MRI	177 cases	Preoperative synchronous distant metastasis	Logistic Regression	AUC:0.827
Badic et al. (2022)	CT	193 cases	Recurrence	Multivariate regression	ACC:0.78
Xue et al. (2022)	CT	121 cases/ 51 cases/ 114 cases	OS	LASSO COX regression	C-index: 0.782/0.721/ 0.677

neoadjuvant chemoradiotherapy and therefore can undergo organ preservation treatment, including local resection and watch-wait. A growing body of literature supports the usefulness of radiomics in providing diagnostic, prognostic, and predictive information. Radiomics models have been used to predict tumour response and pCR after chemoradiotherapy in rectal cancer and have the potential to identify patients suitable for sphincter-sparing surgery. Shaish et al. (2020) utilized a radiomics model of pre-treatment staging MRI to predict neoadjuvant rectal score (NAR), as well as pCR and tumour regression grade (TRG), in LARC patients receiving neoadjuvant therapy. Despite the extremely heterogeneous image data, the model demonstrated moderate accuracy. Zhang et al. (2020) developed and validated a deep learning method based on diffusion kurtosis and T2-weighted MRI to predict the response of rectal cancer to neoadjuvant therapy, including pCR, TRG, and T downstaging. The AUROC curve (ROC) of the pCR model in the test cohort was 0.99. The deep learning model based on diffusion kurtosis MRI exhibited good performance in predicting pathological complete response, aiding radiologists in evaluating locally advanced disease response after neoadjuvant chemoradiotherapy for rectal cancer.

Cellular effects

Targeted therapy can increase selective exposure to cancer cells, improve the precision of cancer cell treatment, and reduce the impact of treatment on normal cells by coupling therapeutic drugs to various antibodies or other ligands that can recognize tumour-related proteins in cancer cells.

Although targeted therapies have achieved amazing results, they are limited to a small number of patients. Therefore, biomarkers with predictive value for treatment response are crucial for introducing targeted therapies into clinical practice. Medical imaging can be used to assess the efficacy of targeted drugs, allowing non-invasive visualization and quantification of individual disease progression. A clinical trial showed that 70% of patients with HER2-amplified or over-expressed metastatic CRC achieved clinical benefit from treatment with trastuzumab plus lapatinib. Unfortunately, patients show heterogeneous responses to this treatment. Giannini et al. (2020) developed and validated a machine learning algorithm to predict response in individuals with HER2-amplified colorectal liver metastases receiving dual HER2-targeted therapy. After three-dimensional manual segmentation of pre-treatment portal vein CT, 24 radiomic features were extracted; a genetic algorithm was then used for feature selection. The sensitivity, specificity, negative predictive value (NPV), and positive predictive value (PPV) per lesion were 89%, 85%, 93%, 78%, and 90%, 42%, 73%, 71%, respectively, in the test and validation datasets. The developed method proved effective in predicting the behaviour of individual metastases in response to targeted therapy in a cohort of HER2-amplified patients. Dercle et al. (2020) attempted to predict tumour sensitivity to irinotecan, 5-fluorouracil, and leucovorin (FOLFIRI) alone or in combination by using on-treatment radiomic signatures to predict survival and enhance treatment decisions in patients with colorectal cancer with liver metastases. Radiomic response signatures are superior to known biomarkers in providing early predictions of treatment sensitivity and can be used to guide decisions regarding the continuation of cetuximab therapy.

Prognosis analysis of colorectal cancer

Once metastatic colon cancer is diagnosed, the patient's prognosis is extremely poor. Predictive factors are urgently needed to identify patients who are likely to benefit from more aggressive treatment. Due to the successful application of radiomics biomarkers in other cancers, many researchers have attempted to study the prognostic value of radiomics analysis in colorectal cancer.

Liu et al. (2019) combined MRI radiomics features and clinical features to construct a radiomics model for predicting synchronous distant metastasis in patients with rectal cancer who received different treatments. The AUC in the validation set reached 0.827, which can help formulate treatment strategies. Badic et al. (2022) assessed the value of radiomics based on contrast-enhanced (CE) diagnostic CT in predicting recurrence of colorectal cancer. This study included 193 patients diagnosed with stage II and stage III colorectal adenocarcinoma and utilized three different machine learning models to develop prediction models for disease-free survival (DFS). The results demonstrated that a multivariable regression model, combining clinical variables with two radiomic features (compactness and minimum axial length), exhibited optimal performance, with a balanced accuracy (BAcc) of 0.78 and an Matthews correlation coefficient (MCC) of 0.6, associated with the required 95% sensitivity. Xue et al. (2022) developed a radiomics model by combining CT images and clinical predictors to determine overall survival after surgery in colorectal cancer patients. Radiomic features were selected using univariate Cox regression and least absolute shrinkage and selection operator regression. The c-index of the nomogram was 0.782, 0.721, and 0.677 in the training cohort, internal validation cohort, and external testing cohort, respectively. Negreros-Osuna et al. (2020) investigated the potential of radiomic texture signatures as biomarkers for detecting the presence of *BRAF* mutations and predicting five-year overall survival in stage IV CRC. Modelling the association between radiomic texture signatures and five-year overall survival (OS) through multivariate Cox proportional hazards regression analysis demonstrated that radiomic texture signatures can serve as potential biomarkers for determining *BRAF* mutation status and predicting overall survival in patients with advanced CRC.

Other applications of radiomics

In addition to its widespread use in cancer diagnosis, such as screening and staging, radiomics can also be utilized for predicting gene mutations and histopathological classification. The specific classification of histopathology and genetic mutations in CRC are closely linked to the effectiveness of targeted therapy and the sensitivity of radiotherapy and chemotherapy. Radiomics-based gene mutation and cancer classification can serve as a non-invasive, real-time, cost-effective, and easily implementable detection method. Some researchers have demonstrated the success of radiomics in classifying cancer histopathology and predicting gene mutations and molecular phenotypes, including the prediction of histopathological grade, mutations in *KRAS/NRAS/BRAF*, and microsatellite instability (MSI), among others (Table 9.4).

Prediction of gene mutation in colorectal cancer

Identifying the status of *KRAS/NRAS/BRAF* and MSI is crucial in developing personalized treatment strategies for colorectal cancer. While pathological testing is the gold standard for detecting gene mutations, it may not fully reflect post-biopsy tumour genotype changes, especially after multiple treatments, due to tumour heterogeneity. Therefore, a non-invasive and reproducible method is needed to reflect intertumoural heterogeneity and identify gene mutation status.

Several studies have shown that medical imaging techniques such as CT and MRI can predict *KRAS* mutations. Cao et al. (2023) used CT-based radiomics features to predict *KRAS* mutation status in 447 patients with colorectal cancer. The study divided patients into a training group (n = 313) and a validation group (n = 134) and found that the clinical-radiomics fusion model had the best predictive performance for *KRAS* mutation status, with an AUC, sensitivity, and specificity of 0.755, 0.724, and 0.724, respectively, in the validation cohort. Shin et al. (2016) used MRI to study imaging predictors of *KRAS* mutations in patients with rectal cancer and found that tumours with *KRAS* mutations had a longer axial length and a greater ratio of axial to longitudinal dimensions.

Negreros-Osuna et al. (2020) utilized a CT-based radiomics model to predict the presence of *BRAF* mutations and five-year overall survival in stage IV CRC. Their study demonstrated that radiomics texture features have the potential to serve as biomarkers for determining *BRAF* mutation status and predicting five-year OS in patients with advanced CRC. Similarly, Yang et al. (2018) investigated the predictive capability of CT-based radiomics features for *KRAS/NRAS/BRAF* mutations in CRC. They extracted a total of 346 radiomics features from the primary tumour region in portal venous phase CT images and used a support vector machine approach to select key features and build a radiomics model. The results showed a significant association between radiomic signatures and *KRAS/NRAS/BRAF* mutations ($P < 0.001$).

In another study, Pei et al. (2022) developed a radiomics nomogram to predict pre-treatment microsatellite instability (MSI) status in CRC patients. They retrospectively included 762 CRC patients whose MSI status was confirmed by surgical pathology and polymerase chain reaction (PCR) method. Radiomic signatures were extracted from routine pre-treatment abdominal and pelvic CT scans, and a radiomics nomogram was constructed using multivariate logistic regression. The results demonstrated that the radiomics model could effectively differentiate between non-MSI-H (non-MSI-high) and MSI-H patients, with an area under the curve (AUC) of 0.77 (95% CI, 0.68–0.85). Similarly, Chen et al. (2022) employed an artificial neural network model enhanced by genetic algorithm to construct MSI-related radiomic features.

Table 9.4 Description of studies in the radiomics analysis in other application of colorectal cancer

Author, year	Modality	Study population	Outcome	Method	AUC/ACC/C-index
Cao et al., (2023)	CT	313 cases/ 134 cases	KRAS	Random Forest	AUC:0.772/0.755
Shin et al. (2016)	MRI	275 cases	KRAS	-	-
Negreros-Osuna et al. (2020)	CT	145 cases	BRAF/OS	-	-
Pei et al. (2022)	CT	534 cases/ 228 cases	MSI	LASSO	AUC:0.74/0.77
Chen et al., (2022)	CT	277 cases/ 119 cases/ 441 cases	MSI	Neural Network	AUC:0.792/0.788/0.775

Future challenges in radiomics

Automatic extraction of quantitative features from medical imaging data represents the latest development direction of radiomics. There is a clear trend among researchers to incorporate more deep learning methods into radiomics as it advances in learning disease-specific features from medical images. However, the development of powerful deep learning models still faces significant obstacles due to the strong need for scalable training data. Additionally, another major trend is multi-modal integration. Most methods are limited to a single data mode, and comprehensive methods across modes are relatively under-developed. Multimodal integration of advanced molecular diagnostics, radiological and histological imaging, and compiled clinical data provides opportunities for precision oncology beyond genomics and standard molecular techniques. However, most medical datasets are still too sparse for training with modern machine learning techniques, and significant challenges remain until this problem can be solved.

Radiomics plays a crucial role in identifying complex information in medical images, transforming qualitative and subjective image analysis into quantitative assessments, and even quantifying image information that humans cannot perceive to supplement clinical decision-making. The current challenges in this field include ensuring clinical utility and model reproducibility across different clinical sites. Only when the results of radiomics research are thoroughly validated and implemented in various hospitals can we fully maximize the clinical value of radiomics research.

REFERENCES

Aerts, H. J. W. L., Velazquez, E. R., Leijenaar, R. T. H., et al. (2014). Decoding tumour phenotype by noninvasive imaging using a quantitative radiomics approach. *Nature Communication*, *5*, 4006. https://doi.org/10.1038/ncomms5006.

Amin, M. B., Greene, F. L., Edge, S. B., et al. (2017). The Eighth Edition AJCC Cancer Staging Manual: continuing to build a bridge from a population-based to a more 'personalized' approach to cancer staging. *CA: A Cancer Journal for Clinicians*, *67*, 93–99. https://doi.org/10.3322/caac.21388.

Badic, B., Da-ano, R., Poirot, K., et al. (2022). Prediction of recurrence after surgery in colorectal cancer patients using radiomics from diagnostic contrast-enhanced computed tomography: a two-center study. *European Radiology*, *32*, 405–414. https://doi.org/10.1007/s00330-021-08104-4.

Balagurunathan, Y., Gu, Y., Wang, H., et al. (2014). Reproducibility and prognosis of quantitative features extracted from CT images. *Translational Oncology*, *7*, 72–87. https://doi.org/10.1593/tlo.13844.

Cao, Y., Zhang, J., Huang, L., et al. (2023). Construction of prediction model for KRAS mutation status of colorectal cancer based on CT radiomics. *Japan Journal of Radiology*, https://doi.org/10.1007/s11604-023-01458-3.

Chen, X., He, L., Li, Q., et al. (2022). Non-invasive prediction of microsatellite instability in colorectal cancer by a genetic algorithm–enhanced artificial neural network–based CT radiomics signature. *European Radiology*, *33*, 11–22. https://doi.org/10.1007/s00330-022-08954-6.

Dercle, L., Lu, L., Schwartz, L. H., et al. (2020). Radiomics response signature for identification of metastatic colorectal cancer sensitive to therapies targeting EGFR pathway. *Journal of the National Cancer institute*, *112*, 902–912. https://doi.org/10.1093/jnci/djaa017.

Dou, Y., Liu, Y., Kong, X., et al. (2022). T staging with functional and radiomics parameters of computed tomography in colorectal cancer patients. *Medicine (Baltimore) 101*, e29244. https://doi.org/10.1097/MD.0000000000029244.

Gessert, N., Wittig, L., Drömann, D., et al. (2019). Feasibility of colon cancer detection in confocal laser microscopy images using convolution neural networks. In H. Handels, T. M. Deserno, A. Maier, et al. (Eds.), *Bildverarbeitung Für Die Medizin 2019, Informatik Aktuell* (pp. 327–332). Springer Fachmedien Wiesbaden. https://doi.org/10.1007/978-3-658-25326-4_72.

Giannini, V., Rosati, S., Defeudis, A., et al. (2020). Radiomics predicts response of individual HER2-amplified colorectal cancer liver metastases in patients treated with HER2-targeted therapy. *International Journal of Cancer*, *147*, 3215–3223. https://doi.org/10.1002/ijc.33271

Gillies, R. J., Kinahan, P. E., & Hricak, H. (2016). Radiomics: Images Are More than Pictures, They Are Data. *Radiology*, *278*, 563–577. https://doi.org/10.1148/radiol.2015151169

Glastonbury, C. M., Bhosale, P. R., Choyke, P. L., et al. (2016). Do radiologists have stage fright? Tumor staging and how we can add value to the care of patients with cancer. *Radiology*, *278*, 11–12. https://doi.org/10.1148/radiol.2015151563

Godkhindi, A. M., & Gowda, R. M. (2017). Automated detection of polyps in CT colonography images using deep learning algorithms in colon cancer diagnosis. [Paper presentation] 2017 International Conference on Energy, Communication, Data Analytics and Soft Computing (ICECDS), IEEE, Chennai. https://doi.org/10.1109/ICECDS.2017.8389744

Grosu, S., Wesp, P., Graser, A., et al. (2021). Machine learning–based differentiation of benign and premalignant colorectal polyps detected with CT colonography in an asymptomatic screening population: a proof-of-concept study. *Radiology*, *299*, 326–335. https://doi.org/10.1148/radiol.2021202363

Huang, X., Cheng, Z., Huang, Y., et al. (2018). CT-based radiomics signature to discriminate high-grade from low-grade colorectal adenocarcinoma. *Academic Radiology*, *25*, 1285–1297. https://doi.org/10.1016/j.acra.2018.01.020

Huang, Y., Liang, C.-H., He, L., et al. (2016). Development and validation of a radiomics nomogram for preoperative prediction of lymph node metastasis in colorectal cancer. *Journal of Clinical Oncology*, *34*, 2157–2164. https://doi.org/10.1200/JCO.2015.65.9128

Kumar, V., Gu, Y., Basu, S., et al. (2012). Radiomics: the process and the challenges. *Magnetic Resonance Imaging*, *30*, 1234–1248. https://doi.org/10.1016/j.mri.2012.06.010

Lambin, P., Rios-Velazquez, E., Leijenaar, R., et al. (2012). Radiomics: extracting more information from medical images using advanced feature analysis. *European Journal of Cancer*, *48*, 441–446. https://doi.org/10.1016/j.ejca.2011.11.036

Liang, C., Huang, Y., He, L., et al. (2016). The development and validation of a CT-based radiomics signature for the preoperative discrimination of stage I-II and stage III-IV colorectal cancer. *Oncotarget*, *7*, 31401–31412. https://doi.org/10.18632/oncotarget.8919

Liu, H., Zhang, C., Wang, L., et al. (2019). MRI radiomics analysis for predicting preoperative synchronous distant metastasis in patients with rectal cancer. *European Radiology*, *29*, 4418–4426. https://doi.org/10.1007/s00330-018-5802-7

Negreros-Osuna, A. A., Parakh, A., Corcoran, R. B., et al. (2020). Radiomics texture features in advanced colorectal cancer: correlation with *BRAF* mutation and 5-year overall survival. *Radiology:*

Imaging Cancer, 2, e190084. https://doi.org/10.1148/rycan.2020190084

Parmar, C., Leijenaar, R. T. H., Grossmann, P., et al. (2015). Radiomic feature clusters and prognostic signatures specific for lung and head & neck cancer. *Science Reports, 5*, 11044. https://doi.org/10.1038/srep11044

Pei, Q., Yi, X., Chen, C., et al. (2022). Pre-treatment CT-based radiomics nomogram for predicting microsatellite instability status in colorectal cancer. *European Radiology, 32*, 714–724. https://doi.org/10.1007/s00330-021-08167-3

Shaish, H., Aukerman, A., Vanguri, R., et al. (2020). Radiomics of MRI for pretreatment prediction of pathologic complete response, tumor regression grade, and neoadjuvant rectal score in patients with locally advanced rectal cancer undergoing neoadjuvant chemoradiation: an international multicenter study. *European Radiology, 30*, 6263–6273. https://doi.org/10.1007/s00330-020-06968-6

Shin, Y. R., Kim, K. A., Im, S., et al. (2016). Prediction of KRAS mutation in rectal cancer using MRI. *Anticancer Research, 36*, 4799–7804. https://doi.org/10.21873/anticanres.11039

Smith, A. J., Driman, D. K., Spithoff, K., et al. (2010). Guideline for optimization of colorectal cancer surgery and pathology: colorectal cancer surgery and pathology. *Journal of Surgical Oncology, 101*, 5–12. https://doi.org/10.1002/jso.21395

Sun, Y., Hu, P., Wang, J., et al. (2018). Radiomic features of pretreatment MRI could identify T stage in patients with rectal cancer: preliminary findings. *Journal of Magnetic Resonance Imaging, 48*, 615–621. https://doi.org/10.1002/jmri.25969

Wang, S., Liu, Z., Chen, X., et al. (2018). Unsupervised deep learning features for lung cancer overall survival analysis. [Paper presentation] 2018 40th Annual International Conference of the IEEE Engineering in Medicine and Biology Society (EMBC), IEEE, Honolulu, HI. https://doi.org/10.1109/EMBC.2018.8512833

Wang, S., Zhou, M., Liu, Z., et al. (2017). Central focused convolutional neural networks: Developing a data-driven model for lung nodule segmentation. *Medical Image Analysis, 40*, 172–183. https://doi.org/10.1016/j.media.2017.06.014

Xue, T., Peng, H., Chen, Q., et al. (2022). A CT-Based radiomics nomogram in predicting the postoperative prognosis of colorectal cancer: a two-center study. *Academic Radiology, 29*, 1647–1660. https://doi.org/10.1016/j.acra.2022.02.006

Yang, L., Dong, D., Fang, M., et al. (2018). Can CT-based radiomics signature predict KRAS/NRAS/BRAF mutations in colorectal cancer? *European Radiology, 28* (2058–2067. https://doi.org/10.1007/s00330-017-5146-8

Yu, D., Zhou, M., Yang, F., et al. (2017). Convolutional neural networks for predicting molecular profiles of non-small cell lung cancer. [Paper presentation]. 2017 IEEE 14th International Symposium on Biomedical Imaging (ISBI 2017), IEEE, Melbourne, Australia. https://doi.org/10.1109/ISBI.2017.7950585

Zhang, X.-Y., Wang, L., Zhu, H.-T., et al. (2020). Predicting rectal cancer response to neoadjuvant chemoradiotherapy using deep learning of diffusion kurtosis MRI. *Radiology, 296*, 56–64. https://doi.org/10.1148/radiol.2020190936

SECTION 3

Multidisciplinary management

10

Controversies in the multidisciplinary management of locally advanced rectal cancer including total neoadjuvant therapy

Sean M. O'Cathail and Timothy O'Brien

Introduction

For almost two decades, the standard of care for locally advanced rectal cancer (LARC) has been neoadjuvant chemoradiotherapy followed by total mesorectal excision (TME) (Sauer et al., 2012). And for good reason. Prior to the incorporation of this paradigm into routine practice, local recurrence rates ranged from 25% at best, to in excess of 50% with surgery alone, leading to significant morbidity and mortality (Gastrointestinal Study Group, 1985). Post the introduction of TME, the rate is now less than 10%.

Despite the improvements in local control, nearly one in three patients with LARC will suffer from a distant metastatic relapse, leading to death in most cases. The exact benefit of adjuvant chemotherapy in reducing distant recurrence is uncertain as many adjuvant trials have suffered from poor accrual, low compliance, and an inconsistent survival benefit (Bosset et al., 2014; Glynne-Jones et al., 2014; Sainato et al., 2014; Breugom et al., 2015) With this in mind, there has been substantial investigation of shifting what would previously have been systemic adjuvant chemotherapy into the neoadjuvant setting, as part of a novel strategy termed total neoadjuvant therapy (TNT).

The principal idea behind TNT is simple: patient compliance increases when chemotherapy is administered pre-operatively. Earlier introduction would, theoretically, be more effective treatment of micro-metastatic disease and reduce the risk of distant recurrence, the main issue currently facing patients with LARC. Another possible benefit of sequencing chemotherapy with chemoradiation is the potential synergy in downsizing the primary tumour. Not only might this improve operability but in select cases TNT might negate the requirement for surgery entirely. Although the principle is a simple one, the reality of applying it is not.

The quickly evolving and increasingly complex management of LARC is typical of modern cancer medicine. In a field awash with data ranging from single-institution, retrospective case series to international, randomized phase 2 and 3 trials, the challenge facing the multidisciplinary team (MDT) is to assimilate and integrate this knowledge into clinical practice to achieve the most effective outcome for the individual patient. This is compounded by a distinct lack of consensus regarding some basic issues such as, what is TNT, which patients to select for TNT, what TNT regimen to use, and whether patients can safely avoid an operation following a complete clinical response to TNT. A greater understanding of rectal tumour biology, such as the DNA mismatch repair status and the intratumoral microbiome composition, might influence these choices in the near future.

This chapter provides a summary of the most influential data relevant to the total neoadjuvant management of LARC, including the timing of surgery and the concept of non-operative management. In addition, other controversial areas are highlighted such as TNT in the elderly; the role, or lack thereof, for adjuvant chemotherapy for LARC; and the evidence for immunotherapy in microsatellite unstable rectal cancer. Abbreviations are defined in Table 10.1.

Selecting the optimal TNT regimen

The emergence of TNT as a potential strategy in the management of LARC is underpinned by several contemporary clinical trials, summarized in Table 10.2. In general, these trials have attempted to improve either the rate of disease recurrence, especially distant metastasis, or else focused on achieving maximal downstaging of the primary tumour to improve operability. This is an important distinction for the multidisciplinary team to consider when employing

Table 10.1 Abbreviations and TNT terminology

5-FU	5-fluorouracil, an antimetabolite chemotherapy agent, a long-standing cornerstone of systemic treatment of colorectal cancer
CAPOX	A combination of capecitabine (a prodrug of 5FU) and oxaliplatin given every 3 weeks
cCR	Clinical Complete Response
Consolidation TNT	Chemotherapy delivered after neoadjuvant radiotherapy
CRM	Circumferential Resection Margin
DFS	Disease-free survival
EMVI	Extra Mural Venous Invasion
FOLFIRINOX	A combination of 5FU, irinotecan and oxaliplatin given every 2 weeks
FOLFOX	A combination of 5FU and oxaliplatin given every 2 weeks
Induction TNT	Chemotherapy delivered before neoadjuvant radiotherapy
LARC	Locally advanced rectal cancer
LCCRT	Long-course Chemoradiotherapy
MDT	Multidisciplinary Team
MMR	DNA mismatch-repair proteins
MRI	Magnetic Resonance Imaging
MSI	Microsatellite Instability
MRF	Mesorectal fascia
NOM	Non-Operative Management
OS	Overall Survival
pCR	Pathological Complete Response
SCRT	Short-course radiotherapy
TME	Total Mesorectal Excision
TNT	Total Neoadjuvant Therapy
WW	Watch and wait

a TNT approach. Here we describe the key trials that have shaped the TNT debate as well as discussing some of the controversies that have arisen in this increasingly complex field.

Reducing distant disease recurrence

Despite the unquestionable improvement in local recurrence rates achieved in recent decades with total mesorectal excision and neoadjuvant chemoradiotherapy, patients with LARC have a significant rate of recurrence, primarily in the form of distant metastases, which are commonly fatal. Therefore, numerous efforts have been made to reduce distant recurrence by incorporating systemic chemotherapy into the neoadjuvant paradigm.

Polish II

Some of the earliest data for TNT was demonstrated in this phase 3 trial, which randomized > 500 patients with fixed, predominantly lower third, cT3 or cT4 rectal tumours to standard of care long-course chemoradiotherapy (LCCRT), using 5-FU and oxaliplatin, or to short-course radiotherapy (SCRT) followed by three cycles of FOLFOX (Bujkoet al., 2016). Whilst this trial failed to improve its primary endpoint of R0 resection rate (77% vs 71%, $p = 0.07$) and made no impact on longer-term disease-free survival (DFS) (43% vs 41%, $p = 0.65$) or overall survival (OS) (49% vs 49%), it demonstrated the feasibility of preoperative hypofractionated radiotherapy, in combination with systemic chemotherapy, and prompted other TNT studies to intensify the dose and duration of the chemotherapy component (Cisel et al., 2019). It also reassured the community that the long-term local recurrence rate in this population was not significantly worse than LCCRT.

RAPIDO

The largest phase 3 TNT trial to date employed a similar experimental arm to Polish II, SCRT followed by chemotherapy, but increased the duration of the consolidation component (nine cycles of FOLFOX or six cycles of CAPOX) (Bahadoer et al., 2021). This approach built on an earlier study of patients with oligometastatic disease undergoing treatment with curative intent, the main advantage being the reduced time interval between radiation and the delivery of systemic chemotherapy (Bisschop et al., 2017). RAPIDO enrolled patients with high-risk disease including cT4, cN2, EMVI- (extra mural venous invasion) positive, MRF- (mesorectal fascia) positive, or lateral lymph node involvement. Reported in 2020, it significantly improved its primary endpoint of three-year disease-related treatment failure (drTF, 24% vs 30%, $p = 0.019$) as well as pathological complete response (pCR) rate (28% vs 14%, $p < 0.0001$). Whilst the composite disease-related treatment failure (drTF) endpoint included local recurrence, new CRC primary or treatment-related death, it was the reduction in distant metastases that drove the improvement in outcomes (20% vs 27% at 3 years, $p = 0.0048$).

Enthusiasm for this ground-breaking trial has been tempered significantly by a recent update of five-year follow up, which has shown an increased risk of locoregional recurrence (10% vs 6%, $p = 0.027$) and no overall survival benefit when compared to LCCRT, although the reduced risk of metastasis was maintained (Dijkstra et al., 2023). There are several theories regarding the higher local recurrence rate. First, less aggressive surgery was performed in patients with complete or near-complete responses, as evidenced by fewer abdominoperineal resections (APRs) in the TNT arm, despite similar baseline tumour characteristics to the control arm. This may have been compounded by the concept of tumour fragmentation whereby clinically undetectable, scattered islands of potentially viable tumour cells exist on the periphery of the post-treatment tumour bed (Glynne-Jones et al., 2023). Considering that two-thirds of patients in RAPIDO had an initially positive MRF, it is conceivable that areas of fragmented tumour existed beyond the resection margin, contributing to an increased local recurrence rate. Additionally, the longer time to surgery in the TNT arm (25 weeks) compared to LCCRT (14–16 weeks) may have allowed intrinsically chemotherapy resistant tumour cells to regrow.

STELLAR

This phase 3 trial conducted in a Chinese population employed a similar approach to RAPIDO, namely SCRT followed by consolidation chemotherapy (Jin et al., 2022). It enrolled a slightly lower risk population (low to mid rectal, T3 or T4 or node-positive tumours) and used a shorter duration of chemotherapy compared to RAPIDO

Table 10.2 Overview of important TNT trials

Trial	MRI inclusion criteria	ECOG	Median Age	TNT Regimen	Control	Primary endpoint	Met primary endpoint?	Complete response? (Control)	3-year DFS (Control)	OS benefit? (Control)	TNT toxicity grade >3 (control)
POLISH II Poland Phase 3 *N* = 515	Palpably fixed T3 T4	0–2	60	SCRT ↓ FOLFOX ×3 ↓ Surgery	LCCRT* ↓ Surgery ↓ +/− FOLFOX ×12 or CAPOX ×8	Improvement in R0 rate	No 77% (71%) *P* = 0.07	pCR rate 16% (12%) *P* = 0.17	53% (52%)	No At 8 years: 49% in both arms	23% (21%)
RAPIDO Europe/US Phase 3 *N* = 920	T4 N2 EMVI+ MRF+ Lateral LNs	0–1	62	SCRT ↓ FOLFOX ×9 or CAPOX ×6 ↓ Surgery	LCCRT ↓ Surgery ↓ +/− FOLFOX ×12 or CAPOX ×8	Improvement in 3 year drTF	Yes	pCR rate 28% (14%)	76%** (70%)	No At 5 years: 82% (80%)	48% (25%)
STELLAR China Phase 3 *N* = 599	T3 T4 N+	0–1	55	SCRT ↓ CAPOX ×4 ↓ Surgery ↓ CAPOX ×2	LCCRT ↓ Surgery ↓ CAPOX ×6	Non-inferior 3-year DFS	Yes	pCR rate 22% (13%)	65% (62%)	Yes*** At 3 years: 87% (75%)	27% (13%)
PRODIGE 23 French Phase 3 *N* = 461	T3 T4	0–1	61–62	FOLFIRINOX ×6 ↓ LCCRT ↓ Surgery ↓ FOLFOX ×6 or CAPOX ×4	LCCRT ↓ Surgery ↓ +/− FOLFOX ×12 or CAPOX ×8	Improvement in 3-year DFS	Yes	pCR rate 28% (12%)	76% (69%)	Yes At 7 years: 82% (76%)	46% (36%)
CAO/ARO/ AIO-12 German Phase 2, 2 arms *N* = 311	T3 if < 6 cm T3 and EMVI if 6–12 cm T4 Lateral LNs	0–1	62	*Induction* FOLFOX ×3 ↓ LCCRT* ↓ Surgery	None	Improvement in pCR rate vs standard 15% with LCCRT	Yes, only for Consolidation arm	pCR rate Induction: 17%	73% in both arms	92% 3-year OS in both arms	Induction: 37%
			61	*Consolidation* LCCRT ↓ FOLFOX ×3 ↓ Surgery				Consolidation: 25%			Consolidation: 27%
OPRA USA Phase 2, 2 arms *N* = 324	T3 T4 N+	0–2	59 56	*Induction* FOLFOX ×8 or CAPOX ×5 ↓ LCCRT ↓ WW or surgery *Consolidation* LCCRT ↓ FOLFOX ×8 or CAPOX ×5 ↓ Surgery	Historical controls LCCRT ↓ Surgery ↓ +/- FOLFOX ×12 or CAPOX ×8	Improved DFS vs historical controls	No	Induction: 72% NOM Consolidation: 76% NOM cCR not published	76% in both arms	88% 5-year OS in both arms	Induction: 46% Consolidation: 40%

*chemoradiation included 5FU and oxaliplatin
**or rather the drTF was 24% (TNT) vs 30% (control)
***unclear if truly an OS benefit as local and distant recurrence rates were similar in both groups

(four rather than six cycles of CAPOX). Instead of aiming to improve DFS, this study was powered to detect non-inferiority of TNT versus LCCRT. It succeeded in this regard, demonstrating a three-year DFS of 64.5% compared to 62.3% for standard of care ($p < 0.001$ for non-inferiority). In contrast to RAPIDO there was no difference in local recurrence rates. Somewhat confusingly, TNT was associated with a considerable survival advantage (three-year OS 86.5% vs 75.1%, $p = 0.033$), despite being unable to significantly improve DFS. This may be better explained by the increased all-cause mortality in the control arm.

PRODIGE-23

Arguably one of the most influential and robust TNT trials, the French PRODIGE-23 trial randomized patients with cT3 or cT4 rectal tumours to TNT or standard LCCRT (Conroy et al., 2021). Although this trial aimed to reduce disease recurrence, it differed from the previously discussed trials in its TNT approach, employing systemic chemotherapy first, termed induction. The PRODIGE-23 regimen, consisted of six cycles of modified FOLFIRINOX (bolus 5-FU omitted to reduce neutropenia), followed by LCCRT, mandatory TME, and adjuvant chemotherapy (six cycles of FOLFOX or four cycles of CAPOX).

The trial met its primary endpoint as TNT improved the three-year DFS (76% vs 69%, hazard ratio 0·69, p = 0·034) compared to LCCRT alone, a feat that was primarily achieved by reducing distant metastasis (hazard ratio 0·64, p = 0·017). The TNT group also benefitted from superior pCR rates (28% vs 12%, $p < 0.0001$) and an improvement in tumour-related symptoms (Bascoul-Mollevi et al., 2023). As expected, there was increased toxicity from the arduous neoadjuvant treatment, however, similar proportions underwent surgery and operative outcomes were not compromised in this fit study population (ECOG 0-1). Furthermore, longer-term follow-up has also confirmed a modest five-year overall survival benefit (76% vs 72%, $p = 0.033$) with the PRODIGE-23 strategy (Etienne et al., 2023).

Despite strong data, PRODIGE-23 has notable drawbacks, most significantly the risk of overtreatment. Although this point applies to all TNT approaches it is especially pertinent to PRODIGE-23 considering the physical, financial, and time toxicity of triplet chemotherapy: 47% experienced Grade 3 or 4 adverse events during this treatment. This would likely be even higher in a 'real-world' population given that participants in this trial were particularly robust (92% completed six cycles of FOLFIRINOX). In addition, the treatment intensification employed in PRODIGE-23 contrasts with the trend of de-escalating chemotherapy where possible, for example, reducing the duration of adjuvant treatment in stage 3 colon cancer (Grothey et al., 2018).

Another concern is whether irinotecan, an agent with no proven benefit in the adjuvant context, contributed to the beneficial outcomes reported in PRODIGE-23. This question is being formally assessed in the JANUS phase 2 trial, which is comparing neoadjuvant consolidation FOLFIRINOX versus FOLFOX (NCT05610163). Interestingly this study was designed with significant input from colorectal cancer patient support groups that recommended a trial with more chemotherapy rather than more radiotherapy (Garcia-Aguilar et al., 2022).

Finally, the risk of overtreatment in PRODIGE-23 was compounded by adjuvant chemotherapy being mandated by the trial sponsors. Supportive data for adjuvant chemotherapy for rectal cancer are inconsistent and flawed, which is reflected in the high variability in clinical practice. Furthermore, the benefit of adjuvant chemotherapy following TNT, particularly in the context of a pCR or near pCR, is even less certain.

Undoubtedly, some patients benefitted substantially from the PRODIGE-23 protocol, whilst others may have fared equally well with neoadjuvant LCCRT alone. Delineating distinct patient populations and tailoring treatment accordingly is an ongoing endeavour not just in rectal cancer but across all oncology.

PROSPECT

In stark contrast to the intense treatment of PRODIGE-23, the minimalist approach of the PROSPECT trial was to de-escalate neoadjuvant treatment without compromising DFS, albeit in a lower risk population (Schrag et al., 2023). This phase 3 trial investigated neoadjuvant FOLFOX with the omission of radiotherapy provided tumour regression was at least 20%, compared to standard of care LCCRT. Patients with cT2N+, cT3N−, or cT3N+ tumours were recruited whilst those with more advanced disease, in whom omitting radiation was not considered to be safe, were excluded (T4 tumours, threatened radial margins, or > four lymph nodes).

PROSPECT demonstrated that neoadjuvant FOLFOX with selective use of LCCRT was non-inferior to conventional treatment in terms of five-year local recurrence (1.8 vs 1.6%), DFS (81% vs 79%), and OS (90% in both). The most significant implication of this study was that more than 90% of participants could safely avoid pelvic radiation, which means many patients were spared from the short- and possible long-term consequences of LCCRT such as pelvic fracture and sexual dysfunction.

Whilst many have hailed PROSPECT as a practice-changing trial, there are several important caveats that render this approach an additional strategy rather than a direct replacement for traditional LCCRT (O'Cathail et al., 2023).

First, although nearly half of all new rectal cancer diagnoses in the United States would meet the staging criteria applied in this trial, in Europe, the majority of these tumours would be regarded as early or intermediate risk and may not receive any form of neoadjuvant treatment (Glynne-Jones et al., 2017). It must be emphasized that participants in PROSPECT did not have T4 tumours or a high burden of lymph node disease and thus represented a lower risk category of rectal cancer that some might not consider to be truly locally advanced. Secondly, the lack of magnetic resonance imaging (MRI) staging in 15% of patients raises a concern of possible overstaging. Thirdly, over 80% of patients in this trial had tumours in the upper two-thirds of the rectum, which may be more suitable for upfront surgery given the lower risk of local recurrence.

Finally, the authors of PROSPECT concluded that overall health-related quality of life did not differ between the intervention and control arms. However, patient-reported outcomes for 12 out of 14 symptoms were worse with neoadjuvant FOLFOX suggesting that LCCRT was better tolerated in this study.

In summary, universally adopting the PROSPECT approach could lead to significant overtreatment and increased toxicity. Nonetheless, it represents an additional approach for certain patients who wish to avoid radiotherapy or in whom it is contraindicated. In the future, translational data may help to determine the best TNT strategy based on distinctive molecular features that predict response to chemotherapy or LCCRT.

Maximizing local response

The other significant aim of TNT is to downsize the primary tumour. This offers numerous potential benefits such as improved resectability, decreasing R1 rates, reduced rates of morbid surgeries such as abdominoperineal resections (APR) and, in certain cases of complete response, the possibility of non-operative management. Compared to the trials discussed previously, it must be noted that the following data are based on lower-level evidence, primarily phase 2 trials. This may be due to the difficulty in randomizing patients with a complete response to a control TME arm.

CAO/ARO/AIO-12

A phase 2 trial undertaken by the German Rectal Cancer Study Group, investigated two TNT regimens head-to-head, with the so-called winner to be taken forward into a phase 3 trial against LCCRT (Fokas et al., 2019). The trial randomized 306 patients with stage 2 or 3 rectal cancer to receive three cycles of a FOLFOX-like regimen either before (induction) or after (consolidation) LCCRT. The timing of surgery was protocol mandated as 123 days from the start of treatment. The primary endpoint was an improved pCR rate of greater than 25%, compared to 15% traditionally obtained with LCCRT. Notably, adjuvant chemotherapy was not recommended.

The clear winner was the consolidation regimen, as 25% of patients developed a pCR ($p > 0.001$) compared to only 17% in the induction arm ($p = 0.21$). The increased response rate in the consolidation arm was most likely a consequence of the increased time interval between radiation and surgery, relative to the induction arm, as has been shown in other studies (Garcia-Aguilar et al., 2015). Reassuringly, surgical outcomes such as rates of R0 resection, sphincter preservation, and post-operative complications were broadly similar in both groups and comparable to historical data.

At three-year follow-up, the improved pCR rate in the consolidation arm did not translate into a difference in DFS (73% in both) or OS (92% in both), which indicates that both regimens may be appropriate in certain clinical situations (Fokas et al., 2022). The authors suggest that a consolidation strategy—that is, radiotherapy then chemotherapy—may be best if the goal is maximal tumour regression. This might include a tumour with a positive MRF or when aiming to avoid an APR in a low-lying tumour. On the other hand, an induction approach, might be preferable in patients with a high risk of metastasis, for example, tumours with EMVI or significant lymph node involvement. This rationale is reinforced by the fact that compliance with the initial TNT component is likely to be higher than the subsequent. In CAO/ARO/AIO-12, 97% of patients received the full radiotherapy dose when administered first compared to 91% after chemotherapy.

OPRA

Whilst good quality rectal cancer surgery is often curative, living with Low Anterior Resection syndrome (LARS), a permanent end-colostomy, or myriad other surgical sequelae can unquestionably reduce quality of life. Therefore, whether surgery can be safely omitted in certain instances when the combination of radiotherapy and chemotherapy alone is sufficient is a vital clinical question and possibly the ultimate goal of TNT.

The provocative phase 2 OPRA trial investigated whether an organ preservation strategy could be achieved without compromising long-term oncologic outcomes (Garcia-Aguilar et al., 2022). Patients with stage 2 or 3 rectal cancer were randomized to either induction or consolidation chemotherapy consisting of eight cycles of FOLFOX or five cycles of CAPOX, sequenced with standard LLCRT. Following the decision to forego surgery in the case of a complete (or near complete) clinical response to TNT, patients underwent a strict surveillance protocol and proceeded to TME if there was tumour regrowth.

OPRA did not significantly improve three-year DFS (76% in both induction and consolidation arms) compared to historical controls (75%), and as such failed to meet its primary endpoint. However, despite being considered a 'negative' trial, OPRA significantly challenged the notion that TME is mandatory for all patients with LARC. Perhaps the most significant findings were that after five-years of follow-up, 54% of patients in the consolidation arm and 39% in the induction arm were alive without having undergone a TME (Verheij et al., 2023). In addition, those who underwent TME following local regrowth had a similar DFS to patients who underwent up front TME, suggesting that a watch and wait (WW) strategy was safe in this cohort of patients.

This trial not only supported the premise that consolidation chemotherapy is a more effective approach for downstaging the primary tumour than induction but also demonstrated that a significant proportion of patients may be safely spared a major operation without detriment to their oncologic outcomes. The main caveat is that not all patients are willing or able to comply with a rigorous and long-term surveillance program, such as that mandated in OPRA, potentially rendering them unsuitable for this organ-preservation strategy. However, data from a large registry study has raised the possibility of de-escalating follow-up in some patients with a sustained complete clinical response (Fernandez et al., 2021).

Non-operative management

Although several definitions exist, a clinical complete response (cCR) is generally considered to be the absence of macroscopic tumour following neoadjuvant treatment. The combination of digital rectal examination, endoscopy, and MRI is 98% accurate in reaching this conclusion (Maas et al., 2015). As the practice of TNT has become more widespread, the proportion of patients developing a cCR has risen. Consequently, the MDT are increasingly confronted with the proposition of subjecting a patient to a major operation in the absence of a clinically identifiable tumour. This paradox has intensified the focus on non-operative management (NOM) or a WW approach, which is a more palatable option for clinicians and patients alike (Gani et al., 2019).

The International Watch & Wait Database (IWWD) comprises > 1,000 patients with baseline cT2-3, cN0-2 rectal cancer who received neoadjuvant therapy and *did not* proceed to TME (van der Valk et al., 2018). In the majority of cases ($n = 880$) this was because they achieved a cCR with LCCRT. The rate of local relapse in this cohort was 25%, with almost all these recurrences occurring within the first two years. The five-year overall survival rate in this cohort was 85% indicating that cCR is a reasonable surrogate for less aggressive tumour biology.

The prognostic benefit of sustaining a cCR for a year or longer was hugely significant in the IWWD cohort. For example, if a cCR was maintained for a year, the risk of local regrowth and distant metastases in the next two years was low, 12% and 8%, respectively. If the cCR continued for three years, these rates dropped to 3% and 2%, respectively, supporting the case for less intensive surveillance in these patients. Finally, patients who had a near complete response at first assessment but went on to develop a cCR at a later date had a similarly good prognosis (Temmink et al., 2023).

Whilst achieving a cCR is undoubtedly a beneficial prognostic indicator, data from this registry study are retrospective and subject to inherent limitations. Importantly, the findings only relate to patients undergoing neoadjuvant LCCRT, as less than 2% received TNT in any form. Another retrospective analysis of 113 patients with a cCR managed with a WW strategy, worryingly demonstrated a higher rate of distant metastases (36% vs 1%, $p < 0.001$) and a worse five-year OS (73% vs 94%) when compared to 136 patients who achieved a pCR (Smith et al., 2019). The most notable bias in this single institution study was that the WW group were significantly older than the pCR group (67 vs 57 years, $p < 0.001$).

Aside from OPRA, there is a lack of high-quality evidence to support a WW strategy for patients achieving a near complete or complete response following TNT. As the use of TNT increases, it is imperative that the safety of non-operative management is validated and indeed many ongoing TNT studies do incorporate a WW protocol. In conclusion, it would be prudent to adopt NOM cautiously, ideally as part of a clinical trial involving a defined surveillance protocol in a sufficiently resourced, high-volume centre.

Timing of surgery

There can be no doubt that good quality total mesorectal excision is indicated for a significant proportion of patients with LARC who will not be cured by radiotherapy, chemotherapy, or the combination. But the optimal timing of surgery following neoadjuvant therapy remains a controversial issue.

Conventional wisdom was to ideally operate within eight to ten weeks, but definitely no later than 12 weeks, from the last day of radiotherapy for LARC. This is supported by a pooled analysis of over 3,000 patients treated with LCCRT, which demonstrated that 95% of pCRs occurred within 10 weeks without compromising local recurrence, DFS, or OS (Gambacorta et al., 2021). In addition, some surgeons fear that beyond this timepoint there is an increase in surgical difficulty and complication rate as a result of radiation-induced pelvic fibrosis (Lefevre et al., 2016). Indeed, this was illustrated by the lower quality TME specimens in the RAPIDO trial investigational arm, where the extended course of chemotherapy resulted in surgery being postponed approximately 25 weeks after pelvic radiotherapy (Glynne-Jones et al., 2023). Furthermore, there were valid concerns about progressive disease if surgery was delayed for too long. The counter-argument to these views is that the full effects of chemoradiation can in fact take many months to be realized.

An influential trial that systematically explored this issue, known colloquially as the 'timing' study, might also be considered a nascent consolidation TNT trial (Garcia-Aguilar et al., 2015). This phase 2 trial sequentially assigned patients with stage 2 or 3 rectal cancer to receive LCCRT alone, or followed by two, four, or six cycles of FOLFOX before surgery. Naturally, the delivery of neoadjuvant chemotherapy extended the time interval to surgery whilst providing a level of protection from distant metastases.

The 'timing' trial demonstrated a strong correlation between the primary endpoint, pCR rate, and a longer time interval: 18% with LCCRT alone increasing to 38% in the group with the longest time to surgery, approximately 20 weeks. Reassuringly, technical difficulty and surgical complication rate was broadly similar across all groups despite surgeons scoring pelvic fibrosis higher as the time interval increased. This study provided evidence that delaying surgery following LCCRT, and administering chemotherapy during this time, was not only safe but also improved the response rate.

Adjuvant chemotherapy

Despite a plethora of randomized trials, the role of adjuvant chemotherapy for rectal cancer remains uncertain in the modern era. This was clearly illustrated in the international TNT study, RAPIDO, in which only 25 of 54 recruiting sites had an agreed policy to administer adjuvant chemotherapy following LCCRT (Bahadoer et al., 2021). Whilst the latest version of the National Comprehensive Cancer Network (NCCN) guidelines recommends adjuvant chemotherapy following neoadjuvant (chemo)radiotherapy regardless of pathological staging, it acknowledges the lack of robust data to support a DFS and OS benefit (NCCN, 2023). In fact, the ambiguity surrounding adjuvant chemotherapy in this context has been a powerful driving force behind the emergence of TNT in recent years.

Much of the literature to support adjuvant chemotherapy for rectal cancer is significantly outdated. For example, although a Cochrane meta-analysis from 2012 concluded that there was a significant benefit of adjuvant 5FU, most of the studies included were conducted before the widespread introduction of TME and neoadjuvant chemoradiation, rendering this conclusion tenuous at best (Petersen et al., 2012). Studies pre-dating the gold standard of MRI assessment could have incorrectly staged rectal tumours and neglected to account for negative prognostic indicators such as EMVI or distance to the MRF when stratifying participants. Finally, extrapolating data from trials that pooled colon and rectal cancer cases is ill advised considering the obvious embryological and molecular differences that have been elucidated in the intervening years.

More contemporary trials of adjuvant chemotherapy following neoadjuvant (chemo)radiotherapy have yielded conflicting results and have suffered from numerous limitations. For example, EORTC 22921, a randomized control trial of 1,011 patients with T3 or T4 rectal cancer, found that adjuvant 5FU-based chemotherapy following neoadjuvant (chemo)radiotherapy made no impact on DFS or OS (Bosset et al., 2014). However, it was unlikely that the chemotherapy component, bolus 5FU every three weeks for four cycles, was sufficient adjuvant therapy. Meanwhile, the CHRONICLE trial used a more modern regimen, six cycles of CAPOX, as adjuvant therapy but suffered from poor accrual and premature closure, making the underpowered results questionable (Glynne-Jones et al., 2014).

One of the most critical issues that has disrupted the interpretation of adjuvant trials in rectal cancer has been poor compliance with chemotherapy, which has generally been in the region of 50%, even after dose modification (Bosset et al., 2014; Hong et al., 2019). This figure is perhaps unsurprising when considering the already arduous and unpleasant journey patients must endure to reach adjuvant treatment. From a pathophysiological perspective, neoadjuvant pelvic radiation impacts bone marrow reserves and can cause small bowel enteritis, both of which can lead to surgical complications and delays in the administration of adjuvant chemotherapy. For further exploration of the intricacies and flaws of individual adjuvant rectal trials, readers are directed to an excellent systematic review (Carvalho & Glynne-Jones, 2017).

As the popularity of TNT for LARC rises, it is likely that adjuvant chemotherapy will become a less frequent clinical consideration in the future. TNT undoubtedly increases the proportion of patients achieving a pCR, a cohort who arguably derive little benefit from further chemotherapy (Cancer Research UK). In addition, patients with a poor response to TNT are likely to be intrinsically resistant to therapy and may also be unlikely to gain from further chemotherapy, although this is yet to be proven definitively.

TNT and the older patient

The incidence of rectal cancer is strongly associated with increasing age. Each year in the United Kingdom, 40% of the 8,000 to 13,000 new cases of rectal cancer are diagnosed in patients 75 years and older (Cancer Research UK).) Whether or not TNT is a safe and effective strategy for older patients is an open question, given their stark under-representation in the landmark trials discussed already.

The median age of participants in contemporary TNT trials has ranged from 55 to 61, whilst PRODIGE-23 excluded patients > 75 years old (Bujko et al., 2016; Bahadoeret al., 2021; Conroy et al., 2021; Jin et al., 2022; Verheijet al., 2023) Although this problem is not unique to TNT trials, it is imperative that trials are more representative of a real-world population. For example, the French phase 2 NACRE trial randomized patients > 75 years old with T3 or T4 rectal cancer to LCCRT or SCRT and indicated that the latter is better tolerated in this unique patient cohort (François et al., 2023). An ongoing Belgian study (NCT06052332) is specifically recruiting patients 70 and older to a randomized study of SCRT versus investigator choice of TNT.

Another major concern relating to TNT in the older patient is overtreatment and toxicity. Whilst a more aggressive approach to LARC may be justifiable in a younger patient aiming to avoid surgery and extend life expectancy, an older patient may not tolerate TNT as well. For example, the 43% rate of grade 3 toxicities observed with FOLFIRINOX in PRODIGE-23 is likely to be even higher in an older population given their reduced physiological reserve. In addition, an older patient's goals of care may focus more on quality of life, which should be the main consideration of the MDT when planning treatment.

The WW approach following a complete or near complete clinical response is particularly relevant to the older patient considering that they are at the highest risk of intra- and post-operative complications. Unfortunately, in the IWWD described earlier, the median age was 65 and the oldest patient 72, again making it difficult to translate this data to older patients with any degree of certainty.

All the modern TNT trials have included oxaliplatin in the chemotherapy regimen, which would represent a significant shift in practice for many oncologists treating older patients considering that, in the adjuvant setting, most colorectal cancer guidelines do not recommend oxaliplatin in adults over age 70 due to a lack of supportive data. Furthermore, the addition of oxaliplatin to 5FU and bevacizumab in an exclusively older population (mean age 79) with metastatic colorectal cancer improved response rates but did not improve PFS or OS (Hamaguchi et al., 2022).

In summary, it is difficult to apply much of the TNT data to an older population with any validity. Whilst they are a cohort that could benefit tremendously from a non-operative strategy, which is achieved to a greater extent with TNT, they are also likely to suffer the most toxicity from doublet or triplet oxaliplatin-based therapy. However, geriatric-focused assessments and multidisciplinary team input could help to select fitter older patients who might benefit from TNT as excluding patients solely on the basis of age would be foolish. Future trials conducted exclusively in older patients will be helpful.

DNA mismatch repair protein deficiency and microsatellite instability as a separate entity in neoadjuvant treatment

Immune checkpoint inhibitors have revolutionized the treatment of many cancer types in recent years including melanoma, lung, and renal cancer. These biologic agents target an inhibitory interaction between tumour cells and T cells, such as the programmed death (PD1) and cytotoxic T-lymphocyte antigen (CTLA) receptors. In some patients, especially those with tumours deficient in DNA mismatch repair proteins (dMMR) or high in DNA microsatellite instability (MSI-H), immunotherapy can trigger powerful and durable anti-tumour immunity resulting in very deep tumour responses to treatment. This strategy has recently shown considerable promise in the neoadjuvant treatment of dMMR/MSI-H rectal cancer.

A phase 2 trial of 12 patients with dMMR or MSI-H, stage 2 or 3 rectal cancer treated with six months of neoadjuvant dostarlimab, an anti-PD1 antibody, demonstrated a 100% complete clinical response rate (Cercek et al., 2022). At one-year follow-up, these patients had avoided both chemoradiotherapy and surgery without disease progression or recurrence. These encouraging data, albeit in a small cohort of biologically distinct patients from a single institution, formed the basis for an ongoing international, single arm study, AZUR-1, which will hopefully confirm these impressive results with longer follow-up (Cercek et al., 2023). At present, neoadjuvant immune checkpoint inhibitors are not the standard of care for dMMR/MSI-H rectal cancer although the NCCN guidelines do list them as their preferred option (NCCN, 2023). Indeed the US FDA has recently given dostarlimab Breakthrough Therapy designation for the treatment of locally advanced rectal cancers which are dMMR/MSI-H, based on a collaborative phase 2 trial between GSK and Memorial Sloan Kettering, which showed a 100% cCR in all 42 patients treated, as evidenced by MRI, positron emission tomography (PET), and endoscopy and digital rectal examination.

Despite understandable excitement within the oncological community and the mainstream media, immunotherapy is certainly not a panacea for all rectal cancer. Deficient MMR/MSI-H rectal cancer represents less than 10% of cases therefore the majority of patients would be ineligible for the single-agent approach (Swets et al., 2022). There are, however, emerging data and ongoing trials investigating the addition of neoadjuvant immunotherapy to the TNT paradigm for patients with proficient MMR rectal cancer. For example, a small Japanese study, VOLTAGE-A, has investigated the benefit of neoadjuvant LCCRT followed by nivolumab in patients with MMR proficient, T3 or T4 rectal cancer, demonstrating a pCR in 12 of 38 patients (Tsukada et al., 2023). Meanwhile, the UK-based PRIME-RT trial is adding durvalumab to both the radiation and chemotherapy components of a consolidation TNT approach (Roxburgh et al.,

Table 10.3 Selected ongoing and future neoadjuvant rectal cancer trials

Trial	Inclusion criteria (MRI defined unless specified otherwise)	Intervention arm(s)	Control arm	Study design	Primary endpoint	Status (as of 12/2023)	Comments
NORAD01 - GRECCAR 16 France NCT03875781	Mid or low T3N0 or T1-3N+ And CRM > 2 mm	mFOLFIRINOX ×6 cycles ↓ Surgery if CRM < 2 mm, otherwise LCCRT	LCCRT	Non-inferiority, randomized controlled trial	3-year Progression-free Survival	Recruiting	Similar to PROSPECT Adjuvant chemotherapy optional
JANUS USA NCT05610163	T4N0 Any T, N+ Or T3N0 requiring APR or coloanal anastomosis Within 12 cm on anal verge	*Group I* LCCRT ↓ FOLFOX or CAPOX ×4/12 ↓ WW or Surgery *Group II* LCCRT ↓ mFOLFIRINOX ×4/12 ↓ WW or Surgery	None	Randomized phase 2	Clinical complete response rate	Recruiting	Watch & wait protocol embedded into trial design Designed with significant input from patient groups
ACO/ARO/AIO-18.1 Germany NCT04246684	Mid or low Any T3 if < 6 cm T3c/d 6–12 cm T4 N+ CRM+ EMVI+	LCCRT* ↓ FOLFOX ×6 or CAPOX ×4 ↓ WW or Surgery	SCRT ↓ FOLFOX ×9 or CAPOX ×6 ↓ WW or Surgery	Randomized phase 3	Organ preservation rate at 3 years	Not yet recruiting	The control arm is the RAPIDO regimen
SHAPERS Belgium NCT06052332	Operable stage 3 or high-risk stage 2 Age ≥ 70	SCRT ↓ WW or Surgery +/− Adjuvant chemotherapy	Investigator choice of TNT: RAPIDO RAPIDO light OPRA induction or consolidation	Randomized, pragmatic	Overall survival	Not yet recruiting	Only patients 70 years and older are eligible
AZUR-1 International NCT05723562	dMMR or MSI-H T3 T4 N+	Dostarlimab × ≤ 9 cycles ↓ WW or Surgery	None	Phase 2	Clinical complete response maintained for > 12 months	Recruiting	Seeks to confirm the impressive 100% response rate seen in the earlier trial
PRIME-RT NCT04621370	> T3b EMVI+ MRF + or < 2 mm Low tumour requiring APR	*Arm A* SCRT ↓ Durvalumab + FOLFOX ×3/12 ↓ WW or Surgery Arm B LCCRT ↓ Durvalumab + FOLFOX ×2/12 ↓ WW or Surgery	None	Randomized phase 2	Clinical complete response rate	Closed, not yet reported	Patients with pMMR or MSI-L were eligible

*chemoradiation includes 5FU and oxaliplatin, standard of care in Germany

2023). Finally, the Chinese TORCH-E study is adding toripalimab to the chemotherapy component of TNT only (Yajie et al., 2023).

Combining neoadjuvant immunotherapy with chemotherapy might be a safer strategy when considering that a trial by André et al. suggested that almost 40% of patients with dMMR/MSI-H metastatic colorectal cancer progressed within six months of pembrolizumab monotherapy (André et al., 2020). This rate of progression would be disastrous in the neoadjuvant treatment of patients with LARC, particularly in those with high-risk, low-lying tumours in whom the intention is significant downstaging.

Finally, in relation to TNT, there is evidence that dMMR/MSI-H rectal tumours do not respond well to chemotherapy alone. In a retrospective study, 25% of patients with dMMR rectal cancer experienced progressive disease with neoadjuvant FOLFOX as opposed to 0% in a matched proficient MMR cohort (Cercek et al., 2020). In contrast, sensitivity to chemoradiation was not influenced by MMR status. Crucially, none of the TNT studies discussed in this chapter required assessment of MMR or MSI status before study enrolment, probably because mandatory testing in newly diagnosed patients was not standard of care at the time. A retrospective analysis of the major TNT trials could delineate whether dMMR/MSI-H patients truly benefited from TNT. At present, the role of TNT in patients with dMMR/MSI-H is unclear and future TNT trials may well exclude or stratify for these patients, depending on the strategy being tested.

Conclusions and future directions

This chapter demonstrates the significant developments, challenges, and controversies in the multidisciplinary management of patients with locally advanced rectal cancer.

Clearly, TNT is an appropriate strategy for carefully selected patients with LARC. The increased compliance with systemic chemotherapy contributes to meaningful benefits in disease-free survival and primary tumour regression. This is supported by a recent meta-analysis of eight TNT studies comprising more than 2,000 patients, which showed improvements in pCR, DFS, OS, and distant metastases when compared to standard chemoradiotherapy (Liu et al., 2021). Importantly, TNT appears safe and does not significantly compromise the delivery of LCCRT or surgery.

Currently, the NCCN recommends TNT for > T3 tumours, any node positive disease or an involved or threatened circumferential margin (NCCN, 2023). Adopting this approach across the board will ultimately lead to the overtreatment of a significant number of patients, whilst on the other hand, the outdated European Society of Medical Oncology (ESMO) rectal cancer guidelines probably under-treats many others (Glynne-Jones et al., 2017). Several ongoing trials, summarized in Table 10.3, will help to answer some key questions such as the optimal radiotherapy platform, the precise benefit of neoadjuvant irinotecan, and the potential benefit of immunotherapy in pMMR tumours.

In the future, a better understanding of the heterogenous molecular biology underpinning rectal cancer will hopefully lead to better risk stratification and predictive biomarkers that enable clinicians to tailor neoadjuvant treatment to the individual patient. But for now, integrating TNT into everyday clinical practice remains complex and should be framed by the ultimate intention of neoadjuvant treatment: downsizing of the primary tumour and/or reducing the risk of distant metastases (Fig. 10.1). As such, an informed multidisciplinary team approach centred on the patients' goals of care, is the best strategy.

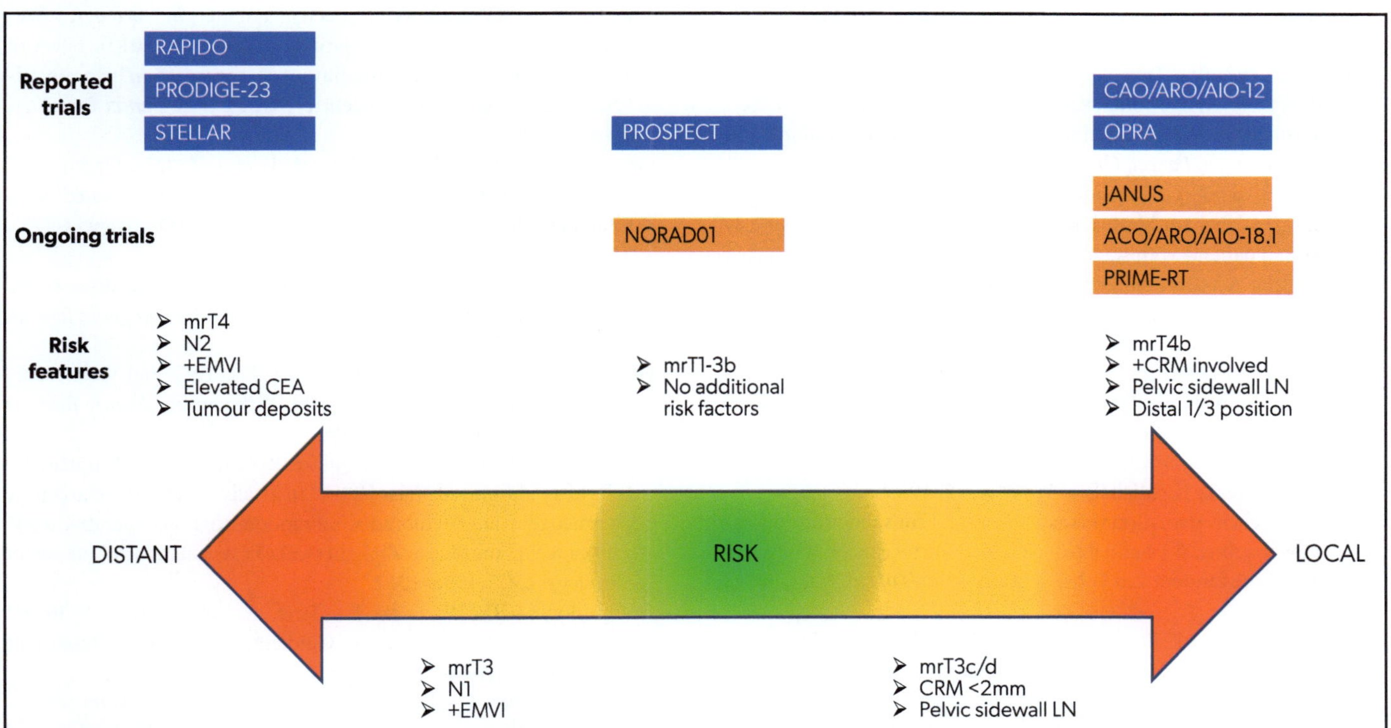

Figure 10.1 Assessing the relative risk of local recurrence versus distant metastases with associated trials, both reported and ongoing.

REFERENCES

André, T., Shiu, K.-K., Kim, T. W., et al. (2020). Pembrolizumab in microsatellite-instability–high advanced colorectal cancer. *New England Journal of Medicine, 383*(23), 2207–2218.

Bahadoer, R. R., Dijkstra, E. A., van Etten, B., et al. (2021). Short-course radiotherapy followed by chemotherapy before total mesorectal excision (TME) versus preoperative chemoradiotherapy, TME, and optional adjuvant chemotherapy in locally advanced rectal cancer (RAPIDO): a randomised, open-label, phase 3 trial. *Lancet Oncology, 22*(1), 29–42.

Bascoul-Mollevi, C., Gourgou, S., Borg, C., et al. (2023). Neoadjuvant chemotherapy with FOLFIRINOX and preoperative chemoradiotherapy for patients with locally advanced rectal cancer (UNICANCER PRODIGE 23): health-related quality of life longitudinal analysis. *European Journal of Cancer, 186*:151–165.

Bisschop, C., van Dijk, T. H., Beukema, J. C., et al. (2017). Short-course radiotherapy followed by neoadjuvant bevacizumab, capecitabine, and oxaliplatin and subsequent radical treatment in primary stage IV rectal cancer: long-term results of a phase II study. *Annals of Surgical Oncology, 24*(9), 2632–2638.

Bosset, J. F., Calais, G., Mineur, L., et al. (2014). Fluorouracil-based adjuvant chemotherapy after preoperative chemoradiotherapy in rectal cancer: long-term results of the EORTC 22921 randomised study. *Lancet Oncology, 15*(2), 184–190.

Breugom, A. J., van Gijn, W., Muller, E. W., et al. (2015). Adjuvant chemotherapy for rectal cancer patients treated with preoperative (chemo)radiotherapy and total mesorectal excision: a Dutch Colorectal Cancer Group (DCCG) randomized phase III trial. *Annals of Oncology, 26*(4), 696–701.

Bujko, K., Wyrwicz, L., Rutkowski, A., et al. (2016). Long-course oxaliplatin-based preoperative chemoradiation versus 5 × 5 Gy and consolidation chemotherapy for cT4 or fixed cT3 rectal cancer: results of a randomized phase III study. *Annals of Oncology, 27*(5), 834–842.

Cancer Research UK. https://www.cancerresearchuk.org/health-professional/cancer-statistics/statistics-by-cancer-type/bowel-cancer/incidence#heading-Two.

Carvalho, C., & Glynne-Jones, R. (2017). Challenges behind proving efficacy of adjuvant chemotherapy after preoperative chemoradiation for rectal cancer. *Lancet, Oncology, 18*(6), e354–363.

Cercek, A., Bachet, J.-B., Capdevila, J., et al. (2023). Phase II, single-arm, open-label study of dostarlimab monotherapy in previously untreated patients with stage II/III dMMR/MSI-H locally advanced rectal cancer. *Journal of Clinical Oncology, 41*(16_suppl), TPS3639.

Cercek, A., Dos Santos Fernandes, G., Roxburgh, C. S., et al. Mismatch repair–deficient rectal cancer and resistance to neoadjuvant chemotherapy. *Clinical Cancer Research*, 2020;*26*(13), 3271–3279.

Cercek, A., Lumish, M., Sinopoli, J., et al. (2022). PD-1 blockade in mismatch repair–deficient, locally advanced rectal cancer. *New England Journal of Medicine, 386*(25), 2363–2376.

Ciseł, B., Pietrzak, L., Michalski, W., et al. (2019). Long-course preoperative chemoradiation versus 5 × 5 Gy and consolidation chemotherapy for clinical T4 and fixed clinical T3 rectal cancer: long-term results of the randomized Polish II study. *Annals of Oncology, 30*(8), 1298–1303.

Conroy, T., Bosset, J. F., Etienne, P. L., et al. (2021). Neoadjuvant chemotherapy with FOLFIRINOX and preoperative chemoradiotherapy for patients with locally advanced rectal cancer (UNICANCER-PRODIGE 23): a multicentre, randomised, open-label, phase 3 trial. *Lancet Oncology, 22*(5), 702–715.

Dijkstra, E. A., Nilsson, P. J., Hospers, G. A. P., et al. (2023). Locoregional failure during and after short-course radiotherapy followed by chemotherapy and surgery compared with long-course chemoradiotherapy and surgery: a 5-year follow-up of the RAPIDO Trial. *Annals of Surgery, 278*(4), e766–772.

Etienne, P.-L., Rio, E., Evesque, L., et al. (2023). Total neoadjuvant therapy with mFOLFIRINOX versus preoperative chemoradiation in patients with locally advanced rectal cancer: 7-year results of PRODIGE 23 phase III trial, a UNICANCER GI trial. *Journal of Clinical Oncology, 41*(17_suppl), LBA3504.

Fernandez, L. M., São, Julião G. P., Figueiredo, N. L., et al. (2021). Conditional recurrence-free survival of clinical complete responders managed by watch and wait after neoadjuvant chemoradiotherapy for rectal cancer in the International Watch & Wait Database: a retrospective, international, multicentre registry study. *Lancet Oncology, 22*(1), 43–50.

Fokas, E., Allgäuer, M., Polat, B., et al. (2019). Randomized phase II trial of chemoradiotherapy plus induction or consolidation chemotherapy as total neoadjuvant therapy for locally advanced rectal cancer: CAO/ARO/AIO-12. *Journal of Clinical Oncology, 37*(34), 3212–3222.

Fokas, E., Schlenska-Lange, A., Polat, B., et al. (2022). Chemoradiotherapy plus induction or consolidation chemotherapy as total neoadjuvant therapy for patients with locally advanced rectal cancer: long-term results of the CAO/ARO/AIO-12 randomized clinical trial. *JAMA Oncology, 8*(1), e215445.

François E., De Bar,i B., Ronchin, P., et al. (2023). Comparison of short course radiotherapy with chemoradiotherapy for locally advanced rectal cancers in the elderly: A multicentre, randomised, non-blinded, phase 3 trial. *European Journal of Cancer, 180*:62–70.

Gambacorta, M. A., Masciocchi, C., Chiloiro, G., et al. (2021). Timing to achieve the highest rate of pCR after preoperative radiochemotherapy in rectal cancer: a pooled analysis of 3085 patients from 7 randomized trials. *Radiotherapy & Oncology, 154*:154–160.

Gani, C., Gani, N., Zschaeck, S., et al. (2019). Organ preservation in rectal cancer: the patients' perspective. *Frontiers in Oncology, 9*:318.

Garcia-Aguilar, J., Chow, O. S., Smith, D. D., et al. (2015). Effect of adding mFOLFOX6 after neoadjuvant chemoradiation in locally advanced rectal cancer: a multicentre, phase 2 trial. *Lancet Oncology, 16*(8), 957–966.

Garcia-Aguilar, J., Patil, S., Gollub, M. J., et al. (2022). Organ preservation in patients with rectal adenocarcinoma treated with total neoadjuvant therapy. *Journal of Clinical Oncology, 40*(23), 2546–2556.

Gastrointestinal Study Group. (1985). Prolongation of the disease-free interval in surgically treated rectal carcinoma. *New England Journal of Medicine, 312*(23), 1465–1472.

Glynne-Jones, R., & Hollingshead, J. (2023). TNT and local recurrence in the RAPIDO trial—untangling the puzzle. *Nature Reviews Clinical Oncology, 20*(6), 357–358.

Glynne-Jones, R., Counsell, N., Quirke, P., et al. (2014). Chronicle: results of a randomised phase III trial in locally advanced rectal cancer after neoadjuvant chemoradiation randomising postoperative adjuvant capecitabine plus oxaliplatin (XELOX) versus control. *Annals of Oncology, 25*(7), 1356–1362.

Glynne-Jones, R., Wyrwicz, L., Tiret, E., et al. (2017). Rectal cancer: ESMO Clinical Practice Guidelines for diagnosis, treatment and follow-up. *Annals of Oncology, 28*(suppl_4), iv22–40.

Grothey, A, Sobrero, A. F., Shields, A. F., et al. (2018). Duration of adjuvant chemotherapy for stage III colon cancer. *New England Journal of Medicine, 378*(13), 1177–1188.

Hamaguchi, T., Takashima, A., Mizusawa, J., et al. (2022). A randomized phase III trial of mFOLFOX7 or CapeOX plus bevacizumab versus 5-FU/l-LV or capecitabine plus bevacizumab as initial therapy in elderly patients with metastatic colorectal cancer: JCOG1018 study (RESPECT). *GI ASCO*; 01/02/2022.

He, F., Ju, H.-Q., Ding, Y., et al. (2020). Association between adjuvant chemotherapy and survival in patients with rectal cancer and pathological complete response after neoadjuvant chemoradiotherapy and resection. *British Journal of Cancer*, *123*(8), 1244–1252.

Hong, Y. S., Kim, S. Y., Lee, J. S., et al. (2019). Oxaliplatin-based adjuvant chemotherapy for rectal cancer after preoperative chemoradiotherapy (ADORE): long-term results of a randomized controlled trial. *Journal of Clinical Oncology*, *37*(33), 3111–3123.

Jin, J., Tang, Y., Hu, C., et al. Multicenter, randomized, phase III trial of short-term radiotherapy plus chemotherapy versus long-term chemoradiotherapy in locally advanced rectal cancer (STELLAR). *Journal of Clinical Oncology*, *40*(15), JCO.21.01667.

Lefevre, J. H., Mineur, L., et al. (2016). Effect of interval (7 or 11 weeks) between neoadjuvant radiochemotherapy and surgery on complete pathologic response in rectal cancer: a multicenter, randomized, controlled Trial (GRECCAR-6). *Journal of Clinical Oncology*, *34*(31), 3773–3780.

Liu, S., Jiang, T., Xiao, L., et al. (2012). Total neoadjuvant therapy (TNT) versus standard neoadjuvant chemoradiotherapy for locally advanced rectal cancer: a systematic review and meta-analysis. *Oncologist*, *26*(9), e1555–e66.

Maas, M., Lambregts, D. M., Nelemans, P. J., et al. (2015). Assessment of clinical complete response after chemoradiation for rectal cancer with digital rectal examination, endoscopy, and MRI: selection for organ-saving treatment. *Annals of Surgical Oncology*, *22*(12), 3873–3880.

NCCN. Rectal Cancer guidelines Version 5.2023 September 2023. https://www.nccn.org/professionals/physician_gls/pdf/rectal.pdf.

O'Cathail, S. M., Adams, R., Hawkins, M. A., et al. (2023). Patient-reported outcomes in PROSPECT trial (Alliance N1048)—FOLFOX is not a panacea. *Clinical and Translational Radiation Oncology*, *43*.

Petersen, S. H., Harling, H., Kirkeby, L.T., et al. (2012). Postoperative adjuvant chemotherapy in rectal cancer operated for cure. *Cochrane Database of Systematic Reviews*, *2012*(3), Cd004078.

Roxburgh, C. S. D., Hanna, C. R., Graham, J., et al. (2023). Durvalumab (MEDI 4736) with extended neoadjuvant regimens in rectal cancer: A randomised phase II trial (PRIME-RT). *Journal of Clinical Oncology*, *41*(4_suppl), TPS282.

Sainato, A., Cernusco Luna Nunzia, V., Valentini, V., et al. (2014). No benefit of adjuvant Fluorouracil Leucovorin chemotherapy after neoadjuvant chemoradiotherapy in locally advanced cancer of the rectum (LARC): long term results of a randomized trial (I-CNR-RT). *Radiotherapy & Oncology*, *113*(2), 223–229.

Sauer, R., Liersch, T., Merkel, S., et al. (2012). Preoperative versus postoperative chemoradiotherapy for locally advanced rectal cancer: results of the German CAO/ARO/AIO-94 randomized phase III trial after a median follow-up of 11 years. *Journal of Clinical Oncology*, *30*(16), 1926–1933.

Schrag, D., Shi, Q., Weiser, M. R., et al. (2023). Preoperative treatment of locally advanced rectal cancer. *New England Journal of Medicine*, *389*(4), 322–334.

Smith, J. J., Strombom, P., Chow, O. S., et al. (2019). Assessment of a watch-and-wait strategy for rectal cancer in patients with a complete response after neoadjuvant therapy. *JAMA Oncology*, *5*(4), e185896.

Swets, M., Graham Martinez, C., van Vliet, S., et al. (2022). Microsatellite instability in rectal cancer: what does it mean? A study of two randomized trials and a systematic review of the literature. *Histopathology*, *81*(3), 352–362.

Temmink, S. J. D., Peeters, K. C. M. J., Bahadoer, R. R., et al. (2023). Watch and wait after neoadjuvant treatment in rectal cancer: comparison of outcomes in patients with and without a complete response at first reassessment in the International Watch & Wait Database (IWWD). *British Journal of Surgery*, *110*(6), 676–684.

Tsukada, Y., Bando, H., Inamori, K., et al. (2023). Survival outcomes and functional results of VOLTAGE-A: preoperative chemoradiotherapy (CRT) and consolidation nivolumab (nivo) in patients (pts) with both microsatellite stable (MSS) and microsatellite instability–high (MSI-H) locally advanced rectal cancer (LARC). *Journal of Clinical Oncology*, *41*(4_suppl), 108.

van der Valk, M. J. M., Hilling, D. E., Bastiaannet, E., et al. (2018). Long-term outcomes of clinical complete responders after neoadjuvant treatment for rectal cancer in the International Watch & Wait Database (IWWD): an international multicentre registry study. *Lancet*, *391*(10139), 2537–2345.

Verheij, F. S., Omer, D. M., Williams, H., et al. (2023). Long-term results of organ preservation in patients with rectal adenocarcinoma treated with total neoadjuvant therapy: the randomized phase II OPRA trial. *Journal of Clinical Oncology*, Jco2301208.

Yajie, C., Yaqi, W., Hui, Z., et al. (2023). Short-course radiotherapy combined with chemotherapy and PD-1 inhibitor in low-lying early rectal cancer: study protocol for a single-arm, multicentre, prospective, phase II trial (TORCH-E). *BMJ Open*, *13*(10), e076048.

11

The multidisciplinary management of colorectal liver metastases

Alex Gordon-Weeks, Daniel Hughes, and Mike Silva

Introduction

The anatomical variability with which CRLM seed within the liver, combined with variation in hepatic vascular and biliary anatomy significantly impact upon the suitability of liver-directed treatments. Whilst some patients present with a relatively small burden of liver disease, others have inoperable metastases at the outset. A proportion of those with inoperable disease may become operable after a period of systemic therapy, whilst other patients may only be rendered operable after measures are taken to increase the predicted post-resection liver volume. The presence of a synchronous primary tumour brings a further dimension to the treatment algorithm and here, additional clinical decisions must be made.

As the number of treatment modalities for CRLM have grown, the complexity of the decision-making process has increased. Whilst some therapeutic approaches have been developed on the back of robust clinical evidence, many do not have a sufficient evidence base to enable an understanding of how they can be best used in a patient-specific manner. The chronology of different modalities is also of paramount importance, as the window of benefit for some is short, and others demonstrate a degree of mutual exclusivity. Given these complexities, it is vital to ensure that treatment decisions for CRLM patients are made through the collaborative efforts of clinicians from a wide range of specialist backgrounds, thus underlining the importance of the multidisciplinary team in the decision-making process. With these issues in mind, this chapter explores the role of the MDT in the management of CRLM though reference to standard clinical scenarios.

Evidence for the value of the MDT in CRLM management

The primary benefit of the MDT is that it brings together clinicians from a range of specialist interests. At a minimum, this should include a radiologist, oncologist, and surgeon. Ideally, a hepatobiliary surgeon, gastrointestinal radiologist, interventional radiologist with expertise in ablative techniques and transcatheter arterial chemoembolization (TACE), clinical oncologist, and a radiation oncologist with expertise in SBRT (stereotactic body radiotherapy) and SIRT (selective internal radiation therapy) With this input, all potential therapeutic modalities can be considered and a rational plan formulated. For cases of synchronous disease, the presence of a colorectal surgeon is important for aiding coordination of order of resection (primary then metastases versus metastases then primary versus synchronous) and the importantly, the team should have access to contemporaneous and all relevant historical cross-sectional imaging such that the response to prior treatments can be accurately assessed. Ideally, the case should be presented by the referring clinician, as this increases diagnostic accuracy, improves communication about the well-being and performance status of the patient, as well as the likelihood of the MDT-prescribed management plan being enacted (Basta et al., 2016). It ensures that unrealistic treatment plans are not suggested through lack of knowledge of patient fitness. Where this is not possible, a standardized proforma should be used so that a minimum set of relevant information is routinely obtained. This prevents cases being deferred until relevant information is available or incorrect decisions being made because inadequate information is presented.

Comparison of local and specialist hepatobiliary MDT assessment demonstrates a clinically significant alteration in the management of up to 41% of patients reviewed at the specialist hepatopancreatobilary (HPB)/liver metastases multidisciplinary team (MDT) (van Hagen et al., 2013; Zhang et al., 2013; Meguid et al., 2016). Interestingly, whilst it is well recognized that the MDT in general alters management plans, this change appears particularly significant in MDTs where decisions surrounding the management of CRLM are made (Meguid et al., 2016), perhaps underlining the additional complexity of clinical decision making in this setting. Patients assessed at a specialist HPB MDT are also more likely to be recruited to clinical trials (Zhang et al., 2013) and are significantly less likely to experience tumour recurrence; findings attributed to greater staging accuracy (Ye et al., 2012) and higher rates of chemotherapy use either before or after surgery in patients reviewed in the MDT (MacDermid et al., 2009).

However, it is also recognized that the MDT decision is not implemented in at least 10% of CRC patients, with the most common reason being lack of appreciation of comorbidity during the MDT discussion (Wood et al., 2008). Equally, it is important to consider that whilst the MDT may be capable of bringing together the broadest expertise possible to formulate the most accurate management plan based on the available information, there are patient-specific factors that it cannot assess, and crucially, it lacks input from the patient's perspective (Taylor et al., 2014). Whilst it may be practically impossible to involve patients in the MDT discussion, it is important that the MDT outcome is not considered absolute and is used as part of a shared decision-making process in a clinic setting post-MDT (Taylor et al., 2014).

Key decisions to be made by the MDT

The primary function of the MDT is to arrive at a consensus agreement on the appropriate management. This primarily focuses around assessment of operability or a plan to achieve operability, given that this is the primary modality capable of providing long-term cure, or the possibility of other 'radical' interventions if surgery is not possible, either through anatomy or fitness of the patient discussed. In cases where surgery is not immediately an option, then the focus is often on whether systemic therapies may be able to down-size disease burden sufficiently to enable potentially curative surgery in the future after a period of treatment Alternatively, there is mounting evidence that liver-directed treatment modalities can be used to limit disease progression/gain maximal control, with a view to prolonging survival whilst maintaining quality of life. An example algorithm that the MDT may work through is demonstrated in Fig. 11.1.

Immediately resectable colorectal liver metastasis

Although not yet supported by robust randomized prospective longitudinal data, surgery is considered the best treatment option for patients with CRLM as removal of all visible metastases provides the greatest chance of long-term cure. The fact that it is now difficult to go back and run a randomized trial is testament to the observation that the oncological community is convinced by past observation that liver metastatectomy provides a meaningful path to long-term cure of CRLMs.

Assessing those for resection and the role of peri-operative chemotherapy in immediately resectable CRLM

The number of liver metastases no longer govern the decision-making process, although it is understood that multiple and widespread CRLM is a surrogate of poor tumour biology (Fong et al., 1999). Instead, leaving sufficient functional liver volume (at least two contiguous liver segments) with adequate vascular (portal venous and hepatic arterial) inflow and hepatic venous outflow along with biliary drainage is a requirement (Guglielmi et al., 2012). Nonetheless, it should be noted that it is the function, rather than the volume, of remnant liver that is most closely related to post-operative outcome, with dynamic assessment of liver function being particularly important for patients with biochemical or radiological evidence of liver dysfunction. Indocyanine green excretion is commonly used in Asia and the far East, but less frequently in Western centres where chronic liver disease is less prevalent amongst patients with CRLMs (Rassam et al., 2017). Scintigraphic tests provide visualization of function, which is helpful where there may be regional variability in function, but this does require specialist equipment and radiochemicals and these methods are infrequently used in the West (de Graaf et al., 2010). Another surrogate of functionality is the ability of the liver to hypertrophy in response to portal vein embolization. Our practice is to offer hepatic vein embolization or a

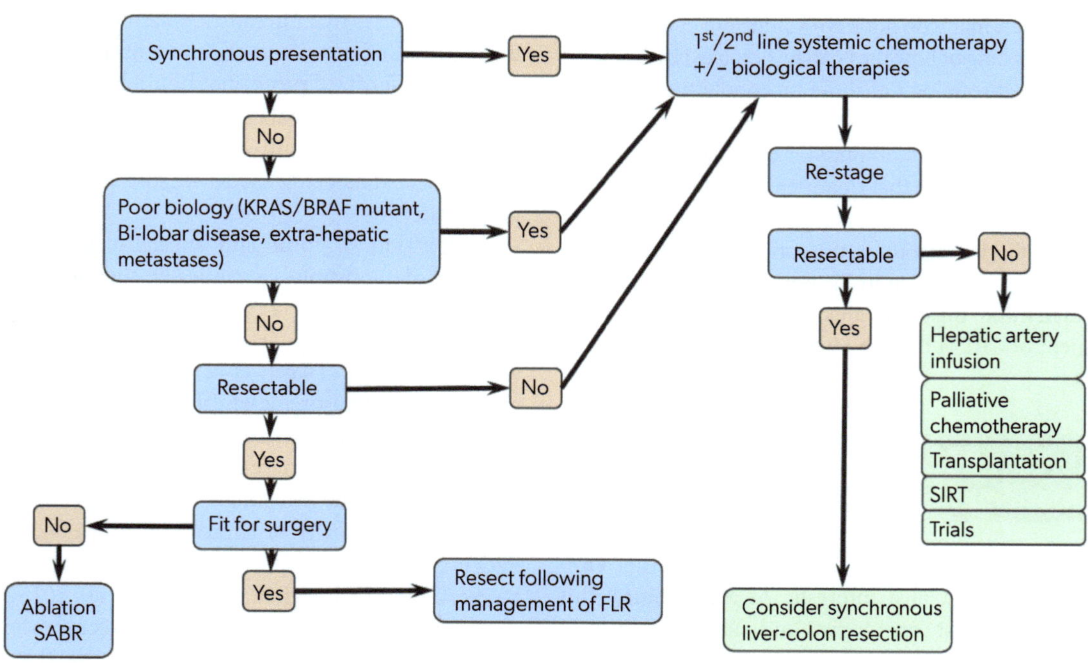

Figure 11.1 MDT-directed pathway for the management of liver-dominant metastatic CRC.

rescue ALPPS (an associating liver partition and portal vein ligation for staged hepatectomy) procedure in patients who do not show adequate hypertrophy within 10 weeks of technically successful portal vein embolization. These assessments are based solely on volume assessment rather than dynamic, quantitative tests.

For patients with operable liver metastases from the outset, some form of peri-operative chemotherapy may improve disease-free survival but with no long-term overall survival benefit (Nordlinger et al., 2013; Kanemitsu et al., 2021). However, morbidity is significantly higher in patients that undergo hepatectomy following chemotherapy (Karoui et al., 2006; Welsh et al., 2007; Konopkeet al., 2009), due to a negative impact on liver function, with sinusoidal congestion, veno-occlusive disease, steatosis and steatohepatitis all recognized histological findings (Rubbia-Brandt et al., 2004; Aloia et al., 2006; Gangi & Lu, 2020). Currently, there is no universally accepted protocol for the use of peri-operative chemotherapy in patients with operable liver metastasis (Krasnodebski et al., 2020) and whilst the National Institute for Health and Care Excellence (NICE) recommends peri-operative chemotherapy for CRLM (Mohamed et al., 2020), the Japanese Society for Cancer of the Colon and Rectum (JSCCR) guidelines do not recommend chemotherapy (Hashiguchi et al., 2020) and the NCCN guidance states equivalence between peri-operative chemotherapy versus no chemotherapy (Xu & Zhou, 2021). This uncertainty again highlights the importance of the MDT in making a patient-tailored decision around the use of peri-operative chemotherapy. Our practice is to offer neoadjuvant chemotherapy to patients with operable CRLM only when we deem them to be of higher oncological risk. This may include patients with *RAS/RAF* mutations, those with multiple liver metastases, where the primary was associated with extensive nodal disease, and synchronous presentation or relapse rapidly after primary removal or the end of adjuvant chemotherapy. We also use chemotherapy as a 'test of time' in these patients to assess whether we are just seeing the 'tip of the iceberg' of their disease, as well as those with potential disease (i.e. unconfirmed nodules) at other sites such as the lung or peritoneum: This is a recognised practice favoured by many MDTs but it is not based on high-level evidence.

Achieving adequate functional liver remnant

Depending on the number and location of CRLM, one stage liver resection based on segmental liver anatomy or wedge resections is the preference. It is well established that patients with a normal liver parenchyma can tolerate a reduction in liver volume down to as little as 20% of the entire hepatic volume. In those with chemotherapy-induced liver injury, a volume of approximately 30% and those with cirrhosis require at least a 40% residual liver volume. For patients who require major liver resection (more than three contiguous segments), especially if liver function is impacted by ongoing or recent chemotherapy, quantification of future liver remnant volume is paramount. This allows some degree of risk stratification with regards occurrence of post-operative liver failure and also helps identify those patients who may require strategies to increase future liver remnant volume.

Following this assessment, there are several options to consider in patients with resectable disease but borderline remnant liver volume, particularly in those patients with extensive bi-lobar liver metastasis: (i) portal vein embolization, and the more recent practice of subsequent hepatic vein embolization (Guiu et al., 2016; Guiu et al., 2017) can be performed safely with minimal morbidity (Fig. 11.2); (ii) combined resection with ablation; and (iii) staged liver resections, or ALPPS (Schnitzbauer et al., 2012) are all recognized strategies to facilitate operability in terms of leaving an adequate volume and functional reserve.

The addition of liver partitioning to portal vein ligation as the first in a two-stage approach results in rapid hypertrophy of the future liver remnant (Schnitzbauer et al., 2012; Schadde et al., 2014). This occurs more rapidly than the volume increase seen in portal vein embolization alone and results in higher resection rates, albeit at the expense of greater morbidity (Eshmuminov et al., 2016). Although there are questions regarding whether volume increase is matched by functional gains (Budai et al., 2019; Yifan et al., 2019), ALPPS has been widely adopted and provides comparable results to standard two-stage hepatectomy (Björnsson et al., 2014). We particularly consider ALPPS in patients deemed likely to progress in

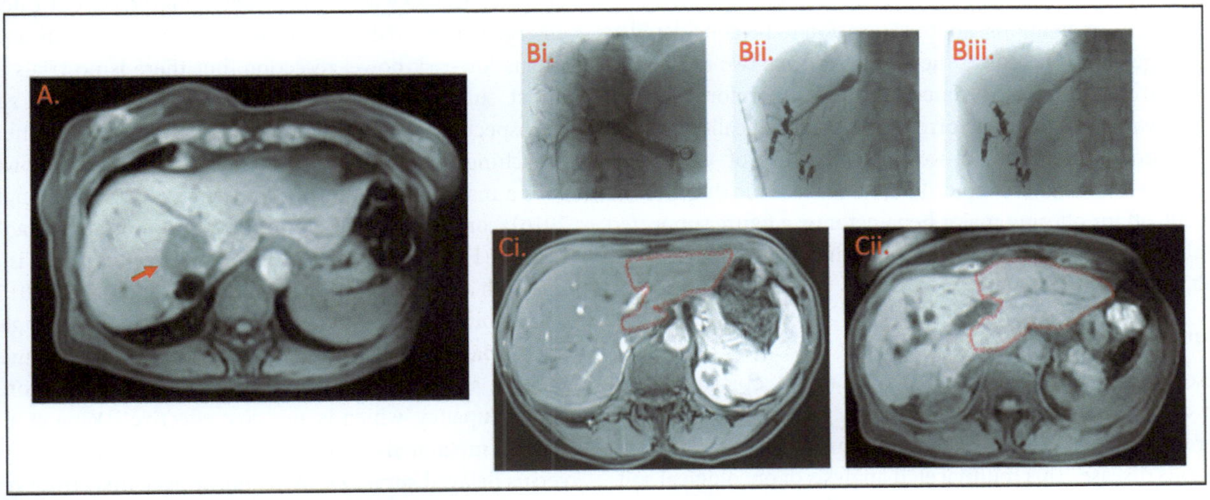

Figure 11.2 Dual vein embolization to improve the FLR. **A.** the patient presented with an awkwardly placed CRLM straddling the right and middle hepatic veins (arrow), with a relatively small left lateral section. **Bi–iii.** The patient underwent embolization of the right portal vein (i) followed 24 hours later by embolization of the right and middle hepatic veins (ii–iii). **Ci–ii.** This resulted in a 35% increase in the FLR (red outline) by four weeks and the patient subsequently underwent an extended right hepatectomy without complication.

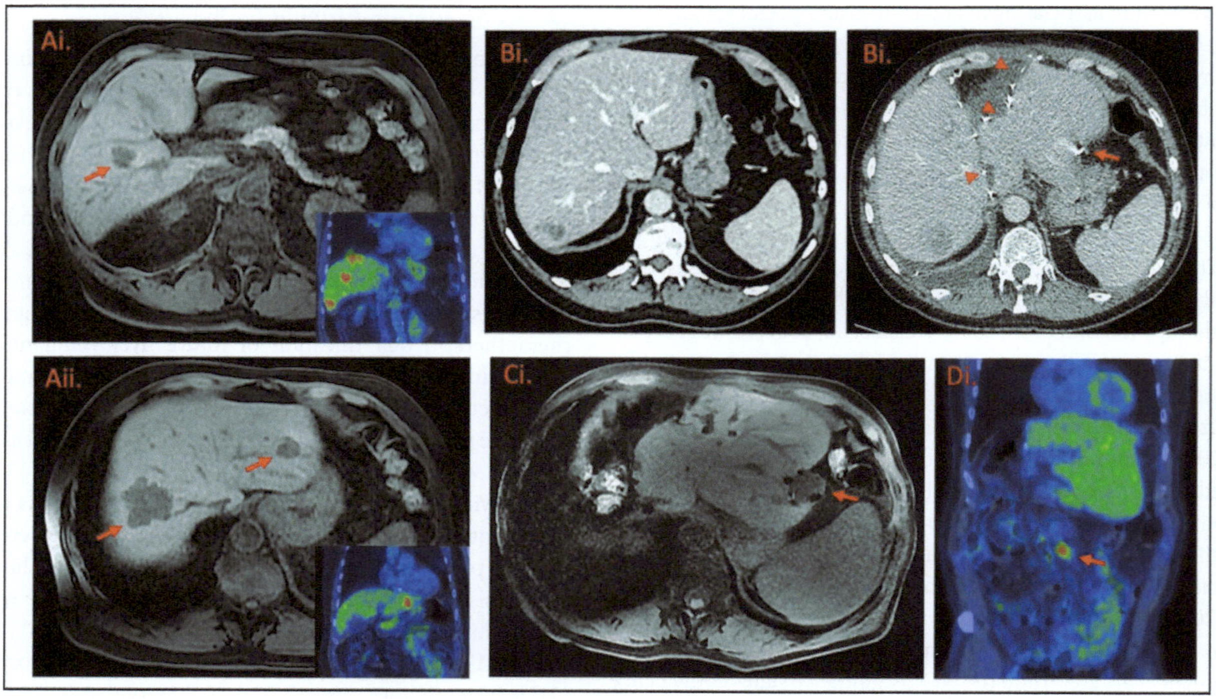

Figure 11.3 ALPPS in a patient with bi-lobar CRLM and insufficient FLR. **Ai–ii.** The patient presented with eight bi-lobar CRLM and a synchronous sigmoid malignancy (CT-PET inset). The MDT advised neoadjuvant chemotherapy which was given but without significant response. After second-line chemotherapy, the patient had still demonstrated minimal response, but the disease remained confined to the liver and with no increase in the number or size of metastases through treatment thus far. Given the indication of reasonable tumour biology, a decision was made to proceed to ALPPS as a preferred management of the insufficient FLR, as portal vein embolization would have resulted in a longer chemotherapy-free period with the chance of interval progression and embolization of the right hemi liver may have increased growth of the segment III metastasis. **Bi–ii.** Imagine pre- (i) and 10 days post stage 1 ALPPS (ii), where the liver parenchyma has been transected to preserve inflow to segments I, II, III (arrow heads), and the segment II CRLM has been resected (arrow). The image demonstrates growth of the FLR which was measured at 42% increase in volume. **Ci.** The patient made an uneventful recovery but developed a solitary hepatic recurrence 18 months following ALPPS (arrow). The MDT decision was for further systemic therapy as a test of tumour biology. This resulted in a period of disease stability followed by resection of the metastasis without complication. **Di.** Two years later the patient developed mesenteric nodal recurrence (arrow), which, following discussion at the MDT was treated with SABR. Ultimately the patient succumbed with widespread metastatic disease a further two years later, having experienced good quality of life for over five years since his initial diagnosis.

the interval between portal vein embolization (PVE) and resection or between first and second stage hepatectomy (Fig. 11.3). Often, at the first stage of an ALPPS procedure, if the future liver remnant has a limited tumour burden, this can be addressed with either wedge resections or ablations; another decision to be considered at the MDT stage. ALPPS requires the patient to have two major surgical procedures within a short time frame and is therefore reserved for patients with adequate performance status, typically assessed through thorough anaesthetic workup inclusive of cardiopulmonary exercise testing. We typically use an anaerobic threshold of 10.5 as a cut-off for offering major hepatectomy; a figure supported by several retrospective series (Kasivisvanathan et al., 2015; Kumar & Garcea, 2018).

Management of synchronous disease

Liver resection may be safely carried out laparoscopically, robotically, or as an open procedure, and before, synchronously, or following, resection of the primary colonic tumour in patients with synchronous disease. This multifaceted analysis of oncological suitability, liver anatomy, and functional residual liver volume is a key consideration for the MDT. This decision is aided if knowledge of patient performance status is known, in addition to the symptomatology of the primary or propensity for imminent obstruction.

Depending on the extent of liver disease and need for major hepatectomy along with the location of the bowel primary; with right-sided disease being comparatively lower risk versus left colon or rectal disease which is considered high risk, four categories have emerged: High-risk versus low-risk liver resection and high-risk versus low-risk bowel resection, but there is no trials evidence to direct surgical order in these patients. Numerous single-centre retrospective studies demonstrate that there is a morbidity approaching 50% with the combination of a high-risk bowel resection with a major hepatectomy (Shubert et al., 2015; Muangkaew et al., 2016), comparable to the morbidity and mortality of an ALPPS resection. However, any type of minor liver resection is considered safe with any type of bowel resection (Shubert et al., 2015).

Combined hepatectomy and colectomy means a single operation for the patient, with benefits in terms of planning adjuvant chemotherapy, single hospital admission, and, overall, a shorter hospital bed occupancy, which is also cost effective (Wang et al., 2020). In several meta-analyses comparing the outcomes of simultaneous versus delayed surgery (colon and/or liver-first) from retrospective case series has concluded that in selected patients with low burden of liver disease, simultaneous surgery results in a shorter hospital stay without a significant increase in morbidity or mortality (Slesser et al., 2013; Kelly et al., 2015; Gavriilidis et al., 2018). Whilst major hepatectomy can be performed simultaneous to colonic resection (Muangkaew et al., 2016), the practice of our MDT is to offer simultaneous resection only to patients requiring minor liver resection alongside non-rectal primary cancers.

Traditional practice was to operate on the primary tumour followed by chemotherapy, restaging of the liver disease, and then liver-directed therapy with surgery as the preference. However, interval disease progression in the liver following surgery for the primary in up to 40% of patients (Yoshidome et al., 2008) and complications following bowel surgery in approximately 30% of patients resulted in frequently incomplete treatment and poor outcomes (Andres et al., 2012). This approach was justified by the assumption that disease progression and inoperability indicated poor tumour biology and thus avoided futile surgery. In the mid part of the last decade, this practice was challenged, especially for patients requiring major hepatectomy or for those with significant burden of liver disease, with the reversed strategy, 'liver first approach' now being popular. This strategy serves patients with borderline resectable liver disease at risk of progression on chemotherapy. In the absence of a colonic primary that requires urgent surgery, we typically offer this approach based on the rationale that the liver metastases will ultimately prove fatal to the patient if not treated first.

Summary

The complexity of liver resection is not governed by anatomical considerations alone. While the need for a central liver resection, posterior, or superior segmental resection along with extended liver resections are considered complex, the additional need for bile duct and vascular reconstruction along with caudate lobe resection also adds to complexity. Additionally, the knowledge that tumour recurrence is common indicates a need to consider parenchymal-sparing surgery such that liver-directed modalities remain should recurrence occur. Local expertise and surgical experience also play a role here and thus supports centralisation of such services. The decision to offer liver surgery and the timing of it therefore is a complex one that requires uniformity in approach. This is best done in an MDT setting on an individual patient basis. There also is evidence that such MDT recommendations are associated with better patient outcomes following treatment (Lan et al., 2016).

Initially non-resectable colorectal liver metastasis

Up to 80% of patients with CRLM are inoperable at the time of diagnosis (Adam, 2003), with inoperability predominantly due to three factors. First, the patient may not be fit enough to undergo surgical resection, either acutely or chronically. For these patients, an assessment of fitness for chemotherapy needs to be undertaken, and if unfit for chemotherapy, then ablative techniques may be considered if it is felt that the patient will never get fit enough for surgery; secondly, the burden of disease within the liver may be too great such that the disease cannot be safely resected at that initial evaluation. In these patients, the aim is to render the disease operable following a period of neoadjuvant chemotherapy and/or through improvement in the functional liver remnant; thirdly, the extent of extra-hepatic disease may be too great for liver resection to be oncologically sensible. Whilst there is some evidence of a survival benefit for patients undergoing liver resection even in the presence of inoperable extra-hepatic (lung) metastases (Albertsmeier et al., 2020), such patients would not routinely be offered liver resection by our MDT. However, interestingly, whilst the mechanism for such an effect is unclear, some believe that resection of liver metastases may positively improve the own host's anti-tumour immune surveillance. This is speculated to be related to T-cell accumulation causing a pooling effect in the hepatic metastases, which, when the hepatic disease is excised (Yu et al., 2021), causes reversal of this phenomenon, improving immune-mediated cancer cell destruction at distant sites; a positive feature that may in the future be harnessed to improve sensitivity of extra-hepatic sites to immune checkpoint therapy.

Technically initially unresectable CRLM with treatable extrahepatic disease

In these patients, the aim is to achieve a state within the liver where surgical resection is technically feasible; so-called conversion therapy. Liver resection improves the survival of patients with CRLM (Raoof et al., 2019), and provides a survival benefit better than with chemotherapy alone, where the expected five-year overall survival from the inception of chemotherapy is less than 5% (Giacchetti et al., 1999; Engstrand et al., 2018). In addition, the oncological outcome following post-chemotherapy resection for patients who were rendered operable following chemotherapy, albeit not as good as up-front resectable patients, is encouraging (Adam et al., 2004; Irving et al., 2012; Villard et al., 2021). As advances in biological treatment continue, the proportion of patients who become operable as a result of downstaging will increase. Furthermore, it should be noted that the definition of what constitutes treatable extrahepatic disease is the subject of current debate (Lievens et al., 2020) and is likely to vary significantly, even between high-volume centres. In general, we would consider liver resection in the presence of treatable pulmonary metastasis and/or peritoneal disease where HIPEC is considered an option (see below), or in patients with nodal disease considered treatable with SBRT.

Extended resection following PVE, two-stage resection, resection/ablation, and ALPPS should all be considered in patients with a high burden of disease; a technical decision at the discretion of the surgical team in concert with the MDT. Importantly, the presence of a dedicated hepatobiliary surgeon is required within the MDT, as there is still a significantly degree of misunderstanding within the general surgical field as to what constitutes operable CRLM.

Systemic chemotherapy for conversion to operability

Systemic chemotherapy is the therapeutic mainstay for down-sizing liver metastases to a state of operability, with combination chemotherapy regimens significantly changing the oncological outlook of these patients (Wang & Li, 2012). Assessment of chemotherapy response in the liver is best carried out with diffusion-weighted MRI as diffusion parameters correlate more strongly with histological chemotherapy response than change in tumour size (Donati et al., 2017; Uutela et al., 2021). Positron emission tomography (PET) imaging following chemotherapy can also be useful to ensure that extra-hepatic metastases have not developed or progressed during chemotherapy. PET imaging is certainly worthwhile before any neo-adjuvant systemic treatment is commenced to look for occult disease not detected by other imaging modalities.

Generally, progression during chemotherapy would be a contra-indication to major hepatectomy, as patients who undergo liver resection following a period of progression on neo-adjuvant chemotherapy have a poor outcome (Adam et al., 2004; Villard et al., 2021). Ideally, post-chemotherapy imaging should be performed within the last four weeks prior to the planned resection to exclude any disease progression in the period between conclusion of chemotherapy and surgery. Timing of surgery following chemotherapy is a further important consideration. Enough time needs to be left for the patients to overcome the physiological stress of systemic chemotherapy, but waiting too long risks further disease progression, especially in borderline patients. Most centres look to operate on patients four to six weeks following the completion of chemotherapy as this has been demonstrated to be a relatively safe period (Welsh et al., 2007; Chen et al., 2020) and this process requires close communication between oncologists and surgeons typically through the MDT.

When assessing chemotherapy response, comparison with historical images is of paramount importance. This is because major hepatectomy may be oncologically futile even in the face of dramatic chemotherapy response. An example would be where pre-chemotherapy imaging demonstrated involvement of all hepatic vascular segments as in such patients, surgical resection is unlikely to ever be beneficial. If following a period of chemotherapy there has been disease progression, then second-line chemotherapy and biological agents should be considered, with the hope of still reaching an operable state. The proportion of initially inoperable patients who achieve adequate conversion to a state of operability on first-line chemotherapy is variable depending upon local definitions of resectability, but response rates are lower for second-line chemotherapy than for first and the greatest proportionate response is seen within the first three to four months cycles of chemotherapy. This depreciating return on successive chemotherapy regimens is a consequence of a degree of therapeutic resistance that evolves over time and during exposure to treatment, and suggests that selection of the optimal regimen for the first line is crucial. Potential chemotherapy regimens are covered elsewhere in this book.

A further consideration in patients with synchronous disease is the degree of response of the primary tumour. Particularly with rectal primaries, it is important to assess the extent to which the circumferential resection margin is threatened, whether this precludes operability, and whether the inclusion of radiotherapy or chemoradiotherapy directed at the primary tumour, within the neo-adjuvant package, is required to achieve operability. Again, this requires close liaison with the colorectal team, preferably through the MDT.

Occasionally, a 'cooling-off' period of imaging surveillance may be warranted following systemic therapy and prior to aggressive surgical intervention. This is particularly true in the case of patients with potential extrahepatic disease such as pulmonary nodules or intra-abdominal lymphadenopathy, which is of an indeterminate nature at the time of post-chemotherapy imaging. If a short period (typically three months) off systemic treatment results in rapid disease progression within extra-hepatic sites at follow-up imaging, then morbid yet ultimately futile liver surgery will have been avoided without significant impact on long-term survival through a short chemotherapy break.

Biological therapy for conversion to operability

The addition of selected biological therapies on a per-patient basis chosen in response to mutational profiling may also be important in achieving adequate successful conversion. Evidence indicates a significant benefit from biological therapies targeting epidermal growth factor receptor (EGFR) and vascular endothelial growth factor (VEGF) and more recently immune checkpoint inhibitors in selected patients. Anti-EGFR therapy in patients with KRAS wild-type tumours (Karapetis et al., 2008; Misale et al., 2012) and anti-VEGF monoclonal antibodies (Salz et al., 2008; Wong et al., 2011; Tang et al., 2020) both demonstrate efficacy in the conversion of non-resectable liver metastasis to resectable states. However, it should be noted that evidence from trials paints a mixed picture regarding the benefit of anti-EGFR therapies of surgery for resectable liver metastases, with the new-EPOC trial in particular demonstrating worse overall and progression-free survival in patients given cetuximab peri-operatively (Primrose et al., 2014; Bridgewater et al., 2020). Immune checkpoint inhibitors can also be used for down-sizing hepatic metastases in patients with microsatellite unstable (dMMR) metastatic CRC (Yu et al., 2020). Because of the clear benefit of such agents, and the potential impact of *RAS* and *RAF* mutations on long-term survival in mCRC, the MDT mandates that the mutational profile (*RAS*, *BRAF*) and microsatellite status of the primary tumour are provided for all patients on referral to the MDT in order to direct appropriate biological therapy.

Emerging methods for addressing non-resectable CRLM

Hepatic artery chemotherapy

An alternative approach for improving operability in initially unresectable patients may be hepatic artery-delivered chemotherapy (Zhang et al., 2021). This can be performed through a surgically (Shin et al., 2020; Thiels & D'Angelica, 2020) or radiologically (Chevallier et al., 2021) placed catheter and has the advantage of delivering chemotherapy directly to the arterially supplied CRLM with the additional benefit of hepatic first-pass metabolism ensuring minimal chemotherapy spill-over to the systemic circulation, therefore allowing much higher locoregional doses with no increase in systemic toxicity. The patient is able to receive continuous chemotherapy over the course of several weeks through a reservoir attached to the catheter. It is worth noting that if extra-hepatic disease is present, then this needs to be given alongside a systemic regimen to reduce the chance of extrahepatic progression during hepatic arterial infusion (HAI) treatment. Case series in high-volume centres have demonstrated that almost 50% of patients with initially inoperable CRLM undergo successful resectional surgery following HAI (Kemeny et al., 2005; Kemeny et al., 2009; Cercek et al., 2016). Importantly, most of these patients were already refractory to systemic chemotherapy regimens (D'Angelica et al., 2015; Cercek et al., 2016) indicating the value of this therapeutic strategy even in the face of aggressive tumour biology. Nonetheless, there remain limited Grade 1 trials-level data to confirm the efficacy of the technique when compared to standardized regimens of combination chemotherapy alongside biological therapies. Also, placement of the catheter system is not without complication and requires significant surgical expertise.

Liver transplantation for CRLM

A more recent concept is liver transplantation for patients with technically inoperable CRLM. This has primarily been offered to patients without evidence of extrahepatic disease and current experience with the approach remains in its infancy (Bonney et al., 2021; Soliva & Figueras, 2021). Liver transplantation was assessed for utility in CRLM many decades ago and it failed. However, it is strongly believed that this failure was due to poor selection of patients in terms of disease restricted to the liver, inadequate knowledge of the importance of certain mutations in oncoproteins and their impact upon prognosis, and wholly inadequate complementary chemotherapy regimes. Nowadays, with increased knowledge in all these spheres, this is a rapidly expanding field, and selected studies have demonstrated five-year overall survival of up to 60% in patients with inoperable CRLM, albeit with recurrence rates of 90% (Hagness et al., 2013). An important caveat to this approach is the effect on the allocation of transplantation resources and organs to patients with acute and chronic liver failure, whilst other unresolved issues include the timing of transplantation in patients with synchronous disease. At the time of writing, a randomized trial comparing chemotherapy alone versus chemotherapy followed by liver transplantation is underway (TRANSMET, NCT02597348), whilst transplantation for inoperable CRLM has recently been granted approval in the United Kingdom under certain strict criteria.

Management of extra-hepatic metastasis in CRLM patients

Both the lung and peritoneum serve as additional sites for metastatic disease in CRC patients, albeit at lower frequencies when compared to hepatic metastasis (van der Geest et al., 2015). A paradigm shift has been observed in the last decade regarding the management of metastatic colorectal cancer with lung and/or peritoneal involvement (van der Geest et al., 2015; Zellweger et al., 2018; Mangiameli et al., 2022). Further understanding of tumour biology, advances in surgical techniques, development of focal ablative strategies, and combination chemotherapy now serve as additional options that increase the potential for long-term survival in this patient cohort.

Lung metastases

The newest generation of computed tomography (CT) machines have vastly improved the detection yield for colorectal lung metastases. The combination of thinner, multi-slice contrast-enhanced images has increased the sensitivity and specificity for the identification of pulmonary metastases such that they are identified with increased frequency (Klippenstein & Lamonica , 2007). However, this can also result in the detection of non-relevant pulmonary nodules which can pose a dilemma for the MDT, a challenge that radiomics, artificial intelligence, and machine learning algorithms may soon be able to address (Hu et al., 2019). PET CT is now widely used to exclude occult pulmonary metastases, with a sensitivity for detecting of 87% in patients with elevated carcino embryonic antigen (CEA) but no visible pulmonary metastasis on CT (Pastorino et al., 2003).

Selection of patients for pulmonary metastatectomy typically occurs within the cardiothoracic MDT setting following an evaluation of disease distribution and pulmonary fitness. Inclusion of a thoracic surgeon in the hepatobiliary MDT is useful, but in most centres, where the number of patients of relevance for the thoracic team is low, this is an unaffordable luxury. The American College of Chest Physicians has established a pre-defined pulmonary fitness criteria for patients undergoing thoracic surgery for colorectal lung metastases (Degani-Costa et al., 2014). This is dependent on physiological assessment through formal pulmonary function testing. In brief, patients are required to have adequate forced expiratory volume, sufficient residual lung volume (> 2 litres (L) for pneumonectomy, > 1.5 L for lobectomy) and carbon monoxide diffusion (DLCO) ≥ 80% or greater of predicted (Degani-Costa et al., 2014). The development of minimally invasive thoracic surgery (video-assisted thoracoscopic surgery (VATS)) has further impacted outcomes by increasing the proportion of eligible patients for surgery and reducing morbidity associated with thoracotomy (Atkins et al., 2007; Guerrini et al., 2017).

Patients are selected for lung resection with consideration given to whether the colorectal primary is treatable/already resected, and the extent to which any other extra-pulmonary metastases are deemed treatable, in addition to any other pulmonary disease factors (Thomford et al., 1965). When hepatic and pulmonary metastases are present, the management pathway and decision-making process require close coordination between multiple MDTs. In our practice, it is typical to treat operable hepatic metastases prior to managing pulmonary metastases, the reason being that pulmonary metastases tend to evolve and grow more slowly than liver metastases. However, in some centres, synchronous liver and lung surgery and/or ablation are also considered. Basal pulmonary metastases can even be resected through a trans-diaphragmatic approach at the time of liver surgery, thereby obviating the need for a second thoracic incision (Mise et al., 2014), although this is likely to be at the cost of greater morbidity and relevant for only a relatively small subset of patients. Specific pulmonary considerations include disease distribution, whether complete resection and R0 status can be achieved and the cardiopulmonary reserve (Thomford et al., 1965). The International Registry of Lung Metastases (IRLM) has previously published long-term results following metastatectomy for CRLM, demonstrating that a R0 resection is associated with a median survival of 35 months, a figure that is halved in the context of R1 disease (Pastorino et al., 1997).

The long-term survival following pulmonary resection for colorectal lung metastases is variable. A comprehensive systematic review of 25 studies concluded that the five-year survival rates varied between 27% and 68% (Gonzalez et al., 2013). Published data from IRLM clearly demonstrated that one of the key factors determining survival is the disease-free interval between diagnosis of the primary CRC and diagnosis of the pulmonary metastasis (Pastorino et al., 1997). For patients who develop metastases within 12 months of their primary cancer diagnosis, the median survival was 29 months (Pastorino et al., 1997) compared with 49 months for patients who develop pulmonary metastasis three years or more following their primary CRC diagnosis (Pastorino et al., 1997). Serum CEA concentration > 10 mg/dl also appears to be a significant prognostic indicator, with patients with high CEA experiencing significantly worse cancer-specific outcomes.

It is worth highlighting that survival estimates following thoracic resection are predominantly from single centres and based on retrospective series. More recently, the Pulmonary Metastasectomy versus Continued Active Monitoring in Colorectal Cancer (PulMiCC) trial evaluated whether surgical resection of pulmonary metastases provides a survival advantage (Treasure et al., 2019). Unfortunately, the trial failed to demonstrate a difference in five-year overall survival between patients undergoing resection and those managed expectantly (38% vs 29% respectively, HR 0.82, 95% CI: 0.43–1.56) (Treasure et al., 2019). However, these results are difficult to interpret because the trial closed to recruitment prior to reaching an adequately powered sample size. Nonetheless, the trial demonstrated higher-than-expected survival amongst patients in the non-resected arm, potentially related to selection of better prognosis patients at the outset. This subject of surgery for pulmonary metastatic colorectal cancer is reviewed more extensively elsewhere in this book.

Ablation with either microwave energy of radiofrequency is increasingly employed in patients with inoperable and operable lung metastases (de Baère et al., 2015). The technique is most affective when dealing with small metastases (< 3 cm) and is well tolerated with low morbidity and mortality (Taylor et al., 2020). Survival outcomes following radiofrequency ablation (RFA) are promising, with three- and five-year overall survival rates 46–60% and 35–45% respectively (Schlijper et al., 2014). The largest single-institution series of patients receiving RFA (566 patients) demonstrated three- and five-year survival rates of 68% and 52% respectively (de Baère et al., 2015). This is not dissimilar to a smaller series of 77 patients who underwent RFA for colorectal lung metastases and experienced three-year overall survival of 84% (Hasegawa et al., 2020).

Other treatment options for colorectal lung metastases include stereotactic ablative body radiotherapy (SBRT). Initial SBRT experience for colorectal cancer lung metastases demonstrated a median overall survival of 38 months and a three-year overall survival of 50.8% (Agolli et al., 2017). However, despite the highly targeted delivery of radiation to the tumour, radiation pneumonitis rates of up to 8% have been described (Ibrahim et al., 2016).

Peritoneal metastases

Peritoneal metastases are noted at the initial diagnosis of colorectal cancer in approximately 8% of patients (Sugarbaker , 2014) and are associated with poor survival (Sugarbaker et al., 2016). When compared to lung and liver metastases, patients with metastatic colorectal cancer to the peritoneum have a significantly worse prognosis (Prasanna et al., 2018). Risk factors for metachronous peritoneal metastases include right-sided colonic cancer, advanced stage at diagnosis (particular T4 staging of the primary tumour), *BRAF* mutation, poor differentiation, and having had an emergency colectomy (Sánchez-Hidalgo et al., 2019).

Selecting patients with peritoneal metastases for surgical management requires a comprehensive assessment focusing on determination of patient fitness and tumour burden. The Peritoneal Cancer Index (PCI) is a validated tool for quantification of peritoneal disease (Jacquet & Sugarbaker , 1996). The PCI is composed of a systematic approach of assessing macroscopic disease within the abdomen performed during either open or laparoscopic surgery. In summary, the abdomen is divided into 13 locations, each scored for the presence and size of disease present, resulting in a score between 0 and 39 (Jacquet & Sugarbaker , 1996), with overall survival directly proportional to score. PCI-based stratification yields a five-year overall survival of 53% for a PCI < 10 and 12% for patients with a PCI > 20 (Sánchez-Hidalgo et al., 2019). This serves as the foundation for several clinical guidelines were a PCI score > 20 is generally considered a contraindication to active surgical treatment (Elias et al., 2010). Only a small cohort of patients with peritoneal metastasis are suitable for radical surgical resection following assessment. Cytoreductive surgery (CRS) is undertaken with the intention of removing all macroscopic disease, but this aggressive approach has a high degree of morbidity, albeit with acceptably low mortality rates when undertaken in high-volume centres (Wu et al., 2017). It is therefore infrequent for the CRLM of such a patient to be the primary determinant of the possibility of radical treatment, given the outcome from the peritoneal disease is so bad. With the increasing use of specific and effective anti-*BRAF* mutation regimens (such as encorafenib and cetuximab), this may change.

Over the last decade, much attention has been drawn to combining CRS with hyperthermic intraperitoneal chemotherapy (HIPEC). This has predominantly been influenced by the evolving literature and experience in the technique gained through the management of pseudomyxoma peritonei (Sugarbaker et al., 1993). HIPEC constitutes delivery of intra-peritoneal chemotherapy heated to 40°C to achieve additional cytotoxicity (van Stein et al., 2021). Variable survival rates have been described in the literature when combining CRS and HIPEC for peritoneal disease with five-year survival ranging from 28% to 44% (Franko et al., 2010; Quénet et al., 2011). However, the recent PRODIGE-7 trial (Quénet et al., 2021) failed to demonstrate any additional survival benefit when HIPEC was added to CRS, in addition to significantly higher post-operative morbidity with the combination therapy (Quénet et al., 2021) indicating that the clinical setting in which to use this aggressive approach remains to be defined. Typically, treatments for peritoneal disease are only offered in supra-specialist centres and so the development of functional links between the MDT and such centres is important to ensure that patients are offered all available therapeutic modalities.

Concluding remarks

The MDT plays a key role in the planning of appropriate management strategies for patients with CRLM. Moving forwards, the MDT will have at its disposal better tools to stratify tumour biology and to predict therapeutic response in addition to novel biological therapies. These will enable tailoring of both the therapeutic modality and the sequence of treatments in a precision-based approach. Development of such tools will rely upon integration of novel technologies and collaboration between clinicians, academics, and patients alike. Nonetheless, the central role of the MDT in bringing together clinicians with wide-reaching expertise, so that the most recent research evidence can be brought to bear on the complex clinical issues that arise in these patients will remain.

REFERENCES

Adam, R. (2003). Chemotherapy and surgery: new perspectives on the treatment of unresectable liver metastases. *Annals of Oncology*, *14*, ii13–ii16.

Adam, R., Delvart, V., Pascal, G., et al. (2004). Rescue surgery for unresectable colorectal liver metastases downstaged by chemotherapy. *Annals of Surgery*, *240*, 644–658.

Adam, R., Pascal, G., Castaing, D., et al. (2004). Tumor progression while on chemotherapy: a contraindication to liver resection for multiple colorectal metastases? *Annals of Surgery*, *240*, 1052–1061; discussion 1061–1064.

Agolli, L., Bracci, S., Nicosia, L., et al. (2017). Lung metastases treated with stereotactic ablative radiation therapy in oligometastatic colorectal cancer patients: outcomes and prognostic factors after long-term follow-up. *Clinical Colorectal Cancer*, *16*, 58–64.

Albertsmeier, M., Riedl, K., Stephan, A.-J., et al. (2020). Improved survival after resection of colorectal liver metastases in patients with unresectable lung metastases. *HPB*, *22*, 368–375.

Aloia, T., Sebagh, M., Plasse, M., et al. (2006). Liver histology and surgical outcomes after preoperative chemotherapy with fluorouracil plus oxaliplatin in colorectal cancer liver metastases. *Journal of Clinical Oncology*, *24*, 4983–4990.

Andres, A., Toso, C., Adam, R., et al. (2012). A survival analysis of the liver-first reversed management of advanced simultaneous colorectal liver metastases: a LiverMetSurvey-based study. *Annals of Surgery*, *256*, 772–778; discussion 778–779.

Atkins, B. Z., Harpole, D. H., Mangum, J. H., et al. (2007). Pulmonary segmentectomy by thoracotomy or thoracoscopy: reduced hospital length of stay with a minimally-invasive approach. *Annals of Thoracic Surgery*, *84*, 1107–1113.

Basta, Y. L., Baur, O. L., van Dieren, S., et al. (2016). Is there a benefit of multidisciplinary cancer team meetings for patients with gastrointestinal malignancies? *Annals of Surgical Oncology*, *23*, 2430–2437.

Björnsson, B., Sparrelid, E., Røsok, B., et al. (2016). Associating liver partition and portal vein ligation for staged hepatectomy in patients with colorectal liver metastases—intermediate oncological results. *European Journal of Surgical Oncology*, *42*, 531–537.

Bonney, G. K., Chew, C. A., Lodge, P., et al. (2021). Liver transplantation for non-resectable colorectal liver metastases: the International Hepato-Pancreato-Biliary Association consensus guidelines. *Lancet Gastroenterology & Hepatology*, *6*, 933–946.

Bridgewater, J. A., Pugh, S. A., Maishman, T., et al. (2020). Systemic chemotherapy with or without cetuximab in patients with resectable colorectal liver metastasis (New EPOC): long-term results of a multicentre, randomised, controlled, phase 3 trial. *Lancet Oncology*, *21*, 398–411.

Budai, A., Horváth, G., Tretter, L., et al. (2019). Mitochondrial function after associating liver partition and portal vein ligation for staged hepatectomy in an experimental model. *British Journal of Surgery*, *106*, 120–131.

Cercek, A., Boucher, T, M., Gluskin, J. S., et al. (2016). Response rates of hepatic arterial infusion pump therapy in patients with metastatic colorectal cancer liver metastases refractory to all standard chemotherapies. *Journal of Surgical Oncology*, *114*, 655–663.

Chen, Q., Mao, R., Zhao, J., et al. (2020). From the completion of neoadjuvant chemotherapy to surgery for colorectal cancer liver metastasis: what is the optimal timing? *Cancer Medicine*, *9*, 7849–7862.

Chevallier, O., Mvouama, S., Pellegrinelli, J., et al. (2021). Percutaneous implantation of a microcatheter-port system for hepatic arterial infusion chemotherapy of unresectable liver tumors: technical feasibility, functionality, and complications. *Diagnostics (Basel)*, *11*, 399.

D'Angelica, M. I., Correa-Gallego, C., Paty, P. B., et al. (2015). Phase II trial of hepatic artery infusional and systemic chemotherapy for patients with unresectable hepatic metastases from colorectal cancer: conversion to resection and long-term outcomes. *Annals of Surgery*, *261*, 353–360.

de Baère, T., Aupérin, A., Deschamps, F., et al. (2015). Radiofrequency ablation is a valid treatment option for lung metastases: experience in 566 patients with 1037 metastases. *Annals of Oncology*, *26*, 987–991.

Degani-Costa, L. H., Faresin, S. M., & dos Reis Falcão, L. F. (2014). Preoperative evaluation of the patient with pulmonary disease. *Brazilian Journal of Anesthesiology*, ***64***, 22–34.

de Graaf, W., Bennink, R. J., Veteläinen, R., et al. (2010). Nuclear imaging techniques for the assessment of hepatic function in liver surgery and transplantation. *Journal of Nuclear Medicine*, *51*, 742–752.

Donati, F., Boraschi, P., Pacciardi, F., et al. (2017). 3T diffusion-weighted MRI in the response assessment of colorectal liver metastases after chemotherapy: correlation between ADC value and histological tumour regression grading. *European Journal of Radiology*, *91*, 57–65.

Elias, D., Gilly, F., Boutitie, F., et al. (2010). Peritoneal colorectal carcinomatosis treated with surgery and perioperative intraperitoneal chemotherapy: retrospective analysis of 523 patients from a multicentric French study. *Journal of Clinical Oncology*, *28*, 63–68.

Engstrand, J., Nilsson, H., Strömberg, C., et al. (2018). Colorectal cancer liver metastases—a population-based study on incidence, management and survival. *BMC Cancer*, *18*, 78.

Eshmuminov, D., Raptis, D. A., Linecker, M., et al. (2016). Meta-analysis of associating liver partition with portal vein ligation and portal vein occlusion for two-stage hepatectomy. *British Journal of Surgery*, *103*, 1768–1782.

Franko, J., Ibrahim, Z., Gusani, N. J., et al. (2010). Cytoreductive surgery and hyperthermic intraperitoneal chemoperfusion versus systemic chemotherapy alone for colorectal peritoneal carcinomatosis. *Cancer*, *116*, 3756–3762.

Franko, J., Shi, Q., Meyers, J. P., Maughan, T. S., et al. (2016). Analysis and Research in Cancers of the Digestive System (ARCAD) Group. Prognosis of patients with peritoneal metastatic colorectal cancer given systemic therapy: an analysis of individual patient data from prospective randomised trials from the Analysis and Research in Cancers of the Digestive System (ARCAD) database. *Lancet Oncology*, *17*, 1709–1719.

Fong, Y., Fortner, J., Sun, R. L., et al. (1999). Clinical score for predicting recurrence after hepatic resection for metastatic colorectal cancer. *Annals of Surgery*, *230*, 309.

Gangi, A., & Lu, S. C. (2020). Chemotherapy-associated liver injury in colorectal cancer. *Therapeutic Advances in Gastroenterology*, *13*, 1756284820924194.

avriilidis, P., Sutcliffe, R. P., Hodson, J., et al. (2018). Simultaneous versus delayed hepatectomy for synchronous colorectal liver metastases: a systematic review and meta-analysis. *HPB*, *20*, 11–19.

Giacchetti, S., Itzhaki, M., Gruia, G., et al. (1999). Long-term survival of patients with unresectable colorectal cancer liver metastases following infusional chemotherapy with 5-fluorouracil, leucovorin, oxaliplatin and surgery. *Annals of Oncology*, *10*, 663–669.

Gonzalez, M., Poncet, A., Combescure, C., et al. (2013). Risk factors for survival after lung metastasectomy in colorectal cancer patients: a systematic review and meta-analysis. *Annals of Surgical Oncology*, *20*, 572–579.

Guerrini, G. P., Lo, F., Vagliasindi, A., et al. (2014). The role of minimally invasive surgery in the treatment of lung metastases. *Journal of Investigative Surgery*, *30*, 110–115.

Guglielmi, A., Ruzzenente, A., Conci, S., et al. (2012). How much remnant is enough in liver resection? *DSU*, ***29***, 6–17.

Guiu, B., Chevallier, P., Denys, A., et al. (2016). Simultaneous trans-hepatic portal and hepatic vein embolization before major hepatectomy: the liver venous deprivation technique. *European Radiology*, *26*, 4259–4267.

Guiu, B., Quénet, F., Escal, L., et al. (2017). Extended liver venous deprivation before major hepatectomy induces marked and very rapid increase in future liver remnant function. *European Radiology*,. *27*, 3343–3352.

Hagness, M., Foss, A., Line, P.-D., et al. (2013). Liver transplantation for nonresectable liver metastases from colorectal cancer. *Annals of Surgery*, *257*, 800–806.

Hasegawa, T., Takaki, H., Kodama, H., et al. (2020). Three-year survival rate after radiofrequency ablation for surgically resectable colorectal lung metastases: a prospective multicenter study. *Radiology, 294*, 686–695.

Hashiguchi, Y., Muro, K., Saito, Y., et al. (2020). Japanese Society for Cancer of the Colon and Rectum (JSCCR) guidelines 2019 for the treatment of colorectal cancer. *International Journal of Clinical Oncology, 25*, 1–42.

Hu, T., Wang, S., Huang, L., et al. (2019). A clinical-radiomics nomogram for the preoperative prediction of lung metastasis in colorectal cancer patients with indeterminate pulmonary nodules. *European Radiology, 29*, 439–449.

Ibrahim, T., Tselikas, L., Yazbeck, C., et al. (2016). Systemic versus local therapies for colorectal cancer pulmonary metastasis: what to choose and when? *Journal of Gastrointestinal Cancer, 47*, 223–231.

Irving, G. R., Tiernan, J. P., Briggs, C. D., et al. (2012). OC-060 Survival after downstaging chemotherapy for initially un-resectable colorectal liver metastases: experience from a UK resection centre. *Gut, 61*, A26–A26.

Jacquet, P., & Sugarbaker, P. H. (1996). Clinical research methodologies in diagnosis and staging of patients with peritoneal carcinomatosis. *Cancer Treatment Research, 82*, 359–374.

Kanemitsu, Y., Shimizu, Y., Mizusawa, J., et al. (2021). Hepatectomy followed by mFOLFOX6 versus hepatectomy alone for liver-only metastatic colorectal cancer (JCOG0603): A phase II or III randomized controlled trial. *Journal of Clinical Oncology, 39*, 3789–3799.

Karapetis, C. A., Khambata-Ford, S., Jonker, D. J. et al. (2008). K-ras mutations and benefit from cetuximab in advanced colorectal cancer. *New England Journal of Medicine, 359*, 1757–1765. https://www.nejm.org/doi/full/10.1056/nejmoa0804385

Karoui, M., Penna, C., Amin-Hashem, M., et al. (2006). Influence of preoperative chemotherapy on the risk of major hepatectomy for colorectal liver metastases. *Annals of Surgery, 243*, 1–7.

Kasivisvanathan, R., Abbassi-Ghadi, N., McLeod, A. D. M., et al. (2015). Cardiopulmonary exercise testing for predicting postoperative morbidity in patients undergoing hepatic resection surgery. *HPB, 17*, 637–643.

Kelly, M. E., Spolverato, G., Lê, G. N., et al. (2015). Synchronous colorectal liver metastasis: a network meta-analysis review comparing classical, combined, and liver-first surgical strategies. *Journal of Surgical Oncology, 111*, 341–351.

Kemeny, N., Jarnagin, W., Paty, P., et al. (2005). Phase I trial of systemic oxaliplatin combination chemotherapy with hepatic arterial infusion in patients with unresectable liver metastases from colorectal cancer. *Journal of Clinical Oncology, 23*, 4888–4896.

Kemeny, N. E., Melendez, F. D. H., Capanu, M., et al. (2009). Conversion to resectability using hepatic artery infusion plus systemic chemotherapy for the treatment of unresectable liver metastases from colorectal carcinoma. *Journal of Clinical Oncology, 27*, 3465–3471.

Klippenstein, D. L., & Lamonica, D. M. (2007). Preoperative imaging for metastasectomy. *Surgical Oncology Clinics of North America, 16*, 471–492, vii.

Konopke, R., Kersting, S., Bunk, A., et al. (2009). Colorectal liver metastasis surgery: analysis of risk factors predicting postoperative complications in relation to the extent of resection. *International Journal of Colorectal Disorders, 24*, 687–697.

Krasnodebski, M., Kim, B. J., Wei, S. H., et al. (2020). Chemotherapy in combination with resection for colorectal liver metastases—current evidence. *Surgery in Practice and Science, 3*, 100021.

Kumar, R., & Garcea, G. (2018). Cardiopulmonary exercise testing in hepato-biliary & pancreas cancer surgery—a systematic review: are we any further than walking up a flight of stairs? *International Journal of Surgery, 52*, 201–207.

Lan, Y.-T., Jiang, J.-K., Chang, S.-C., et al. (2016). Improved outcomes of colorectal cancer patients with liver metastases in the era of the multidisciplinary teams. *International Journal of Colorectal Disorders, 31*, 403–411.

Lievens, Y., Guckenberger, M., Gomez, D., et al. (2020). Defining oligometastatic disease from a radiation oncology perspective: An ESTRO—ASTRO consensus document. *Radiotherapy & Oncology*, ***148***, 157–166.

MacDermid, E., Hooton, G., MacDonald, M., et al. (2009). Improving patient survival with the colorectal cancer multi-disciplinary team. *Colorectal Disorders, 11*, 291–295.

Mangiameli, G., Cioffi, U., Alloisio, M., et al. (2022). Pulmonary metastases: surgical principles, surgical indications, and innovations. *Exon Publications, 3*, 49–62.

Meguid, C., Schulick, R. D., Schefter, T. E., et al. (2016). The multidisciplinary approach to GI cancer results in change of diagnosis and management of patients. multidisciplinary care impacts diagnosis and management of patients. *Annals of Surgical Oncology, 23*, 3986–3990.

Misale, S., Yaeger, R., Hobor, S., et al. (2010). Emergence of KRAS mutations and acquired resistance to anti-EGFR therapy in colorectal cancer. *Nature, 486*, 532–536.

Mise, Y., Mehran, R. J., Aloia, T. A., et al. (2014). Simultaneous lung resection via a transdiaphragmatic approach in patients undergoing liver resection for synchronous liver and lung metastases. *Surgery, 156*, 1197–1203.

Mohamed, F., Kallioinen, M., Braun, M., et al. (2020). Management of colorectal cancer metastases to the liver, lung or peritoneum suitable for curative intent: summary of NICE guidance. *British Journal of Surgery, 107*, 943–945.

Muangkaew, P., Cho, J. Y., Han, H.-S., et al. (2016). Outcomes of simultaneous major liver resection and colorectal surgery for colorectal liver metastases. *Journal of Gastrointestinal Surgery, 20*, 554–563.

Nordlinger, B., Sorbye, H., Glimelius, B., et al. (2013). Perioperative FOLFOX4 chemotherapy and surgery versus surgery alone for resectable liver metastases from colorectal cancer (EORTC 40983): long-term results of a randomised, controlled, phase 3 trial. *Lancet Oncology, 14*, 1208–1215.

Pastorino, U., Buyse, M., Friedel, G., et al. (1997). International Registry of Lung Metastases. Long-term results of lung metastasectomy: prognostic analyses based on 5206 cases. *Journal of Thoracic and Cardiovascular Surgery, 113*, 37–49.

Pastorino, U., Veronesi, G., Landoni, C., et al. (2003). Fluorodeoxyglucose positron emission tomography improves preoperative staging of resectable lung metastasis. *Journal of Thoracic and Cardiovascular Surgery, 126*, 1906–1910.

Prasanna, T., Karapetis, C. S., Roder, D., et al. (2018). The survival outcome of patients with metastatic colorectal cancer based on the site of metastases and the impact of molecular markers and site of primary cancer on metastatic pattern. *Acta Oncologica, 57*, 1438–1444.

Primrose, J., Falk, S., Finch-Jones, M., Valle, J., et al. (2014). Systemic chemotherapy with or without cetuximab in patients with resectable colorectal liver metastasis: the New EPOC randomised controlled trial. *Lancet Oncology, 15*, 601–611.

Quénet, F., Elias, D., Roca, L., et al. (2021). Cytoreductive surgery plus hyperthermic intraperitoneal chemotherapy versus cytoreductive surgery alone for colorectal peritoneal metastases (PRODIGE 7): a multicentre, randomised, open-label, phase 3 trial. *Lancet Oncology, 22*, 256–266.

Quénet, F., Goéré, D., Mehta, S. S., et al. (2011). Results of two bi-institutional prospective studies using intraperitoneal oxaliplatin with or without irinotecan during HIPEC after cytoreductive surgery for colorectal carcinomatosis. *Annals of Surgery*, *254*, 294–301.

Raoof, M., Haye, S., Ituarte, P. H. G., et al. (2019). Liver resection improves survival in colorectal cancer patients: causal-effects from population-level instrumental variable analysis. *Annals of Surgery*, *270*, 692–700.

Rassam, F., Olthof, P. B., Bennink, R. J., et al. (2017). Current modalities for the assessment of future remnant liver function. *Visceral Medicine*, *33*, 442–448.

Rubbia-Brandt, L., Audard, V., Sartoretti, P., et al. (2004). Severe hepatic sinusoidal obstruction associated with oxaliplatin-based chemotherapy in patients with metastatic colorectal cancer. *Annals of Oncology*, *15*, 460–466.

Saltz, L. B., Clarke, S., Díaz-Rubio, E., et al. (2008). Bevacizumab in combination with oxaliplatin-based chemotherapy as first-line therapy in metastatic colorectal cancer: a randomized phase III study. *Journal of Clinical Oncology*, *26*, 2013–2019.

Sánchez-Hidalgo, J. M., Rodríguez-Ortiz, L., Arjona-Sánchez, Á., et al. (2019). Colorectal peritoneal metastases: optimal management review. *World Journal of Gastroenterology*, *25*, 3484–3502.

Schadde, E., Ardiles, V., Robles-Campos, R., et al. (2014). Early survival and safety of ALPPS: first report of the International ALPPS Registry. *Annals of Surgery*, *260*, 829–836; discussion 836–838.

Schlijper, R. C. J., Grutters, J. P. C., Houben, R., et al. (2014). What to choose as radical local treatment for lung metastases from colorectal cancer: surgery or radiofrequency ablation? *Cancer Treatment Reviews*, *40*, 60–67.

Schnitzbauer, A. A., Lang, S. A., Goessmann, H., et al. (2012). Right portal vein ligation combined with in situ splitting induces rapid left lateral liver lobe hypertrophy enabling 2-staged extended right hepatic resection in small-for-size settings. *Annals of Surgery*, *255*, 405–414.

Shin, P. J., & Kingham, T. P. (2020). Minimally invasive approaches to hepatic arterial infusion pump placement in metastatic colorectal cancer. *Laparoscopic Surgery*, *4*. https://ls.amegroups.com/article/view/5548

Shubert, C. R., Habermann, E. B., Bergquist, J. R., et al. (2015). A NSQIP review of major morbidity and mortality of synchronous liver resection for colorectal metastasis stratified by extent of liver resection and type of colorectal resection. *Journal of Gastrointestinal Surgery*, *19*, 1982–1994.

Slesser, A. A. P., Simillis, C., Goldin, R., et al. (2013). A meta-analysis comparing simultaneous versus delayed resections in patients with synchronous colorectal liver metastases. *Surgical Oncology*, *22*, 36–47.

Soliva, R., & Figueras, J. (2021). Liver transplant oncology: is it time to revisit our ideas? *Hepatobiliary Surgery and Nutrition*, *10*, 864–867.

Sugarbaker, P. H. (2014). Colorectal cancer: prevention and management of metastatic disease. *Biomedical Research International*, 782890.

Sugarbaker, P. H., Zhu, B. W., Sese, G. B., et al. (1993). Peritoneal carcinomatosis from appendiceal cancer: results in 69 patients treated by cytoreductive surgery and intraperitoneal chemotherapy. *Diseases of the Colon & Rectum*, *36*, 323–329.

Tang, W., Ren, L., Liu, T., et al. (2020). Bevacizumab plus mFOLFOX6 versus mFOLFOX6 alone as first-line treatment for RAS mutant unresectable colorectal liver-limited metastases: the BECOME randomized controlled trial. *Journal of Clinical Oncology*, *38*, 3175–3184.

Taylor, C., Finnegan-John, J., & Green, J. S. (2014). 'No decision about me without me' in the context of cancer multidisciplinary team meetings: a qualitative interview study. *BMC Health Services Research*, *14*, 488.

Taylor, M., Abah, U., & Shah, R. (2020). A review of interventional treatments for colorectal lung metastases: is it time for a change in practice? *Quantitative Imaging in Medicine and Surgery*, *10*, 1413–1417.

Thiels, C. A, & D'Angelica, M. I. (2020> Hepatic artery infusion pumps. *Journal of Surgical Oncology*, *122*, 70–77.

Thomford, N. R., Woolner, L. B., & Clagett, O. T. (1965). The surgical treatment of metastatic tumors in the lungs. *Journal of Thoracic and Cardiovascular Surgery*, *49*, 357–363.

Treasure, T., Farewell, V., Macbeth, F., et al. (2019). Pulmonary Metastasectomy versus Continued Active Monitoring in Colorectal Cancer (PulMiCC): a multicentre randomised clinical trial. *Trials*, *20*, 718.

Uutela, A., Ovissi, A., Hakkarainen, A., et al. (2021). Treatment response of colorectal cancer liver metastases to neoadjuvant or conversion therapy: a prospective multicentre follow-up study using MRI, diffusion-weighted imaging and 1H-MR spectroscopy compared with histology (subgroup in the RAXO trial). *ESMO Open*, *6*, 100208.

van der Geest, L. G. M., Lam-Boer, J., Koopman, M., et al. (2015). Nationwide trends in incidence, treatment and survival of colorectal cancer patients with synchronous metastases. *Clinical & Experimental Metastasis*, *32*, 457–465.

van Hagen, P., Spaander, M. C. W., van der Gaast, A., et al. (2013). Impact of a multidisciplinary tumour board meeting for upper-GI malignancies on clinical decision making: a prospective cohort study. *International Journal of Clinical Oncology*, *18*, 214–219.

van Stein, R. M., Aalbers, A. G. J., Sonke, G. S., et al. (2021). Hyperthermic intraperitoneal chemotherapy for ovarian and colorectal cancer: a review. *JAMA Oncology*, *7*, 1231–1238.

Villard, C., Habib, M., Nordenvall, C., et al. (2021). Conversion therapy in patients with colorectal liver metastases. *European Journal of Surgical Oncology*, *47*, 2038–2045.

Wang, C.-C., & Li, J. (2012). An update on chemotherapy of colorectal liver metastases. *World Journal of Gastroenterology*, *18*, 25–33.

Wang, J., Griffiths, C., Simunovic, M., et al. (2020). Simultaneous versus staged resection for synchronous colorectal liver metastases: a population-based cost analysis in Ontario, Canada—health economic evaluation. *International Journal of Surgery*, *78*, 75–82.

Welsh, F. K. S., Tilney, H. S., Tekkis, P. P., et al. (2007). Safe liver resection following chemotherapy for colorectal metastases is a matter of timing. *British Journal of Cancer*, *96*, 1037–1042.

Wong, R., Cunningham, D., Barbachano, Y., et al. (2011). A multicentre study of capecitabine, oxaliplatin plus bevacizumab as perioperative treatment of patients with poor-risk colorectal liver-only metastases not selected for upfront resection. *Annals of Oncology*, *22*, 2042–2048.

Wood, J. J., Metcalfe, C., Paes, A., et al. (2008). An evaluation of treatment decisions at a colorectal cancer multi-disciplinary team. *Colorectal Disorders*, *10*, 769–772.

Wu, W., Yan, S., Liao, X., et al. (2017). Curative versus palliative treatments for colorectal cancer with peritoneal carcinomatosis: a systematic review and meta-analysis. *Oncotarget*, *8*, 113202–113212.

Xu, L., & Zhou, J. (2021). Interpretation of NCCN guidelines for hepatobiliary tumors V3 update in 2021. *Hepatobiliary Surgery and Nutrition*, *10*, 682–685.

Ye, Y.-J., Shen, Z.-L., Sun, X.-T., et al. (2012). Impact of multidisciplinary team working on the management of colorectal cancer. *Chinese Medical Journal (English)*, *125*, 172–177.

Yifan, T., Ming, X., Yifan, W., et al. (2019). Hepatic regeneration by associating liver partition and portal vein ligation for staged hepatectomy (ALPPS) is feasible but attenuated in rat liver with thioacetamide-induced fibrosis. *Surgery*, *165*, 345–352.

Yoshidome, H., Kimura, F., Shimizu, H., et al. (2008). Interval period tumor progression: does delayed hepatectomy detect occult metastases in synchronous colorectal liver metastases? *Journal of Gastrointestinal Surgery*, *12*, 1391–1398.

Yu, J., Green, M. D., Li, S., et al. (2021). Liver metastasis restrains immunotherapy efficacy via macrophage-mediated T cell elimination. *Nature Medicine*, *27*, 152–164.

Yu, X., Zhu, L., Liu, J., et al. (2020). Emerging Role of Immunotherapy for Colorectal Cancer with Liver Metastasis. *OncoTargets and Therapy*, *13*, 11645–11658.

Zellweger, M., Abdelnour-Berchtold, E., Krueger, T., et al. (2018). Surgical treatment of pulmonary metastasis in colorectal cancer patients: Current practice and results. *Critical Reviews in Oncology/Hematology*, *127*, 105–116.

Zhang, J., Mavros, M. N., Cosgrove, D., et al. (2013). Impact of a single-day multidisciplinary clinic on the management of patients with liver tumours. *Current Oncology*, *20*, e123–131.

Zhang, Y., Wang, K., Yang, T., et al. (2021). Meta-analysis of hepatic arterial infusion for liver metastases from colorectal cancer. *Frontiers in Oncology*, *11*. https://www.frontiersin.org/articles/10.3389/fonc.2021.628558

12

Multidisciplinary management of pulmonary metastases

Elizabeth Belcher and Michael Shackcloth

Introduction

In 1944, Alfred Blalock first described the experience of resection of a colorectal cancer (CRC) pulmonary metastasis by right pneumonectomy four years after resection of a large bowel carcinoma (Blalock, 1944). Over the following decades, several authors have proposed criteria for undertaking pulmonary metastasectomy to ensure operative intervention occurs in a setting where a survival benefit is possible (Ehrenhaft et al., 1958). Thomford et al. proposed surgical tenets that the patient should be at reasonable risk for surgical intervention, the primary malignancy should be under control, there should be no evidence of metastatic disease elsewhere, and metastasis should be limited to one lung (Thomford et al., 1965). These criteria have undergone various modifications to encompass bilateral lung lesions and the concept of oligometastatic disease, described as an intermediate state between purely localized lesions and widespread metastatic disease (Hellman & Weichselbaum, 1995).

Incidence and presentation

Pulmonary metastases (PMs) are a common occurrence in colorectal cancer (CRC), seen in approximately 10–30% of patients diagnosed with metastatic disease (Parnaby et al., 2012): Only liver metastases are seen more frequently (Desch et al., 2005). PMs are more frequently associated with rectal tumours, occurring at twice the rate in this group compared to those with a colonic primary (Parnaby et al., 2012). They are also associated with mutated *RAS* in the primary colorectal cancer (CRC).

Most PMs are found within the lung parenchyma and are asymptomatic however, around 15% of patients will develop symptoms. For example, invasion of PMs into the chest wall may produce chest pain, and stridor and breathlessness are seen with endobronchial disease; furthermore endobronchial metastases and invasion of metastases into the pulmonary artery can lead to haemoptysis. Such symptoms are unlikely to be associated with radical options for treatment and therefore most PMs that are put forward for radical treatment have been picked up purely on radiological staging during the course of the disease.

Overall role of surgery in colorectal pulmonary metastatic disease

Most patients with PMs as part of the spectrum of CRC receive palliative systemic therapy as their definitive treatment. Surgical palliation in intrathoracic disease may be indicated in selected cases. Bronchoscopy and debulking, with or without stenting, provide symptomatic relief for airway obstruction and haemoptysis. However, in addition to intervention aimed solely at palliation, patients with oligometastatic disease are candidates for lung-directed therapies. In such patients, pulmonary metastasectomy offers definitive diagnosis and local control and may improve survival in selected patients.

Work-up for patients with PMs from CRC

Differential diagnosis

PMs often present as solitary or multiple nodules distributed throughout the lung fields, frequently identified through routine follow-up computed tomography (CT) scans. The differential diagnosis of PM is that of any other solitary or multiple lung nodules. The differential diagnosis requires a multidisciplinary approach, integrating clinical, radiological, and sometimes histopathological data. Accurate identification and characterization of metastatic lesions are imperative for guiding appropriate therapeutic strategies and optimizing patient outcomes.

In a patient with a solitary lung lesion in conjunction with CRC or a CRC history, consideration should be given to it being a primary lung cancer. The differentiation between primary lung cancers and PMs is crucial due to the distinct therapeutic approaches and prognostic implications associated with each. The gold standard treatment for resection of primary lung cancer is an anatomical resection, while that of a PM is a wedge resection if possible. Factors that would make one suspicious of a primary lung cancer include a solitary lesion, if the lesion is spiculated on CT scan, upper lobe lesions, and if the patient is a heavy smoker. If primary lung cancer is suspected as a differential, then a CT-guided biopsy should be performed where possible (NG151, 2020). This is preferable to performing a frozen section as immunohistochemistry (with its two to three days of processing time) is often needed to distinguish between an adenocarcinoma of lung versus bowel origin. A metastatic lesion originating from CRC may express markers such as CK20 and CDX2, while a primary lung adenocarcinoma is more likely to show positivity for TTF-1 and Napsin A. With careful multidisciplinary assessment, an accurate diagnosis of PM can be made. In the PulMiCC trial (Milosevic et al., 2020), only two out of the 93 patients randomized (one in each arm) were subsequently found not to have metastasis.

Investigations

Suspected CRC PMs necessitate a thorough and methodical approach to confirm the diagnosis and guide subsequent management. Patients will need multiple investigations to determine the diagnosis, assess whether other sites of metastatic disease are present, and then to assess the patient's fitness to undergo treatment. Most patients with PMs are asymptomatic. They are usually found on routine follow-up or initial staging CT scans of the chest, abdomen, and pelvis. The Association of Coloproctology of Great Britain and Northern Ireland has promoted an active policy of monitoring, detecting, and team discussions to offer further treatment if lung metastases are present. A chest CT scan will determine the number, size, and exact anatomical location of the suspected PM. Pulmonary metastases tend to be well-circumscribed and located more commonly in the lower lobes, while primary lung cancers are often spiculated and more common in the upper lobes. With modern CT scans slice thicknesses of 2 mm or less can be viewed in multiple planes, with nodule detection software available. This has led to the detection of more and more nodules. Nodules up to 2–3 mm can now be detected. Not all of these nodules will turn out to be malignant. Using 1-mm slice thickness multidetector row CT, Kang et al. found no more nodules at the time of surgery (Kang et al., 2008). The CT scan should be performed within the previous four weeks prior to surgery (Detterbeck et al., 2010) to avoid missing new nodules at the time of operation.

If the PMs are considered resectable, most clinicians would advocate a [18F]2-fluoro 2-deoxy-D-glucose positron emission tomography (FDG PET) scan to identify any lymph node involvement and other sites of metastatic disease. Pastorino et al. found that a PET scan excluded 21% of patients from undergoing pulmonary metastasectomy due to detection of extrapulmonary metastasis, primary site recurrence, mediastinal lymphadenopathy, or benign disease (Pastorino et al., 2003). However, it should be noted that PET scans cannot reliably determine whether small lung lesions are malignant (Bury et al., 1996). This is especially the case in lesions less than 1 cm (Reinhardt et al., 2006) where sensitivity is low. Therefore the PET scan is more likely to be looking for occult lesions that have not come to light on CT scanning, but that are outside of the lungs.

If there is suspicion of liver metastasis, an MRI scan of the liver should be performed. This may be more pertinent in right-sided primary CRC, where isolated PMs are less common. Brain imaging is not routinely performed prior to the treatment of PM, unless there is clinical suspicion, due to the low rate of brain metastasis in CRC. Where brain metastases do occur, they are usually a late feature that come to light later and metachronously to other sites of metastatic spread.

Although assessment of the patient's clinical features and the radiological characteristics of a lesion will help to determine the diagnosis, it is often not possible to reliably determine whether a solitary nodule is primary lung cancer or PM. In this situation, a CT biopsy should be attempted to determine an accurate tissue diagnosis. However, it is important to realize that the size of some of these nodules makes accurate biopsy impossible and a false negative may be gleaned.

Pulmonary function tests, including gas transfer factor, should be performed to assess the patient's fitness for surgery. An echocardiogram may be helpful if there is a history of cardiovascular disease. In borderline patients, a cardiopulmonary exercise test (CPET) can be used to determine the patient's fitness for surgery.

Indications for surgery and what defines resectability and operability

The aim of pulmonary metastasectomy is to remove all lung metastases with clear margins to improve the patient's survival. The indications for pulmonary metastasectomy are constantly evolving with the development of new effective chemotherapy and targeted therapies (Rusch, 2010). The majority of the indications for pulmonary metastasectomy are based on evidence from retrospective case series and population-based studies.

Generally accepted indications for pulmonary metastasectomy are if:

- All metastases are potentially resectable with clear margins (resectability)
- The patient is able to tolerate the procedure (operability)
- The primary site is either already resected or there is a plan to resect it or control it in some other way
- There are no extra-thoracic metastases except resectable liver metastasis

Assessing a patient's suitability for surgery can be divided into operability and resectability. Operability refers to the patient's overall ability to withstand surgery, which is influenced by factors such as age, comorbidities, and pulmonary function. Resectability, on the other hand, pertains to the technical feasibility of completely removing all detectable lung metastases while preserving sufficient lung function. Pre-operative pulmonary function tests are crucial to ensure patients have adequate respiratory reserve post-surgery. Patients with lesions amenable to complete resection without compromising critical structures are considered good candidates for metastasectomy.

Resection of one or more of a number of lesions may also be indicated in certain other situations. These include:

- When tissue needs to be obtained to confirm metastatic disease and provide tissue for molecular and genetic testing to guide treatment
- Symptomatic metastases. Metastasis may cause bronchial obstruction with distal infection that cannot be managed non-operatively

- A new primary lung cancer is a possibility
- Oligoprogression: If there are a large number of metastases that are controlled by systemic chemotherapy but progression in one or two metastases, then resection may improve survival

When considering whether to resect a PM, one must consider other available treatment options. These include other local ablative techniques or systemic therapy. This is where discussion in the MDT is essential. Factors that may influence the assessment of resectability are those that have been shown to be associated with prolonged survival in patients who have undergone pulmonary metastasectomy. Favourable prognostic factors include a long disease-free interval from the last intervention (e.g. primary removal), presence of a solitary metastasis, low serum CEA level, and the absence of lymph nodes in association with the primary.

Role of the MDT in determining optimal treatment of colorectal pulmonary metastases

The treatment of CRC PMs requires a sophisticated and coordinated approach. Multidisciplinary teams (MDTs) play a pivotal role in evaluating and managing these complex cases, ensuring patients receive individualized and optimal care. The MDT will assess the resectability and operability as defined above. The timing of metastasectomy vis-à-vis systemic therapy is complex and requires expert input, as does the risk/benefit assessment of local therapies, including surgical resection versus stereotactic body radiotherapy (SBRT) versus percutaneous ablation versus systemic therapy alone. Referring people to MDTs that specialize in primary lung disease may not be appropriate as they do not specialize in the management of PMs from CRC and therefore a specialist PMs MDT is optimal, or at least a section of the main MDT being dedicated to these complex cases.

A PMs MDT typically comprises specialists from various fields, including colorectal surgeons, medical and clinical oncologists, radiologists, thoracic surgeons, specialists in non-surgical ablation, pathologists, specialist nurses and sometimes palliative care experts. Each member brings a unique perspective and expertise, contributing to a comprehensive assessment of the patient's condition. The MDT meets regularly to discuss new cases, review diagnostic findings, and formulate individualized treatment plans.

As well as deciding on which patients undergo pulmonary metastasectomy, the MDT also plays a crucial role in integrating adjunctive therapies into the treatment plan. This includes neoadjuvant and adjuvant chemotherapy, targeted therapies, and immunotherapy. For instance, patients with *KRAS*-mutated versus *KRAS*-wt tumours may benefit from specific targeted therapies, as highlighted in studies by Fiorentino et al. (2010) and Pfannschmidt et al. (2007). The coordination of these treatments helps to maximize the therapeutic benefit and improve overall survival.

Although the proportion of patients offered surgery has increased over time, significant regional variations in rates of pulmonary metastasectomy persist (Fenton et al., 2021). This is not surprising given the absence of universally accepted guidelines, the lack of equipoise due to poor quality evidence, and the inequity of access for patients to specialized MDTs. The IMPACT initiative addresses these themes and recommends a focus on equitable access to specialist advanced CRC MDTs. Discussions with patients should include information regarding the need for more high-quality evidence. Pulmonary metastasectomy, where low morbidity and mortality must be balanced with uncertain benefits, can mean treatment decisions are finely balanced. Acknowledgement of these issues is a prerequisite for informed consent before pulmonary metastasectomy.

Evidence for benefit from pulmonary metastasectomy

Most of the evidence for pulmonary metastasectomy in CRC comes from retrospective case series and population-based studies. These studies are hampered by selection bias. As there often is no control arm, they do not clarify the role of metastasectomy in prolongation of overall survival. The literature is further hampered by inconsistent or absent description of other local or systemic therapies and variable length of follow-up.

One of the largest series is the International Registry of Lung Metastases (Pastorino et al., 1997). The five-year survival of 4,572 patients who underwent complete resection of lung metastases was 36%. This study contained multiple tumour types. Factors associated with a better prognosis were the presence of a solitary metastasis and a disease-free interval from primary resection of greater than 36 months.

One of the largest population-based studies is by Fenton et al. (2021). They used HES (Hospital Episode Statistics) data to investigate pulmonary metastasectomy in England. Pulmonary metastasectomy occurred in 2% of patients with CRC within three years of the initial colorectal resection. Operative mortality was low at 0.6%, and five-year survival in patients undergoing pulmonary metastasectomy was 50.8% which compares well with contemporaneous patients undergoing chemotherapy alone.

A meta-analysis by Gonzalez et al. (2013) reported a five-year survival rate of approximately 40–50% following pulmonary metastasectomy in CRC patients, also compared to a significantly lower survival rate in patients managed with systemic therapy alone. This survival benefit is particularly pronounced in patients with fewer metastases, longer disease-free intervals, and the absence of liver metastases.

Another study by Pfannschmidt et al. (2007) systematically reviewed published series on pulmonary metastasectomy, demonstrating consistent survival benefits across various patient cohorts. The analysis emphasized that patients who underwent complete resection of lung metastases experienced markedly improved survival outcomes, reinforcing the importance of achieving clear surgical margins. The study also highlighted those patients with metachronous metastases (metastases appearing after the primary tumour) had better outcomes than those with synchronous metastases (metastases present at the same time as the primary tumour).

Fiorentino et al. (2010) conducted a qualitative synthesis of reported outcomes, highlighting the heterogeneity of patient selection criteria and surgical techniques across different studies. Despite this variability, the overarching conclusion was that pulmonary metastasectomy could lead to favourable survival outcomes in well-selected patients, underscoring the need for standardized criteria and protocols in clinical practice. This synthesis also emphasized the importance of considering the disease-free interval, the number of metastases, and the absence of extra-thoracic disease as critical factors in patient selection.

Additionally, a study by Mitry et al. (2010) explored the long-term outcomes of patients undergoing pulmonary metastasectomy and identified several prognostic factors associated with improved survival. These factors included the complete resection of metastases, a long disease-free interval between the primary cancer and the appearance of lung metastases, and the absence of lymph node involvement alongside the primary tumour. This study underscored the importance of thorough pre-operative assessment and careful patient selection to maximize the benefits of surgery.

The Pulmonary Metastasectomy in Colorectal Cancer (PulMiCC) trial was a randomized controlled trial designed to evaluate the efficacy of pulmonary metastasectomy in improving survival outcomes for CRC patients (Treasure et al., 2019). This trial aimed to provide high-level evidence to support or refute the benefits of metastasectomy, primarily supported by retrospective studies and non-randomized data. Despite its importance, the PulMiCC trial struggled with patient recruitment and was ultimately unable to enrol enough participants to meet its original objectives.

Several factors contributed to this challenge:

1. Patient and clinician preferences: There was a strong preference among both patients and clinicians for surgical intervention based on existing beliefs and observational data suggesting benefits. This preference made randomization difficult, as there was not ethical equipoise, and many were reluctant to forego surgery and be assigned to the control arm.
2. Multidisciplinary decision-making: The involvement of multidisciplinary teams often led to a consensus for surgery, making it challenging to convince both the patient and the treating team to consider randomization into a trial that might not include surgical intervention.
3. Timing and logistics: The logistical challenges of coordinating trial enrolment across multiple centres, combined with the timing of surgeries and follow-up assessments, further complicated recruitment efforts.

The trial did not meet the target recruitment of 300 patients. It was closed after six years. Results were published with only 65 patients randomized (Treasure et al., 2019) and again with the data from a further 28 patients that were randomized in a centre in Serbia (Milosevic et al., 2020). Unsurprisingly, due to the low number of patients randomized, there was no significant difference in survival between the groups. Five-year survival for those randomized to surgery was 36.4% compared with to 29.6% with no surgery, and median survival was also similar (3.78 vs 3.53, respectively). Conclusions that can be drawn from this trial are that the survival for patients with PM who do not undergo metastasectomy is higher than expected. The five-year survival in the control group of 29.6% is significantly higher than the 5% or less five-year survival that is often quoted in case series without a control arm.

Despite the recruitment issues, the PulMiCC trial provided valuable insights and underscored the need for continued high-quality research in this area. The challenges faced by the trial highlighted the complexities of conducting randomized controlled trials in pulmonary metastasectomy and the importance of designing studies that can effectively address these hurdles.

Guidelines

Several guidelines have been published on the role of pulmonary metastasectomy in CRC. When reading these guidelines, one must consider that most of the recommendations are based on expert opinion, not evidence-based medicine. A summary of the more commonly used guidelines follows.

National Institute for Health and Care Excellence (NICE), UK

The National Institute for Health and Clinical Excellence (NICE) published guidance on the management of CRC in 2020 (NG151, 2020). These guidelines contained a section on the management of metastatic disease (Section 1.5). They recommend that one should perform pulmonary metastasectomy, ablation, or stereotactic body radiation therapy for people with lung metastases that are suitable for local treatment after discussion by an MDT that includes a thoracic surgeon and a specialist in non-surgical ablation. They made the recommendation, acknowledging there was limited clinical evidence, and recommendations were based on clinical knowledge. They concluded there was not enough evidence to recommend surgery over stereotactic radiotherapy or image-guided ablation.

Based on clinical experience, they recommend patients with a solitary lesion should undergo a biopsy to rule out primary lung cancer. In reality, this biopsy may need to be an excision biopsy to confirm the differential diagnosis.

European Society of Medical Oncology (ESMO)

The European Society of Medical Oncology (ESMO) published guidelines on the management of metastatic CRC in 2023 (Cervantes et al., 2023). Recommendation 10 of the guidelines suggests chemotherapy should be considered the initial part of any treatment strategy of metastatic CRC except in patients with a single/few liver or lung metastases. They acknowledge that in the absence of randomized control trials, surgery has remained the treatment of choice for patients with oligometastatic CRC. They state that treatment should aim to achieve complete resection of all tumour masses using surgical resection and/or non-surgical interventions. For patients with resectable oligometastatic disease confined to a single organ (most frequently liver or lung) and/or a few organs (and even localized peritoneal spread), the guidelines state surgery remains the standard and best (potentially) curative treatment approach. Operative resection of metastases must be seen in the context of prognostic information and technical limitations.

National Comprehensive Cancer Network (NCCN)

The National Comprehensive Cancer Network (NCCN) provides evidence-based guidelines for the treatment of CRC (Benson et al., 2024), including the management of lung metastases. Most of the evidence in these guidelines is classed as level 2b evidence (low level of evidence without a uniform consensus, but with no major disagreement).

They emphasize the importance of a comprehensive initial assessment and staging process for patients with suspected lung metastases from CRC. This involves detailed imaging studies, including high-resolution CT and PET scans, to evaluate the extent of metastatic disease accurately.

The NCCN guidelines advocate for a multidisciplinary approach in the management of CRC lung metastases. An MDT, comprising surgical oncologists, medical oncologists, radiologists, pulmonologists, and pathologists, should collaboratively evaluate each case. They advise that a team-based approach ensures a comprehensive review of the patient's condition, enabling personalized treatment plans that integrate surgical, systemic, and supportive therapies.

Society of Thoracic Surgeons

The Society of Thoracic Surgeons (STS) issued a consensus statement on the role of pulmonary metastasectomy in the treatment of patients with metastatic cancer (Handy et al., 2019). They acknowledge the level of evidence for pulmonary metastasectomy is poor. The consensus statement was therefore generated using a modified Delphi methodology. This consensus statement includes PMs from all cancer types, although some recommendations are specific to CRC. It outlines the importance of a multidisciplinary approach and individualized patient care.

These are the only guidelines that describe the surgical technique. They recommend minimally invasive surgery due to its shorter recovery time and discourage the use of pneumonectomy. They state that pulmonary metastasectomy is best suited to patients with three or fewer metastases and recommend lymph node sampling or dissection to help predict survival.

Technical aspects of pulmonary metastasectomy

Diagnostic biopsy

A pre-operative biopsy is unnecessary where imaging is consistent with PMs and operative risks, including the risk of resection for benign disease, are acceptable to the patient. Biopsy should be considered where the diagnosis is in doubt; an alternative diagnosis may change management or higher risk extended resection contemplated.

Choice of approach

Thoracotomy has traditionally been the approach of choice for metastases limited to a single lung. In the case of bilateral disease, median sternotomy has the advantage of a single procedure; however, it provides limited access to left lower lobe lesions and for systematic nodal dissection. Most surgeons, therefore, favour a staged bilateral approach in such cases. Open surgery allows bimanual palpation of the entire lung and may enable the detection of previously undiagnosed nodules, which is an important consideration as CT and FDG-PET are limited in detecting all colorectal PMs (Guerrera et al., 2017). However, evidence of the superiority of thoracotomy over a minimal access approach in detecting unexpected metastases has not been confirmed. Over the last two decades, there has been a move to video-assisted thoracoscopic surgery (VATS) to resect PMs (Gonzalez et al., 2021; van Dorp et al., 2020). Prenafeta Claramunt et al. (2020) compared ipsilateral recurrence after open or VATS resection of colorectal PMs. In a matched sample, there was no difference in ipsilateral recurrence rates between VATS and open cases (23.6% vs 26.2% respectively ((95% CI for risk reduction with VATS: −22.6% to 17.5%; $p = 0.80$)) (Prenafeta Claramunt et al., 2020).

Whilst the demographics of patients with colorectal PMs differ from those of the primary lung cancer population, the proven short-term benefits of VATS in primary lung cancer, with less pain, fewer in-hospital complications, shorter hospital stay, and superior early functional recovery, have been extrapolated to its routine use in pulmonary metastasectomy (Lim et al., 2022). The increasing focus on Robotic-assisted Thoracic Surgery (RATS) in primary lung cancer resection will lead to an increase in CRC PMs resected via this approach.

Resection margin and tumour size

Most lung metastases are amenable to local excision. This requires a resection margin to be determined, balancing the adequacy of resection to prevent local recurrence, with lung conservation to preserve pulmonary function for possible future intervention. The size of metastases has been examined as a predictor of local recurrence. In an evaluation of 459 resected lung metastases, margins < 7 mm were associated with local recurrence. Larger metastases were associated with more aggressive growth patterns suggesting resection margins should generally increase with the metastasis size (Welter et al., 2017). Nelson et al. showed that a margin length of at least half the tumour size resulted in a local recurrence risk of < 11% at two years and similarly identified that larger tumour size was associated with increased risk, with an adverse hazard ratio of 1.5 per additional cm (Nelson et al., 2019a).

Takeda-Miyata et al. identified spread through air spaces (STAS) in 41.6% of colorectal lung metastases. The extent of STAS was an independent risk factor for surgical margin relapse. Patients with STAS also show significantly worse overall five-year survival than those without (30.3% vs 76.9%; $p = 0.002$). An elevated pre-metastasectomy serum carcinoma embryonic antigen (CEA) level was independently correlated with STAS. Metastasis size and STAS should be considered when evaluating the optimal resection margin of metastases suitable for local excision.

What is the role of anatomical resection?

The importance of complete resection with adequate margins is evident; however, the requirement for anatomical resection, shown in most studies of primary lung cancer to reduce the risk of local recurrence, is less certain in pulmonary metastasectomy. Anatomical resection consisting of segmentectomy, lobectomy, or, rarely, pneumonectomy has generally been reserved for large or central lesions or multiple lesions within one anatomical region. Local excision via wedge resection has remained the procedure of choice. International data on pulmonary metastasectomy show that rates of wedge excision versus anatomical resection have remained stable over time, at around two-thirds: one-third of cases respectively (Gonzalez et al., 2021; van Dorp et al., 2020). There are several justifications for this approach; operative morbidity and mortality of local excision are low, and the lung-sparing advantage of local excision facilitates future metastasectomy.

In primary lung cancer, there has been a move from lobectomy to anatomic segmentectomy for smaller lesions (Saji et al., 2022). Whether an increase in segmentectomy will be applied to pulmonary metastasectomy at the expense of local excision is yet to be determined. A systematic review of over 1,300 patients showed a tendency to perform anatomical resections for larger metastases. Anatomical resections were associated with improved recurrence-free survival

(RFS), while the impact of such procedures on overall survival (OS) remained uncertain. A significantly higher incidence of resection-margin recurrences was observed in patients who underwent non-anatomical resections (Prisciandaro et al., 2022). However, the specific role of anatomic segmentectomy versus local excision in pulmonary metastasectomy requires prospective studies.

Role of lymph node sampling and systematic nodal dissection

The adverse prognostic outcomes associated with intrathoracic nodal involvement in association with PMs are viewed by most MDTs as a contraindication to surgery. Whether there is a role for lymph node sampling or systematic nodal dissection in addition to pulmonary metastasectomy as a routine adjunct in patients without pre-operative evidence of lymph node involvement is yet to be determined. Nodal excision may facilitate more accurate pathological staging and potentially provide therapeutic benefits however, it increases operative time and is associated with a risk of chyle leak. Furthermore, avoiding lymph node dissection preserves hilar planes, which can simplify future operations.

Lymph node metastases in surgical series are reported to occur in 20–43% of patients undergoing pulmonary metastasectomy for CRC. Higher rates of lymph node involvement are seen in patients with larger or multiple metastases and patients with rectal tumours (Bolukbas et al., 2014). The Society of Thoracic Surgeons consensus statement recommends that lymph node sampling or dissection concomitant with pulmonary metastasectomy be considered (Handy et al., 2019), and rates of lymph node sampling during pulmonary metastasectomy in Europe have increased over time, with 67% of respondents in the European Society of Thoracic Surgeons survey performing mediastinal lymph node sampling or dissection (van Dorp et al., 2023a).

In a review of 518 patients undergoing pulmonary metastasectomy for CRC, systematic nodal dissection was not a significant factor for prolonged survival in the lymph node-positive group (Hamaji et al., 2012). The RCT NCT03118818 will test the hypothesis that systematic mediastinal lymph node dissection in conjunction with pulmonary metastasectomy in CRC is associated with improved survival compared to pulmonary metastasectomy alone.

Special considerations in pulmonary metastasectomy

Synchronous and metachronous hepatic metastases

The successful outcomes associated with the resection of colorectal liver metastases have led to patients presenting for pulmonary resection with synchronous or metachronous hepatic metastases. Andres et al. (2015) interrogated the LiverMetSurvey prospective registry to assess outcomes of patients with CRC simultaneously diagnosed with liver and lung metastases. Survival of patients who underwent resection of all metastases was similar to a control group undergoing resection of isolated liver secondaries (overall five-year survival 51.5% and 44.5% respectively), but worse for the group undergoing liver resection alone without resection of their PMs (14.35%, $p = 0.001$), suggesting that where resectable, simultaneous liver and lung metastases should not be considered a contraindication to surgery (Andres et al., 2015).

The highly selective nature of patients who have undergone both liver and lung resections for CRC, the differential prognostic features they are likely to exhibit, and the variable reporting of outcomes confounds simple comparisons between studies. The focus of studies on whether patients who undergo liver and lung resection have inferior outcomes compared to those undergoing pulmonary resection alone may be less important to individual patients making informed treatment decisions.

Redo pulmonary metastasectomy

Despite the good survival rates associated with the resection of CRC PMs, pulmonary recurrence remains common and accounts for up to 50% of the mortality in this group (Van Cutsem et al., 2014). Consequently, repeat pulmonary metastasectomy has gained traction amongst thoracic surgeons and patients. Patients for repeat pulmonary metastasectomy should be considered by the same criteria as first-time pulmonary metastasectomy. Notably, several repeat metastasectomy series show no associated in-hospital mortality (Hachimaru et al., 2016; Welter et al., 2007). Moreover, repeat metastasectomy is associated with a morbidity rate comparable to that seen at first-time resection regarding complications such as air leak, atrial fibrillation, and pneumonia (Hachimaru et al., 2016; Menna et al., 2018).

Regarding long-term outcomes, re-operation is associated with five-year survival rates of 33–64%, with no difference in survival rates compared with the first metastasectomy (Hachimaru et al., 2016; Menna et al., 2018). Outcomes from the Dutch Lung Cancer audit found that five-year OS was 53% after pulmonary metastasectomy for colorectal metastases and 52% after repeat metastasectomy (van Dorp et al., 2023b).

Adverse prognostic factors for patients undergoing repeat metastasectomy are similar to first-time pulmonary resection. In the meta-analysis by Salah et al., more than two metastatic pulmonary nodules and a maximum diameter of the largest pulmonary nodule of 3 cm or greater were independent factors associated with inferior survival following repeated resection (Salah et al., 2013).

Patients undergoing repeat procedures are likely to have been offered surgery based on favourable prognostic factors compared to those deemed unsuitable for further metastasectomy. Indeed, this is the nature of selection for surgery. The purported benefit of repeat resection may be due to such favourable factors. What is clear is that such patients are generally at low operative risk. Openness with patients reflecting on these issues allows those with favourable prognostic features to access surgery, having understood the risks and benefits, including areas of uncertainty.

Prognostic and predictive clinical indicators

Several clinical and biological factors have been described concerning outcomes after pulmonary metastasectomy. The terms 'prognostic' and 'predictive' have often been used interchangeably, although it is important to distinguish a factor's prognostic effect from its ability to predict a differential outcome after treatment. There remains uncertainty regarding these factors and whether the prognosis of such patients is altered by undergoing metastasectomy.

- Disease-free interval (DFI), defined as the time between resection of the primary tumour and detection of metastases, is considered a predictor of tumour biology and prognosis. Short DFI is independently associated with an adverse risk of recurrence and lower survival, although no cut-off period has been defined (Gonzalez et al., 2013; Onaitis et al., 2009).
- The number of metastases is an independent prognostic factor of recurrence and survival in pulmonary metastasectomy. Most studies have identified a single metastasis associated with more favourable outcomes than multiple metastases (Cho et al., 2015; Onaitis et al., 2009). The findings of isolated studies have been confirmed in meta-analyses where the presence of multiple metastases was an independent adverse prognostic indicator for survival (HR 2.05 95% CI 1.583–2.648, $p < 0.001$) (Salah et al., 2012). Gonzalez et al. found a similar magnitude of influence in their meta-analysis (HR 2.04 95% CI 1.72–2.41) (Gonzalez et al., 2013).
- Hilar or mediastinal lymph node involvement is associated with reduced survival following pulmonary metastasectomy (Welter et al., 2007; Zampino et al., 2014). In a series of 165 patients, all of whom underwent complete resection, Saito et al. found that five-year survival was 53.6% for patients without intrathoracic nodal metastases versus 6.2% at four years for patients with nodal disease ($p < 0.001$) (Saito et al., 2002). The findings of retrospective series are confirmed by the meta-analysis by Gonzalez et al., where hilar and/or mediastinal lymph node involvement was associated with an adverse HR of 1.65 for survival (95% CI 1.38–2.02) (Gonzalez et al., 2013). Whilst mediastinal nodal involvement portends a worse outcome than hilar disease in primary lung cancer (Rami-Porta, 2016), the impact of mediastinal location on survival did not differ from that of the hilar position following lung metastasectomy in CRC (Renaud et al., 2014).
- Kim et al. found that a rectal (as opposed to colonic) primary was an independent adverse risk factor associated with disease-free survival after pulmonary metastasectomy (HR 2.04 (CI 1.09-3.79; $p = 0.03$) (Kim et al., 2017). Cho and colleagues confirmed this in a larger series (Cho et al., 2014). Distinct prognostic factors exist for patients with PMs from lower rectal compared with upper rectal or colon cancer. Completeness of resection, lymph node involvement, gender, and stage predicts survival in patients with lower and middle rectal cancer, compared to the completeness of resection and number of metastases in patients with upper rectal or colon cancer (Meimarakis et al., 2014).
- Elevated pre-metastasectomy serum CEA is an independent parameter of poor survival (HR 1.91, 95% CI 1.57–2.32) (Gonzalez et al., 2013). Salah et al. found a CEA > 5 g/mL to be one of the most important predictors of survival in their prognostic model (Salah et al., 2012).
- Renaud et al. examined the role of neutrophil to lymphocyte ratio, a biomarker that influences prognosis in several tumour types (Sarraf et al., 2009). A neutrophil-to-lymphocyte ratio of ≤ = 4.05 (as opposed to > 4.05) was an independent favourable prognostic factor for both OS (HR 0.29 95% CI 0.167–0.503; $p < 0.0001$) and time to pulmonary recurrence (HR 0.346 95% CI 0.221–0.54; $p < 0.0001$) (Renaud et al., 2019b).

Whether these factors represent predictive or prognostic factors uninfluenced by the decision to undergo pulmonary metastasectomy is uncertain. However, the cumulative effect of these individual factors may be utilized to assess the potential benefit of pulmonary metastasectomy. Salah et al. identified three independent poor prognostic factors of CEA > 5 g/mL, > 1 metastasis, and DFI < 36 months in a pooled analysis and developed a prognostic model of OS. They proposed three groups based on zero or one risk factor, two risk factors, or three. The authors recommended that in the absence of randomized studies, surgical resection of lung metastases should be offered to low and intermediate-risk groups whose five-year survival was 68.2% and 46.4%, respectively, given this is unlikely to be achieved by other modalities (Salah et al., 2012).

Alternative treatments to pulmonary metastasectomy

Whilst surgery remains the gold standard for patients with radically treatable colorectal PMs, alternative options for patients who are not fit for or do not wish to undergo surgery include stereotactic radiotherapy (SBRT) or percutaneous or endobronchial ablative techniques.

Nelson et al. analysed 381 patients with CRC PMs who underwent surgery or SRBT over a 10-year period. The two-year risk of local recurrence for each nodule was 14.1% after surgery versus 29.4% after SRT ($p = 0.023$), with the risk of local recurrence increasing with increasing tumour size (Nelson et al., 2019b). PMs from CRC have greater radio-resistance compared to other secondary tumours. SAFRON II, a phase 2 study examining single-fraction vs multi-fraction SRT for the treatment of patients with pulmonary oligometastases, suggested local failure events in the single-fraction arm of the study were driven by patients with colorectal disease (Siva et al., 2021). In the LaIT-SABR study, the largest series to date, two-year freedom from local progression-free survival (FLP) was 75.4%. Dose escalation reduced the risk of local progression (Nicosia et al., 2022). SBRT is a feasible approach to lung metastases in patients unsuitable for surgical resection.

High-quality studies comparing surgery and percutaneous radiofrequency ablation (RFA) are lacking, however most evidence supports surgery as the most effective treatment option. In a review of studies of either surgery or RFA for CRC PMs, five-year survival rates for surgery vs RFA were 29–71% versus 35–45%, respectively. Treatment-related mortality rates for RFA and surgery were 0% and 1.4–2.4%, respectively, whereas morbidity rates seemed lowest for surgery (Schlijper et al., 2014). Morbidity rates are commonly related to chest drainage requirement, seen in up to 47% of treatments, however major complications are rare (Delpla et al., 2021).

Percutaneous microwave ablation (MWA) may be superior to RFA in the treatment of CRC lung metastases in terms of local control rates, the favoured outcome measure of interventional radiologists. In a study of 109 patients with colorectal PMs undergoing 231 CT-guided ablative treatments, local control rates in patients receiving MWA were 88.3% vs 69.2% in patients treated with RFA. There was no difference in time to progression or survival rates between RFA and MWA (Vogl et al., 2016).

To date, no clinical trial has compared surgery, SRT, and ablative techniques, however some important insights from the Danish national registry are worth highlighting. In the 14 years covered by the study, there was an increase in the utility of all treatment modalities, from 3.4% in the first interval to 15.4% in the last interval, whilst the number of resected primary tumours only increased slightly over time. Median survival was 3.7 years for patients undergoing metastasis-directed therapy, A higher survival for patients who underwent a surgical local treatment compared to RFA or SRT was seen, however this should be interpreted with caution given the inherent selection bias to offer ablation and SBRT to patients who are not judged fit to major surgery (Boysen et al., 2018).

While surgical resection remains the gold standard, ablative techniques can produce acceptable outcomes. They should be considered in patients who are not fit for or do not wish to undergo pulmonary metastasectomy alone or in conjunction with surgical resection for resectable lung metastases. The ESMO guidelines emphasize a multidisciplinary approach to local therapy modalities. For lung-only metastases or oligometastatic disease, including lung lesions, ablation may be considered along with resection according to tumour size, number and location of metastases, extent of parenchymal loss, comorbidities, or other factors. Whilst SBRT is recognized as a treatment option with a low morbidity profile, it is unclear which patients benefit most from this approach (Cervantes et al., 2023).

The advent of navigational bronchoscopy, combined with cone-beam CT, has facilitated accurate real-time visualization of peripheral lung lesions. Precision application of probes and confirmation of treatment zones have enabled bronchoscopic ablation of peripheral lesions. In addition, the ability to obtain biopsy samples, not usually provided during percutaneous ablation, will be increasingly important in an era of individualized management. In a study of CT-guided bronchoscopic RFA in patients with medically inoperable lung cancer, the local control rate was 82.6%, and five-year OS was 61.5% (95% confidence interval: 36–87%) (Koizumi et al., 2015).

The NAVABLATE study investigated bronchoscopic microwave ablation, verified with cone-beam CT in malignant lung nodules, one-third of which were oligometastatic. One-month technique efficacy was 100%, with low complication rates and local recurrence rates like those observed in percutaneous lung ablation at a median follow-up of approximately 18 months (Chan et al., 2021; Lau et al., 2023). If larger studies confirm longer-term efficacy and low complication rates, bronchoscopic microwave ablation has the potential to compete with current treatments in the setting of CRC PMs (Lau et al., 2021). The development of robotic-assisted bronchoscopy platforms can potentially increase reach within the lung and the ability to target lesions more accurately (Agrawal et al., 2020; Fielding et al., 2019).

MDT recommendations of treatment options and patient preferences will ultimately determine pathways. Treatment modalities may increasingly be combined in a complementary fashion to offer more radical options for patients with multiple metastases.

Endobronchial disease

Whilst endobronchial metastases are less frequently encountered than parenchymal metastases, colorectal metastases represent one of the most common causes of metastatic endobronchial disease. Endobronchial disease arises from direct endobronchial deposits or invasion into the airway from parenchymal or nodal metastases. Symptoms include stridor, dyspnoea, cough, and haemoptysis, although one-quarter of patients remain asymptomatic (Marchioni et al., 2014). Symptomatic patients require endobronchial intervention to maintain airway patency where possible. Mechanical debulking, cryotherapy, diathermy, laser therapy, argon plasma coagulation, brachytherapy, and photodynamic therapy are employed according to unit preference. Stenting with either silicone or covered expandable metal stents may maintain airway patency for longer following disobliteration. Most patients have limited life expectancy at the point of diagnosis of endobronchial disease, however some patients may undergo repeated interventions over time. Reintervention will likely be of diminishing benefit, as distal airway involvement limits success over time.

Future directions

The established selection criteria and predictive factors are, in the main, clinical factors and are limited in determining the benefits of radical treatment in individual patients. There is increasing evidence that biomarkers may play an important role via precision analysis in supporting individualized patient management and may identify patients likely to benefit most from pulmonary metastasectomy (Lang et al., 2019).

KRAS (Kirsten rate sarcoma virus) mutations are seen in almost half of all CRC PMs. They are associated with early recurrence and reduced OS after pulmonary metastasectomy, both in association with the KRAS mutation in the primary tumour and in the lung metastases (Renaud et al., 2017a; Schweiger et al., 2014). The identification of such markers may offer the opportunity to tailor management. Renaud et al. found that anatomical resection was associated with significantly improved OS in KRAS patients (101 vs 45 months, $p = 0.02$) but did not impact survival in wild-type patients (Renaud et al., 2019a). Perioperative bevacizumab was associated with longer OS and time to recurrence in the presence of exon 2 codon 12 KRAS mutation following PMs (Renaud et al., 2017b), but this is not part of routine practice.

BRAF (V-raf Murine sarcoma viral oncogene homologue B1) mutations in the primary tumour have been shown to correlate with significantly worse survival in patients undergoing resection of PMs compared to the wild-type (five-year survival 0% vs 100%) (Renaud et al., 2015). Overexpression of c-MET/STAT3, a transmembrane tyrosine-protein kinase receptor and its signalling effector, was associated with reduced median OS in the context of PMs for CRC (Schweiger et al., 2016b). Density and distribution of tumour infiltrating lymphocytes (TILs) and tertiary lymphoid structures (TLSs), markers of host immune response and their overexpression of PD-L1 are associated with reduced OS after PMectomy (Okada et al., 2018; Schweiger et al., 2016a).

CRC PMs are likely to harbour various conserved and *de novo* mutations such that targeted next-generation sequencing can provide a rationale for targeted therapies for patients with CRC lung metastases (Schweiger et al., 2018). Treatments directed to mutations are currently limited with anti-EGFR receptor antibodies targeted at patients with KRAS wild-type, however these biomarkers can potentially individualize patients' management beyond that which clinical prognostic factors currently permit. Also, if a patient has dMMR PM from CRC, the question would be whether to give immunotherapy or to purely resect the disease if it is limited in nature. This will be no doubt a question for future trials.

Putative circulating biomarkers have been identified in patients with CRC PMs, including glycoproteins, circulating tumour cells, acute phase proteins, and neutrophils (Lang et al., 2019). Studies to date are small and further validation is required to verify these markers' prognostic role and establish them in clinical practice.

Conclusion

The mortality of oligometastatic colorectal cancer has reduced over time. This reflects improvements in many aspects of multidisciplinary management. Recent advances in systemic therapies and biological treatments, combined with lung-targeted therapies of pulmonary metastasectomy, ablation, and SBRT, allow more patients the opportunity for prolonged disease control and improved prognosis. The challenge of decision-making in the absence of significant randomized controlled trial evidence relies on multidisciplinary consideration of tumour and patient factors on a case-by-case basis.

REFERENCES

Agrawal, A., Hogarth, D. K., & Murgu, S. (2020). Robotic bronchoscopy for pulmonary lesions: a review of existing technologies and clinical data. *Journal of Thoracic Disease, 12*, 3279–3286.

Andres, A., Mentha, G., Adam, R., et al. (2015). Surgical management of patients with colorectal cancer and simultaneous liver and lung metastases. *British Journal of Surgery, 102*, 691–699.

Benson, A. B., Venook, A. P., Adam, M., et al. (2024). Colon Cancer, Version 3.2024, NCCN Clinical Practice Guidelines in Oncology. *Journal of the National Comparative Cancer Network*, 22.

Blalock, A. (1944. Recent advances in surgery. *New England Journal of Medicine, 231*, 261–267.

Bolukbas, S., Sponholz, S., Kudelin, N., et al. (2014). Risk factors for lymph node metastases and prognosticators of survival in patients undergoing pulmonary metastasectomy for colorectal cancer. *Annals of Thoracic Surgery, 97*, 1926–1932.

Boysen, A. K., Spindler, K. L., Hoyer, M., et al. (2018). Metastasis directed therapy for liver and lung metastases from colorectal cancer-A population-based study. *International Journal of Cancer, 143*, 3218–3226.

Bury, T., Dowlati, A., Paulus, P., et al. (1996). Evaluation of the solitary pulmonary nodule by positron emission tomography imaging. *European Respiratory Journal, 9*, 410–414.

Cervantes, A., Adam, R., Rosello, S., et al. (2023). Metastatic colorectal cancer: ESMO Clinical Practice Guideline for diagnosis, treatment and follow-up. *Annals of Oncology, 34*, 10–32.

Chan, J. W. Y., Lau, R. W. H., Ngai, J. C. L., et al. (2021). Transbronchial microwave ablation of lung nodules with electromagnetic navigation bronchoscopy guidance-a novel technique and initial experience with 30 cases. *Translational Lung Cancer Research, 10*, 1608–1622.

Cho, J. H., Hamaji, M., Allen, M. S., et al. (2014). The prognosis of pulmonary metastasectomy depends on the location of the primary colorectal cancer. *Annals of Thoracic Surgery, 98*, 1231–1237.

Cho, J. H., Kim, S., Namgung, M., et al. (2015). The prognostic importance of the number of metastases in pulmonary metastasectomy of colorectal cancer. *World Journal of Surgical Oncology, 13*, 222.

Delpla, A., De Baere, T., Varin, E., et al. (2021). Role of thermal ablation in colorectal cancer lung metastases. *Cancers (Basel)*, 13.

Desch, C. E., Benson, A. B., 3rd, Somerfield, M. R., et al. (2005). Colorectal cancer surveillance: 2005 update of an American Society of Clinical Oncology practice guideline. *Journal of Clinical Oncology, 23*, 8512–8519.

Detterbeck, F. C., Grodzki, T., Gleeson, F., et al. (2010). Imaging requirements in the practice of pulmonary metastasectomy. *Journal of Thoracic Oncology, 5*, S134–139.

Ehrenhaft, J. L., Lawrence, M. S., & Sensenig, D. M. (1958). Pulmonary resections for metastatic lesions. *AMA Archives of Surgery, 77*, 606–612.

Fenton, H. M., Finan, P. J., Milton, R., et al. (2021). National variation in pulmonary metastasectomy for colorectal cancer. *Colorectal Disease, 23*, 1306–1316.

Fielding, D. I. K., Bashirzadeh, F., Son, J. H., et al. (2019). First human use of a new robotic-assisted fiber optic sensing navigation system for small peripheral pulmonary nodules. *Respiration, 98*, 142–150.

Fiorentino, F., Hunt, I., Teoh, K., et al. (2010). Pulmonary metastasectomy in colorectal cancer: a systematic review and quantitative synthesis. *Journal of the Royal Society of Medicine, 103*, 60–66.

Gonzalez, M., Brunelli, A., Szanto, Z., et al. (2021). Report from the European Society of Thoracic Surgeons database 2019: current surgical practice and perioperative outcomes of pulmonary metastasectomy. *European Journal of Cardiothoracic Surgery, 59*, 996–1003.

Gonzalez, M., Poncet, A., Combescure, C., et al. (2013). Risk factors for survival after lung metastasectomy in colorectal cancer patients: a systematic review and meta-analysis. *Annals of Surgical Oncology, 20*, 572–579.

Guerrera, F., Renaud, S., Schaeffer, M., et al. (2017). Low accuracy of computed tomography and positron emission tomography to detect lung and lymph node metastases of colorectal cancer. *Annals of Thoracic Surgery, 104*, 1194–1199.

Hachimaru, A., Maeda, R., Suda, T., et al. (2016). Repeat pulmonary resection for recurrent lung metastases from colorectal cancer: an analysis of prognostic factors. *Interactive Cardiovascular and Thoracic Surgery, 22*, 826–830.

Hamaji, M., Cassivi, S. D., Shen, K. R., et al. (2012). Is lymph node dissection required in pulmonary metastasectomy for colorectal adenocarcinoma? *Annals of Thoracic Surgery, 94*, 1796–800.

Handy, J. R., Bremner, R. M., Crocenzi, T. S., et al. (2019). Expert Consensus Document on Pulmonary Metastasectomy. *Annals of Thoracic Surgery, 107*, 631–649.

Hellman, S., & Weichselbaum, R. R. (1995). Oligometastases. *Journal of Clinical Oncology, 13*, 8–10.

Kang, M. C., Kang, C. H., Lee, H. J., et al. (2008). Accuracy of 16-channel multi-detector row chest computed tomography with thin sections in the detection of metastatic pulmonary nodules. *European Journal of Cardiothoracic Surgery, 33*, 473–479.

Kim, J. Y., Park, I. J., Kim, H. R., et al. (2017). Post-pulmonary metastasectomy prognosis after curative resection for colorectal cancer. *Oncotarget, 8*, 36566–36577.

Koizumi, T., Tsushima, K., Tanabe, T., et al. (2015). Bronchoscopy-guided cooled radiofrequency ablation as a novel intervention therapy for peripheral lung cancer. *Respiration, 90*, 47–55.

Lang, C., Hoetzenecker, K., & Schweiger, T. S. (2019). Emerging biomarkers in pulmonary metastasectomy. *Journal of Visualized Surgery, 5*.

Lau, K., Lau, R., Baranowski, R., et al. (2021). Late Breaking Abstract - Bronchoscopic microwave ablation of peripheral lung tumors. *European Respiratory Journal, 58*, OA230.

Lau, K. K. W., Lau, R. W. H., Baranowski, R., et al. (2023). Transbronchial microwave ablation of peripheral lung tumors: the NAVABLATE study. *Journal of Bronchology & Interventional Pulmonology.*

Lim, E., Harris, R. A., Mckeon, H. E., et al. (2022). Impact of video-assisted thoracoscopic lobectomy versus open lobectomy for lung cancer on recovery assessed using self-reported physical function: VIOLET RCT. *Health Technology Assessments, 26*, 1–162.

Marchioni, A., Lasagni, A., Busca, A., et al. (2014). Endobronchial metastasis: an epidemiologic and clinicopathologic study of 174 consecutive cases. *Lung Cancer, 84*, 222–228.

Meimarakis, G., Spelsberg, F., Angele, M., et al. (2014). Resection of pulmonary metastases from colon and rectal cancer: factors to predict survival differ regarding to the origin of the primary tumor. *Annals of Surgical Oncology, 21*, 2563–2572.

Menna, C., Berardi, G., Tierno, S. M., et al. (2018). Do repeated operations for recurrent colorectal lung metastases result in improved survival? *Annals of Thoracic Surgery, 106*, 421–427.

Milosevic, M., Edwards, J., Tsang, D., et al. (2020). Pulmonary metastasectomy in colorectal cancer: updated analysis of 93 randomized patients—control survival is much better than previously assumed. *Colorectal Disease, 22*, 1314–1324.

Mitry, E., Guiu, B., Cosconea, S., et al. (2010). Epidemiology, management and prognosis of colorectal cancer with lung metastases: a 30-year population-based study. *Gut, 59*, 1383–1388.

National Institute for Health and Care Excellence (2020). Colorectal cancer (NICE Guidelines NG151). Available at: https://www.nice.org.uk/guidance/ng151 [Date accessed: 24 June 2024].

Nelson, D. B., Tayob, N., Mitchell, K. G., et al. (2019a). Surgical margins and risk of local recurrence after wedge resection of colorectal pulmonary metastases. *Journal of Thoracic and Cardiovascular Surgery, 157*, 1648–1655.

Nelson, D. B., Tayob, N., Nguyen, Q. N., et al. (2019b). Local failure after stereotactic body radiation therapy or wedge resection for colorectal pulmonary metastases. *Journal of Thoracic and Cardiovascular Surgery, 158*, 1234–1241 e16.

Nicosia, L., Franceschini, D., Perrone-Congedi, F., et al. (2022). A multicenter large retrospective database on the personalization of stereotactic ablative radiotherapy use in lung metastases from colon-rectal cancer: The LaIT-SABR study. *Radiotherapy & Oncology, 166*, 92–99.

Okada, S., Itoh, K., Ishihara, S., et al. (2018). Significance of PD-L1 expression in pulmonary metastases from head and neck squamous cell carcinoma. *Surgical Oncology, 27*, 259–265.

Onaitis, M. W., Petersen, R. P., Haney, J. C., et al. (2009). Prognostic factors for recurrence after pulmonary resection of colorectal cancer metastases. *Annals of Thoracic Surgery, 87*, 1684–1688.

Parnaby, C. N., Bailey, W., Balasingam, A., et al. (2012). Pulmonary staging in colorectal cancer: a review. *Colorectal Disease, 14*, 660–670.

Pastorino, U., Buyse, M., Friedel, G., et al. (1997). Long-term results of lung metastasectomy: prognostic analyses based on 5206 cases. *Journal of Thoracic and Cardiovascular Surgery, 113*, 37–49.

Pastorino, U., Veronesi, G., Landoni, C., et al. (2003). Fluorodeoxyglucose positron emission tomography improves preoperative staging of resectable lung metastasis. *Journal of Thoracic and Cardiovascular Surgery, 126*, 1906–1910.

Pfannschmidt, J., Dienemann, H., & Hoffmann, H. (2007). Surgical resection of pulmonary metastases from colorectal cancer: a systematic review of published series. *Annals of Thoracic Surgery, 84*, 324–338.

Prenafeta Claramunt, N., Hwang, D., De Perrot, M., et al. (2020). Incidence of ipsilateral side recurrence after open or video-assisted thoracic surgery resection of colorectal lung metastases. *Annals of Thoracic Surgery, 109*, 1591–1597.

Prisciandaro, E., Ceulemans, L. J., Van Raemdonck, D. E., et al. (2022). Impact of the extent of lung resection on postoperative outcomes of pulmonary metastasectomy for colorectal cancer metastases: an exploratory systematic review. *Journal of Thoracic Disease, 14*, 2677–2688.

Rami-Porta, R. (2016). *IASLC staging manual in thoracic oncology.* Editorial Rx Press.

Reinhardt, M. J., Wiethoelter, N., Matthies, A., et al. (2006). PET recognition of pulmonary metastases on PET/CT imaging: impact of attenuation-corrected and non-attenuation-corrected PET images. *European Journal of Nuclear Medicine and Molecular Imaging, 33*, 134–139.

Renaud, S., Alifano, M., Falcoz, P. E., et al. (2014). Does nodal status influence survival? Results of a 19-year systematic lymphadenectomy experience during lung metastasectomy of colorectal cancer. *Interactive Cardiovascular and Thoracic Surgery, 18*, 482–487.

Renaud, S., Guerrera, F., Seitlinger, J., et al. (2017a). KRAS exon 2 codon 13 mutation is associated with a better prognosis than codon 12 mutation following lung metastasectomy in colorectal cancer. *Oncotarget, 8*, 2514–2524.

Renaud, S., Romain, B., Falcoz, P. E., et al. (2015). KRAS and BRAF mutations are prognostic biomarkers in patients undergoing lung metastasectomy of colorectal cancer. *British Journal of Cancer, 112*, 720–728.

Renaud, S., Schaeffer, M., Falcoz, P. E., et al. (2017b). Perioperative bevacizumab improves survival following lung metastasectomy for colorectal cancer in patients harbouring v-Ki-ras2 Kirsten rat sarcoma viral oncogene homologue exon 2 codon 12 mutationsdagger. *European Journal of Cardiothoracic Surgery, 51*, 255–262.

Renaud, S., Seitlinger, J., Lawati, Y. A., et al. (2019a). Anatomical resections improve survival following lung metastasectomy of colorectal cancer harboring KRAS mutations. *Annals of Surgery, 270*, 1170–1177.

Renaud, S., Seitlinger, J., St-Pierre, D., et al. (2019b). Prognostic value of neutrophil to lymphocyte ratio in lung metastasectomy for colorectal cancer. *European Journal of Cardiothoracic Surgery, 55*, 948–955.

Rusch, V. W. (2010). Pulmonary metastasectomy: a moving target. *Journal of Thoracic Oncology, 5*, S130–131.

Saito, Y., Omiya, H., Kohno, K., et al. (2002). Pulmonary metastasectomy for 165 patients with colorectal carcinoma: a prognostic assessment. *Journal of Thoracic and Cardiovascular Surgery, 124*, 1007–1013.

Saji, H., Okada, M., Tsuboi, M., et al. (2022). Segmentectomy versus lobectomy in small-sized peripheral non-small-cell lung cancer (JCOG0802/WJOG4607L): a multicentre, open-label, phase 3, randomised, controlled, non-inferiority trial. *Lancet, 399*, 1607–1617.

Salah, S., Watanabe, K., Park, J. S., et al. (2013). Repeated resection of colorectal cancer pulmonary oligometastases: pooled analysis and prognostic assessment. *Annals of Surgical Oncology, 20*, 1955–1961.

Salah, S., Watanabe, K., Welter, S., et al. (2012). Colorectal cancer pulmonary oligometastases: pooled analysis and construction of a clinical lung metastasectomy prognostic model. *Annals of Oncology, 23*, 2649–2655.

Sarraf, K. M., Belcher, E., Raevsky, E., et al. (2009). Neutrophil/lymphocyte ratio and its association with survival after complete resection in non-small cell lung cancer. *Journal of Thoracic and Cardiovascular Surgery, 137*, 425–428.

Schlijper, R. C., Grutters, J. P., Houben, R., et al. (2014). What to choose as radical local treatment for lung metastases from colorectal cancer: surgery or radiofrequency ablation? *Cancer Treatment Reviews*, *40*, 60–67.

Schweiger, T., Berghoff, A. S., Glogner, C., et al. (2016a). Tumor-infiltrating lymphocyte subsets and tertiary lymphoid structures in pulmonary metastases from colorectal cancer. *Clinical & Experimental Metastasis*, *33*, 727–39.

Schweiger, T., Hegedus, B., Nikolowsky, C., et al. (2014). EGFR, BRAF and KRAS status in patients undergoing pulmonary metastasectomy from primary colorectal carcinoma: a prospective follow-up study. *Annals of Surgical Oncology*, *21*, 946–54.

Schweiger, T., Liebmann-Reindl, S., Glueck, O., et al. (2018). Mutational profile of colorectal cancer lung metastases and paired primary tumors by targeted next generation sequencing: implications on clinical outcome after surgery. *Journal of Thoracic Disease*, *10*, 6147–6157.

Schweiger, T., Starkl, V., Glueck, O., et al. (2016b). Clinical impact of c-MET expression and mutational status in patients with colorectal cancer lung metastases. *European Journal of Cardiothoracic Surgery*, *49*, 1103–1111; discussion 1111.

Siva, S., Bressel, M., Mai, T., et al. Stereotactic ablative fractionated radiotherapy versus radiosurgery for oligometastatic neoplasia to the lung, I. I. S. I. (2021). Single-fraction vs multifraction stereotactic ablative body radiotherapy for pulmonary oligometastases (SAFRON II): The Trans Tasman Radiation Oncology Group 13.01 phase 2 randomized clinical trial. *JAMA Oncology*, *7*, 1476–1485.

Thomford, N. R., Woolner, L. B., & Clagett, O. T. (1965). The surgical treatment of metastatic tumors in the lungs. *Journal of Thoracic and Cardiovascular Surgery*, *49*, 357–363.

Treasure, T., Farewell, V., Macbeth, F., et al. (2019). Pulmonary Metastasectomy versus Continued Active Monitoring in Colorectal Cancer (PulMiCC): a multicentre randomised clinical trial. *Trials*, *20*, 718.

Van Cutsem, E., Cervantes, A., Nordlinger, B., et al. (2014). Metastatic colorectal cancer: ESMO Clinical Practice Guidelines for diagnosis, treatment and follow-up. *Annals of Oncology*, *25*(Suppl 3), iii1–9.

Van Dorp, M., Beck, N., Steup, W. H., et al. (2020). Surgical treatment of pulmonary metastases in the Netherlands: data from the Dutch Lung Cancer Audit for Surgery. *European Journal of Cardiothoracic Surgery*, *58*, 768–774.

Van Dorp, M., Gonzalez, M., Daddi, N., et al. (2023a). Metastasectomy for colorectal pulmonary metastases: a survey among members of the European Society of Thoracic Surgeons. *Interdiscip Cardiovasc Thorac Surg*. 2023 Feb 6;36(2):ivad002. doi: 10.1093/icvts/ivad002. PMID: 36847670; PMCID: PMC9932002.

van Dorp M, Gonzalez M, Daddi N, Batirel HF, Brunelli A, Schreurs WH. Metastasectomy for colorectal pulmonary metastases: a survey among members of the European Society of Thoracic Surgeons. Interdiscip Cardiovasc Thorac Surg. 2023 Feb 6;36(2):ivad002. doi: 10.1093/icvts/ivad002. PMID: 36847670; PMCID: PMC9932002.

Van Dorp, M., Wolfhagen, N., Torensma, B., et al. (2023b). Pulmonary metastasectomy and repeat metastasectomy for colorectal pulmonary metastases: outcomes from the Dutch Lung Cancer Audit for Surgery. *BJS Open*, 2023 May 5;7(3):zrad009. doi: 10.1093/bjsopen/zrad009. PMID: 37146204; PMCID: PMC10162679

Vogl, T. J., Eckert, R., Naguib, N. N., et al. (2016). Thermal Ablation of colorectal lung metastases: retrospective comparison among laser-induced thermotherapy, radiofrequency ablation, and microwave ablation. *American Journal of Roentgenology*, *207*, 1340–1349.

Welter, S., Arfanis, E., Christoph, D., et al. (2017). Growth patterns of pulmonary metastases: should we adjust resection techniques to primary histology and size? *European Journal of Cardiothoracic Surgery*, *52*, 39–46.

Welter, S., Jacobs, J., Krbek, T., et al. (2007). Long-term survival after repeated resection of pulmonary metastases from colorectal cancer. *Annals of Thoracic Surgery*, *84*, 203–210.

Zampino, M. G., Maisonneuve, P., Ravenda, P. S., et al. (2014). Lung metastases from colorectal cancer: analysis of prognostic factors in a single institution study. *Annals of Thoracic Surgery*, *98*, 1238–1245.

13

Multidisciplinary management of peritoneal metastases

Vasanth Mark Samuel, Glen R. Guerra, and Brendan Moran

Introduction

The term 'peritoneal carcinomatosis' was probably first used by John A. Sampson in 1931 while describing the pathophysiology of metastatic spread of ovarian cancer to the peritoneum. Carcinomatosis involves malignant invasion of both the parietal and visceral peritoneum, the two component parts of the peritoneal cavity. Subsequently carcinomatosis has been used to describe peritoneal metastatic deposits from gastrointestinal cancers, in addition to spread from ovarian cancer. Colorectal cancer is common globally and metastasizes through three different routes: haematogenous, lymphatic, and trans-coelomic to peritoneal surfaces. Though haematogenous spread to the liver and lungs results in the commonest metastatic sites of colorectal cancer spread, peritoneal involvement is frequent and may be synchronous or metachronous to the diagnosis of the primary. At the turn of this century, several studies reported on the natural history of colorectal peritoneal metastasis (CPM), revealing poor outcomes with a median survival of around seven months (Sugarbaker, 2004). A better understanding of the aetiology and natural progression of patients with CPM has led to the development, and refinement, of complex treatment strategies.

Traditionally the term peritoneal carcinomatosis implied a terminal condition, which, irrespective of treatment, led to the patient's death. Best outcomes involved palliative treatment or best supportive care. The landscape in treating peritoneal malignancy began to change with the pioneering work at the National Institute of Health in the 1980s by Paul Sugarbaker and colleagues, who evaluated intraperitoneal administration of 5-fluorouracil (5FU) compared with systemic 5FU in a randomized controlled trial in advanced colorectal cancer (Sugarbaker et al., 1985). Though patient recruitment numbers were low, the trial showed no disease-free or overall survival benefit but did report a reduction in peritoneal carcinomatosis at second-look laparotomy in those treated by intra-peritoneal 5FU. The concept of a loco-regional approach to peritoneal malignancy was proposed, and subsequently evolved over the ensuing decades. Sugarbaker proposed that removal of disease by cytoreductive surgery (CRS) and the addition of hyperthermic intraperitoneal chemotherapy (HIPEC) might benefit patients with pseudomyxoma peritonei (PMP) (Sugarbaker et al., 1993). Pseudomyxoma peritonei is characterized by progressive mucinous ascites, generally originates from a low grade appendiceal neoplasm, and most cases recur and progress within the peritoneal cavity after surgery unless intra-peritoneal chemotherapy is used in combination with CRS. Cytoreductive surgery and HIPEC are now well established in the curative treatment of PMP and appendiceal tumours (Ansari et al., 2016; Chua et al., 2012). Now the principles and strategy of CRS and HIPEC for PMP are being applied to patients with other peritoneal malignancies, including patients with peritoneal spread from colorectal cancer. In this context, CPM has been proposed as nomenclature to differentiate resectable peritoneal disease from peritoneal carcinomatosis to help select patients most likely to benefit from CRS and HIPEC (Moran & Cecil, 2014).

Epidemiology

It is difficult to determine accurately the incidence, and prevalence, of CPM as small-volume peritoneal metastases may be millimetres in size, and even when larger have similar contrast resolution compared with abdominal soft tissues. This results in an inability to detect CPM accurately by any form of modern imaging, and small-volume, limited disease may be undetected at primary tumour presentation or at follow-up. Therefore, CPM is an under-diagnosed disease and an under-represented entity in clinical trials (Tseng et al., 2017). Although autopsy series have reported an incidence of peritoneal metastatic disease in 40–50% of patients with, by definition, advanced and often lethal colorectal cancer (Hugen et al., 2014), the true incidence and prevalence in living patients is unknown. Data from a few case series have shown that CPM is detected in approximately 7% of patients at primary surgery for colorectal cancer (Jayne et al., 2002). CPM has been reported in 2–19% of patients on follow-up after curative surgery for colorectal cancer and in 44% of patients requiring laparotomy for recurrence (Koppe et al., 2006). Traditionally, patients with CPM on systemic 5-fluorouracil based chemotherapy had a median survival of 5.2–12.6 months, whereas patients aggressively managed with CRS and HIPEC had a median survival of 12–32 months, although one must be aware of the potential selection bias in gathering these statistics (Koppe et al., 2006).

Aetiology and pathogenesis of CPM

The peritoneum is derived from the mesoderm and consists of a single layer of mesothelial cells which are supported by a basement membrane. Intra-abdominal reflections and attachments of the peritoneum lead to the formation of ligaments and potential spaces that make this monolayer of cells a complex structure, enough for the peritoneum to be considered an organ in its own right. The peritoneum is the largest serous membrane in the body consisting of two component parts, with the thicker, loosely fixed, parietal peritoneum forming the inner lining of the abdominopelvic cavity and the thinner, more firmly adherent, visceral peritoneum enveloping intraperitoneal organs. The peritoneal cavity is a potential space between the visceral and parietal peritoneum which is subdivided into the greater sac and the lesser sac, enveloped by the greater and lesser omentum (Fig. 13.1). This cavity contains approximately 50 millilitres of serous fluid produced by the mesothelial cells which acts as a lubricant, reducing the friction between mobile peritoneal organs. The distribution of the fluid within the peritoneal cavity depends on factors. These include fluid circulation and absorption, pressure differences within the abdomen, mesenteric partitions, and gravity dependent on body position, for example standing or lying. Peritoneal fluid is distributed within the peritoneal cavity, filtered of any abnormal contents, and absorbed, predominantly on the under surface of the right diaphragm and by the greater and lesser omentum. Deposition, and growth, of intraperitoneal tumour deposits depends on, and correlates with, the natural pathways of flow and the sites of absorption of peritoneal fluid within the peritoneal cavity. In the early stages of virtually all locally advanced, non-mucinous, colorectal cancers, dissemination is random and usually adjacent to the primary tumour, in the absence of ascitic intraperitoneal fluid. Mucinous tumours, or more advanced tumours with ascites, result in widespread peritoneal involvement. The peritoneal compartments, and flow and absorption sites of intraperitoneal fluid, and gravity, results in the 'redistribution' pattern of dissemination with tumour deposits on predictable sites such as the under surface of the right hemi-diaphragm, the omentum, paracolic gutters and in the pelvis. Fig. 13.2 outlines the peritoneal spread of an appendix tumour, but the concept of intraperitoneal spread is similar for any motile cell within the peritoneal cavity (Sugarbaker, 1994).

There are two instances in the natural history and treatment of colorectal cancer where intraperitoneal seeding of tumour cells may occur. First, peritoneal spread may occur pre-operatively as a result of full thickness invasion through the bowel wall by an invasive cancer as the cancer progresses (T4 disease). Secondly, intraperitoneal spread may result by iatrogenic release of tumour cells intra-operatively during surgery (Koppe et al., 2006).

In the earlier stage of colorectal cancer progression, cancerous implants are contained by the peritoneum and capacity to penetrate throughout the peritoneum is limited as the peritoneum is an excellent defence barrier (Sugarbaker, 2007). Peritoneal invasion by cancer cells and subsequent progression to macroscopic lesions follows a biological cascade of events including the shedding and transit of cells followed by colonization of the peritoneum by micro-metastases. Common sites for disease aggregation, as described above in the 'redistribution' phenomenon, include the right subphrenic space, the mesenteric border of the small bowel, the lower part of the left paracolic sulcus, the recto-vesical cul-de-sac, the greater and lesser omentum, and the ileocecal region. These regions correspond to areas of reabsorption of peritoneal fluid, areas

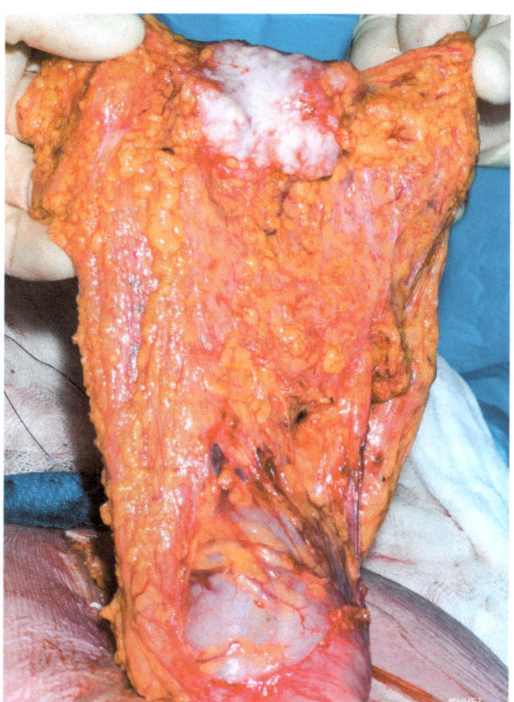

Figure 13.1 Colorectal peritoneal metastases to the greater omentum.

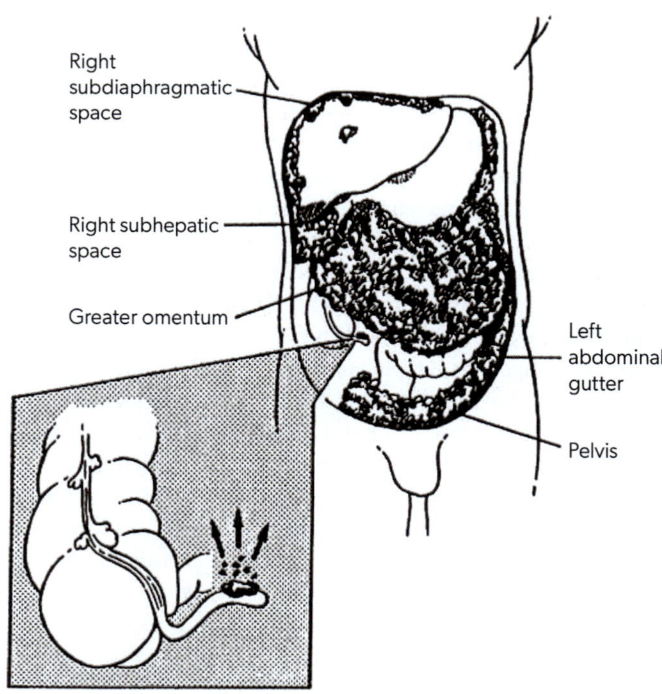

Figure 13.2 Ruptured appendiceal neoplasm highlighting the "redistribution phenomenon" (Sugarbaker, 1994).

rich in lymphoid aggregates, and dependant areas where cancer cells tend to gravitate and accumulate. Natural or iatrogenic raw surfaces within the abdomen and pelvis, for example surgical incisions, are also weak points for peritoneal defences against cancer implants. A Krukenberg tumour (metastatic spread to the ovary) is an example of adherence of cancer cells to a naturally occurring raw surface associated with the corpus haemorrhagicum. Similarly, cancer cells are entrapped in raw areas of surgical trauma, partly explaining the increased incidence of cancerous implants at anastomotic sites (Sugarbaker, 2004). The motility of an intra-abdominal organ also determines the volume of tumour deposit on its peritoneal surface. Constant peristaltic movement of the small bowel offers relative protection from tumour involvement though this may be overcome in more invasive tumours, and at adhesion sites from previous surgery, where eventual small bowel involvement can lead to luminal obstruction.

Risk assessment and diagnosis

Peritoneal metastases are synchronous at first diagnosis of colorectal cancer in approximately 7% of patients. Metachronous peritoneal metastases are detected in 10–20% of patients in the months or years after curative resection of the primary tumour. Population based studies have reported that TNM stage T4, right-sided colon tumours, obstructing tumours, particularly if managed initially by an intraluminal stent, tumour perforation, signet ring cell or mucinous histology, and poorly differentiated tumours are strong risk factors for peritoneal metastases (Hompes et al., 2012).

There is a high incidence of peritoneal metastases, ranging from 10% to 45%, in BRAF-mutant colorectal cancers and the propensity to metastasize to sites like the peritoneum, which is associated with a poor prognosis, could explain the poor survival outcomes in this subgroup of patients (Prasanna et al., 2018). Based on gene expression profiling, colorectal cancer can be categorized into four consensus molecular sub-types (CMS1–4). A profound desmoplastic reaction and a high stromal cell content is seen in CMS 4 patients. In a study on patients undergoing CRS and HIPEC for colorectal peritoneal metastases at the Netherlands Cancer Institute, Amsterdam, a reverse transcriptase-quantitative polymerase chain reaction (PCR) test was used to assess CMS4 status of fresh-frozen tissue from the primary tumour and from the peritoneal metastases. There was a significant higher level of CMS 4 positivity in this group of patients when compared to the reported CMS4 levels in unselected stage 1 to 4 colorectal cancers (Ubink et al., 2018). Therefore, it is likely that the CMS 4 sub-type of CRC also has a propensity to manifest as peritoneal metastases.

However, a validated approach to accurately select patients at high risk of peritoneal metastases for aggressive treatment strategies is currently not available. There is a need for novel biomarkers to predict peritoneal metastases in patients with colorectal cancer. Detection of tumour-derived biological material, such as tumour-derived cell-free DNA (cfDNA) shed by metastatic tumour deposits, has potential in this field. Although low levels of cfDNA are seen in the plasma of colorectal cancer patients with isolated peritoneal metastases, high levels of cfDNA are detectable in peritoneal fluid suggesting that the peritoneal fluid might be a more reliable source in predicting peritoneal metastases (van't Erve et al., 2021).

Parallel to the challenges in predicting risk of peritoneal metastases in patients with colorectal cancer, the detection of low-volume peritoneal disease, having limited soft tissue contrast resolution, is also problematic. It is virtually impossible to detect peritoneal metastases which are smaller than 3–5 mm in size by current non-invasive imaging modalities such as computed tomography (CT), positron emission tomography-CT (PET-CT), or magnetic resonance imaging (MRI). Recently, diffusion-weighted MRI (DW-MRI), has shown a marginal increase in sensitivity and specificity compared with other imaging techniques. In addition to anatomical details of the highly vascular small tumour deposits, DW-MRI can also detect intra-abdominal metastases to other intraperitoneal sites (van't Sant et al., 2019). The increasing use of diagnostic laparoscopy in colorectal surgery, and in staging patients suspected to have CPM, helps detect low-volume CPM not identified at pre-operative staging, but complete assessment of the peritoneal cavity may not be feasible, particularly after previous abdominal surgery (Moran & Cecil, 2014).

Peritoneal Cancer Index (PCI) and Completeness of Cytoreduction Scoring (CCS) system

The main determinants of outcome in the treatment of peritoneal malignancies are the extent of the disease and whether all the disease is surgically resectable, and CPM is no exception. The extent of the peritoneal disease is measured by what is called the Peritoneal Carcinoma Index (PCI) as described by Sugarbaker and Jacquet (Fig. 13.3) (Jacquet & Sugarbaker, 1996). The Completeness of Cytoreduction Score (CCS) incorporates a documentation of the size and extent of any residual disease after optimal surgery. Pre-operative assessment of whether the disease can be resected surgically, intra-operative planning of extent of surgical resection and the long term post-operative prognosis are all determined by the extent and distribution of peritoneal disease and the ability to resect disease by cytoreductive surgery. PCI is a comprehensive and widely used standard intra-operative staging system for peritoneal malignancy but it is pertinent to note that PCI was described and can only be accurately measured at laparotomy (Jacquet & Sugarbaker, 1996). PCI consolidates abdominopelvic regional assessment and anatomic site assessment as a single score which has been clinically validated and allows comparative statistical evaluation and comparison between groups. The abdomen and pelvis are divided into 13 regions, comprising nine abdominal and pelvic regions anatomically by two transverse and two sagittal planes (Fig. 13.1) and four regions specifically for the small bowel. The size of the lesion in each region is assigned a score of 0 to 3 where 0 signifies no disease, and 3 a maximum tumour mass size of > 5 cm. The PCI therefore can range from 0 to 39 (Jacquet & Sugarbaker, 1996). This intra-operative quantification of tumour is a valuable tool in estimating the probability of completeness of cytoreduction in patients with colorectal peritoneal metastases and for assessing prognosis (Bijelic et al., 2021). The higher the PCI, even if CPM is completely removable by CRS, the worse the outcome. In general, a PCI score of > 20 is associated with a five-year survival rate of < 10% and therefore should be considered a relative contraindication to CRS and HIPEC (Elias et al., 2010).

Peritoneal Cancer Index

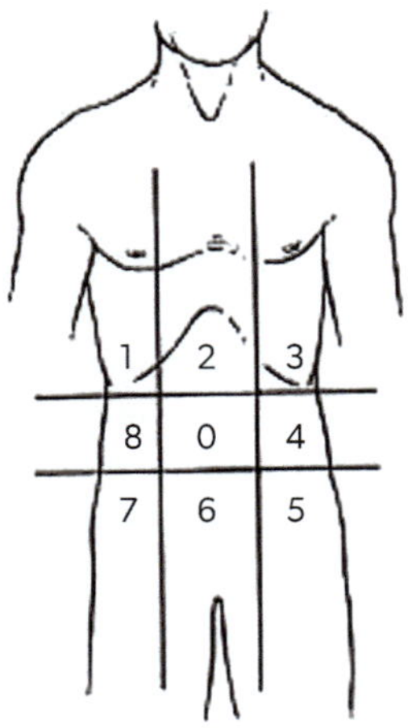

Regions	Lesion Size
0 Central	____
1 Right Upper	____
2 Epigastrium	____
3 Left Upper	____
4 Left Flank	____
5 Left Lower	____
6 Pelvis	____
7 Right Lower	____
8 Right Flank	____
9 Upper Jejunum	____
10 Lower Jejunum	____
11 Upper Ileum	____
12 Lower Ileum	____
PCI	☐

Lesion Size Score

LS 0	No tumour seen
LS 1	Tumour up to 0.5 cm
LS 2	Tumour up to 5.0 cm
LS 3	Tumour > 0.5 cm or confluence

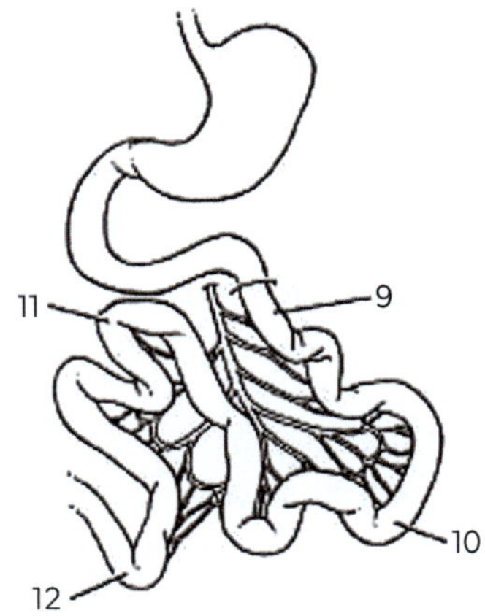

Figure 13.3 Peritoneal Cancer Index (PCI) (Sugarbaker, 2004).

The major limitation with PCI is that accurate assessment can only be performed at full exploration during a laparotomy. Alternate methods to estimate PCI such as radiological PCI using cross-sectional imaging, or laparoscopic PCI at laparoscopy, are helpful. However, radiological and laparoscopic PCI both commonly under-estimate, and therefore under-stage, the actual PCI and disease extent.

A further limitation of PCI as a selection tool for CRS is that PCI does not take into account other important factors that influence survival, such as pathology of the tumour, for example, signet ring cell or poorly differentiated tumours. A number of alternative scoring systems have been proposed but have not been widely accepted and PCI remains the most used as a validated, simple, and reliable measurement of peritoneal malignancy (Bijelic et al, 2021; Sugarbaker, 2004).

The other main prognostic indicator is the completeness of tumour removal as measured by the Completion of Cytoreduction scoring (CCS) system. Completeness of cytoreduction is measured intra-operatively by the surgeon's assessment of the extent of visible residual macroscopic disease at the end of CRS. The CC score ranges from CC0 to CC3 where CC0 denotes patients in whom there is no visible residual tumour, CC1 where there are residual tumour nodules of < 2.5 mm in diameter, CC2 residual tumour nodules between 2.5 mm and 25 mm and CC3 with residual lesions > 25 mm in diameter. Theoretically tumour nodules smaller than 2.5 mm may respond to intraperitoneal chemotherapy and, for PMP in particular, CC0 and CC1 are classified as complete cytoreduction.

Several studies have demonstrated a survival advantage in patients with a low PCI score. One of the largest reports of patients with CPM, a French multicentre retrospective study, highlighted the inverse relationship between the five-year survival rate and a higher PCI score (Elias et al., 2010). Two recent meta-analyses have shown that limited PCI and complete cytoreduction are the most important predictors of survival and recurrence in CPM (Hallam et al., 2019; Narasimhan et al., 2020).

Rationale for CRS and HIPEC

The performance status of the patient, the extent of metastatic disease, and the risk-benefit ratio of treatment form the basis for decision-making during the comprehensive management of metastatic colorectal cancer. The treatment options for these patients include systemic agents (cytotoxic, targeted, and immunotherapy) and regional therapies (Franko, 2018). Historically, peritoneal metastasis in patients with colorectal cancer was regarded as inevitably fatal and extensive involvement of the peritoneum still precludes curative surgical treatment.

When compared with colorectal metastases to other sites such as the liver or lungs, patients with CPM have a worse prognosis. A pooled analysis of two trials which examined various first-line systemic chemotherapy agents in patients with metastatic colorectal cancer showed significant shorter survival among patients with CPM compared with other sites of metastatic disease (Franko et al., 2012). Patients with CPM often present with features of declining performance status, progressive worsening gastrointestinal dysfunction, and malnutrition. Many present or progress to gastro-intestinal obstruction. Response to systemic therapies is diminished, partly due to poor performance status and inability to tolerate toxic treatments, but an additional problem is limitations in intraperitoneal concentrations of systemic therapies due to the plasma-peritoneal barrier (Mirnezami et al., 2014). Palliative and best supportive care is often the optimal option for these patients to ensure best possible quality of life (Kranenburg et al., 2021).

Cytoreductive surgery (CRS), first advocated for ovarian cancer in the 1930s, demonstrated better survival rates by more extensive surgery with a key prognostic factor being the size of tumour masses and extent of the residual disease after completion of CRS (Koppe et al., 2006). Over the next few decades the improved results of radical cytoreductive surgery in patients with ovarian cancer stimulated an interest in considering CRS for other peritoneal malignancies including CPM. In 1979, the technique of hyperthermic peritoneal perfusion was evaluated in animal studies, and soon thereafter Spratt et al. first reported CRS followed by intraperitoneal chemotherapy perfusion in a patient with PMP (Spratt et al., 1980). Until then, systemic chemotherapy alone was considered standard of care for CPM. During the 1990s, multiple cohort studies from various institutions had reported encouraging surgical resection rates and improved five-year survival, following CRS. This combined modality treatment of CPM, including CRS, and what is now termed HIPEC, has been refined and used all over the world, spearheaded by the ceaseless enthusiasm of Paul Sugarbaker, to deliver the optimal management of patients with primary peritoneal malignancy or peritoneal metastases.

An important milestone in the management of CPM was a randomized controlled trial (RCT) from the Netherlands Cancer Institute comparing CRS and HIPEC with systemic chemotherapy and palliative surgery as needed. The paper was published initially in 2003, with a significant difference in overall survival (OS) at a median follow-up of 21.6 months (22.3 months in the CRS and HIPEC arm vs 12.6 months in the standard therapy arm) (Verwaal et al., 2003). A publication on long-term follow-up in 2008 reported that patients who underwent a complete cytoreduction (CC0) with HIPEC had a five-year survival of 43% (Verwaal et al., 2008).

A multicentre cohort study on 506 patients by the French Renape group confirmed the benefits of CRS and HIPEC and the beneficial prognostic effects of a lower PCI and complete cytoreduction (Glehen et al., 2004). Criticisms of this trial were that it was from a large number of centres over a long period of time (1987–2002) with no overall denominators as to how patients were selected as the only entry criterion was that a patient with CPM had to have CRS and HIPEC. Nevertheless, excellent results were reported in subsets of selected patients.

Cytoreductive surgery

Management of CPM is complex, and treatment decisions require experienced surgical and anaesthetic teams with a multidisciplinary, multimodality approach. Advances in anaesthesia, critical care, surgical techniques, and diagnostic and interventional radiology have ensured better results in the initial management as well as the management of post-operative complications. The goal of cytoreductive surgery in patients with CPM is to remove all visible disease, if possible, and to minimize the associated morbidity and occasional post-operative deaths. Surgery generally involves peritonectomy and organ resection procedures, to achieve complete cytoreduction by removal of all macroscopic disease. An understanding of the 'redistribution' of tumour within the peritoneal cavity, as outlined above, is key in achieving this goal. The key sites are assessed and radiological, laparoscopic, and laparotomy assessment of the greater and lesser omentum, the under-surface of the diaphragm and the pelvis and paracolic gutters are key to staging and managing CPM.

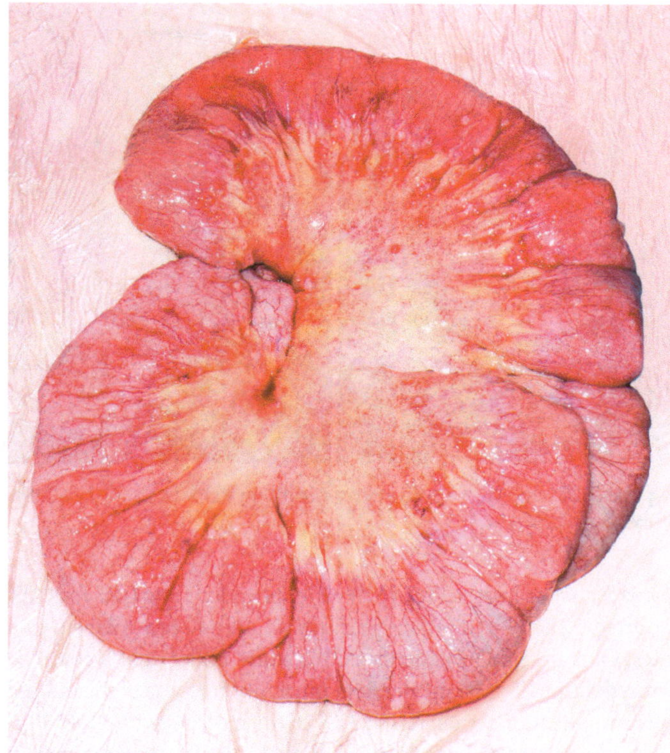

Figure 13.4 Extensive small bowel involvement in a patient with colorectal peritoneal metastases.

The principles of CRS for CPM have been developed and evolved from experience with the surgical treatment of PMP, with some fundamental differences with CPM management. First, due to the more invasive nature of CPM, small bowel and mesenteric involvement is more common compared with PMP, and colorectal cancer frequently disseminates to involve lymph nodes and other systemic metastatic sites. Secondly, metachronous CPM may develop in previously dissected tissue planes and scar tissue and adhesions may entrap cancer cells. Additionally, unlike PMP, where CC0 and CC1 are considered complete cytoreduction, in CPM a significant survival benefit is only seen in patients undergoing a CC0 cytoreduction (Elias et al., 2009). The nature of CPM means that many patients have extensive small bowel involvement (Fig. 13.4) resulting in suboptimal cytoreduction and, unlike PMP, there is little evidence to support surgical debulking with the exception of symptomatic ovarian metastases, where a palliative bilateral salpingo-oophorectomy may be necessary as ovarian metastases may grow rapidly and may not respond to systemic chemotherapy (Fig. 13.5).

Institutional experience influences outcomes with morbidity, and survival varying by case volume and experience and a significant 'learning curve' effect as with most complex interventional procedures (Glehen et al., 2010).

Outcomes of CRS and HIPEC for patients with CPM

In a highly selected group of patients with CPM, a complete cytoreduction and HIPEC was associated with five-year survival rates of 40–60% (Elias et al., 2009). A French, multicentre,

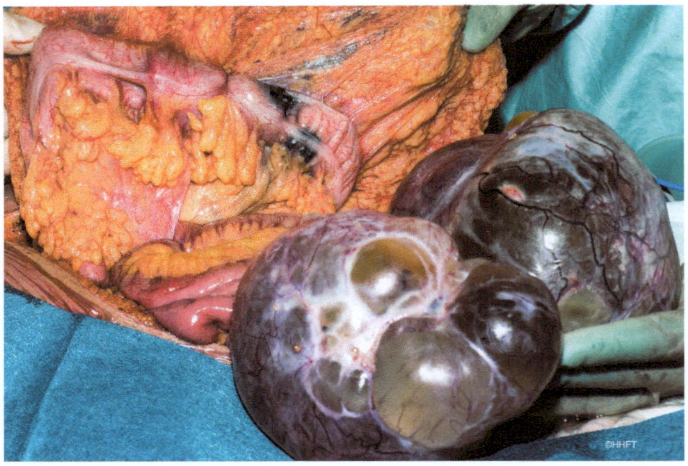

Figure 13.5 Transverse colon cancer forming a stricture with bilateral Krukenberg tumours.

retrospective cohort study of 523 patients undergoing CRS for CPM reported 27% and 10%, five-year overall and disease-free survival rates. Overall, 84% of patients in this study underwent a complete cytoreduction. The post-operative mortality rate was 3.3% and serious complications occurred in 31% of the patients with 11% of patients requiring a re-operation (Elias et al., 2010). Unfortunately, in many patients with CPM, due to either volume of disease or disease distribution, a complete cytoreduction is not achievable in an estimated 20% of patients (Moran et al., 2015). Therefore, careful selection of patients for CRS based on PCI, resectability of intra-abdominal disease, and presence of distant metastases outside the peritoneum is essential as CRS is a lengthy, high-cost procedure associated with considerable morbidity and mortality. Despite these selection criteria, approximately half the patients undergoing CRS and HIPEC experience disease progression in the first year following treatment. This increases to 70% at two years following treatment (Kranenburg et al., 2021).

In 2014, Mirnezami et al. reported on a meta-analysis of four studies (three case-control, one RCT) comparing survival following CRS and HIPEC versus chemotherapy alone for CPM. Treatment associated morbidity and mortality rates attributed to CRS and HIPEC were provided by two of the four studies. The only randomized study in this field reported a major morbidity rate of 7% and a mortality rate of 7%. A morbidity rate of 72% and a mortality rate of 0% was reported by one of the other three case control studies in the meta-analysis (Mirnezami et al., 2014). There is no doubt that the combined approach involving two aggressive loco-regional therapeutic options can lead to increased morbidity and mortality rates. Experienced surgical judgement is key to achieve a balance between postoperative risks associated with extensive surgery and potential survival benefit and quality of life in patients with CPM undergoing CRS and HIPEC.

Details of Hyperthermic Intra-Peritoneal Chemotherapy (HIPEC)

Systemic chemotherapy is a standard component of treatment for patients with advanced colorectal cancer either as an adjuvant to surgical resection or in the treatment of patients with metastatic disease. Intraperitoneal chemotherapy is a relatively new concept, designed to overcome the plasma peritoneal barrier and increases the concentration loco-regionally (Sugarbaker, 2004). This is given with the intention of treating any residual microscopic disease after the cytoreductive phase, by exposing the entire peritoneal cavity to hyperthermic chemotherapy. The most commonly used intraperitoneal chemotherapeutic agents are mitomycin C and oxaliplatin. At the end of the last century there were a number of different terminologies for heated intraperitoneal chemotherapy including HIPC, IPHC, CHIP, and HIPEC. Global agreement on the Dutch term HIPEC was suggested by Moran in 2002 and adopted by PSOGI (Peritoneal Surface Oncology Group International), such that today HIPEC (hyperthermic intraperitoneal chemotherapy) is now global terminology (Moran et al., 2006). Animal and human studies have confirmed the safety and efficacy of chemotherapy perfusion at 42–43°C. Heat enhances chemotherapeutic drug penetration into tumour nodules by passive diffusion and hyperthermia increases the cytotoxic effects of a number of chemotherapeutic agents. In addition, hyperthermia has direct anti-tumour effects. HIPEC is administered after completion of CRS and is administered by either an open, semi-open, or closed technique. There is little evidence to support the use of one technique over another and likewise ongoing debate as to the specific drug used and the dose or duration of HIPEC. There is no current standard regimen for HIPEC for CPM, though opinion has moved away from the use of oxaliplatin, and mitomycin C is now the most widely used globally.

Decision re definitive management of CPM

Diffuse low-volume peritoneal dissemination of cancer may only be detected at laparotomy, or laparoscopy, and a decision as to whether to proceed to primary tumour resection or to defer surgical excision and commence systemic chemotherapy can only be made on a case-by-case basis. Clearly, an actual or impending bowel obstruction requires resection, bypass, or a proximal stoma if feasible. It is easier to consider deferral at laparoscopy and more difficult at laparotomy where post-operative recovery is more problematic and thus commencement of treatment may be delayed.

Ideally advice should be sought from a peritoneal malignancy unit if there is a possibility that the patient is, or maybe rendered amenable to, CRS and HIPEC. Safe and effective CRS is easier if there has been minimal surgical intervention with minimal disruption of anatomical planes. Unfortunately, cancer cells within scar tissue is a concern after any laparotomy, or resection, in a patient with peritoneal malignancy and scars are relatively avascular diminishing the penetration and effectiveness of subsequent systemic chemotherapy. For this reason, an impending bowel obstruction secondary to a colorectal cancer may be best managed by proximal defunctioning, subsequent chemotherapy, further imaging and then reassessment with a view to definitive CRS and HIPEC (Moran and Cecil, 2003). Guidelines for initial management and proposed definitive treatment algorithms are outlined in Figs. 13.6 and 13.7.

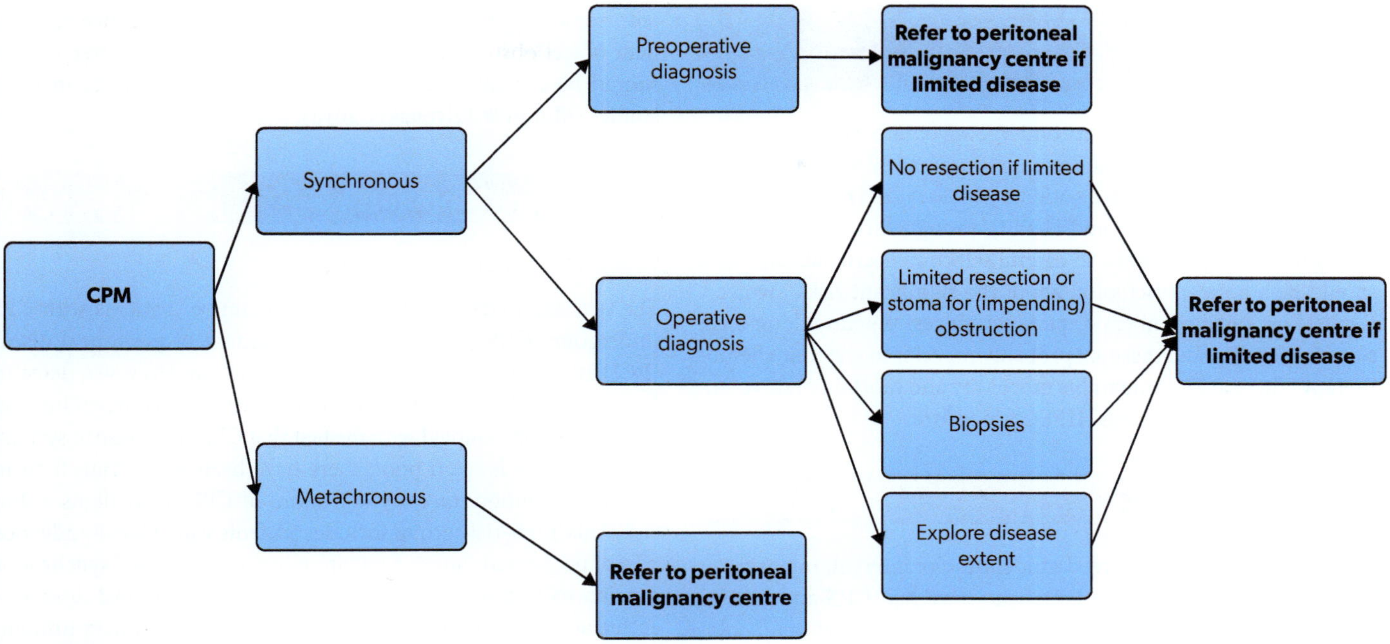

Figure 13.6 Initial management of colorectal peritoneal metastases.

How is systemic chemotherapy integrated in to the treatment pathway

The indication, timing, and efficacy of systemic chemotherapy for CPM is currently debatable. The hypothesis supporting systemic chemotherapy is that up to 50% of patients with CPM undergoing CRS and HIPEC subsequently develop extra-peritoneal metastatic disease. For patients with metachronous CPM, most have had adjuvant chemotherapy following their index operation. There is currently little evidence for the role of adjuvant systemic chemotherapy following complete resection of CPM by CRS and HIPEC and treatment decisions tend to be individualized based on prior systemic chemotherapy, extent of CPM, and both fitness and agreement by the patient.

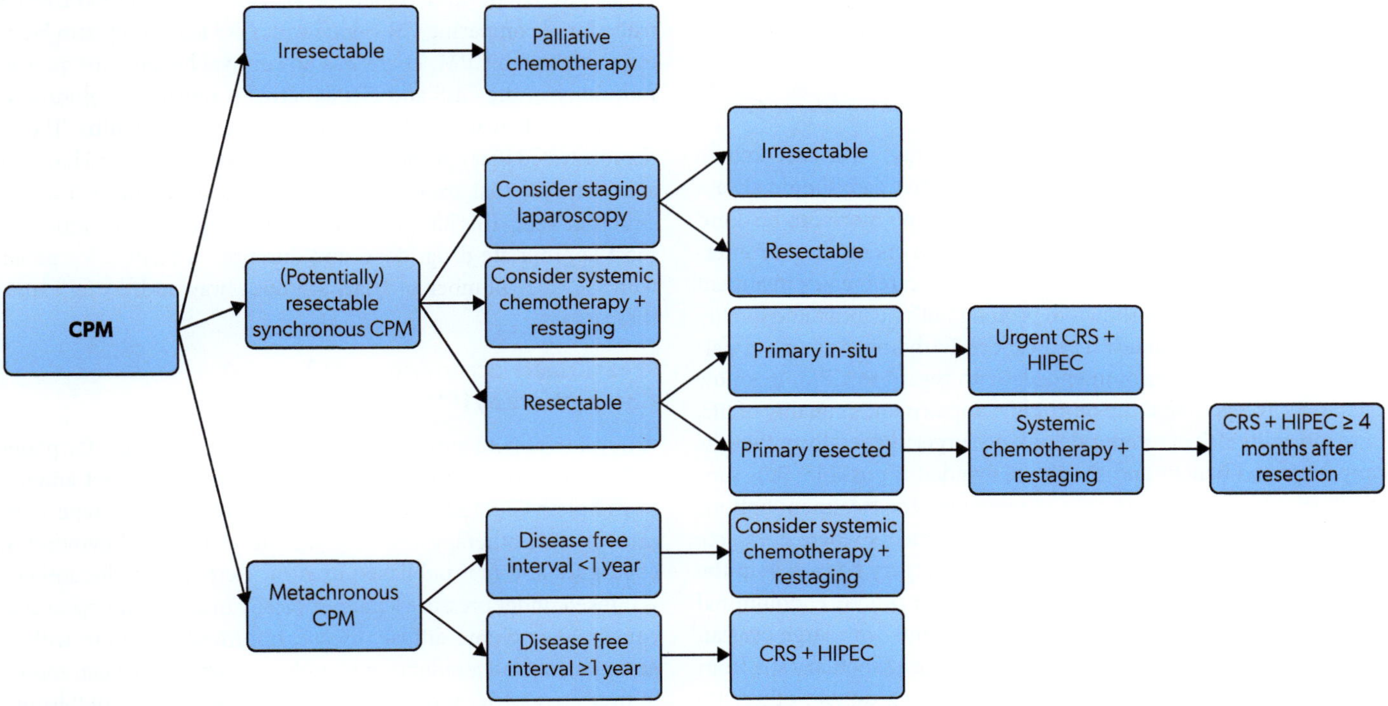

Figure 13.7 Definitive management of colorectal peritoneal metastases in peritoneal malignancy centres.

Re-operative CRS and HIPEC for recurrence after CRS and HIPEC

Approximately 70% of patients undergoing curative intent CRS and HIPEC develop recurrent disease, predominantly within the peritoneal cavity. Highly selected patients with localized recurrence may be amenable to redo CRS and HIPEC, though surgical complexity may outweigh any benefits, so careful selection is crucial, and there should be a honest discussion about the significant risks involved. Reports on small numbers of patients suggest potential long-term survival benefits, and these are probably superior to systemic chemotherapy. There are a comparable morbidity and mortality rates compared to the index CRS and HIPEC procedure.

Follow-up

Currently, there are no agreed guidelines for interval, intensity, or duration of follow-up in patients who have had CRS and HIPEC for CPM. Of course, this is a similar scenario to follow-up of colorectal cancer in general, where there is debate as to whether intensive follow-up after curative surgery for colorectal cancer improves outcomes and survival, compared with minimal follow-up or follow-up based on patient symptoms. Most units recommend surveillance with a chest abdominal and pelvic CT every six to 12 months for five years as there is a 70% risk of recurrence after CRS and HIPEC for CPM. In patients who are tumour marker secretors, then CEA, CA19-9, and CA 125 measurements may be useful in identifying recurrence and characterizing radiological abnormalities. The role of PET currently remains unclear and the main use in the context of CPM is in identifying sites of recurrent disease in patients with abnormal tumour markers and normal conventional cross-sectional imaging.

Palliative treatment and best supportive care: a key treatment modality

Most patients with advanced colorectal cancer will succumb to their disease, and palliative and best supportive care should always be part of the management. The phrase that 'no more can be done' should not be used just because surgery and chemotherapy interventions are no longer feasible, and palliative care is a key treatment modality that has been shown to prolong both quantity and quality of life in patients with advanced cancer. Early involvement of palliative care teams is recommended. With regard to CPM, it is now generally accepted that the morbidity, impairment in quality of life, and mortality risk of tumour debulking surgery generally outweighs any projected benefit and should be avoided if possible. Best supportive care and systemic chemotherapy are the treatment options that provide optimal outcomes in most patients where complete cytoreduction is not achievable. Palliative surgery has a role in the management of gastrointestinal obstruction where endoluminal stenting is not possible or fails, and in patients with large ovarian metastases as the ovarian metastases often are a sanctuary site from systemic chemotherapy, commonly progressing despite otherwise effective systemic treatment. The role of HIPEC in the context of palliative surgery is controversial but may help in the control of ascites with some suggestion that HIPEC reduces the incidence of malignant bowel obstruction. This concept of obstruction-free survival should be evaluated as an important outcome measure in future studies (Moran & Tzivanakis, 2018).

Recent developments

Prophylactic CRS and HIPEC

The two main factors determining outcome of patients with CPM undergoing CRS and HIPEC are the extent of peritoneal disease (PCI) and achieving a complete cytoreduction. However, detecting low-volume CPM is problematic and difficult with current imaging. For this reason, coupled with the fact that CPM response to systemic chemotherapy is often poor, there have been some trials focusing on the prevention, or early detection, of CPM in patients at high risk. This 'high-risk' group includes patients with a locally advanced pT4 or perforated cancer, a mucinous primary, isolated synchronous ovarian metastases, or limited synchronous peritoneal disease resected at the index operation when removing the primary tumour.

PROPHYLOCHIP (Goéré et al., 2020) focussed on assessing the role of second-look surgery compared with routine surveillance in high-risk patients with normal imaging at one year after primary colorectal cancer surgery. This trial failed to demonstrate a survival benefit with second-look CRS and HIPEC. However, the study highlighted the limitations of imaging in that over a third of patients had histological evidence of peritoneal disease despite both normal imaging and tumour markers prior to second-look surgery.

The COLOPEC trial (Klaver et al., 2019) assessed the role of adjuvant HIPEC in a similar high-risk patient group at the time of resection of the primary tumour or very early in the post-operative period. This trial also failed to demonstrate a survival benefit compared with adjuvant systemic chemotherapy alone.

The PRODIGE 7 trial (Quénet et al., 2021) was a randomized controlled trial comparing CRS alone with CRS and oxaliplatin HIPEC in patients with CPM. There was no survival benefit, but increased morbidity in the CRS and HIPEC arm. A remarkable finding was that the median survival in both groups was 42 months. The trial demonstrated that optimal CRS alone does result in good long-term survival; and that oxaliplatin HIPEC had no additional demonstrable benefit. This has prompted further consideration around the most appropriate drug, dose, and duration of HIPEC for patients with CPM. A number of trials are underway addressing some of these issues.

Pressurized Intraperitoneal Aerosol Chemotherapy (PIPAC)

A novel treatment strategy has recently been proposed for patients with diffuse low-volume peritoneal carcinomatosis, not amenable to complete CRS (Alyami et al., 2019). Pressurized intraperitoneal aerosol chemotherapy (PIPAC) was developed by Reymond and colleagues and first published in 2011. Aerosolized chemotherapy is infused under pressure laparoscopically in an attempt to treat and control low-volume diffuse disease. Improved palliation with disease control, and a reduction in ascitic volume, have been reported in ovarian, gastric, and colorectal carcinomatosis and in peritoneal mesothelioma (Grass et al., 2017). PIPAC seems relatively safe with infrequent complications, though generally previous extensive surgery interferes with safe access and diffusion around the peritoneum. Research on PIPAC is ongoing including a possible role as a neoadjuvant therapy in selected patients, aiming to reduce the volume and extent of disease in patients with borderline resectable disease.

Molecular and immune therapies

With the increasing accessibility of genomic sequencing and the evolution of personalized medicine, an array of molecular targeted therapies and immunotherapy have made their way into the armamentarium of treatment options, particularly for patients with metastatic disease. Whilst enormously exciting, the reality is that these therapies are at an embryonic stage and few patients benefit currently from this futuristic approach. It is uncertain where these therapies will fit into the management of CPM and again may have application in neoadjuvant therapy prior to CRS and HIPEC.

Conclusion

There has been significant evolution over the last three decades in the management of patients with colorectal peritoneal metastasis. From a uniformly palliative approach, CRS and HIPEC now offer improved overall survival and quality of life, with the potential of cure in a select few. Complete cytoreduction has now been firmly established as the key component in achieving best outcomes for patients with CPM. Despite advances in imaging, CPM continues to be under-staged by all modern forms of imaging and careful selection by experienced surgical teams is pivotal to maximize benefits, minimize complications, and deliver cost-effective treatments. The combination of CRS and HIPEC is a high-risk strategy with considerable operative morbidity and mortality. Despite optimal surgery and HIPEC, many patients' disease recurs, and palliative and best supportive care should always form part of the management strategy for patients with CPM. Research is ongoing in this complex and rewarding field of cancer care. Surgical decision making and technical skill is crucial and decisions are more important than incisions.

REFERENCES

Alyami, M., Hübner, M., Grass, et al. (2019). Pressurised intraperitoneal aerosol chemotherapy: rationale, evidence, and potential indications. *Lancet Oncology*, *20*(7), e368–377. https:// doi: 10.1016/ S1470-2045(19)30318-3

Ansari, N., Chandrakumaran, K., Dayal, S., et al. (2016). Cytoreductive surgery and hyperthermic intraperitoneal chemotherapy in 1000 patients with perforated appendiceal epithelial tumours. *European Journal of Surgical Oncology*, *42*(7), 1035–1041.

Bijelic, L., Ramos, I., & Goeré, D. (2021). The Landmark Series: surgical treatment of colorectal cancer peritoneal metastases. *Annals of Surgical Oncology*, *28*(8), 4140–4150.

Chua, T. C., Moran, B. J., Sugarbaker, P. H., et al. (2012). Early- and long-term outcome data of patients with pseudomyxoma peritonei from appendiceal origin treated by a strategy of cytoreductive surgery and hyperthermic intraperitoneal chemotherapy. *Journal of Clinical Oncology*, *30*(20), 2449–2456.

Elias, D., Gilly, F., Boutitie, F., et al. (2010). Peritoneal colorectal carcinomatosis treated with surgery and perioperative intraperitoneal chemotherapy: retrospective analysis of 523 patients from a multicentric French study. *Journal of Clinical Oncology*, *28*(1), 63–68.

Elias, D., Lefevre, J. H., Chevalier, J., et al. (2009). Complete cytoreductive surgery plus intraperitoneal chemohyperthermia with oxaliplatin for peritoneal carcinomatosis of colorectal origin. *Journal of Clinical Oncology*, *27*(5), 681–685.

Franko, J. (2018). Therapeutic efficacy of systemic therapy for colorectal peritoneal carcinomatosis: Surgeon's perspective. *Pleura and Peritoneum*, *3*(1), 1–9. https:// doi: 10.1515/pp-2018-0102

Franko, J., Shi, Q., Goldman, C. D., et al. (2012). Treatment of colorectal peritoneal carcinomatosis with systemic chemotherapy: A pooled analysis of North Central Cancer Treatment Group phase III trials N9741 and N9841. *Journal of Clinical Oncology*, *30*(3), 263–267.

Glehen, O., Gilly, F. N., Boutitie, et al. (2010). Toward curative treatment of peritoneal carcinomatosis from nonovarian origin by cytoreductive surgery combined with perioperative intraperitoneal chemotherapy: a multi-institutional study of 1290 patients. *Cancer*, *116*(24), 5608–5618.

Glehen, O., Kwiatkowski, F., Sugarbaker, P. H., et al. (2004). Cytoreductive surgery combined with perioperative intraperitoneal chemotherapy for the management of peritoneal carcinomatosis from colorectal cancer: a multi-institutional study. *Journal of Clinical Oncology*, *22*(16), 3284–3292.

Goéré, D., Glehen, O., Quenet, F., et al. BIG-RENAPE group, (2020). Second-look surgery plus hyperthermic intraperitoneal chemotherapy versus surveillance in patients at high risk of developing colorectal peritoneal metastases (PROPHYLOCHIP-PRODIGE 15): a randomised, phase 3 study. *Lancet Oncology*, *21*(9), 1147–1154.

Grass, F., Vuagniaux, A., Teixeira-Farinha, H., et al. (2017). Systematic review of pressurized intraperitoneal aerosol chemotherapy for the treatment of advanced peritoneal carcinomatosis. *British Journal of Surgery*, *104*(6), 669–678.

Hallam, S., Tyler, R., Price, M., et al. (2019). Meta-analysis of prognostic factors for patients with colorectal peritoneal metastasis undergoing cytoreductive surgery and heated intraperitoneal chemotherapy. *British Journal of Surgery Open*, *3*(5), 585–594.

Hompes, D., Tiek, J., Wolthuis, A., et al. (2012). HIPEC in T4a colon cancer: a defendable treatment to improve oncologic outcome? *Annals of Oncology*, *23*(12), 3123–3129.

Hugen, N., van de Velde, C., de Wilt, J., et al. (2014). Metastatic pattern in colorectal cancer is strongly influenced by histologic subtypes. *Annals of Oncology*, *25*(3), 651–657.

Jacquet, P., & Sugarbaker, P. H. (1996). 23. Clinical research methodologies in diagnosis and staging of patients with peritoneal carcinomatosis. *Cancer Treatment and Research Communications*, *82*, 359–374.

Jayne, D., Fook, S., Loi, C., et al. (2002). Peritoneal carcinomatosis form colorectal cancer. *British Journal of Surgery*, *89*(12), 1545–1550.

Klaver, C. E. L., Wisselink, D. D., Punt, C. J. A., et al. (2019). Adjuvant hyperthermic intraperitoneal chemotherapy in patients with locally advanced colon cancer (COLOPEC): a multicentre, open-label, randomised trial. *Lancet Gastroenterology & Hepatology*, *4*(10), 761–770.

Koppe, M. J., Boerman, O. C., Oyen, W. J. G., et al. (2006). Peritoneal carcinomatosis of colorectal origin: Incidence and current treatment strategies. *Annals of Surgery*, *243*(2), 212–222.

Kranenburg, O., Speeten, K., & van der, Hingh, I. de. (2021). Peritoneal metastases from colorectal cancer: defining and addressing the challenges. *Frontiers in Oncology*, *16*, 1–11. 650098.://doi: 10.3389/ fonc.2021.650098

Mirnezami, R., Mehta, A. M., Chandrakumaran, K., et al. (2014). Cytoreductive surgery in combination with hyperthermic intraperitoneal chemotherapy improves survival in patients with colorectal peritoneal metastases compared with systemic chemotherapy alone. *British Journal of Cancer, 111*(8), 1500–1508.

Moran, B., Cecil, T., Chandrakumaran, K., et al. (2015). The results of cytoreductive surgery and hyperthermic intraperitoneal chemotherapy in 1200 patients with peritoneal malignancy. *Colorectal Disease, 17*(9), 772–778.

Moran, B. J., & Cecil, T. D. (2003). The etiology, clinical presentation, and management of pseudomyxoma peritonei. *Surgical Oncology Clinics of North America, 12*(3), 585–603.

Moran, B. J., & Cecil, T. D. (2014). Treatment of surgically resectable colorectal peritoneal metastases. *British Journal of Surgery, 101*(2), 5–7.

Moran, B. J., Meade, B., & Murphy, E. (2006). Hyperthermic intraperitoneal chemotherapy and cytoreductive surgery for peritoneal carcinomatosis of colorectal origin: A novel treatment strategy with promising results in selected patients. *Colorectal Disease, 8*(7), 544–550.

Moran, B., & Tzivanakis, A. (2018). The concept of 'obstruction-free survival' as an outcome measure in advanced colorectal cancer management. *Pleura and Peritoneum, 3*(1), 20180101. https://doi.org/10.1515/pp-2018-0101

Narasimhan, V., Tan, S., Kong, et al. (2020). Prognostic factors influencing survival in patients undergoing cytoreductive surgery with hyperthermic intraperitoneal chemotherapy for isolated colorectal peritoneal metastases: a systematic review and meta-analysis. *Colorectal Disease, 22*(11), 1482–1495.

Prasanna, T., Karapetis, C. S., Roder, et al. (2018). The survival outcome of patients with metastatic colorectal cancer based on the site of metastases and the impact of molecular markers and site of primary cancer on metastatic pattern. *Acta Oncologica, 57*(11), 1438–1444.

Quénet, F., Elias, D., Roca, L., et al. (2021). Cytoreductive surgery plus hyperthermic intraperitoneal chemotherapy versus cytoreductive surgery alone for colorectal peritoneal metastases (PRODIGE 7): a multicentre, randomised, open-label, phase 3 trial. *Lancet Oncology, 22*(2), 256–266.

Spratt, J. S., Adcock, R. A., Muskovin, M., et al. (1980). Clinical delivery system for intraperitoneal hyperthermic chemotherapy. *Cancer Research, 40*(2), 256–260.

Sugarbaker, P., Zhu, B., Sese, G., et al. (1993). Peritoneal carcinomatosis form appendiceal cancer: results in 69 patients treated by cytoreductive surgery and intraperitoneal chemotherapy. *Diseases of the Colon and Rectum, 36*(4), 323–329.

Sugarbaker, P. H. (2007). Peritoneum as the first-line of defense in carcinomatosis. *Journal of Surgical Oncology, 95*(2), 93–96.

Sugarbaker, P. H. (2004). Carcinomatosis from gastrointestinal cancer. *Annals of Medicine, 36*(1), 9–22.

Sugarbaker, P. H. (1994). Pseudomyxoma peritonei. A cancer whose biology is characterized by a redistribution phenomenon. *Annals of Surgery, 219*(2), 109–111.

Sugarbaker, P. H., Gianola, F. J., Speyer, J. C., et al. (1985). Prospective, randomized trial of intravenous versus intraperitoneal 5-fluorouracil in patients with advanced primary colon or rectal cancer. *Surgery, 98*(3), 414–422.

Tseng, J., S Bryan, D., Poli, E., et al. (2017). Under representation of peritoneal metastases in published clinical trials of metastatic colorectal cancers. *Lancet Oncology, 18*(6), 711–712.

Ubink, I., van Eden, W. J., Snaebjornsson, P., et al. (2018). Histopathological and molecular classification of colorectal cancer and corresponding peritoneal metastases. *British Journal of Surgery, 105*(2), e204–e211.

van't Sant, I., van Eden, W. J., Engbersen, M. P., et al. (2019). Diffusion-weighted MRI assessment of the peritoneal cancer index before cytoreductive surgery. *British Journal of Surgery, 106*(4), 491–498.

van't Erve, I., Rovers, K. P., Constantinides, A., et al. (2021). Detection of tumor-derived cell-free DNA from colorectal cancer peritoneal metastases in plasma and peritoneal fluid. *Journal of Pathology: Clinical Research, 7*(3), 203–208.

Verwaal, V. J., Bruin, S., Boot, H., et al. (2008). 8-year follow-up of randomized trial: cytoreduction and hyperthermic intraperitoneal chemotherapy versus systemic chemotherapy in patients with peritoneal carcinomatosis of colorectal cancer. *Annals of Surgical Oncology, 15*(9), 2426–2432.

Verwaal, V. J., van Ruth, S., de Bree, et al. (2003). Randomized trial of cytoreduction and hyperthermic intraperitoneal chemotherapy versus systemic chemotherapy and palliative surgery in patients with peritoneal carcinomatosis of colorectal cancer. *Journal of Clinical Oncology, 21*(20), 3737–3743.

14

Integrating stereotactic ablative body radiotherapy into the multidisciplinary management of recurrent colorectal cancer

Rebecca Muirhead and Rebecca Johnson

Introduction to the history and development of SABR/SBRT

Stereotactic ablative body radiotherapy (SABR) or stereotactic body radiotherapy (SBRT) are interchangeable terms which define a precise form of image-guided radiotherapy in which extracranial lesions receive an ablative dose of radiotherapy, delivered in a small number of fractions (less than 10). The origins of SABR can be traced back to the early 1950s, when the pioneering fields of stereotaxy and radiotherapy were merged (Leksell, 1951). In 1967 the first Gamma Knife technique was developed, which used a cage to immobilize the head, while individual cobalt-60 sources delivered an ablative dose of radiotherapy to an intracranial target, in a technique that was termed 'radiosurgery' (Fig. 14.1). However, extracranially, there is significant motion of both the malignant lesions and the normal organs we are trying to avoid, known as organs at risk (OARs). Motion can be both between different radiotherapy fractions (interfraction) or occur during a single radiotherapy fraction (intrafraction). Examples of causes of tumour and OAR motion are respiratory and cardiac motion (intrafraction); variations in patient set-up both while on the bed (intrafraction) and day to day (interfraction); and changing position and size of organs such as the rectum and bladder over minutes (intrafraction), hours, days, and weeks (interfraction). Despite the early development of stereotaxy to cranial lesions, for many years, the technology did not exist to safely deliver ablative doses to mobile extracranial targets.

Fast forward two decades, image-guided radiotherapy (IGRT) has revolutionized radiotherapy planning and delivery. Different IGRT technologies allow us to improve our accuracy in different stages of radiotherapy, facilitating the introduction of SABR. We can quantify four-dimensional (4D) motion during planning with a 4D computed tomography (4DCT) rather than estimating it according to population-based data. We routinely incorporate diagnostic magnetic resonance imaging (MRI) and positron emission tomography (PET)/CT into the planning system to optimize our target and OAR volumes. On the treatment couch we can visualize the tumour and the adjacent OARs using cone beam CT images (CBCT), so that we can match our radiotherapy plan to the tumour rather than relying on bony surrogates. With CBCT we can assess the changes in bladder or rectal shape and position to calculate if there is any resultant change to the dose delivered. We can check or allow for respiratory motion with 4D cone beam CT (4DCBCT) or a gating technique, where radiotherapy is delivered on certain phases of the respiratory cycle to maximize coverage and minimize damage. We use abdominal compression devices to reduce respiratory motion. We have the ability to adapt the treatment on a fraction-to-fraction basis to deal with interfraction motion. The CyberKnife (Accuray Incorporated) platform has a robotic arm that uses kilovolt (kV) X-rays to track and follow target motion in order to treat the malignant lesion while it moves.

More recent technological advances include magnetic resonance image guided radiotherapy, using high field strength MR imaging with a linear accelerator, constructed within a single system (MR-LINAC). MR-LINAC systems integrate MR imaging before, during, and after radiotherapy delivery, permitting real-time visualization of both the target lesion and the surrounding normal tissue, without the exposure of additional radiation from CT imaging. The superior soft tissue differentiation of MR imaging results in improved liver tumour visualization compared with traditional CT imaging and obviates the need for multiphase CT imaging. This may further improve our accuracy and may facilitate safe treatment in more patients; indeed, the superior soft tissue imaging permits the adaptive contouring of both the target lesion and the OARs on a per fraction basis. In addition, the enhanced images achievable with MR

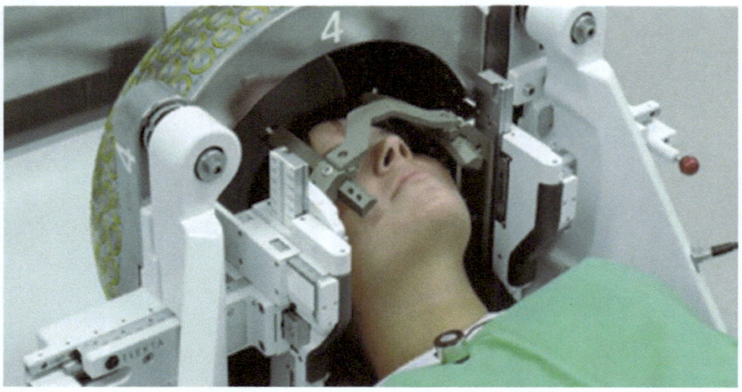

Figure 14.1 Gamma knife radiosurgery to an intracranial lesion.

scanning eliminates the need for fiducial markers which are used on some platforms to track the tumour motion.

Another exciting development is the use of protons as the radiation source. There are several potential advantages of proton-SABR which may be applicable to the targeted treatment of metastatic colorectal cancer (CRC) deposits, particularly lesions which may be deemed too close to critical structures for conventional SABR. A proton beam has different physical properties when compared with photon beams; a proton loses almost all its energy immediately before it comes to stop, which results in a Bragg peak with sharp distal fall-off. By forming a particular arrangement of beams, a spread-out Bragg peak (SOBP) can be created which results in a high, uniform dose being delivered to the target lesion, with an incredibly sharp dose fall-off and subsequent sparing of surrounding normal tissues. This characteristic may be exploited when treating lesions close to critical structures, for example central lung lesions. Proton-SABR remains very experimental but as proof of principle, a recent series report of 46 patients with stage 1 non-small cell lung cancer were treated with proton-SABR; the overall three-year survival rate was 71.8% and progression free survival was 66.9%, with a three-year local control rate of 91.5%, which is similar to photon-SABR outcomes in this patient group. The treatment was well tolerated, with no grade 4 or 5 toxicities reported; three patients experienced grade 3 dyspnoea (Bayasgalan et al., 2021).

Although the hardware and software for SABR delivery vary across centres, a number of international guidelines have been produced by American Society for Radiation Oncology (ASTRO) and American Association of Physicists in Medicine (AAPM), amongst others (Das et al., 2022), highlighting the requirements for the safe delivery of ablative doses in the body. As such, SABR is now routinely delivered for oligometastatic disease in CRC.

How does SABR vary from conventional radiotherapy?

With conventional external beam radiotherapy, the volume irradiated comprises the visible tumour, the space once occupied by the tumour in the context of adjuvant radiotherapy, or areas of potential microscopic spread such as elective lymph nodes. We then add a series of margins to account for microscopic spread, tumour motion and set up uncertainties. The planned target volume (PTV) is the final volume the physicists are provided in order to create a radiotherapy plan (Hodapp, 2012). In conventional radiotherapy the PTV tends to be large (500–1000 cm^3) and include normal tissues. To preserve the normal tissues, the dose delivered is homogenous across the whole PTV and fractionated over four to six weeks to allow for recovery of the irradiated normal tissues between fractions. The homogeneous delivery over the PTV results in the dose outside the PTV falling very slowly, so adjacent OARs receive doses close to the prescription dose.

In SABR, the volumes must be significantly smaller to be delivered safely. We achieve this through patient selection, immobilization and using our IGRT techniques before and during radiotherapy to minimize the margins required for microscopic disease, motion and set up variations. Standard SABR volumes are approximately 5–150cm^3 and they do not generally include any OARs. We deliver a peaked dose to allow the dose to rapidly fall-off outside the PTV to minimize the dose to adjacent OARs. Fig. 14.2 demonstrates a conventional plan and SABR plan to highlight these differences.

Conventional external beam radiotherapy in CRC delivers doses of approximately 40–55 Gy in equivalent 2 Gy/fraction (EQD2) with the intention to destroy as many tumour cells as possible but allow normal tissues to recover. With SABR we deliver EQD2 doses up to 160 Gy with the aim of ablating all tissue within the PTV.

The SABR pathway

Patients are referred to a SABR team, usually by the CRC team. A review of imaging may have already taken place in a specialist

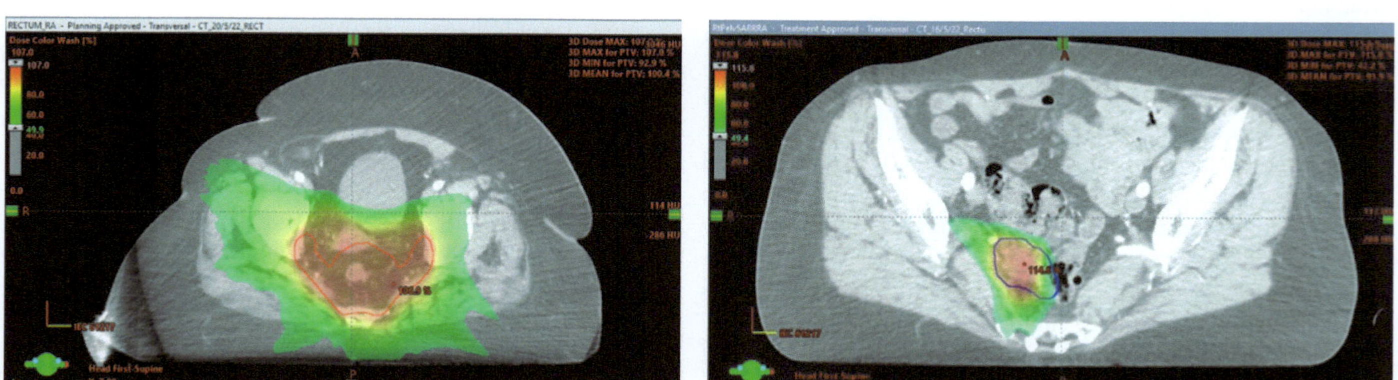

Figure 14.2 On the left a conventional radiotherapy plan, with the PTV in red and the dose wash highlighted for between 50% and 107% of the planned dose of 50 Gy in 25 fractions. On the right is a SABR plan, with the PTV in blue and the dose wash highlighted for between 50% and 115.8% of the planned dose of 50Gy in five fractions. The equivalent dose in 2 Gy/fraction is approximately 90 Gy.

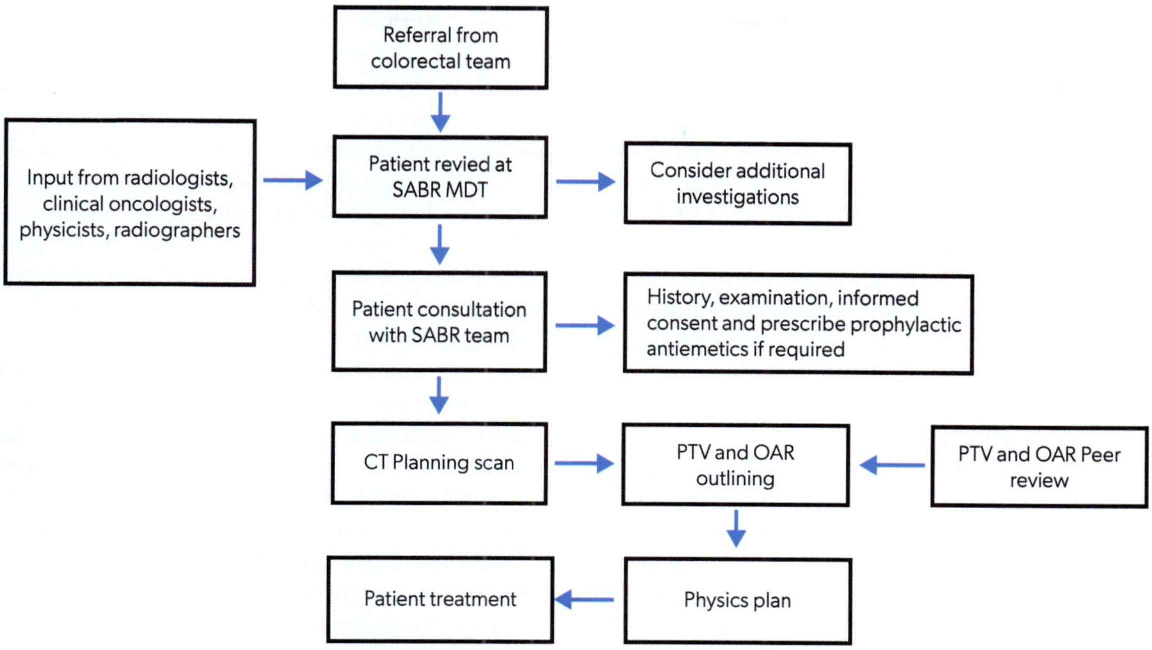

Figure 14.3 A schematic illustrating a typical patient pathway for SABR treatment.

Multidisciplinary Team (MDT) such as a Liver Metastases MDT or Lung Metastases MDT, where other treatment modalities may have been discussed such as surgery or microwave ablation. Thereafter there would ideally be further specific discussion in a SABR MDT with input from radiologists, clinical oncologists, physicists, and radiographers. At this review, consideration would be given to all technical aspects such as additional investigations required. Such examples include PET/CT to ensure no other disease, MRI to aid delineation of target or OARs, differential kidney scan for lesions close to kidney, lung function for patients with lung metastasis, or baseline cortisol for those with adrenal metastasis. Additional patient set-up requirements should be determined, for example is 4DCT, and/or abdominal compression required, intravenous (IV) or oral contrast, timing of contrast, full or empty bladder ,and enemas for rectal size and position. Following this MDT, a consultation between the patient and a member of the treating team will occur. A good comprehensive history would include details such as underlying lung, liver, or inflammatory bowel disease, identification of radiosensitizing medication, or potential for difficulties in positioning or immobilization. The SABR team will then describe the treatment, and the short- and long-term potentially serious adverse effects of the treatment. It is also an appropriate timepoint to prescribe any prophylactic medications required, such as omeprazole if the lesion is close to the oesophagus, antiemetics if irradiating the liver, analgesia to cover a pain flare, or steroids to avoid a pain flare in bony metastasis. A baseline carcinoma embryonic antigen (CEA) (or other relevant tumour marker) is a useful addition to assess response if representative. The patient will then attend for a CT planning scan, which is then used by the clinicians and radiographers to delineate the PTV and OAR volumes. There is significant evidence that peer review of volumes improves outcomes and, as such, most centres will perform peer review in some capacity (Brunskill et al., 2017). The physics team will then create a radiotherapy plan which is approved by the clinician if appropriate. The plan is then quality assured by the radiotherapy physics team before final checks. The patient then attends for usually three, five, or eight outpatient visits where they lie, immobilized on the treatment bed for 10–60 minutes. Patients are usually well during treatment and often drive themselves to and from appointments. Follow-up is centre dependant, however an assessment of toxicities and repeat tumour markers represents good practice four to eight weeks following treatment. A new baseline imaging scan three months after treatment can be used for follow-up thereafter. Fig. 14.3 illustrates the pathway.

Technical considerations

The most common sites of metastatic deposits for colorectal cancer include the liver, lung, peritoneum, and lymph nodes (van Cutsem et al., 2016), and SABR can be delivered to all these sites. In terms of whether SABR is technically possible, each case has different potential adverse effects depending on the adjacent OARs. All these toxicities can be limited by careful patient selection, accurate OAR contouring, and planning according to published dose constraints.

In the short term, SABR is very well tolerated with less than 1.5% of oligometastatic patients experiencing grade 3 and above side effects (Lehrer et al., 2021). The main toxicity experienced is fatigue, which is self-limiting. Depending on the adjacent OARs the other short-lived acute toxicities may be mild shortness of breath, cough, chest wall pain, skin redness, bowel upset, dysphagia, or pain flare for bony lesions.

In terms of more serious potential toxicity, constraints are designed to carry no more than a 5% risk of a grade 3 toxicity. In the lung, this is pneumonitis and clinically relevant chest wall pain if the lesion is adjacent to the chest wall. The constraints for normal liver usually prevent any significant radiation hepatitis, provided there is no underlying liver disease. If the lesion is adjacent to the gastrointestinal tract, particularly the oesophagus, stomach, small bowel, or duodenum, the risk is of perforation, haemorrhage, or stricture. The great vessels such as the aorta have dose constraints to prevent aneurysms. At the upper end of OAR constraints, large bowel, bladder, or vagina have approximately 5% risk of fistulas, perforation, or haemorrhage. Equally, skin lesions must stay within tolerance to avoid long-term ulceration of the skin. Irradiating cauda equina, cord, brachial plexus, or lumbosacral plexus carries a risk of irreversible myelopathy or neuropathy. In the heart, there is a theoretical risk of pericarditis and increased ischaemic heart disease, however data are based on lung cancer population with high rates of background lung disease and smoking, which is not representative of the general CRC population, therefore this is likely to be less than 3%. Following irradiation of a bone there is up to a 30% fracture risk, however, often the fracture risk due to malignancy is similar. Stabilization should be considered in patients with a high Mirel's score prior to SABR (Tatar et al., 2014).

There are few instances where SABR cannot be delivered. The main absolute contraindication is in cases where disease is infiltrating the lumen of the gastrointestinal tract, such as an anastomotic recurrence, as the ablative nature would result in a perforation. There is also significant controversy over SABR to central or ultra-central lung metastasis, defined as lesions where the PTV touches or overlaps the central bronchial tree, oesophagus, pulmonary vein, or pulmonary artery. This concern follows the publication of the HILUS study, a phase 2 study of ultra-central primary lung cancers treated with SABR which reported a 15% death rate due to broncho-pulmonary haemorrhage and fistulas (Lindberg et al., 2021). Advocates for the use of SABR would highlight that these were primary lung cancers, therefore arising and infiltrating the lumen of the bronchial tree, and the radiotherapy technique did not optimally avoid/compromise dose to the central structures. Many groups have published retrospective series of ultra-central SABR with more acceptable mortality rates. A systematic review of 10 retrospective studies of ultra-central SABR for both primary lung and metastatic lesions reported to central lung lesions; reported median mortality rates of 5% (0–22%) (Chen et al., 2019). The median grade 3 or greater toxicity rate was 10% (range 0–50%). The features that correlated with SABR-related mortality included dose to proximal bronchial tree ≥ 180 Gy, peri-SABR bevacizumab, and anti-coagulant or antiplatelet medication use. If considering SABR for central and ultra-central lesions, careful radiotherapy planning and consideration of the magnitude of benefit versus the risk of a serious adverse effect must be discussed fully with the patient.

Evidence base for SABR and how it compares to other oligometastasis directed modalities

Oncologists are constantly trying to determine which treatment choice is best for their patient. There are many facets to this, and detailed information is required to make the best decision, including patient, tumour, and disease factors, all discussed in more detail elsewhere in this book. In everyday practice, oncologists have to ask themselves 'will oligometastatic directed therapy; improve quality of life (QoL), disease free survival or overall survival for my patient?' For all three major modalities of metastasis-directed therapy (surgery, ablation, and SABR), there are multiple single and multi-centre cohort studies reporting the features that correlate with improved patient outcome. These are metachronous presentation of metastasis compared to primary; lower tumour burden in terms of size, number of sites, and number of organs involved; lung metastasis versus liver; absence of synchronous peritoneal or nodal disease; RAS/RAF wild-type disease; this being the first episode of metastasis; favourable pathology from primary resection (Hoyer et al., 2006; Margalit et al., 2019; Nicosia et al., 2020). However, these are also biological factors to select favourable tumour biology, which in turn correlates with improved outcomes. So, in essence, are we just selecting patients that would do well irrelevant of whether or not they receive oligometastatic-directed treatment, and patting ourselves on the back when they do?

The only way of knowing the true worth of an intervention is with randomized trials. SABR-COMET is one of the few trials of oligometastatic-directed therapy demonstrating improved survival that has remained positive in each subsequent publication. The SABR-COMET trial was a randomized phase 2 trial for patients with one to five sites of oligometastatic disease from a variety of different primary sites. Patients were randomized 2:1 between SABR versus standard of care and the primary endpoint was overall survival (OS). 99 patients were recruited with 18 (18%) being metastases from colorectal malignancies. The initial publication has follow-up of 25 months and reported an OS of 28 months (95% CI 19–33) in the standard of care arm versus 41 months (95% CI 26–not reached) with SABR (Palma et al., 2019). The follow-up publication had extended follow up to 51 months and confirmed the five-year OS was 17.7% (95% CI, 6–34%) and 42.3% (95% CI, 28–56%; stratified log-rank p = 0.006) with best supportive care and SABR respectively (Palma et al., 2020). Median OS was 28 months (95% CI, 18–39 months) versus 50 months (95% CI, 29–83 months; stratified log-rank test p = 0.006; HR, 0.47; 95% CI, 0.27–0.81) in the best supportive care and SABR arm respectively. The local control rate of the lesions that underwent SABR was 63% (65 of 104 assessable lesions) in the SABR arm (p = 0.039). The local control rate differed between treatment sites, adrenal 100%; bone, 72%; lung, 51%; liver, 50%. There was no difference between the patient reported outcome measures and SABR arm reported a 29% risk of grade ≥ 2 and a 5% grade 5 toxicity rate. The three patient deaths occurred due to radiation pneumonitis, pulmonary abscess, and a subdural haemorrhage after surgery to repair a SABR-related perforated gastric ulcer.

This trial has been criticized for a number of reasons. A major criticism is that the patients were not stratified by tumour type, and there were more prostate cancer patients, who by virtue of their disease have better survival rates than other tumour types, in the SABR arm (21% vs 6%). In addition, the trial was powered with a two-sided α of 0.20 and a power of 80%, acknowledging that any outcome is be likely to need to be confirmed in a phase 3 trial. However, the sensitivity analysis did not suggest that the results were because of tumour type bias. The authors state: 'Despite the reduced power after excluding patients with prostate cancer, a benefit was still demonstrated that would meet the cut-off for a randomized phase 2 screening trial.' Interestingly, the trial also highlighted that it is likely that most patients with oligometastatic disease had undetectable micrometastasis at the time of enrolment due to the similar new metastasis rate in both arms. They hypothesized that subsequent SABR is likely to have contributed to the significant survival benefit, rather than just the single SABR delivery. The hypothesis is that with a relatively small progression-free survival (PFS) difference (5.4 vs 11.6 months), the treatment received after the trial is likely to have had an effect on survival. As there was no difference in the use of systemic therapy or palliative radiotherapy following the trial intervention, it would suggest the use of repeat SABR, which occurred in 14% in the SABR arm, had a further impact on overall survival (OS). Despite the criticism, a 24% absolute improvement in five-year overall survival and 22-month improvement in median survival has provided enough evidence for SABR to be increasingly offered to appropriate patients all around the world. Further trials are planned by the same group including SABR-COMET 3 (NCT03862911) and SABR-COMET 10 (NCT03721341) which are assessing outcomes after SABR in patients with one to three, and four to – 10 metastases respectively. Importantly there is a focus on identifying predictive biomarkers, which could help determine future patient selection for SABR.

A large cohort publication including colorectal patients was prospectively performed in the United Kingdom within an NHS England commissioning through evaluation scheme (Chalkidou et al., 2021). In this scheme, 1,422 patients were recruited from 17 hospitals in England, of which 397 (27.9%) were CRC patients. In colon cancer (n = 233) the one- and two-year OS was 92.0% and 80.3% respectively, and in rectal cancer (n = 164) the one- and two-year OS was 93.7% and 77.8% respectively. The local control rate in colon cancer was 80.8% and 62.3% at one- and two-years and 83.3% and 59.3% at one- and two-years in rectal cancer. The sites with best local control were adrenal, bone, spine, and lymph nodes; those with the worse local control rates were liver. There was a 3% grade ≥ 3 toxicity and no treatment-related deaths.

Comparison with other modalities

It is unlikely that any of the targeted treatment options, be it surgical resection, microwave ablation, or SABR will be compared in head-to-head randomized control trials. There have been, however, a limited series of publications which compared treatment options for specific metastatic sites of other tumour types.

Tetta et al. published a systematic review which evaluated the outcomes of SABR and metastatectomy for the treatment of lung metastases from soft tissue sarcomas (Tetta et al., 2020). The data analysed was from 1,306 patients; 1,104 who underwent metastatectomy and 202 who were treated with SABR. The SABR group, as expected, contained an older population with a shorter disease-free interval so significant selection bias. Despite this, the cumulative mean OS was 46.7 months for the surgical group and 47.6 months for the SABR group. Additionally, the cumulative rate of patients alive with disease was 5% for the surgical group and 15% for the SABR group, which is a really great outcome. Whilst surgery is still generally considered to be the gold standard of care for lung metastases, with SABR more traditionally reserved for patients who are deemed unsuitable for surgery, the authors concluded from this systematic review that for soft tissue sarcoma metastases, SABR is a viable alternative for patients.

In order to be able to compare SABR with radiofrequency ablation (RFA), we can look at literature from hepatocellular carcinoma (HCC). There is wide variation in reported effectiveness, but long-term follow-up studies have reported a five-year survival of > 50% and a local control rate which varies between 59% and 97%, when solitary HCC lesions < 5 cm were treated with RFA (reviewed in Minami & Kudo, 2011). A recently published series has compared outcomes of RFA with SABR for HCC. Patients with unresectable, non-metastatic HCC (224 patients) underwent RFA or SABR; one- and two-year local control rates were reported as 83.6% and 80.2% for RFA, and 97.4% and 83.8% for SABR. Further analysis revealed that RFA was associated with decreased local control (HR 3.84, $p = 0.00$). There have been other meta-analyses of SABR versus ablation. For example, Wang et al. looked at 7,928 patients and reported an improved local control with SABR, particularly for lesions > 2 cm and equivalent survival (Wang et al., 2020).

With this low-level evidence, we must accept there is uncertainty about which oligometastatic directed therapy is most appropriate, and all appropriate options should be presented to the patient so an informed decision can be made. In some cases it may come down to a choice between avoiding multiple visits to hospital (in which case surgery or ablation may be better) or avoiding a general anaesthetic (in which case SABR may be preferred).

Evolving indications for SABR

Elsewhere in this book are details highlighting the heterogeneity of colorectal cancer. Particularly with targeted agents, this can result in oligoprogression, oligoresistance, or oligopersistance (Guckenberger et al., 2020). This is where the majority of the metastatic disease is controlled by a systemic agent, but one biologically unique clone progresses while the rest of the disease is stable on systemic therapy, failing to respond while the rest of the disease is responding on systemic therapy, or appears while the rest of the disease remains stable or responding on systemic therapy. SABR for oligoprogression is being investigated within trials in other tumour types such as in non-small cell lung cancer HALT (NCT03256981) and STOP-NSCLC (NCT02756793); in prostate cancer the TRAP trial (NCT03644303); and in renal cell carcinoma a phase 2 trial (NCT 02019576). A recent publication by Lee et al. have reported a cohort of 55 oligoprogressive and 36 oligopersistent colorectal patients who underwent metastasis-directed radiotherapy, 86% of which was SABR (Lee et al., 2021). The one-year local control and overall survival rates were 69% and 99% respectively. Considering that 50%, 15%, and 5% of these patients were on second-, third-, and fourth-line chemotherapy respectively, these outcomes are encouraging. Further work is required in this area.

SABR for locally recurrent rectal cancer

Locally recurrent rectal cancer (LRRC) results in significant morbidity resulting in a very poor quality of life (QoL). A minority of patients undergo exenterative surgery, which results in median OS improvements from 14–16 months without surgery, to 39–60 months with the use of surgery. The biggest predictor of median OS is the resection status (R0, R1, R2) which falls from 36 months, 27 months, to 16 months respectively (PelvEx Collaborative, 2018). Unfortunately, even in highly selected tertiary referral centres, the R0 resection rate is only 55–79.9% and the surgical complication rate is 38% (PelvEx Collaborative, 2018). More recently pelvic SABR re-irradiation has been used as an alternative to surgery. In a retrospective analysis of a series of 69 patients with 81 lesions, median PFS and OS were 12.1 months (95% CI, 10.4–17.7) and 38.7 months (95% CI, 28.9–not reached) respectively. Two-year OS was 0.77, that is 77% (95% CI, 0.66–0.89), very similar results to those reported with surgery for recurrence (Johnstone et al., 2021). A national UK audit is now underway to collect prospective data on the use of SABR in this setting with PROMS (patient-reported outcome measures) to establish a benchmark to inform clinical decisions and research in this area.

SABR in combination with immunotherapy

The term 'abscopal' effect was first coined over six decades ago, and was used to describe the effect following radiotherapy of regression of metastatic cancer at sites that were not irradiated. The basis of this phenomenon is believed to be the local radiation induced anti-tumour effect through modulation of the immune response, and the distant effects 'off-target' of immunostimulatory cytokines. Whilst a well-known and much discussed phenomenon, it has proven relatively elusive to harness, with only just over 40 cases of radiation-induced abscopal effect reported in the literature since its original definition (Abuodeh et al., 2015). The biology underpinning the abscopal effect is thought to be that cells injured through radiation release novel tumour-associated antigens. These neoantigens in turn stimulate a tumour specific immune response via antigen presenting cells, which go on to stimulate mature CD8+ T cells that can then attack cancer cells at both the irradiated and non-irradiated sites. There are preliminary data to suggest that the combination of radiotherapy and immunotherapy may enhance the abscopal effect. The combination of immunotherapy and SABR is still in its infancy, but encouragingly there have been several studies which have demonstrated that SABR in combination with PD-1/PDL-1 block results in improved clinical outcomes in metastatic cancers from different primary sites (Lieverse et al., 2020; Welsh et al., 2019). Further studies are required to define the positive predictive factors from both patient and tumour characteristics more precisely, but the emerging field of immuno-radiotherapy, in particular with SABR as the radiation treatment modality, gives much promise for future use.

SABR follow-up specifics

Following SABR, a local tissue reaction occurs, which can result in a lesion identifiable on imaging. This can often be a source of concern for any practitioners that are not well versed in SABR, as it can be interpreted as progression. However it needs to be communicated that this can be thought of as a treatment scar and it is likely that it does not contain any viable cancer cells and does not represent treatment failure. CT-PET scans can also be problematic following SABR, with lesions remaining FDG-avid for many months and years following treatment due to the ongoing necrosis of the treated lesion (Hoopes, et al. 2007). Currently relapses are diagnosed if there is convincing evidence of serial growth on cross-sectional imaging across multiple timepoints, although there is ongoing work using combinations of different imaging techniques.

Summary

There is increasing evidence that SABR is an effective treatment choice for recurrent colorectal cancer, with initial studies showing outcomes comparable to alternative treatment modalities with acceptable side effect profiles. Definitive results from phase 3 randomized control trials are awaited.

In future, we hope with combinations of molecular profiling and liquid biopsies we will be able to predict which patients stand to gain from oligometastatic-directed therapy and which management strategy is likely to offer the best outcome. We may be able to select patients with a higher burden of metastatic disease who can gain from oligometastatic-directed therapy. Until then, all suitable strategies should be presented to patients so an informed decision can be made.

REFERENCES

Bayasgalan, U., Moon, S. H., Jeong, J. H., et al. (2021). Treatment outcomes of passive scattering proton beam therapy for stage I non-small cell lung cancer. *Radiation Oncology*, *16*(1), 155. https://doi.org/10.1186/s13014-021-01855-w

Brunskill, K., Nguyen, T. K., Boldt, R. G., et al. (2017). Does peer review of radiation plans affect clinical care? A systematic review of the literature. *International Journal of Radiation Oncology, Biology, Physics*, *97*(1), 27–34. https://doi.org/10.1016/j.ijrobp.2016.09.015

Chalkidou, A., Macmillan, T., Grzeda, M. T., et al. (2021). Stereotactic ablative body radiotherapy in patients with oligometastatic cancers: a prospective, registry-based, single-arm, observational, evaluation study. *Lancet Oncology*, *22*(1), 98–106. https://doi.org/10.1016/S1470-2045(20)30537-4

Chen, H., Laba, J. M., Zayed, S., et al. (2019). Safety and effectiveness of stereotactic ablative radiotherapy for ultra-central lung lesions: a systematic review. *Journal of Thoracic Oncology*, *14*(8), 1332–1342. https:// doi.org/10.1016/j.jtho.2019.04.018

Das, I. J., Dawes, S. L., Dominello, M. M., et al. (2022). Quality and safety considerations in stereotactic radiosurgery and stereotactic body radiation therapy: An ASTRO Safety White Paper Update. *Practical Radiation Oncology*. https://doi.org/10.1016/j.prro.2022.03.001

Guckenberger, M., Lievens, Y., Bouma, A. B., et al. (2020). Characterisation and classification of oligometastatic disease: a European Society for Radiotherapy and Oncology and European Organisation for Research and Treatment of Cancer consensus recommendation. *Lancet Oncology*, *21*(1), e18–28. https://doi.org/10.1016/S1470-2045(19)30718-1

Hodapp, N. (2012). The ICRU Report 83: prescribing, recording, and reporting photon-beam intensity-modulated radiation therapy (IMRT). *Strahlentherapie und Onkologie*, *188*(1), 97–99. https://doi.org/10.1007/s00066-011-0015-x

Hoopes, D. J., Tann, M., Fletcher, J. W., et al. FDG-PET and stereotactic body radiotherapy (SBRT) for stage I non-small-cell lung cancer. *Lung Cancer*, *59*, 229—234. https:// doi:10.1016/j.lungcan.2006.12.009

Hoyer, M., Roed, H., Traberg Hansen, A., et al. (2006). Phase II study on stereotactic body radiotherapy of colorectal metastases. *Acta Oncologica*, *45*(7), 823–830. https://doi.org/10.1080/02841860600904854

Johnstone, P., Okonta, L., Aitken, K., et al. (2021). A multicentre retrospective review of SABR reirradiation in rectal cancer recurrence. *Radiotherapy and Oncology*, *162*, 1–6. https://doi.org/10.1016/j.radonc.2021.06.030

Lee, J., Koom, W. S., Byun, H. K., et al. (2021). Metastasis-directed radiotherapy for oligoprogressive or oligopersistent metastatic colorectal cancer. *Clinical Colorectal Cancer*, *21*(2), e78–86. https://doi.org/10.1016/j.clcc.2021.10.009

Lehrer, E. J., Singh, R., Wang, M., et al. (2021). Safety and survival rates associated with ablative stereotactic radiotherapy for patients with oligometastatic cancer: a systematic review and meta-analysis. *JAMA Oncology*, *7*(1), 92–106. https://doi.org/10.1001/jamaoncol.2020.6146

Leksell, L. (1951). The stereotaxic method and radiosurgery of the brain. *Acta Chirurgica Scandinavica*, *102*(4), 316–319.

Lieverse, R. I. Y., van Limbergen, E. J., Oberije, C. J. G., et al. (2020). Stereotactic ablative body radiotherapy (SABR) combined with immunotherapy (L19-IL2) versus standard of care in stage IV NSCLC patients, ImmunoSABR: a multicentre, randomised controlled open-label phase II trial. *BMC Cancer*, *20*(1), 557. https://doi.org/10.1186/s12885-020-07055-1

Lindberg, K., Grozman, V., Karlsson, K., et al. (2021). The HILUS Trial: a prospective Nordic multicenter phase 2 study of ultracentral lung tumors treated with stereotactic body radiotherapy. *Journal of Thoracic Oncology*, *16*(7), 1200–1210. https://doi.org/10.1016/j.jtho.2021.03.019

Margalit, O., Shacham-Shmueli, E., Lawrence, Y. R., et al. (2019). Lung metastasis predicts better prognosis in metastatic colorectal cancer with mutated KRAS. *Clinical Colorectal Cancer*, *18*(3), e300–307. https://doi.org/10.1016/j.clcc.2019.06.001

Minami, Y., & Kudo, M. (2011). Radiofrequency ablation of hepatocellular carcinoma: a literature review. *International Journal of Hepatology*, *2011*, 104685.

Nicosia, L., Cuccia, F., Mazzola, R., et al. (2020). Disease course of lung oligometastatic colorectal cancer treated with stereotactic body radiotherapy. *Strahlentherapie Und Onkologie*, *196*(9), 813–820. https://doi.org/10.1007/s00066-020-01627-7

Palma, D. A., Olson, R., Harrow, S., et al. (2019). Stereotactic ablative radiotherapy versus standard of care palliative treatment in patients with oligometastatic cancers (SABR-COMET): a randomised, phase 2, open-label trial. *Lancet*, *393*(10185), 2051–2058. https://doi.org/10.1016/S0140-6736(18)32487-5

Palma, D. A., Olson, R., Harrow, S., et al. (2020). Stereotactic ablative radiotherapy for the comprehensive treatment of oligometastatic cancers: long-term results of the SABR-COMET phase II randomized trial. *Journal of Clinical Oncology*, *38*(25), 2830–2838. https://doi.org/10.1200/JCO.20.00818

PelvEx Collaborative. (2018). Factors affecting outcomes following pelvic exenteration for locally recurrent rectal cancer. *British Journal of Surgery*, *105*(6), 650–657. https://doi.org/10.1002/bjs.10734

Tatar, Z., Soubrier, M., Dillies, A. F., et al. (2014). Assessment of the risk factors for impending fractures following radiotherapy for long bone metastases using CT scan-based virtual simulation: a retrospective study. *Radiation Oncology*, *9*, 227. https://doi.org/10.1186/s13014-014-0227-1

Tetta, C., Londero, F., Micali, L. R., et al. (2020). Stereotactic body radiotherapy versus metastasectomy in patients with pulmonary metastases from soft tissue sarcoma. *Clinical Oncology*, *32*(5), 303–315. https://doi.org/10.1016/j.clon.2020.01.005

van Cutsem, E., Cervantes, A., Adam, R., et al. (2016). ESMO consensus guidelines for the management of patients with metastatic colorectal cancer. *Annals of Oncology*, *27*(8), 1386–1422. https://doi.org/10.1093/annonc/mdw235

Wang, L., Ke, Q., Huang, Q., et al. (2020). Stereotactic body radiotherapy versus radiofrequency ablation for hepatocellular carcinoma: a systematic review and meta-analysis. *International Journal of Hyperthermia*, *37*(1), 1313–1321. https://doi.org/10.1080/02656736.2020.1843719

Welsh, J. W., Tang, C., de Groot, P., et al. (2019). Phase II trial of ipilimumab with stereotactic radiation therapy for metastatic disease: outcomes, toxicities, and low-dose radiation-related abscopal responses. *Cancer Immunology Research*, *7*(12), 1903–1909. https://doi.org/10.1158/2326-6066.CIR-18-0793

15

Preventive agents in colorectal cancer

Ernest Hawk and Eduardo Vilar-Sanchez

Introduction

Colorectal cancer (CRC), the third most common cause of cancer and second most common cause of cancer-related death worldwide, accounts for approximately 10% of all cancer diagnoses and 9.4% of all cancer deaths (Sung et al., 2021). In the United States, an estimated 151,030 new CRC diagnoses and 52,580 deaths were expected to occur in 2022 (Siegel et al., 2022). US deaths from the disease have slowly declined over the past 70 years due to well-established screening programmes and surgical techniques (Gupta et al., 2014) plus an early surge in the year 2000 driven by the 2001 Medicare extension of colonoscopy screening coverage (Siegel et al., 2020). However, deaths from CRC remain unacceptably high due to low levels of participation in screening programmes, particularly among medically underserved populations (Gupta et al., 2014). This calls for both better and more systematic participation in proven screening programmes as well as identification of additional, complementary strategies to reduce incidence and mortality of the disease (Wolf et al., 2018).

One such strategy is to intercept the cancer process by administering natural or synthetic preventive agents that block, reverse, or delay carcinogenesis (Katona & Weiss, 2020). This requires a detailed understanding of the molecular and tissue microenvironmental derangements that contribute to cancer formation and growth (Yarla et al., 2020). Interventions that slow these processes may be helpful at any timepoint during the transformation of normal epithelium to histologically distinct precursor adenomatous lesions and before an advanced stage is reached. The best available evidence suggests that CRC usually develops over at least a 10- to 15-year period (Dekker et al., 2019); this provides time to identify the cancer and interrupt its progression before it poses a clinical threat.

Mechanisms underlying colorectal carcinogenesis: the targets of molecular prevention

Carcinogenesis results from a chronic interplay between susceptibility genes and environmental factors that progressively transform the colorectal epithelium in a multistep, multipath, multifocal process requiring sequential or cumulative damage to multiple genes within and across cell generations (Hawk et al., 2004). The diverse breadth and scope of molecular derangements underlying carcinogenesis are daunting and are affected not only by inherent genetics resulting in susceptibilities but also by the tissue's responses to varied environmental insults over time that impinge on normal cell and tissue biology, resulting in unique neoplastic pathologies with differing responses to interventions applied in either preventive or treatment contexts (Hanahan, 2022).

Colorectal tumours have one of the highest mutational burdens and are affected by combinations of roughly 100 different somatic mutations (Kim & Bodmer, 2022; Nguyen et al., 2020). In addition to the signature mutations of the *APC*, *KRAS*, *TP53*, and *SMAD* genes, lower-frequency gene mutations and gene expression profiles have revealed disease heterogeneity: unique histopathologic features, correlation with progression, and divergent clinical outcomes (Li et al., 2021). To illustrate this point, an international consortium of experts aiming to fuel more highly targeted interventions came together to correlate aggregated, gene expression-based, transcriptomics data from multiple cohorts with patient outcomes to characterize key biological features of four consensus molecular subtypes of CRC: microsatellite instability immune (14%), canonical (37%), metabolic (13%), and mesenchymal (23%) (Guinney et al., 2015). Epigenetically, the primary modifications implicated in CRC are DNA methylation, histone modifications, long non-coding RNAs, and microRNAs (Jung et al., 2020). At the cellular or tissue level, specific derangements of key molecular processes and tissue microenvironments occur via acquired derangements in CRC ontogeny: inflammation, genome instability and mutation, avoiding immune destruction, sustaining proliferative signalling, deregulating cellular energetics and metabolism, telomere dysfunction and telomerase reactivation, resisting cell death, evading growth suppressors, tumour-promoting inflammation, inducing angiogenesis, and activating invasion and metastasis (Hanahan, 2022).

While most adenomas do not progress to cancer, 70–90% of CRC cancers arise from precancerous polyps or adenomas that develop when regulatory mechanisms for DNA repair and cell proliferation are altered (Dekker et al., 2019). These include both sporadic cancers, triggered by a DNA alteration after conception and which account for the vast majority of adenoma-producing cancers (Carethers & Jung, 2015), and heritable cancers such as familial adenomatous polyposis (FAP)—a germline mutation characterized by the early onset of hundreds to thousands of precancerous colorectal polyps (adenomatous polyps) (National Organization for Rare Disorders, 2014), with most affected individuals developing CRC far earlier compared to those in the sporadic setting. Because the intestinal epithelium is constantly being renewed, proliferation of the crypt (mucus-producing) cell to produce aberrant crypt foci (ACF) only occurs at the epithelial base (Dekker et al., 2019). Adenoma emergence coincides with inactivating mutations or deletion of the *APC* gene; any resulting adenocarcinoma sustains further inactivating mutations or deletion of *TP53*, telomere dysfunction, and DNA breakage that drives chromosomal instability and invasive/metastatic disease via *KRAS* mutations (Li et al., 2021). Investigations into the natural history of these events and their responses to cancer-preventive agents are simplified because the colorectum is readily accessible to prospective and serial observation, biopsy, and adenoma-directed interventions via endoscopy (Hawk et al., 2004). By identifying relevant biomarkers (e.g. mutation, copy number, methylation, microRNA, and proteomics) that cue tissue and cellular dysplasia, researchers improve current cancer risk prediction models to update guidance for applying preventive interventions and improving the clinical precision of treatment (Guinney et al., 2015; Hawk et al., 2004).

Advancing molecular prevention by establishing clinical effectiveness

Efficacy endpoints, objectively measurable indicators that show if a treatment works, are predetermined before a clinical trial is initiated. The strongest endpoints include improved disease-specific mortality, improved survival, reduced disease incidence, and/or lower cancer burden (Food and Drug Administration, 2018; Hawk & Levin, 2005), but demonstrating these endpoints for preventive agents, through randomized, placebo-controlled trials may require hundreds to thousands of participants over prolonged intervals (e.g. seven to 10 years). As such, they are often considered as too costly, impractical, and risky for drug developers (Kelloff et al., 2004). Fortunately, however, dozens of preclinical, epidemiological, experimental, and clinical studies now support the use of changes in adenomas (e.g. number, size, grade, timing) as a reasonably valid preliminary surrogate endpoint for CRC prevention trials (Hawk & Levin, 2005). As one example, correlations between preventive-agent effects on adenomas, cancer, and cancer-associated mortality in a large number of studies have shown that aspirin and other nonsteroidal anti-inflammatory drugs (NSAIDs) are associated with consistent reductions in disease across the entire spectrum of colorectal neoplasia (ACF, adenomas, CRC, and CRC-associated mortality) (Hawk et al., 2004). As such, colorectal adenomas have become the primary target for screening, surveillance, intervention, and reimbursement according to current national standards of clinical practice (see Table 15.1) (Peterson & Disario, 2002).

Of course, demonstration of improved disease-specific mortality remains the ultimate goal of any cancer preventive or interceptive strategy but demonstrating that objective is no longer considered to be a mandatory requirement for all agent development.

Identifying cancer preventive agents

Before a preventive agent enters the time-consuming and costly clinical trials arena, it must acquire a portfolio of investigative data derived from multiple sources: mechanistically based drug screens, preclinical efficacy tests conducted in several different animal models, toxicology assessments, and often human observational or epidemiological studies (e.g. retrospective, case-control, or cohort) if the agent has been previously used for other indications (Hawk & Levin, 2005). In the past, drug candidates frequently gained entry solely based on epidemiological data collected for agents applied for another indication, as was the case when aspirin's effectiveness against CRC first came to light from secondary data analyses of large observational studies (American Cancer Society, 1992; Kune et al., 1988). Other observational leads were identified following secondary analyses of data from randomized, controlled trials (RCTs) focused on cardiovascular endpoints. For example, data from the Women's Health Initiative suggested that the prophylactically administered oestrogen-plus-progestin compound was a potential CRC preventive agent (Rossouw et al., 2002). Nevertheless, because many agents identified with observational data provided disappointing RCT results, candidate agents are more often prioritized after a breadth of complementary lines of evidence are secured (Hawk & Levin, 2005).

Another way to identify promising cancer preventive agents is to test them using carcinogen- or genetically induced animal models of carcinogenesis wherein changes in incidence, multiplicity, or volume of ACF, adenomas, and/or CRC can be evaluated more rapidly. Findings from studies of *APC*-mutant zebrafish (Eisinger et al., 2006) and *in vitro* human colon cancer cell lines (Coffey et al., 1997) spotlighted that cyclooxygenase-2 (COX-2) expression and development of intestinal neoplasia are promoted by *APC* inactivation and epidermal growth factor receptor (EGFR) signalling. These initial data led to trials of sulindac or celecoxib (Steinbach et al., 2000) and sulindac (Giardiello et al., 1993) in the colorectum of patients with FAP and sulindac with erlotinib versus placebo in FAP patients to examine development of duodenal neoplasia (National Organization for Rare Disorders, 2014). In a recent trial of the sulindac and erlotinib combination, duodenal polyp burden was reduced by 71% (Samadder et al., 2016).

Ideally, a compelling cancer preventive target will meet the following criteria first in *in vivo* settings, and subsequently in clinical studies: (1) varying expression in neoplasia versus normal tissue; (2) functional significance, typically demonstrated by genetic manipulations or RNA-interference approaches; (3) overexpression rather than under-expression because down-modulation of a biologic signal is generally more easily achieved than replacement of an absent function; (4) pharmacologic accessibility; and (5) modulation by an interceptive agent which results in reductions in cancer incidence, burden, or mortality (Hawk & Levin, 2005). Preventive or interceptive agents designed to hit such targets, in turn, are typically identified from *in vitro* studies of compounds wherein careful experiments can elucidate relevant mechanisms of actions,

Table 15.1 Randomized, double-blind trials demonstrating significant ($p < 0.05$) preventive effects in cohorts at risk for CRC

Intervention*	Study	Cohort†	Primary Results	Conclusions
Non-steroid anti-inflammatory agents				
Aspirin, 325 mg/d for 3–4 years	Sandler et al., 2003	635 patients with history of CRC, disease free for > 5 years after curative resection, no history of FAP	Aspirin reduced mean number of large bowel adenomas	Aspirin use was associated with reduced incidence of adenomas in patients with history of CRC
Aspirin, 81 mg/d or 325 mg/d for 3 years	Baron et al., 2003	1121 patients with recent history of adenomas	Aspirin reduced risk of adenomas only with 81 mg dose	Low-dose aspirin moderately affected risk of adenomas
Aspirin, 300 mg/d for 3 years	Logan et al., 2008	945 patients with recent resection of all adenomas	Aspirin reduced risk of recurrent and advanced adenomas	Aspirin may prevent development of advanced adenomas
Aspirin, 100 mg/d as enteric-coated tablet for 2 years	Ishikawa et al., 2014	311 patients with recently resected adenomas and adenocarcinomas	Aspirin reduced incidence of adenomas or adenocarcinoma recurrence	Low-dose, enteric-coated aspirin tablets reduced colorectal tumor recurrence in an Asian population
Aspirin, 600 mg/d for 2 years	Burn et al., 2020	861 patients with Lynch syndrome	Aspirin reduced CRC incidence	Results support use of aspirin to prevent CRC in patients with Lynch syndrome
Aspirin, 100 mg/d for 8 months	Ishikawa et al., 2021	104 patients ages 16 to 70 years with history of > 100 colon adenomatous polyps but no history of colectomy	Aspirin reduced incidence of colorectal polyps of at least 5.0 mm	Low-dose aspirin suppressed polyp recurrence in patients with FAP; may provide alternative to colectomy
Celecoxib, 100 mg or 400 mg, twice daily for 6 months	Steinbach et al., 2000	77 patients ages 18 to 65 years with FAP	Celecoxib at 800 mg/d reduced the mean number of colorectal polyps compared to baseline; SAEs were similar among groups	Twice-daily 400 mg for 6 months significantly reduced number of colorectal polyps in patients with FAP
Celecoxib, 200 mg or 400 mg, twice daily for 3 years	Bertagnolli et al., 2009	2035 patients with recent resection of all sporadic colorectal adenomas	Celecoxib at each dose reduced incidence of adenomas and was associated with increased risk for cardiovascular events	Celecoxib effectively prevented colorectal adenomas, but was not recommended for routine use due to increased risk for cardiovascular events
Celecoxib, 400 mg for 3 years	Arber et al., 2006	1561 patients with prior resection of all adenomas	Celecoxib reduced detection of adenomas at year 3 by colonoscopy	Celecoxib use reduced colorectal adenomas within 3 years after polypectomy
Sulindac, 150 mg, twice daily for 9 months	Giardiello et al., 1993	22 patients with FAP, 18 with no colectomy	Sulindac reduced number and size of polyps by end of treatment	Sulindac is unlikely to replace colectomy as primary treatment for patients with FAP
Other agents				
Metformin, 250 mg/d for 1 years	Higurashi et al., 2016	151 non-diabetic patients with previously resected polyps/adenomas	Metformin lowered polyp/adenoma prevalence with no SAE	Larger, long-term trials needed to confirm results
UDCA, 8–10 mg/kg of body weight for 3 years	Alberts et al., 2005	1285 patients with recent adenoma removal	UDCA did not reduce adenoma recurrence, but did reduce adenomas with high-grade dysplasia	Because highly dysplastic lesions can progress to invasive CRC, future trials with UDCA should be considered

CRC, colorectal cancer; d, day; FAP, familial adenomatous polyposis; SAE, serious adverse event; UDCA, ursodeoxycholic acid.

*All placebo-controlled.

†Includes number randomized.

intracellular concentrations, essential co-factors, and downstream signalling implications.

Cancer preventive agents

Over the last four decades, multiple cancer preventive agents have been evaluated in RCTs focused on preventing colorectal neoplasia. These trials are most often conducted in individuals with greater than average risk for CRC. Most of the studies to date have provided null results: the agent neither significantly increased nor decreased the risk of colorectal neoplasia during the predetermined period of observation. However, several studies have reported preventive effects that illustrate the promise of this approach.

Dietary agents

Dietary components have held strong appeal over the years as preventive agents for colorectal neoplasms because diet has been thought to exert a significant influence on CRC development and because of the direct physical contact between foodstuff and the bowel mucosa In over-the-counter supplemental and often pharmacological doses, nutrients and other compounds are readily accessible as inexpensive substances widely purported to improve or prevent a number of conditions (Ashar & Rowland-Seymour, 2008). However, each person's diet uniquely comprises a complex set of food- and processing-based chemicals (e.g. nutrients, phytochemicals, preservatives, and other additives) that not only interact synergistically but also change with each meal and evolve over time. At best, attributing benefits to single nutrient components within population-based studies is highly challenging (Martínez, 2008). Early ecologic studies suggested strong associations between dietary fat intake and colorectal cancer incidence (Walker & Burkitt, 1976). Additionally, later observational studies suggested that various dietary agents might prevent cancer (Slattery, 2000; Steinmetz & Potter, 1996) and animal studies speculated that dietary changes might reduce cancer risk (Corpet & Pierre, 2003; Lamson & Brignall, 2001a; b). However, observational studies of vitamin and mineral supplements are particularly prone to participants' recall bias and difficulties in accurately measuring and assessing highly varied dietary intakes over time (Gerber, 2012). Other potential confounders include healthy behaviours common to regular supplement consumers and low vitamin levels in people with various comorbid conditions (Katona & Weiss, 2020). Despite preliminary research, clinical trials of most dietary agents, whether extracted from dietary patterns or calculated using individual supplements, have not demonstrated significant efficacy.

Antioxidants

Found in fruits, vegetables, and over-the-counter dietary supplements, antioxidants act as reactive-oxygen-species scavengers to protect cells from oxidative stress. Excess oxidation initiates and promotes carcinogenesis by inducing gene mutations, DNA damage, genome instability, cell proliferation, and inflammation (Song et al., 2015). Beta-carotene and vitamins C and E have potent antioxidative and anti-inflammatory properties; selenium alone provides no such activities but is required for anti-oxidant activity of certain enzymes (Song et al., 2015). A meta-analysis of 12 RCTs concluded that selenium, beta-carotene, and vitamins A, C, and E supplements, taken by the general population alone or in combination with other antioxidants or cancer preventive agents, do not prevent colorectal neoplasia (Papaioannou et al., 2011). The US Preventive Services Task Force (USPSTF) concurs: insignificant evidence is available to recommend single or combined nutrient supplements as cancer preventive agents (Mangione et al., 2022).

Folate

Fruits and vegetables are also good sources of folate (folic acid), which is part of the one-carbon metabolic pathway for DNA synthesis, repair, and methylation (Kim, 2016), a process which, if disrupted, can contribute to carcinogenesis (Katona & Weiss, 2020). However Kim (2016) reported that animal studies and clinical trials collectively suggest a dual modulatory effect of folic acid supplementation depending on the stage of cell transformation at the time of the intervention. Thus folic acid supplementation may prevent neoplastic initiation in the colorectum but may also promote progression of precancerous lesions that are already established: very much a double-edged sword. On the other hand, however, a large body of evidence suggests that folate deficiency predisposes normal tissues to neoplastic transformation while supplementation in the setting of baseline deficiency may suppress neoplastic initiation (Kim, 1999; Kim, 2007). Not surprisingly, conflicting results have emerged from RCTs examining folate supplementation to reduce the recurrence of colorectal adenomas (Katona & Weiss, 2020). As such, no convincing evidence exists that folic acid should be recommended as a preventive agent for CRC or adenomas in average- or high-risk populations (Liang et al., 2021).

Calcium carbonate and vitamin D

These two essential nutrients are often linked for study as vitamin D plays a key role in maintaining calcium homeostasis by increasing intestinal absorption of the mineral (Christakos et al., 2011). Early animal studies suggested that calcium and vitamin D may have antineoplastic effects in the colon (Katona & Weiss, 2020): calcium, due to its bile-acid binding capacity and direct effect on calcium-sensing receptors on colonocytes; and vitamin D, because colonocytes express vitamin D receptors and activation of these receptors inhibits proliferation and angiogenesis, induces differentiation, and promotes apoptosis in epithelial tissues. Data from RCTs have been inconsistent—possibly due to short duration of follow-up or too-low doses of calcium and vitamin D (Katona & Weiss, 2020). One RCT randomly assigned participants with recently diagnosed adenomas to receive daily vitamin D_3 (1000 IU), calcium carbonate (1200 mg), both, or placebo (a partial 2×2 factorial design) and found no reduction in the risk of recurrent colorectal adenomas over three to five years (Baron et al., 2015). A secondary analysis added data from participants who agreed to be followed for an extra cycle of surveillance colonoscopy. At a mean of 4.6 years, results still did not support association between calcium and/or vitamin D and risk of recurrent colorectal adenomas (Calderwood et al., 2019). More recently, a very large, multicentre RCT (the Vitamin D and Omega-3 Trial) provided vitamin D_3 (2000 IU) versus placebo for a median of 5.3 years and found no difference in incidence of any invasive cancer (Manson et al., 2018). Therefore, current literature does not support the routine use of calcium or vitamin D to prevent CRC or adenomas (Mangione et al., 2022).

Dietary fibre

Increased fibre intake may lead to a dilution of faecal carcinogens, reduce intestinal transit time, and increase bacterial fermentation of fibre to produce potentially anticarcinogenic short-chain fatty acids (Ma et al., 2018). Fibre supplements, either as daily wheat bran or ispaghula husk (or psyllium) have failed to reduce colorectal adenomas in high- to moderate-risk patients (Burn et al., 2011; Peleg et al., 1996). In two studies, additional dietary fibre appeared to increase recurrent adenomas in population subsets (Faivre & Bonithon-Kopp, 2022; Schatzkin et al., 2000).

Long-chain omega-3 polyunsaturated fatty acid supplements

The fish- and seafood-derived long-chain omega-3 polyunsaturated fatty acids, eicosapentaenoic acid (EPA) and docosahexaenoic acid (DHA), taken in a pharmacologic, supplemental form have become a popular, yet unproven, strategy to reduce chronic disease (Kantor et al., 2016). Antineoplastic effects proposed for EPA and DHA include anti-inflammatory, antiproliferative, apoptotic, and anti-angiogenic properties (Katona & Weiss, 2020). In the Vitamins and Minerals prospective cohort study, more than 68,000 participants aged 50–76 and without a history of CRC provided questionnaire data to estimate supplemental and dietary intake of EPA/DHA from the prior 10 years (Kantor et al., 2014). Compared to non-users, the group with estimated supplementary EPA/DHA intake of four or more days per week for at least three years was associated with a 49% lower CRC risk. However, subsequent data from two RCTs did not support those preliminary results. The first was a multicentre trial that assigned 709 participants to one of four groups: daily supplemental EPA (2 g), aspirin (300 mg), both treatments, or placebo for 12 months. After a one-year surveillance colonoscopy, neither treatment was associated with reduced colorectal adenomas (Hull, et al., 2018). In the second, the Vitamin D and Omega-3 Trial, participants received 840 mg EPA/DHA versus placebo; at a median follow-up of 5.3 years, no differences were found in the primary endpoint of invasive cancer of any type (Manson et al., 2019). More studies are underway (Table 15.2).

Metabolic agents

The agents highlighted herein first drew attention as potential antineoplastic agents in CRC prevention because of their secondary effects identified after treatment for other disorders.

Statins

Commonly prescribed for their lipid-lowering properties, statins (or 3-hydroxy-3-methylglutaryl-coenzyme A reductase inhibitors) are taken by roughly 25% of Americans aged 40 or older for cardiovascular-disease prevention (Gu et al., 2014). The drugs competitively inhibit 3-hydroxy-3-methylglutaryl-coenzyme A reductase, the rate-limiting enzyme of mevalonate pathway, disruptions in which may reduce tumour initiation, growth, or metastasis (Chan et al., 2003). Interest in examining effects of statins on CRC and related neoplasia ensued after an observational study reported that five-plus years of self-reported statin use, verified in a subgroup using available prescription records, was associated with a large reduction in CRC risk after adjustment for other known risk factors (Poynter et al., 2005). However, several meta-analyses of observational studies have shown smaller or no association, inconsistencies that could have stemmed from confounders such as healthier behaviours in statin users, hard-to-capture use of NSAIDs, or selection- or immortal-time biases (Katona & Weiss, 2020). A planned secondary analysis of the correlation between statin use and colorectal adenoma risk found that, compared with non-statin users, participants in the placebo arm who used statins *at any time* had no benefit over five years, while those who used statins for more than three years had an *increased* adenoma risk over five years (Bertagnolli et al., 2010). As the cancer preventive efficacy of statins has not yet been established, further study is warranted (Liang et al., 2021).

Metformin

A primary treatment for type 2 diabetes, the guanidine-containing agent metformin decreases insulinemia and insulin-like growth factor 1, both of which promote cellular proliferation (Liang et al., 2021) and directly activate the AMP-activated protein kinase (AMPK) pathway to inhibit colon cancer cell proliferation (Algire

Table 15.2 Ongoing prevention trials in colorectal neoplasia

Agent	Control	Population (sample size)	Primary goal	Phase	ClinicalTrials.gov identifier
Eicosapentaenoic acid	N/A	Prior screening or surveillance colonoscopy + removal of ≥ one adenoma (80)	Change from baseline in marine omega-3 polyunsaturated fatty acid composition in colorectal tissues	2	NCT04216251
Omega-3 fatty acids	N/A	Has Lynch syndrome (34)	Retention rate of participants	2	NCT03831698
Metformin and/or aspirin (100 mg/d)	Placebo	Has completely resected stage 1–3 primary CRC (160)	Change in immunochemistry expression of nuclear factor kappa-B	2	NCT03047837
Aspirin (160 mg/d)	Placebo	• Has colorectal tumor with somatic alterations in PIK3CA, PIK3R1, or PTEN (600)	Time to recurrence	3	NCT02647099
Aspirin (100 mg/d or 300 mg/d)	Placebo	• Has Lynch syndrome (852)	Number of patients with at least one adenoma seen on chromo-endoscopy 48 months after complete withdrawal of polyps and initiation of treatment	3	NCT02813824
Aspirin (100 mg/d, 300 mg/, or 600 mg/d)	Dose non-inferiority trial	Has Lynch syndrome	Determine whether the cancer preventive properties of enteric-coated aspirin are dose dependent	3	NCT02497820
Aspirin (80 mg/d)	Placebo	Has stage 2 or 3 colon cancer; may or may not have received chemotherapy (1588)	5-year overall survival	3	NCT02301286
Sulindac and eflornithine (2 × 2 factorial design)	Placebo	Previously treated for stages 0–3 colon or rectal cancer; primary resection within 1 year (1340)	Reduction in 3-year event rate of adenomas and second primary CRCs (NCT)	3	NCT01349881

CRC, colorectal cancer; d, day; N/A, not applicable; OS, overall survival; DFS, disease-free survival.
Table from Clinicaltrials.gov Access date August 19, 2022.

et al., 2010). In rodent models, metformin reduced ACF and adenoma formation (Hosono et al., 2010; Tomimoto et al., 2008), but multiple epidemiological studies that evaluated risk of CRC associated with metformin produced mixed results (Katona & Weiss, 2020). After accounting for potential cancer-modifying effects of other diabetes treatment medications, a larger meta-analysis found a more modest reduction in CRC incidence among metformin users with diabetes (Singh et al., 2013). A second meta-analysis evaluated preventive effects of the drug against colorectal adenomas and found an inverse association between metformin use and adenoma risk in patients with diabetes (Jung et al., 2017). To explore the action of metformin in patients who were not diabetic but who previously had resected colorectal adenomas or polyps, a small, multicentre RCT examined the safety and preventive effect of metformin use versus placebo. After one year, metformin use reduced the prevalence and number of metachronous colorectal adenomas or polyps (Higurashi et al., 2016). While promising, the study was intended as a precursor to phase 3 trials of metformin as a preventive agent against adenomas or polyps. Overall, some experts feel that sufficient data support metformin use in patients with diabetes and high risk for CRC (Liang et al., 2021). However, others feel that more definitive clinical trial results are warranted in all populations (i.e. those with diabetes, those without diabetes, and those at average or high risk for CRC) prior to making such a recommendation (Katona & Weiss, 2020).

Non-steroidal anti-inflammatory drugs and selective COX-2 inhibitors

Among the agents currently being investigated for the prevention of CRC, the volume, variety, and consistency of supportive data on NSAIDs are the most compelling (Hawk et al., 2004). The NSAID aspirin (acetylsalicylic acid) irreversibly inhibits cyclooxygenase-1 (COX-1) and COX-2 to suppress inflammation and several CRC-related pathways including prostaglandin synthesis, platelet activation, and Wnt signalling to β-catenin (Drew et al., 2016). Other non-aspirin NSAIDs like sulindac, ibuprofen, and naproxen inhibit COX-1 and COX-2, but the inhibition is competitive (Mohammed et al., 2018). COXIBs like celecoxib selectively inhibit COX-2 and may reduce the gastrointestinal bleeding associated with non-selective NSAIDs (Gu & Li, 2020; Ross et al., 2017). COX-2 appears to be a likely target against neoplasia as it is commonly over-expressed in precancers and cancers and has been shown to be pathologically relevant in multiple models (Liu et al., 2017). As one example, its over-expression has been associated with poorer survival among patients with colorectal cancer (Chan et al., 2009).

Aspirin

Aspirin use has substantial data to support its CRC preventive effects including extended follow-up from RCTs (Drew et al., 2016). Interest in the agent stemmed from a 1988 case-control study that showed fewer cases of CRC in people who were taking aspirin-containing medications for other indications (Kune et al., 1988). Animal studies that followed found that aspirin reduced the development of tumours that were chemically induced or genetically engineered (Katona & Weiss, 2020), while dozens of observational studies of aspirin with CRC prevention as an endpoint showed that aspirin use over a duration of at least five years and at a variety of doses and follow-up times was associated with decreased risk for CRC (Katona & Weiss, 2020). Secondary analyses of trials examining cardiovascular disease as the primary endpoint have provided much of the RCT data about aspirin. Two large trials of the drug, the Woman's Health Study (low dose, alternate days), and the Physicians' Health Study (standard dose, alternate days), showed no effect on risk of CRC during 10- and 12-year follow-up, respectively (Cook et al., 2005; Stürmer et al., 1998). However, data from longer (10-year) follow-up of the Woman's Health Study (Cook et al., 2013) found a statistically significant 20% reduction in CRC incidence following aspirin use that reinforced the findings from observational studies. Rothwell et al. (2010) performed long-term follow-up of three large trials of daily low-dose aspirin and pooled those data with other long-term follow-up data from two trials of high-dose aspirin to determine that taking at least 75 mg of daily aspirin for several years reduced long-term incidence and mortality due to CRC. These results were supported by two meta-analyses (Algra & Rothwell, 2012; Chubak et al., 2016). Conversely, and quite by surprise, the ASPREE trial recently reported an *increased* risk of CRC with low-dose aspirin use in older healthy individuals aged 65 years or older (McNeil et al., 2018).

Randomized placebo-controlled trials aimed at reducing colonic adenomas in large populations have also demonstrated significant (15–30%) reductions in recurrent adenomas in most trials that employed aspirin. The Aspirin Folate Polyp Prevention Study found that daily aspirin doses of 81 mg (but not 325 mg) decreased risk of adenomas including advanced adenomas (Baron et al., 2003) while the APACC (Association pour la Prevention par l'Aspirine du Cancer Colorectal) study found that daily soluble aspirin in individuals with prior colonic adenomas decreased the risk of having three-plus adenomas, or one of ≥ 5 mm, after one year (Benamouzig et al., 2003); after four years, that risk decrease was not maintained (Benamouzig et al., 2012). Results from the Colorectal Adenoma Prevention Study showed that early-stage CRC survivors randomly assigned to receive 325 mg/day of aspirin (versus placebo) had fewer adenomas and developed the first adenoma at a later time (Sandler et al., 2003). In both the UKCAP and J-CAPP (Japan Colorectal Aspirin Polyps Prevention) trials, patients with endoscopically removed colonic adenomas had a reduced risk of developing colonic adenomas following daily intake of aspirin for two or three years (Ishikawa et al., 2014; Logan et al., 2008).

The use of aspirin to prevent CRC has also been studied in high-risk groups including persons with either FAP or Lynch syndrome (Al-Sukhni et al., 2008), the most common type of hereditary CRC, and whose patients are at high risk for multiple-site tumours (Sinicrope, 2018). The CAPP1 (Colorectal Adenoma/Carcinoma Prevention Programme) study found that aspirin *did not* decrease polyp number in FAP patients, but after one or more years of use *did* decrease the largest polyp size (Burn et al., 2011). Another randomized trial found that daily low-dose aspirin (100 mg) safely suppressed recurrence of polyps ≥ 5 mm in patients with FAP (Ishikawa et al., 2021). With regard to Lynch syndrome carriers, a 10 year follow-up of a randomized placebo-controlled trial of daily aspirin (600 mg) with CRC as the primary endpoint (the CAPP2 study) found that taking aspirin for two years resulted in a significant reduction in CRC incidence (HR 0.65 [95% CI 0.43–0.97; $p = 0.035$]) that persisted for more than 10 years but did not become evident until roughly five years after initiation (Burn et al., 2020). To corroborate the CAPP2 results, the Colon Cancer Family Registry also found reduced risk in patients with Lynch syndrome following aspirin use

(Ait Ouakrim et al., 2015). Indeed, three associations comprising gastroenterology experts recommend that individuals with the syndrome should be advised of the benefit of taking daily aspirin, at an undermined dose, to reduce risk (Monahan et al., 2020; National Comprehensive Cancer Network, 2022; Sammour et al., 2015). The primary drawback of prolonged and continuous use of aspirin is the concern about its associated increased risk for gastrointestinal bleeding (Dehmer et al., 2022). To extend the data for aspirin use in persons with Lynch syndrome, the CAPP3 trial investigates whether cancer preventive properties of aspirin are dose sensitive, in order to define optimal dosing further (NCT02497820, Table 15.2).

Overall, studies of aspirin have demonstrated its effectiveness as a CRC preventive agent that provides a modest reduction in adenoma and CRC risk and the agent appears to be closest to clinical application. Currently, the USPSTF recommends that adults aged 40 to 59 years who have a 10% or greater 10-year risk for cardiovascular disease should each decide whether or not to start low-dose aspirin use for the primary prevention of CRC (Davidson et al., 2022). As well, the recommendation notes that those not at increased risk for bleeding who are willing to take daily low-dose aspirin are most likely to benefit. Clarification about the optimal dose and duration of use is still warranted.

Non-aspirin NSAIDs: sulindac and celecoxib

The evidence for use of sulindac or celecoxib is somewhat less compelling not due to the absence of efficacy but to the occurrence of serious cardiovascular events with prolonged use of non-aspirin NSAIDs and COXIBs. In patients with FAP, sulindac significantly reduced colorectal polyp number and diameter and decreased formation of ACF; in patients post-polypectomy, it decreased risk for future colonic adenomas (Cruz-Correa et al., 2002; Giardiello et al., 1993; Takayama et al., 2011). However, long-term use of sulindac confers a high risk of gastrointestinal bleeding, most likely related to COX-1 inhibition, that limits its clinical use in these patients (Ishikawa et al., 1997).

To retain efficacy while reducing GI bleeding risks, high-dose celecoxib, which selectively inhibits COX-2, was administered to patients with FAP, and it effectively decreased colorectal polyp formation by 31% after six months (Steinbach et al., 2000). In two other trials, the Prevention of Colorectal Sporadic Adenomatous Polyps trial and the Adenoma Prevention with Celecoxib (APC) trial, the drug reduced adenoma detection after three and five years (Arber et al., 2006; Bertagnolli et al., 2009). Unfortunately, use of celecoxib in the APC trial was also associated with a two- to threefold increase in serious cardiovascular events (Solomon et al., 2005). A review by the USPSTF concluded that while non-aspirin NSAIDs reduced the risk of colonic adenomas and CRC, the associated increased risk for cardiovascular events and gastrointestinal bleeding disallowed their use (Rostom et al., 2007). As such, these agents have not been widely accepted as CRC preventive agents except in high-risk populations, such as those with FAP (Katona & Weiss, 2020).

Other agents

Other promising CRC preventive agents which have not yet been as extensively studied include eflornithine (the oral form of difluoromethylornithine or DFMO), EGFR inhibitors, and ursodeoxycholic acid (ursodiol).

Eflornithine

Eflornithine inhibits ornithine decarboxylase to block the synthesis of polyamines, ubiquitous in almost all biological systems (Basuroy & Gerner, 2006). When small doses of eflornithine were administered in combination with sulindac, individuals with previously resected colorectal adenomas had dramatic 70%, 91.5%, and 94.5% reductions in adenoma recurrence, advanced adenomas, and multiple adenomas, respectively (Meyskens et al., 2008). As a result, a confirmatory phase 3 trial of the combination regimen sponsored by the NCI is ongoing (Table 15.2).

Erlotinib

The EGFR inhibitor, erlotinib, which can promote COX-2 expression and therefore also the subsequent development of neoplasia, may sensitize precancerous cells to the effects of COX-2 inhibitors by the upregulation of COX-2. As such, researchers administered erlotinib with sulindac, versus placebo, to evaluate the drugs' combined effect on duodenal neoplasia in patients with FAP after six months. Duodenal polyp burden was significantly reduced (71%) and colorectal adenoma count was significantly reduced (69%) compared to baseline in patients who received the drug combination (Samadder et al., 2016; Samadder et al., 2018). However, due to the high rate of grade 1 and 2 adverse events, dose modifications led to a range of prescribed doses. As such, lower doses applied for longer durations were recommended for future study.

Ursodeoxycholic acid (Ursodiol)

Ursodeoxycholic acid is a tertiary bile acid that prevents colon carcinogenesis in preclinical models and inhibits cell proliferation and signal transduction pathways (Im & Martinez, 2004). However it did not reduce overall recurrence of colorectal adenomas in patients with recent colorectal adenoma resection. On a more positive note, it did significantly reduce (by 39%) recurrent adenomas with high-grade dysplasia which may be a more important clinical indication (Alberts et al., 2005). These and other preventive agents are reviewed more fully elsewhere (Chapelle et al., 2020; Hawk et al., 2004; Laukaitis & Gerner, 2011; Liang et al., 2021; Pabla et al., 2015; Zhang et al., 2021).

Immunoprevention in colorectal cancer

Vaccines and other immune-based approaches (e.g. immune checkpoint inhibitors (ICIs), cytokine modulators) represent a highly promising strategy to prevent CRC. The identification of tumour-associated antigens (TAAs) in various premalignant lesions, including colorectal adenomas, has contributed to new vaccination approaches that hold several potential advantages over drug-based preventive methods: safety, ease of delivery, long-term memory of the immune system, and their ability to be combined with other preventive approaches (Umar, 2014). The tremendous efficacy and public health impact of vaccines that prevent virally induced cancers *without* significant toxicity (e.g. for cervical cancer due to chronic human papillomavirus (HPV) infection; for liver cancer due to hepatitis B infection) illustrates the potential for vaccines in the non-viral setting. In this section, we describe both the rationale underlying the use of immunoprevention in CRC as well as specific clinical trials, completed and ongoing, to test preventive vaccines.

Rationale supporting immunoprevention in CRC

The use of immune-interception strategies in CRC is supported by numerous lines of evidence. First, recent studies demonstrate that immunosurveillance (the immune system's search for foreign pathogens) serves as a barrier to CRC progression when ongoing throughout the adenoma–carcinoma sequence (Galon et al., 2006; Mclean et al., 2011). Galon et al. showed that the type, density, and location of tumour-infiltrating lymphocytes in colorectal tumours predicted recurrence and survival better than, and independent of TNM (tumour, nodes, and metastases) staging (Galon et al., 2006). This work eventually led to the clinical development of an immune-based assay that measures CRC tumour infiltration by T lymphocytes, demonstrating that the immune system's role in predicting medium- and late-stage carcinogenesis is as important as are histopathologic characteristics (Bruni et al., 2020). Later, McLean et al. examined the adaptive immune response in 65 colonic adenomas and 35 adjacent normal mucosal biopsies to demonstrate that macrophages, neutrophils, helper T cells, activated T cells, and natural killers were significantly increased in adenomas compared to normal mucosa, and that macrophages and neutrophils increased significantly as the adenomas progressed from low- to high-grade dysplasia and then to invasive cancer (Mclean et al., 2011). Infiltration of macrophages, neutrophils, and activated T cells also significantly correlated with adenoma size. Additional work has shown that adaptive immunity genes are highly expressed in adenomas from patients with hereditary CRC (Chang et al., 2018). TAAs and specific T-cell responses to these antigens have also been found in adenomas. MUC1, a well-known tumour antigen aberrantly expressed in CRCs and adenomas (Finn, 2008), is a current target of preventive vaccine approaches for sporadic CRC (Kimura et al., 2013). Together, these data suggest the presence of an active anti-tumour immune response in early colorectal neoplasia that can be leveraged to prevent the development of frank malignancy.

Second, indirect evidence supporting immunoprevention is provided by research investigating the 15% of CRCs that are secondary to an inherited mutation (e.g. Lynch syndrome) or are highly responsive to immune checkpoint blockade due to an acquired deficiency in the mismatch repair (MMR) system. MMR deficiency (dMMR) leads to the accumulation of hundreds to thousands of somatic mutations in microsatellite regions of the genome, and consequently, to the generation of thousands of frameshift peptides, created by the insertion or deletion of nucleotide bases in numbers that are not multiples of 3. These peptides serve as mutated TAAs (or *neoantigens*) capable of triggering a potent anti-tumour immune response. In a small phase 2 study, Le et al. tested the activity of pembrolizumab, an anti-PD-1 antibody, in 41 patients with metastatic cancer, 32 of whom (78%) had CRC (Le et al., 2015). Results demonstrated that dMMR status predicted response. Moreover, patients with dMMR CRC showed an immune-related *objective-response* rate and immune-related progression-free survival rate of 40% (four of 10 patients) and 78% (seven out of nine patients), respectively; the corresponding rates for the 18 patients with MMR-proficient tumours were 0% and 11%, respectively. A subsequent study expanded these results across 12 tumour types and confirmed that dMMR status is a predictive factor of solid-tumour response to PD-1 blockade (Le et al., 2017). This work, along with clinical observations that the efficacy of ICIs was restricted to certain tumour types, eventually led to the identification of tumour mutational burden (i.e. mutational rate) as an important predictor of response to this immunotherapy (Samstein et al., 2019; Yarchoan et al., 2017). It also led to the FDA's approval of pembrolizumab for its first tissue/site-agnostic indication: unresectable or metastatic dMMR cancers that progressed after treatment. More recently, another anti-PD-1 inhibitor, dostarlimab, has proved to be highly efficacious in the first-line treatment of patients diagnosed with dMMR, locally advanced, rectal cancers. All 12 patients who received the full course of treatment had a complete response, sparing them from receiving treatment with radiation or subsequent aggressive surgeries (Cercek et al., 2022). The successes of ICIs in treating advanced and locally advanced dMMR cancers highlights the ability of immune modulation to significantly impact tumour development and patient outcomes and suggests the possibility of using these agents at an earlier point in the disease process to prevent cancer development. While the use of ICIs is associated with important side effects mainly due to autoimmunity, their use in a preventive setting may be justified in high-risk populations, such as those carrying inherited mutations leading to dMMR cancers (e.g. Lynch syndrome). However, the benefit ratio of this approach is controversial and remains to be tested.

Finally, increasing evidence suggests that many cancer preventive agents that demonstrate efficacy in CRC prevention trials are mediated by mechanisms that enhance immunosurveillance and/or reverse immune-escape mechanisms operating in premalignant lesions. More specifically, these mechanisms include enhancing the immunologic activity of antigen presenting cells (APCs), stimulating the adaptive immune response, and inhibiting the function of immune-suppressor cells such as regulatory T cells and myeloid derived suppressor cells (MDSCs) (Fletcher et al., 2018; Marzbani et al., 2013). NSAIDs appear to have multiple immune-modulatory effects on immature dendritic cells and MDSCs through inhibition of prostaglandin E2 (PGE_2). PGE_2 is over-expressed in colorectal adenomas (Pugh & Thomas, 1994) and can alter the balance of the immune milieu to favor a T helper cell (Th2) response, which contributes to tumour growth rather than regression and facilitates the differentiation of monocytes into immunosuppressive MDSCs (Wang et al., 2021). By inhibiting PGE_2, NSAIDs both ensure a protective Th1 (helper cell) response in the lesion and keep immunosuppression at bay.

Most recently, a phase 1b trial in 80 patients with Lynch syndrome, a genetic syndrome predisposing to the development of dMMR CRC, demonstrated that the NSAID naproxen was able to activate different types of immune cells within the normal colorectal mucosa (Reyes-Uribe et al., 2021). Metformin, another promising CRC preventive agent, enhanced the generation of memory T cells through modulation of fatty acid metabolism and promotion of CD8 + T cell survival in mice (Pearce et al., 2009). Other preclinical studies suggest that metformin may increase expression of MHC I in transformed cells, increasing their immunogenicity (Oliveras-Ferraros et al., 2012). Preclinical data support other agents' ability to modulate the adaptive immune response: bexarotene may increase the lifespan of T cells and inhibit their apoptosis; curcumin may attenuate tumour-induced suppression of cell-mediated immune responses through a variety of mechanisms (Bhattacharyya et al., 2010).

Immunopreventive clinical trials

Vaccination is perhaps the most promising immunoprevention strategy given its long, established track record of safety. Vaccines are currently being developed for both sporadic and hereditary forms of CRC.

The first phase 2 clinical trial of a CRC-preventive vaccine examined the effectiveness of a MUC1-poly-ICLC vaccine that immunizes against the TAA MUC1 expressed by colorectal epithelial cells. The trial aimed to prevent polyp recurrence and progression of advanced adenomatous polyps in 46 individuals with previous advanced colorectal adenomas (NCT00773097) by demonstrating immunogenicity with the presence of anti-MUC1 antibodies (Kimura et al., 2013). The vaccine elicited an immune response against MUC1 with no associated toxicity in 17 of 39 (44%) vaccinated participants. Those not responsive to the vaccine had high levels of circulating myeloid-derived suppressor cells, known to contribute to an immunosuppressive environment, prior to vaccination. Implications were twofold. First, the TAA-based vaccine was immunogenic and safe in the setting of CRC prophylaxis; and second, either the optimal time for vaccination might be earlier in the carcinogenic process (before immunosuppression has occurred) or the vaccine should be given to non-immunosuppressed individuals. The vaccine was also tested in a second phase 2 trial of 102 individuals with newly diagnosed, advanced colon polyps (NCT02134925). Results confirmed the immunogenicity of the vaccine and demonstrated its ability to elicit long-term memory following a booster dose at one year (Finn et al., 2019). Follow-up colonoscopies to determine the effect of the vaccine on polyp recurrence rates are ongoing.

Regarding hereditary CRC, significant research has occurred in vaccine development for patients with Lynch syndrome, the heritable form of dMMR cancers. Lynch syndrome affects an estimated 1 million Americans who are at high risk for a range of malignancies (Win et al., 2017), particularly colorectal and endometrial (Sinicrope, 2018). Studying this population provides a tremendous opportunity for vaccine development by identifying recurrent frameshift neoantigens that can be incorporated into a vaccine to stimulate the immune system. Lessons learned from developing this vaccine may facilitate its development for the sporadic CRC population, which comprises most CRC cases.

Kloor et al. reported the *first in-human* clinical trial of a vaccine that combined three recurrent mutated neoantigens (derived from mutant versions of *AIM2*, *HT001*, and *TAF1B* genes) frequently shared by inherited and sporadic dMMR colorectal and endometrial cancers (Kloor et al., 2020). This phase 1/2a trial assessed immunogenicity and safety of the vaccine in 22 participants (59% with a confirmed Lynch syndrome germline mutation) with current or past dMMR CRC. All patients who received three cycles of this peptide vaccine in combination with a polymeric adjuvant developed both humoral and cellular immunity with no serious adverse advents, supporting the general feasibility of a neoantigen-based vaccine in patients with dMMR CRC, particularly those with Lynch syndrome.

A second neoantigen vaccine for the dMMR setting selected 209 shared and recurrent mutated neoantigens and leveraged sophisticated, bioinformatic, cloning-based approaches to harness genomic and transcriptomic data from a total of 320 dMMR colorectal, endometrial, and gastric tumours (most, arising in a sporadic context) from the Cancer Genome Atlas database (Leoni et al., 2020). These frameshift peptides were cloned into non-human, great ape adenoviral- and modified vaccinia Ankara vectors to create an off-the-shelf vaccine, Nous-209. Preclinical work using this strategy of vaccine design and development in the context of prevention has demonstrated complete prevention of tumour development using a murine CRC cell line xenografted into immune-competent mice (D'alise et al., 2019). Nous-209 has already been tested in a first-in-human clinical trial for treatment of patients with stage 4 dMMR tumours in combination with the checkpoint inhibitor pembrolizumab (NCT04041310). Preliminary communications have indicated that this vaccine is safe and immunogenic (Fakih et al., 2022). A phase 1b/2 clinical trial is evaluating its safety and immunogenicity in 45 Lynch syndrome patients (NCT05078866) who will be given two doses and monitored for up to 12 months for adverse events. The vaccine represents a novel preventive approach for patients with Lynch syndrome—a high-risk population urgently in need of such interventions.

In addition to vaccines, immune modulators, including ICIs and cytokine blockers, offer an alternative and potentially complementary approach to immunoprevention. As discussed earlier, the success of ICIs in advanced cancers with a high-mutational burden, whether driven by dMMR or another mechanism, suggests their promise in preventive settings with ongoing immunosurveillance. Once more, the Lynch syndrome population represents an ideal cohort in which to test ICIs as these patients have elevated risks for multiple malignancies and may more readily accept the toxicity risks associated with use of immunotherapy. Two trials have tested PD-1 antibodies in patients with Lynch syndrome. The first, a phase 2 trial was designed to see if nivolumab could prevent polyps in those with a history of partial colectomy (NCT03631641): This was abandoned due to unknown reasons after the first three patients were enrolled. The second, a phase 3 trial in China, aims to see if toripalimab can prevent polyps and second primaries in 260 patients (NCT04711434).

Cytokines are also being investigated as potential targets for immunoprevention. Preclinical work in mice suggests that antibodies that block the inhibitory cytokines IL-6, IL-17, IL-23, or IL-22 could be effective in reducing CRC hyperplasia and tumour burden. To date, cytokine modulators have not been tested in clinical trials of either sporadic or hereditary CRC, however results are forthcoming for a phase 1b trial that evaluated the safety and efficacy of a 12-week regimen of guselkumab, an IL-23 inhibitor, in 72 adults with FAP who had undergone colectomy (NCT03649971).

The combination of vaccines and immune modulators may be a particularly effective method of immunoprevention as each agent targets different components of the immune system making synergistic effects possible. This strategy is currently being tested in a phase 2b trial examining a trivalent adenoviral vaccine that targets the CEA, MUC1, and Brachyury TAAs along with an IL-15 agonist in 158 patients with Lynch syndrome (NCT05419011). Additionally, combining different classes of agents, such as a traditional cancer preventive agent with an immuno-preventive vaccine, may be particularly potent for cancer prevention. As an example, preclinical work in a Lynch syndrome mouse model found that the combination of peptide vaccination combined with daily naproxen delayed tumour growth and prolonged survival more effectively compared to the vaccine alone (Gebert et al., 2021).

Conclusions and future directions

Multiple arms of research have examined promising cancer preventive agents over the last four decades. Among single chemical agents, aspirin and other NSAIDs have the most evidence to support future clinical use in preventing CRC. Combining these with other promising agents like eflornithine have demonstrated benefits of synergistic activity. Yet to be determined, however, are the optimal dose and duration of use for each agent to minimise toxicities.

The future of immunoprevention to reduce the burden of CRC is extremely promising. Many of these agents are recent entries into clinical investigations; most work to date has been done in the setting of hereditary CRC. Moving forward, it will be critical to investigate more deeply the use of the MUC1 vaccine in the largest population of CRC patients, those with sporadic pMMR CRC, and to identify potential novel TAAs that can be targeted with vaccines. Given their associated toxicities, the use of immune-modulatory drugs may be less appealing to the sporadic-CRC population, but are an attractive option to prevent hereditary CRC. The drugs should be thoroughly tested in high-risk cohorts with Lynch syndrome as the next step in their development. Combining vaccines with these agents, or with traditional cancer preventive agents, are compelling strategies requiring further clinical testing.

REFERENCES

Ait Ouakrim, D., Dashti, S. G., Chau, R., et al. (2015). Per publication: JNCI J Natl Cancer Inst (2015) 107(9): djv170. *Journal of the National Cancer Institute, 107*(9).

Al-Sukhni, W., Aronson, M., & Gallinger, S. (2008). Hereditary colorectal cancer syndromes: familial adenomatous polyposis and Lynch syndrome. *Surgical Clinics of North America, 88*(4), 819–844, vii.

Alberts, D. S., Martínez, M. E., Hess, L. M., et al. (2005). Phase III trial of ursodeoxycholic acid to prevent colorectal adenoma recurrence. *Journal of the National Cancer Institute, 97*(11), 846–853.

Algire, C., Amrein, L., Zakikhani, M., Panasci, L., et al. (2010). Metformin blocks the stimulative effect of a high-energy diet on colon carcinoma growth in vivo and is associated with reduced expression of fatty acid synthase. *Endocrine-Related Cancer, 17*(2), 351–360.

Algra, A. M., & Rothwell, P. M. (2012). Effects of regular aspirin on long-term cancer incidence and metastasis: a systematic comparison of evidence from observational studies versus randomised trials. *Lancet Oncology, 13*(5), 518–527.

American Cancer Society (1992). Cancer Prevention Study II. The American Cancer Society Prospective Study. *Metropolitan Insurance Company, Statistical Bulletin, 73*(4), 21–29.

Arber, N., Eagle, C. J., Spicak, J., et al. (2006). Celecoxib for the prevention of colorectal adenomatous polyps. *New England Journal of Medicine, 355*(9), 885–895.

Ashar, B. H., & Rowland-Seymour, A. (2008). Advising patients who use dietary supplements. *American Journal of Medicine, 121*(2), 91–97.

Baron, J. A., Barry, E. L., Mott, L. A., et al. (2015). A trial of calcium and vitamin D for the prevention of colorectal adenomas. *New England Journal of Medicine, 373*(16), 1519–1530.

Baron, J. A., Cole, B. F., Sandler, R. S., et al. (2003). A randomized trial of aspirin to prevent colorectal adenomas. *New England Journal of Medicine, 348*(10), 891–899.

Basuroy, U. K., & Gerner, E. W. (2006). Emerging concepts in targeting the polyamine metabolic pathway in epithelial cancer chemoprevention and chemotherapy. *Journal of Biochemistry, 139*(1), 27–33.

Benamouzig, R., Deyra, J., Martin, A., et al. (2003). Daily soluble aspirin and prevention of colorectal adenoma recurrence: one-year results of the APACC trial. *Gastroenterology, 125*(2), 328–336.

Benamouzig, R., Uzzan, B., Deyra, J., et al. (2012). Prevention by daily soluble aspirin of colorectal adenoma recurrence: 4-year results of the APACC randomised trial. *Gut, 61*(2), 255–261.

Bertagnolli, M. M., Eagle, C. J., Zauber, A. G., et al. (2009). Five-year efficacy and safety analysis of the Adenoma Prevention with Celecoxib Trial. *Cancer Prevention Research, 2*(4), 310–321.

Bertagnolli, M. M., Hsu, M., Hawk, E. T., et al. (2010). Statin use and colorectal adenoma risk: results from the adenoma prevention with celecoxib trial. *Cancer Prevention Research, 3*(5), 588–596.

Bhattacharyya, S., Md Sakib Hossain, D., Mohanty, S., et al. (2010). Curcumin reverses T cell-mediated adaptive immune dysfunctions in tumor-bearing hosts. *Cellular & Molecular Immunology, 7*(4), 306–315.

Bruni, D., Angell, H. K., & Galon, J. (2020). The immune contexture and Immunoscore in cancer prognosis and therapeutic efficacy. *Nature Reviews Cancer, 20*(11), 662–680.

Burn, J., Bishop, D. T., Chapman, P. D., et al. (2011). A randomized placebo-controlled prevention trial of aspirin and/or resistant starch in young people with familial adenomatous polyposis. *Cancer Prevention Research, 4*(5), 655–665.

Burn, J., Sheth, H., Elliott, F., et al. (2020). Cancer prevention with aspirin in hereditary colorectal cancer (Lynch syndrome), 10-year follow-up and registry-based 20-year data in the CAPP2 study: a double-blind, randomised, placebo-controlled trial. *Lancet, 395*(10240), 1855–1863.

Calderwood, A. H., Baron, J. A., Mott, L. A., et al. (2019). No Evidence for Posttreatment Effects of Vitamin D and Calcium Supplementation on Risk of Colorectal Adenomas in a Randomized Trial. *Cancer Prevention Research, 12*(5), 295–304.

Carethers, J. M., & Jung, B. H. (2015). Genetics and Genetic Biomarkers in Sporadic Colorectal Cancer. *Gastroenterology, 149*(5), 1177–1190.e3.

Cercek, A., Lumish, M., Sinopoli, J., et al. (2022). PD-1 Blockade in Mismatch Repair-Deficient, Locally Advanced Rectal Cancer. *New England Journal of Medicine, 386*(25), 2363–2376.

Chan, A. T., Ogino, S., & Fuchs, C. S. (2009). Aspirin use and survival after diagnosis of colorectal cancer. *JAMA, 302*(6), 649–658.

Chan, K. K., Oza, A. M., & Siu, L. L. (2003). The statins as anticancer agents. *Clinical Cancer Research, 9*(1), 10–19.

Chang, K., Taggart, M. W., Reyes-Uribe, L., et al. (2018). Immune profiling of premalignant lesions in patients with Lynch syndrome. *JAMA Oncology, 4*(8), 1085–1092.

Chapelle, N., Martel, M., Toes-Zoutendijk, E., et al. (2020). Recent advances in clinical practice: colorectal cancer chemoprevention in the average-risk population. *Gut, 69*(12), 2244–2255.

Christakos, S., Dhawan, P., Porta, A., et al. (2011). Vitamin D and intestinal calcium absorption. *Molecular and Cellular Endocrinology, 347*(1-2), 25–29.

Chubak, J., Whitlock, E. P., Williams, S. B., et al. (2016). Aspirin for the prevention of cancer incidence and mortality: systematic evidence reviews for the U.S. Preventive Services Task Force. *Annals of Internal Medicine, 164*(12), 814–825.

Coffey, R. J., Hawkey, C. J., Damstrup, L., et al. (1997). Epidermal growth factor receptor activation induces nuclear targeting of cyclooxygenase-2, basolateral release of prostaglandins, and mitogenesis in polarizing colon cancer cells. *Proceedings of the National Academy of Sciences of the USA, 94*(2), 657–662.

Cook, N. R., Lee, I. M., Gaziano, J. M., et al. (2005). Low-dose aspirin in the primary prevention of cancer: the Women's Health Study: a randomized controlled trial. *JAMA, 294*(1), 47–55.

Cook, N. R., Lee, I. M., Zhang, S. M., et al. (2013). Alternate-day, low-dose aspirin and cancer risk: long-term observational follow-up of a randomized trial. *Annals of Internal Medicine, 159*(2), 77–85.

Corpet, D. E., & Pierre, F. (2003). Point: From animal models to prevention of colon cancer. Systematic review of chemoprevention in min mice and choice of the model system. *Cancer Epidemiology, Biomarkers & Prevention*, *12*(5), 391–400.

Cruz-Correa, M., Hylind, L. M., Romans, K. E., et al. (2002). Long-term treatment with sulindac in familial adenomatous polyposis: a prospective cohort study. *Gastroenterology*, *122*(3), 641–645.

D'Alise, A. M., Leoni, G., Cotugno, G., et al. (2019). Adenoviral vaccine targeting multiple neoantigens as strategy to eradicate large tumors combined with checkpoint blockade. *Nature Communications*, *10*(1), 2688.

Davidson, K. W., Barry, M. J., Mangione, C. M., et al. (2022). Aspirin use to prevent cardiovascular disease: US preventive services task force recommendation statement. *JAMA*, *327*(16), 1577–1584.

Dehmer, S. P., O'Keefe, L. R., Evans, C. V., et al. (2022). Aspirin use to prevent cardiovascular disease and colorectal cancer: updated modeling study for the US preventive services task force. *JAMA*, *327*(16), 1598–1607.

Dekker, E., Tanis, P. J., Vleugels, J. L. A., et al. (2019). Colorectal cancer. *Lancet*, *394*(10207), 1467–1480.

Drew, D. A., Cao, Y., & Chan, A. T. (2016). Aspirin and colorectal cancer: the promise of precision chemoprevention. *Nature Reviews Cancer*, *16*(3), 173–186.

Eisinger, A. L., Nadauld, L. D., Shelton, D. N., et al. (2006). The adenomatous polyposis coli tumor suppressor gene regulates expression of cyclooxygenase-2 by a mechanism that involves retinoic acid. *Journal of Biological Chemistry*, *281*(29), 20474–20482.

Faivre, J., & Bonithon-Kopp, C. (2002). Effect of fibre and calcium supplementation on adenoma recurrence and growth. *IARC Science Publications*, *156*, 457–461.

Fakih, M., Le, D. T., Pedersen, K. S., et al. (2022). First clinical and immunogenicity results including all subjects enrolled in a phase I study of Nous-209, an off-the-shelf immunotherapy, with pembrolizumab, for the treatment of tumors with a deficiency in mismatch repair/microsatellite instability (dMMR/MSI). *Journal of Clinical Oncology*, *40*(16_suppl), 2515–2515.

Finn, O. J. (2008). Cancer immunology. *New England Journal of Medicine*, *358*(25), 2704–2715.

Finn, O. J., Boardman, L., Cruz-Correa, M., et al. (2019). Randomized, double-blind, placebo-controlled trial of preventative MUC1 vaccine in patients with newly diagnosed advanced adenomas: Results from one-year booster. *Cancer Research*, *29*(9), 1678–1688.

Fletcher, R., Wang, Y. J., Schoen, R. E., et al. (2018). Colorectal cancer prevention: Immune modulation taking the stage. *Biochimia et Biophysica Acta Cancer*, *1869*(2), 138–148.

Food and Drug Administration (2018). *Clinical trial endpoints for the approval of cancer drugs and biologics guidance for industry*. U.S. Department of Health and Human Services.

Galon, J., Costes, A., Sanchez-Cabo, F., et al. (2006). Type, density, and location of immune cells within human colorectal tumors predict clinical outcome. *Science*, *313*(5795), 1960–1964.

Gebert, J., Gelincik, O., Oezcan-Wahlbrink, M., et al. (2021). Recurrent frameshift neoantigen vaccine elicits protective immunity with reduced tumor burden and improved overall survival in a Lynch syndrome mouse model. *Gastroenterology*, *161*(4), 1288–1302 e13.

Gerber, M. (2012). Omega-3 fatty acids and cancers: a systematic update review of epidemiological studies. *British Journal of Nutrition*, *107*(Suppl 2), S228–239.

Giardiello, F. M., Hamilton, S. R., Krush, A. J., et al. (1993). Treatment of colonic and rectal adenomas with sulindac in familial adenomatous polyposis. *New England Journal of Medicine*, *328*(18), 1313–1316.

Gu, K. J., & Li, G. (2020). An Overview of Cancer Prevention: Chemoprevention and Immunoprevention. *Journal of Cancer Prevention*, *25*(3), 127–135.

Gu, Q., Paulose-Ram, R., Burt, V. L., & Kit, B. K. (2014). Prescription cholesterol-lowering medication use in adults aged 40 and over: United States, 2003-2012. *NCHS Data Brief*, *177*), 1–8.

Guinney, J., Dienstmann, R., Wang, X., et al. (2015). The consensus molecular subtypes of colorectal cancer. *Nature Medicine*, *21*(11), 1350–1356.

Gupta, S., Sussman, D. A., Doubeni, C. A., et al. (2014). Challenges and possible solutions to colorectal cancer screening for the underserved. *Journal of the National Cancer Institute*, *106*(4), dju032.

Hanahan, D. (2022). Hallmarks of Cancer: New Dimensions. *Cancer Discovery*, *12*(1), 31–46.

Hawk, E. T., & Levin, B. (2005). Colorectal cancer prevention. *Journal of Clinical Oncology*, *23*(2), 378–391.

Hawk, E. T., Umar, A., & Viner, J. L. (2004). Colorectal cancer chemoprevention--an overview of the science. *Gastroenterology*, *126*(5), 1423–1447.

Higurashi, T., Hosono, K., Takahashi, H., et al. (2016). Metformin for chemoprevention of metachronous colorectal adenoma or polyps in post-polypectomy patients without diabetes: a multicentre double-blind, placebo-controlled, randomised phase 3 trial. *Lancet Oncology*, *17*(4), 475–483.

Hosono, K., Endo, H., Takahashi, H., et al. (2010). Metformin suppresses azoxymethane-induced colorectal aberrant crypt foci by activating AMP-activated protein kinase. *Molecular Carcinogenesis*, *49*(7), 662–671.

Hull, M. A., Sprange, K., Hepburn, T., et al. (2018). Eicosapentaenoic acid and aspirin, alone and in combination, for the prevention of colorectal adenomas (seAFOod Polyp Prevention trial): a multicentre, randomised, double-blind, placebo-controlled, 2 × 2 factorial trial. *Lancet*, *392*(10164), 2583–2594.

Im, E., & Martinez, J. D. (2004). Ursodeoxycholic acid (UDCA) can inhibit deoxycholic acid (DCA)-induced apoptosis via modulation of EGFR/Raf-1/ERK signaling in human colon cancer cells. *Journal of Nutrition*, *134*(2), 483–486.

Ishikawa, H., Akedo, I., Suzuki, T., et al. (1997). Adverse effects of sulindac used for prevention of colorectal cancer. *Journal of the National Cancer Institute*, *89*(18), 1381.

Ishikawa, H., Mutoh, M., Sato, Y., et al. (2021). Chemoprevention with low-dose aspirin, mesalazine, or both in patients with familial adenomatous polyposis without previous colectomy (J-FAPP Study IV): a multicentre, double-blind, randomised, two-by-two factorial design trial. *Lancet Gastroenterology & Hepatology*, *6*(6), 474–481.

Ishikawa, H., Mutoh, M., Suzuki, S., et al. (2014). The preventive effects of low-dose enteric-coated aspirin tablets on the development of colorectal tumours in Asian patients: a randomised trial. *Gut*, *63*(11), 1755–1759.

Jung, G., Hernández-Illán, E., Moreira, L., et al. (2020). Epigenetics of colorectal cancer: biomarker and therapeutic potential. *Nature Reviews Gastroenterology & Hepatology*, *17*(2), 111–130.

Jung, Y. S., Park, C. H., Eun, C. S., et al. (2017). Metformin use and the risk of colorectal adenoma: a systematic review and meta-analysis. *Journal of Gastroenterology and Hepatology*, *32*(5), 957–965.

Kantor, E. D., Lampe, J. W., Peters, U., et al. (2014). Long-chain omega-3 polyunsaturated fatty acid intake and risk of colorectal cancer. *Nutrition and Cancer*, *66*(4), 716–727.

Kantor, E. D., Rehm, C. D., Du, M., et al. (2016). Trends in dietary supplement use among US adults from 1999–2012. *JAMA*, *316*(14), 1464–1474.

Katona, B. W., & Weiss, J. M. (2020). Chemoprevention of colorectal cancer. *Gastroenterology*, *158*(2), 368–388.

Kelloff, G. J., Schilsky, R. L., Alberts, D. S., et al. (2004). Colorectal adenomas: a prototype for the use of surrogate end points in the development of cancer prevention drugs. *Clinical Cancer Research*, *10*(11), 3908–3918.

Kim, J. C., & Bodmer, W. F. (2022). Genomic landscape of colorectal carcinogenesis. *Journal of Cancer Research and Clinical Oncology*, *148*(3), 533–545.

Kim, Y. I. (1999). Folate and carcinogenesis: evidence, mechanisms, and implications. *Journal of Nutritional Biochemistry*, *10*(2), 66–88.

Kim, Y. I. (2007). Folate and colorectal cancer: an evidence-based critical review. *Molecular Nutrition & Food Research*, *51*(3), 267–292.

Kim, Y. I. (2016). Current status of folic acid supplementation on colorectal cancer prevention. *Current Pharmacology Reports*, *2*(1), 21–33.

Kimura, T., McKolanis, J. R., Dzubinski, L. A., et al. (2013). MUC1 vaccine for individuals with advanced adenoma of the colon: a cancer immunoprevention feasibility study. *Cancer Prevention Research*, *6*(1), 18–26.

Kloor, M., Reuschenbach, M., Pauligk, C., et al. (2020). A frameshift peptide neoantigen-based vaccine for mismatch repair-deficient cancers: a phase I/IIa clinical trial. *Clinical Cancer Research*, *26*(17), 4503–4510.

Kune, G. A., Kune, S., & Watson, L. F. (1988). Colorectal cancer risk, chronic illnesses, operations, and medications: case control results from the Melbourne Colorectal Cancer Study. *Cancer Research*, *48*(15), 4399–4404.

Lamson, D. W., & Brignall, M. S. (2001a). Natural agents in the prevention of cancer, part two: preclinical data and chemoprevention for common cancers. *Alternative Medicine Review*, *6*(2), 167–187.

Lamson, D. W., & Brignall, M. S. (2001b). Natural agents in the prevention of cancer. Part 1: human chemoprevention trials. *Alternative Medicine Review*, *6*(1), 7–19.

Laukaitis, C. M., & Gerner, E. W. (2011). DFMO: targeted risk reduction therapy for colorectal neoplasia. *Best Practice & Research Clinical Gastroenterology*, *25*(4-5), 495–506.

Le, D. T., Durham, J. N., Smith, K. N., et al. (2017). Mismatch repair deficiency predicts response of solid tumors to PD-1 blockade. *Science*, *357*(6349), 409–413.

Le, D. T., Uram, J. N., Wang, H., et al. (2015). PD-1 Blockade in Tumors with Mismatch-Repair Deficiency. *New England Journal of Medicine*, *372*(26), 2509–2520.

Leoni, G., D'Alise, A. M., Cotugno, G., et al. (2020). A Genetic Vaccine Encoding Shared Cancer Neoantigens to Treat Tumors with Microsatellite Instability. *Cancer Research*, *80*(18), 3972–3982.

Li, J., Ma, X., Chakravarti, D., Shalapour, S., et al. (2021). Genetic and biological hallmarks of colorectal cancer. *Genes & Development*, *35*(11-12), 787–820.

Liang, P. S., Shaukat, A., & Crockett, S. D. (2021). AGA clinical practice update on chemoprevention for colorectal neoplasia: expert review. *Clinical Gastroenterology and Hepatology*, *19*(7), 1327–1336.

Liu, Y., Sun, H., Hu, M., et al. (2017). The role of cyclooxygenase-2 in colorectal carcinogenesis. *Clinical Colorectal Cancer*, *16*(3), 165–172.

Logan, R. F., Grainge, M. J., Shepherd, V. C., et al. (2008). Aspirin and folic acid for the prevention of recurrent colorectal adenomas. *Gastroenterology*, *134*(1), 29–38.

Ma, Y., Hu, M., Zhou, L., et al. (2018). Dietary fiber intake and risks of proximal and distal colon cancers: A meta-analysis. *Medicine*, *97*(36), e11678.

Mangione, C. M., Barry, M. J., Nicholson, W. K., et al. (2022). Vitamin, mineral, and multivitamin supplementation to prevent cardiovascular disease and cancer: US Preventive Services Task Force Recommendation Statement. *JAMA*, *327*(23), 2326–2333.

Manson, J. E., Cook, N. R., Lee, I.-M., et al. (2018). Vitamin D supplements and prevention of cancer and cardiovascular disease. *New England Journal of Medicine*, *380*(1), 33–44.

Manson, J. E., Cook, N. R., Lee, I.-M., et al. (2019). Marine n-3 fatty acids and prevention of cardiovascular disease and cancer. *New England Journal of Medicine*, *380*(1), 23–32.

Martínez, M. E., Marshall, J. R., & Giovannucci, E. (2008). Diet and cancer prevention: the roles of observation and experimentation. *Nature Reviews Cancer*, *8*(9), 694–703.

Marzbani, E., Inatsuka, C., Lu, H., et al. (2013). The invisible arm of immunity in common cancer chemoprevention agents. *Cancer Prevention Research*, *6*(8), 764–773.

McLean, M. H., Murray, G. I., Stewart, K. N., et al. (2011). The inflammatory microenvironment in colorectal neoplasia. *PLoS One*, *6*(1), e15366.

McNeil, J. J., Nelson, M. R., Woods, R. L., et al. (2018). Effect of aspirin on all-cause mortality in the healthy elderly. *New England Journal of Medicine*, *379*(16), 1519–1528.

Meyskens, F. L., Jr., McLaren, C. E., Pelot, D., et al. (2008). Difluoromethylornithine plus sulindac for the prevention of sporadic colorectal adenomas: a randomized placebo-controlled, double-blind trial. *Cancer Prevention Research*, *1*(1), 32–38.

Mohammed, A., Yarla, N. S., Madka, V., et al. (2018). Clinically relevant anti-inflammatory agents for chemoprevention of colorectal cancer: new perspectives. *International Journal of Molecular Science*, *19*(8). Per publication: Int. J. Mol. Sci. 2018, 19, 2332; doi:10.3390/ijms19082332

Monahan, K. J., Bradshaw, N., Dolwani, S., et al. (2020). Guidelines for the management of hereditary colorectal cancer from the British Society of Gastroenterology (BSG)/Association of Coloproctology of Great Britain and Ireland (ACPGBI)/United Kingdom Cancer Genetics Group (UKCGG). *Gut*, *69*(3), 411–444.

National Comprehensive Cancer Network. (2022). NCCN Guidelines Version 1.2022. Lynch syndrome.

National Organization for Rare Disorders. (2014). *Familial adenomatous polyposis* https://rarediseases.org/rare-diseases/familial-adenomatous-polyposis/#:~:text=Familial%20adenomatous%20polyposis%20(FAP)%20is,at%20a%20relatively%20young%20age

Nguyen, L. H., Goel, A., & Chung, D. C. (2020). Pathways of colorectal carcinogenesis. *Gastroenterology*, *158*(2), 291–302.

Oliveras-Ferraros, C., Cufi, S., Vazquez-Martin, A., et al. (2012). Metformin rescues cell surface major histocompatibility complex class I (MHC-I) deficiency caused by oncogenic transformation. *Cell Cycle*, *11*(5), 865–870.

Pabla, B., Bissonnette, M., & Konda, V. J. (2015). Colon cancer and the epidermal growth factor receptor: current treatment paradigms, the importance of diet, and the role of chemoprevention. *World Journal of Clinical Oncology*, *6*(5), 133–141.

Papaioannou, D., Cooper, K. L., Carroll, C., et al. (2011). Antioxidants in the chemoprevention of colorectal cancer and colorectal adenomas in the general population: a systematic review and meta-analysis. *Colorectal Disease*, *13*(10), 1085–1099.

Pearce, E. L., Walsh, M. C., Cejas, P. J., et al. (2009). Enhancing CD8 T-cell memory by modulating fatty acid metabolism. *Nature*, *460*(7251), 103–107.

Peleg, I. I., Lubin, M. F., Cotsonis, G. A., et al. (1996). Long-term use of nonsteroidal antiinflammatory drugs and other chemopreventors and risk of subsequent colorectal neoplasia. *Digestive Diseases and Sciences*, *41*(7), 1319–1326.

Peterson, K. A., & DiSario, J. A. (2002). Secondary prevention: screening and surveillance of persons at average and high risk for colorectal cancer. *Hematology/Oncology Clinics of North America*, *16*(4), 841–865.

Poynter, J. N., Gruber, S. B., Higgins, P. D., et al. (2005). Statins and the risk of colorectal cancer. *New England Journal of Medicine*, *352*(21), 2184–2192.

Pugh, S., & Thomas, G. A. (1994). Patients with adenomatous polyps and carcinomas have increased colonic mucosal prostaglandin E2. *Gut*, *35*(5), 675–678.

Reyes-Uribe, L., Wu, W., Gelincik, O., et al. (2021). Naproxen chemoprevention promotes immune activation in Lynch syndrome colorectal mucosa. *Gut*, *70*(3), 555–566.

Ross, S. J., Elgendy, I. Y., & Bavry, A. A. (2017). Cardiovascular Safety and Bleeding Risk Associated with Nonsteroidal Anti-Inflammatory Medications in Patients with Cardiovascular Disease. *Current Cardiology Reports*, *19*(1), 8.

Rossouw, J. E., Anderson, G. L., Prentice, R. L., et al. (2002). Risks and benefits of estrogen plus progestin in healthy postmenopausal women: principal results From the Women's Health Initiative randomized controlled trial. *JAMA*, *288*(3), 321–333.

Rostom, A., Dubé, C., Lewin, G., et al. (2007). Nonsteroidal anti-inflammatory drugs and cyclooxygenase-2 inhibitors for primary prevention of colorectal cancer: a systematic review prepared for the U.S. Preventive Services Task Force. *Annals of Internal Medicine*, *146*(5), 376–389.

Rothwell, P. M., Wilson, M., Elwin, C. E., et al. (2010). Long-term effect of aspirin on colorectal cancer incidence and mortality: 20-year follow-up of five randomised trials. *Lancet*, *376*(9754), 1741–1750.

Samadder, N. J., Kuwada, S. K., Boucher, K. M., et al. (2018). Association of sulindac and erlotinib vs placebo with colorectal neoplasia in familial adenomatous polyposis: secondary analysis of a randomized clinical trial. *JAMA Oncology*, *4*(5), 671–677.

Samadder, N. J., Neklason, D. W., Boucher, K. M., et al. (2016). Effect of Sulindac and erlotinib vs placebo on duodenal neoplasia in familial adenomatous polyposis: a randomized clinical trial. *JAMA*, *315*(12), 1266–1275.

Sammour, T., Hayes, I. P., Hill, A. G., et al. (2015). Familial colorectal cancer syndromes: an overview of clinical management. *Expert Review of Gastroenterology & Hepatology*, *9*(6), 757–764.

Samstein, R. M., Lee, C. H., Shoushtari, A. N., et al. (2019). Tumor mutational load predicts survival after immunotherapy across multiple cancer types. *Nature Genetics*, *51*(2), 202–206.

Sandler, R. S., Halabi, S., Baron, J. A., et al. (2003). A randomized trial of aspirin to prevent colorectal adenomas in patients with previous colorectal cancer. *New England Journal of Medicine*, *348*(10), 883–890.

Schatzkin, A., Lanza, E., Corle, D., et al. (2000). Lack of effect of a low-fat, high-fiber diet on the recurrence of colorectal adenomas. Polyp Prevention Trial Study Group. *New England Journal of Medicine*, *342*(16), 1149–1155.

Siegel, R. L., Miller, K. D., Fuchs, H. E., et al. (2022). Cancer statistics, 2022. *CA Cancer Journal for Clinicians*, *72*(1), 7–33.

Siegel, R. L., Miller, K. D., Goding Sauer, A., et al. (2020). Colorectal cancer statistics, 2020. *CA Cancer Journal for Clinicians*, *70*(3), 145–164.

Singh, S., Singh, H., Singh, P. P., et al. (2013). Antidiabetic medications and the risk of colorectal cancer in patients with diabetes mellitus: a systematic review and meta-analysis. *Cancer Epidemiology, Biomarkers & Prevention*, *22*(12), 2258–2268.

Sinicrope, F.A. (2018). Lynch syndrome-associated colorectal cancer. *New England Journal of Medicine*, *379*(8), 764–773.

Slattery, M. L. (2000). Diet, lifestyle, and colon cancer. *Seminars in Gastrointestinal Disease*, *11*(3), 142–146.

Solomon, S. D., McMurray, J. J., Pfeffer, M. A., et al. (2005). Cardiovascular risk associated with celecoxib in a clinical trial for colorectal adenoma prevention. *New England Journal of Medicine*, *352*(11), 1071–1080.

Song, M., Garrett, W. S., & Chan, A. T. (2015). Nutrients, foods, and colorectal cancer prevention. *Gastroenterology*, *148*(6), 1244–1260. e16.

Steinbach, G., Lynch, P. M., Phillips, R. K., et al. (2000). The effect of celecoxib, a cyclooxygenase-2 inhibitor, in familial adenomatous polyposis. *New England Journal of Medicine*, *342*(26), 1946–1952.

Steinmetz, K. A., & Potter, J. D. (1996). Vegetables, fruit, and cancer prevention: a review. *Journal of the American Dietetics Association*, *96*(10), 1027–1039.

Stürmer, T., Glynn, R. J., Lee, I. M., et al. (1998). Aspirin use and colorectal cancer: post-trial follow-up data from the Physicians' Health Study. *Annals of Internal Medicine*, *128*(9), 713–720.

Sung, H., Ferlay, J., Siegel, R. L., et al. (2021). Global cancer statistics 2020: GLOBOCAN estimates of incidence and mortality worldwide for 36 cancers in 185 countries. *CA Cancer Journal for Clinicians*, *71*(3), 209–249.

Takayama, T., Nagashima, H., Maeda, M., et al. (2011). Randomized double-blind trial of sulindac and etodolac to eradicate aberrant crypt foci and to prevent sporadic colorectal polyps. *Clinical Cancer Research*, *17*(11), 3803–3811.

Tomimoto, A., Endo, H., Sugiyama, M., et al. (2008). Metformin suppresses intestinal polyp growth in ApcMin/+ mice. *Cancer Science*, *99*(11), 2136–2141.

Umar, A. (2014). Cancer immunoprevention: a new approach to intercept cancer early. *Cancer Prevention Research*, *7*(11), 1067–1071.

Walker, A. R., & Burkitt, D. P. (1976). Colonic cancer—hypotheses of causation, dietary prophylaxis, and future research. *American Journal of Digestive Disease*, *21*(10), 910–917.

Wang, D., Cabalag, C. S., Clemons, N. J., et al. (2021). Cyclooxygenases and prostaglandins in tumor immunology and microenvironment of gastrointestinal cancer. *Gastroenterology*, *161*(6), 1813–1829.

Win, A. K., Jenkins, M. A., Dowty, J. G., et al. (2017). Prevalence and penetrance of major genes and polygenes for colorectal Cancer. *Cancer Epidemiology, Biomarkers & Prevention*, *26*(3), 404–412.

Wolf, A. M. D., Fontham, E. T. H., Church, T. R., et al. (2018). Colorectal cancer screening for average-risk adults: 2018 guideline update from the American Cancer Society. *CA Cancer Journal for Clinicians*, *68*(4), 250–281.

Yarchoan, M., Hopkins, A., & Jaffee, E. M. (2017). Tumor mutational burden and response rate to PD-1 inhibition. *New England Journal of Medicine*, *377*(25), 2500–2501.

Yarla, N. S., Madka, V., Pathuri, G., et al. (2020). Molecular targets in precision chemoprevention of colorectal cancer: an update from pre-clinical to clinical trials. *International Journal of Molecular Science*, *21*(24). Per publication: Int. J. Mol. Sci. 2020, 21, 9609; doi:10.3390/ijms21249609.

Zhang, H., Xu, H., Zhang, C., et al. (2021). Ursodeoxycholic acid suppresses the malignant progression of colorectal cancer through TGR5-YAP axis. *Cell Death Discovery*, *7*(1), 207.

SECTION 4

Novelty interventions and personalizing the CRC pathway

16

Adjuvant treatment of colorectal cancer

Valentinos Kounnis and Rachel Kerr

Introduction

Since the important role of adjuvant chemotherapy was first recognized in 1990, oncologists have striven to achieve the best outcomes, with the least toxicity, and to tailor, where possible, the adjuvant treatment to the characteristics of the individual patient and of their tumour. This chapter describes the evidence for adjuvant treatment of colorectal cancer and explores the upcoming challenges in this area. It will largely concentrate upon colon cancer as rectal cancer with its unique geographical position, and possibly different molecular genesis, is often a target for peri-operative radiotherapy in preference to chemotherapy, and many of the adjuvant trials described below have not included rectal cancer patients. Total neoadjuvant treatment of rectal cancer is also separately covered in Chapter 10 of this book.

Fluoropyrimidine single agent adjuvant therapy

After a disappointing meta-analysis of adjuvant chemotherapy published by Buyse et al. (1988), it was a great relief when subsequent pivotal trials established the disease-free survival (DFS) and overall survival (OS) benefits of post-operative fluoropyrimidine (FP)-based chemotherapy, specifically 5-fluorouracil (5-FU), compared with surgery alone in resected non-metastatic colon cancer. These were the North Central Cancer Therapy Group (NCCTG) trial and the INT-0035 trial. They demonstrated unequivocally that 5-FU plus levamisole, given for one year, versus surgery alone for stage 3 colon cancer, improved survival. However, their results for patients with stage 2 disease were less impressive.

Levamisole is an antihelminthic agent that was postulated to be potentially useful as part of adjuvant therapy for cancer because it was recognized to modulate the human cellular immune system and it was believed that this may contribute to preventing macroscopic recurrence. The relatively small NCCTG study conducted in the United States included 401 patients (Laurie et al., 1989). The results demonstrated that the combination of 5-FU plus levamisole increased disease-free survival ($p = 0.02$) and was associated with a small but significant ($p = 0.03$) survival benefit in stage 3 patients. The trial also showed that levamisole alone did not increase survival in stage 3 patients. No benefit from any adjuvant chemotherapy for stage 2 colon cancer patients was demonstrated, although numbers recruited were very small.

This trial formed the basis of a second clinical trial, Intergroup (INT)-0035, which was much better powered (1,300 patients) and was carried out to confirm results of the smaller study. This was a broader geographic gathering, comprising a collaborative effort of the NCCTG, the Southwest Oncology Group (SWOG), and the Eastern Cooperative Oncology Group (ECOG). The results of this study were initially published (Moertel et al., 1990) and further updated in 1992 at the American Society of Clinical Oncology (ASCO) meeting (Moertel et al., 1992) with final mature data being presented three years later (Moertel et al., 1995). The pivot point in terms of practice came with that initial report in 1990 where, after median follow-up of 3.5 years, 5-FU plus levamisole had decreased relapse by 41% ($p < 0.0001$) and decreased death from colorectal cancer by 33% ($p = 0.006$). As in the NCCTG published results, the levamisole alone appeared to deliver no beneficial effect.

As the contribution of levamisole to the 5-FU/levamisole regimen appeared likely to be small, attention turned to other potential modifiers and leucovorin (LV), also known as folinic acid, was chosen because of its known role in terms of stabilizing the ternary complex of the metabolite of 5-FU (FdUMP) with its target enzyme (thymidylate synthase) within the cell, with the anticipated consequence that it may prolong and potentiate the inhibitory effect. Table 16.1 below summarizes the major phase 3 trials which tested the combination of LV with 5-FU, which soon displaced levamisole as the 5-FU potentiator of choice in clinical practice.

The INT-0089 trial (Haller et al., 2005) was a four-arm study ($n = 3759$) that randomized high risk stage 2 plus stage 3 resected colon cancer patients to receive either control (5-FU levamisole for one year) or one of the experimental arms alongside the 5-FU: LDLV arm—low-dose LV plus the 5-FU (the Mayo Clinic regimen of LV 20 mg/m ^{2} and 5-FU 425 mg/m^2 on days 1 to 5 by intravenous (IV) push, repeated at week 4, week 8, and then every five weeks, for a total of six courses); HDLV arm—high-dose LV plus 5-FU (Roswell Park regimen; consisting of LV 500 mg/m^2 by a two-hour infusion and 5-FU 500 mg/m^2 by IV push at one hour after the start of the LV infusion, repeated once per week for six weeks, followed by a two-week week rest period, for a total of four × eight week courses);

Table 16.1 Four trials that established the use of 5-FU/leucovorin/capecitabine in the adjuvant treatment of colorectal cancer

Name of Trial	N	Comparison	Take home message	First author and year of publication
INT-0089	3759	5-FU/LEV vs 5FU/LDLV vs 5FU/HDLV vs 5FU/LDLV/LEV	• Early signal that addition of LV is superior • After 10 years, no arm superior	Haller et al., 2005
NSABP-CO4	2151	5-FU/HDLV vs 5-FU/LEV vs 5-FU/HDLV/LEV	• 5-FU/HDLV superior to 5-FU/LEV • 5-FU/HDLV equiv to 5-FU/HDLV/LEV so LEV added no extra benefit	Wolmark et al., 1999
GERCOR c96.1	905	LV5FU2 (infusional) vs mFU/LV (slow bolus)	• Regimes similar in efficacy • Infusion better tolerated	Andre et al., 2007
X-ACT	1987	Bolus 5-FU/LV vs capecitabine	• Trend towards improvement in outcomes with capecitabine • Decreased neutropenia and mucositis with capecitabine	Twelves et al., 2012

LDLV + LEV arm—low-dose LV plus levamisole plus 5-FU (consisting of levamisole 50 mg orally every eight hours for three days, repeated every 14 days for six months, which was given with the same chemotherapy as the Mayo Clinic regimen as above). The trial was complex and cross-arm comparison was hampered by the differences in the 5-FU backbone regimen. Most patients had stage 3 disease (80.5%), and the remainder had high-risk stage 2 disease. Although there looked to be superiority of the LDLV + LEV arm compared to the LEV control at interim analysis, after a median follow-up of 10 years, none of the four treatment arms was statistically superior in DFS or OS for patients with resected stage 2 or 3 colon cancer.

However, the NSABP C-04 trial (Wolmark et al., 1999) also randomized 2151 patients to one of three arms: six cycles of either 5-FU plus high-dose LV (HDLV) or 5-FU plus levamisole (LEV) or 5-FU plus HDLV plus LEV, in patients with stage 2 and 3 colon cancer. This trial did demonstrate that 5-FU plus HDLV delivered better DFS (64% vs 60%; $P < 0.05$) and five-year OS (74% vs 69%; $P < 0.05$) compared to 5-FU plus LEV both in stage 2 and stage 3 colon cancer. There were however no significant differences in DFS and OS between the combination of FU plus HDLV versus 5-FU plus HDLV plus LEV, suggesting that levamisole was adding nothing to the combination.

While the NSABP C-04 trial was ongoing, clinicians were starting to recognize that the acute life-threatening complications of bolus 5-FU may be worse than those seen with infusional 5-FU, both in terms of risk of neutropenia and severe oral mucositis. Therefore, shortly after fortnightly 48 hour infusional 5-FU regimes became established in the metastatic colorectal cancer armamentarium, they were tested in the adjuvant setting. The final results of the GERCOR C96.1 trial were published 12 years ago (Andre et al., 2007). This was a randomized phase 3 study comparing a fortnightly prolonged infusional regime (LV5FU2) with a four-weekly bolus (mFU/LV) regimen of FU plus LV, as adjuvant treatment for stage 2 and 3 colon cancer patients. The LV5FU2 regime was given over two days: first an LV infusion over four hours (200 mg/m^2 if dl-leucovorin; 100 mg/m^2 if l-leucovorin), followed by 400 mg/m^2 FU bolus and a 600 mg/m^2 5-FU over 22 hours continuous infusion, all repeated on day 2. Patients in the weekly mFU/LV group received an infusion of dl-leucovorin LV 200 mg/m^2 (or l-leucovorin LV 100 mg/m^2) over 15 minutes, followed by a 15-minute slow bolus FU 400 mg/m^2 every day on days 1 to 5, repeated every 28 days. The weekly mFU/LV was the control arm. mFU/LV differs slightly from the four-weekly Mayo Clinic regimen outlined above, as it has a higher dose of LV (200 vs 20 mg/m^2), a different period of administration (15 minutes vs bolus), and a slightly lower dose per day of FU (400 vs 425 mg/m^2). A total of 905 patients with stage 2 (43%) and 3 (57%) colon cancer was enrolled. The median follow-up was six years. There was no statistically significant difference between mFU/LV and LV5-FU2 in terms of DFS and OS, but the infusional regimen was better tolerated. These beneficial results were observed across stage 2 and 3 colon cancer.

Although the tolerability of infusional regimes was improved compared to the bolus regimes, this did raise difficulties for many chemotherapy units, who did not have access the implantable pumps, and PICC (peripherally inserted central catheter) lines were not commonplace at this time. So this transition to infusional regimes brought huge capacity pressures upon many units who had to hospitalize these patients for their adjuvant treatment, increasing oncology bed occupancy and decreasing overall quality of life for these patients. It is of no surprise then that there was a huge drive to defining whether the newer oral fluoropyrimidines could replace the 5-FU infusional regimes in terms of effectiveness, while increasing cost effectiveness and efficiency.

The X-ACT trial sought to answer this very question (Twelves et al., 2012). X-ACT was a randomized phase 3 trial of oral capecitabine (a prodrug of 5-FU) versus 5-FU/folinic acid in resected stage 3 colon cancer. Patients were randomized to receive capecitabine 1250 mg/m^2 twice daily on days 1–14 every three weeks for a total of eight cycles or 24 weeks, or the Mayo Clinic regimen (rapid IV infusion of LV 20 mg/m^2 followed immediately by IV bolus 5-FU 425 mg/m^2 on days 1–5 of a 28-day cycle (for six cycles). With a median follow-up of 6.9 years, capecitabine was found to be statistically equivalent to 5-FU/LV in terms of DFS and OS, with a trend towards improvement in DFS and OS. There was significantly less mucositis and neutropenia. The results followed the same pattern irrespective of gender of the patient, nodal status (N1 vs N2), CEA at diagnosis, and age. Capecitabine for six months therefore became a standard of care single agent regime in the adjuvant treatment of colon cancer across many countries of the world. The only potential negative of this transition is the increase in diarrhoea seen with capecitabine compared to the infusional regimes given over two days, which can be troublesome for patients who were left with an ileostomy post resection.

Dual agent adjuvant chemotherapy

Oxaliplatin is a third-generation platinum derivative which, when combined with 5-FU and LV, is a very effective chemotherapy for metastatic colorectal cancer, doubling the response rate compared to 5-FU and LV alone, and extending duration of progression-free and overall survival by approximately 50% (Andre et al., 1999; deGramont et al., 2000). Therefore, investigators set out to establish whether these benefits could be translated into the adjuvant setting to reduce further the chances of recurrence.

First, Andre et al. (2004), in the European MOSAIC trial, explored whether adding oxaliplatin to 5-FU and LV would improve outcomes. They randomized patients to receive either standard LV5-FU2 or the same with oxaliplatin. For LV5-FU2, each cycle comprised a two-hour infusion of 200 mg/m^2 of leucovorin, followed by a bolus of 400 mg/m^2 of fluorouracil then a 22-hour infusion of 600 mg/m^2 of 5-FU, given on two consecutive days every 14 days, for 12 cycles (six months total). In the experimental arm, patients were given the same LV5U2 regime plus a two-hour infusion of 85 mg/m^2 on day 1. Again, the intention was that all patients were treated for six months.

A total of 2,246 patients were randomly assigned in total. After a median follow-up of 37.9 months, 237 patients in the group given LV5-FU2 plus oxaliplatin had had a cancer-related event, as compared with 293 patients in the LV5-FU2 alone group (21.1% vs 26.1%; hazard ratio for recurrence, 0.77; $P = 0.002$). The rate of disease-free survival (DFS) at three years was 78.2% (95% CI, 75.6–80.7) in the experimental + OX group, and 72.9% (95% CI, 70.2–75.7) in the LV5FU2 alone group ($P = 0.002$ by the stratified log-rank test). In the + OX group, the incidence of grade 3 sensory neuropathy was 12.4% during treatment, decreasing to 1.1% at one year of follow-up. Toxic death rate was 0.5% in each arm.

In a follow-up publication from 2009 (Andre et al., 2009), six-year overall survival (OS) rates were 78.5% and 76.0% in the FOLFOX4 and LV5FU2 groups, respectively (HR = 0.84; 95% CI, 0.71–1.00; $P = 0.046$); corresponding six-year OS rates for patients with stage 3 disease were 72.9% and 68.7%, respectively (HR = 0.80; 95% CI, 0.65–0.97; $P = 0.023$). No statistically significant difference in OS was seen in the stage 2 population. However, this analysis may have been impeded by the relatively small number of high risk stage 2 patients, and specifically, the limited number of patients with stage 2 T4 disease which does confer a significantly poorer prognosis.

In the North American counterpart to the MOSAIC trial, the randomized phase 3 trial NSABP C-07 revealed similar results. These investigators assessed how the effectiveness of FLOX compared with FL alone (Kuebler et al., 2007). The control arm FL comprised LV 500 mg/m^2 over two hours, plus 5-FU 500 mg/m^2 administered as an intravenous bolus one hour after the LV infusion was begun. These were repeated weekly for six consecutive weeks followed by a two-week rest period. Patients received three × eight-week cycles of therapy for a total treatment duration of 24 weeks (six months). In the FLOX regime, 5FU and LV were administered exactly as described for the FL alone arm. In addition, oxaliplatin 85 mg/m^2 was administered as a two-hour infusion before LV and 5FU on days 1, 15, and 29 of the eight-week treatment cycle. Again, patients received three cycles of therapy for a total treatment duration of six months.

Analysis of 2,407 patients with stage 2 or 3 colon cancer was undertaken. In the initial publication, the hazard ratio (FLOX vs FULV) was 0.80 (95% CI, 0.69–0.93), a 20% relative risk reduction in favour of the addition of OX ($P < 0.004$). The three- and four-year DFS rates were 71.8% and 67.0% for FULV and 76.1% and 73.2% for FLOX, respectively, so absolute survival improvements of approximately 5–6%. Grade 3 neurosensory toxicity was noted in 8.2% of patients receiving FLOX and in 0.7% of those receiving FULV ($P < 0.001$). In a later publication (Yothers et al., 2011) with longer follow-up (eight years median), OS was similar between treatment groups (hazard ratio (HR), 0.88; 95% CI, 0.75–1.02; $P = 0.08$). FLOX remained superior for DFS (HR, 0.82; 95% CI, 0.72–0.93; $P = 0.002$). The effect of oxaliplatin on OS did not differ by stage of disease (interaction $P = 0.38$ for OS; interaction $P = 0.37$ for DFS) but did vary by age for OS (younger than age 70 vs 70 + interaction $P = 0.039$). There was a similar trend for DFS (interaction $P = 0.073$). Thus, oxaliplatin did significantly improve OS in patients younger than age 70 (HR, 0.80; 95% CI, 0.68–0.95; $P = 0.013$), but no positive additional benefit from OX was evident in older patients. This may be in part due to other comorbidities affecting survival probability in older populations.

A final study worth mentioning in terms of defining the role of oxaliplatin in the adjuvant treatment of colorectal cancer is the XELOXA NO16968 trial (Schmoll et al., 2007). Capecitabine was assessed in combination with oxaliplatin (XELOX) for resected stage 3 colon cancer. Adjuvant treatment was assigned to 1,886 patients with either XELOX or intravenous (IV) bolus 5-FU/LV, given as either Mayo Clinic regime or Roswell Park regime. The XELOX regimen consisted of a two hour IV infusion of oxaliplatin 130 mg/m^2 on day 1 and oral capecitabine 1000 mg/m^2 twice daily given for 14 days of a three-week cycle, for a total of eight cycles (24 weeks). The Mayo Clinic regimen consisted of a rapid IV infusion of LV 20 mg/m^2 followed by an IV bolus of FU 425 mg/m^2 on days 1–5 of a four-week cycle, for a total of six cycles (24 weeks). The Roswell Park regimen consisted of a two hour IV infusion of LV 500 mg/m^2 plus an IV bolus injection of FU 500 mg/m^2 on day 1 of weeks 1–6 of an eight-week cycle, for a total of four cycles (32 weeks). The final results of this trial (Schmoll et al., 2015) showed an improved seven-year DFS rate (66% vs 58%; HR 0.78; $P = 0.002$) and a improved seven-year OS (73% vs 67%; HR 0.83; $P = 0.04$) in the XELOX arm compared with the bolus 5-FU/LV arm. There has been some criticism of the bolus regimes being chosen as the control arm in this study as single agent capecitabine would have given a 'clearer' read-out of the benefit of the addition of oxaliplatin, but at the time of development of the study, bolus 5-FU/LV regimes were more commonly being used.

Overall these studies established that the addition of oxaliplatin to 5-FU or capecitabine in adjuvant regimes is likely to improve disease-free and overall survival for patients under the age of 70 with stage 3 colon cancer. But what about the additional benefits of oxaliplatin for those patients with stage 2 cancer, and older patients?

Selecting patients for adjuvant treatment based on age and stage

Nil versus single versus doublet agent adjuvant chemotherapy for stage 2 CRC

For many years adjuvant trials in colorectal cancer did not include sufficient numbers of stage 2 colon cancer patients to be able to elucidate whether there was any benefit at all to adjuvant chemotherapy.

The QUASAR collaborative group changed this by randomizing 2963 with stage 2 disease to chemotherapy versus observation after resection. The chemotherapy they received was according to the QUASAR protocol, but was essentially bolus 5FU/LV. After a median follow-up of 5.5 (range 0–10.6) years, there were 311 deaths in the chemotherapy group and 370 in the observation group; the relative risk of death from any cause with chemotherapy versus observation alone was 0.82 (95% CI 0.70–0.95; $p = 0.008$). There were 293 recurrences in the chemotherapy group and 359 in the observation group; the relative risk of recurrence with chemotherapy versus observation alone was 0.78 (0.67–0.91; $p = 0.001$). Overall the authors described that this translated into an absolute improvement in survival of 3.6% (95% CI 1.0–6.0) (QUASAR Collaborative Group, 2007), so there became an acceptance that having a discussion with stage 2 CRC patients about chemotherapy, the risks and benefits for them as an individual, was important. Attention then turned to whether the addition of oxaliplatin in these lower-risk patients may garner some additional benefit. Two of the trials above (NSABP C-07 and MOSAIC) recruited patients with stage 2 as well as stage 3 colon cancer. Both carried out *post hoc* exploratory analyses of effect by stage.

In the MOSAIC trial, stage 3 disease 10-year OS in patients receiving FOLFOX compared to LV5-FU2 was statistically significantly increased (67.1% vs 59.0%; HR 0.80; $P = 0.016$). In patients with stage 2 disease (n approximately 450 in each group), six year OS rates were 86.9% and 86.8%, respectively (HR = 1.00; 95% CI 0.70–1.41; $P = 0.986$). In an exploratory analysis, the probability of OS at six years in high-risk stage 2 patients was slightly greater with FOLFOX compared to LV5-FU2 but this did not reach statistical significance (85.0% and 83.3%; HR 0.91; 95% CI 0.61–1.36; $P = 0.648$). However, the underpowered nature of this analysis needs to be recognized. In terms of disease-free survival in the MOSAIC trial, among patients with stage 3 disease, five-year DFS rates were 66.4% and 58.9% in the FOLFOX and LV5-FU2 groups respectively (HR 0.78; 95% CI 0.65–0.93; $P = 0.005$). Among stage 2 patients, the probability of being disease free at five years was 83.7% and 79.9% in the FOLFOX and LV5FU2 groups respectively (HR = 0.84; 95% CI 0.62–1.14; $P = 0.258$). In an exploratory analysis, the probability of disease-free survival at five years in high-risk stage 2 patients were 82.3% and 74.6% in the FOLFOX4 and LV5-FU2 groups, respectively (HR = 0.72; 95% CI, 0.50–1.02). This led the authors to conclude that in high-risk stage 2 disease, the addition of oxaliplatin should still be considered (Andre et al., 2009).

The exploratory subset analysis by stage of the NSABP C-07 trial (Yothers et al., 2011) showed significant differences for DFS in stage 3 (increase of 6.6% for five-year DFS in the FLOX arm; 64.4% vs 57.8%) and a five-year OS improvement estimated at 2.7% with the addition of OX (76.5% vs 73.8%). In stage 2 patients there was a trend towards some benefit from the addition of OX in terms of five-year DFS (2% increase with FLOX; 82.1% vs 80.1%) but five-year OS was not improved (89.7% vs 89.6%; $P = 0.84$). Those data support the lack of benefit to the addition of oxaliplatin to adjuvant regimens in stage 2 disease. Although these results did not corroborate the subgroup analyses from the MOSAIC study, the community agreed that the choice of dual versus single agent chemotherapy in stage 2 patients, especially those with high-risk features, would be likely to be made after close discussion with the patient about their individual characteristics. And all agree that these results and marginal improvements are driving the need to develop better prognostic and predictive markers to refine patient selection for adjuvant treatment.

Age and its impact upon choice of adjuvant treatment

One of the difficult things about extrapolating clinical trial results to patients attending clinic is that the age characteristics of the two populations varies significantly. Thus the median age of a patient in a trial is 62 years and the median age of a new patient with colon cancer is 72 years. However, some trials have attempted retrospective subgroup analyses to assess the beneficial effect in different age groups. In the NSABP C-07 trial, the effect of the addition of oxaliplatin did appear to vary by age for OS (younger than age 70 vs 70+ interaction $P = 0.039$). There was a similar trend for DFS (interaction $P = 0.073$). Oxaliplatin significantly improved OS in patients younger than age 70 (HR, 0.80; 95% CI 0.68–0.95; $P = 0.013$), but no positive effect was reported in older patients (Yothers et al., 2011).

The XELOXA study (NO16968) also carried out exploratory analyses of DFS and OS by age and showed that XELOX improved outcomes vs FU/FA not only in patients younger than 70 years ($n = 1477$) but also in patients age 70 years or older ($n = 409$) although the effect size was diminished in the older patient group. For DFS, the HR was 0.86 (95% CI, 0.64–1.16) in patients age 70 years or older, and 0.80 (95% CI, 0.67 to 0.94) in patients younger than 70 years. For OS, the HR was 0.91 (95% CI, 0.66–1.26) in patients age 70 years or older and 0.82 (95% CI, 0.67–1.01) in patients younger than 70 years. Although the authors point out that, like their counterparts, these analyses were not powered for secure outcomes, oxaliplatin should not be totally disregarded in patients over the age of 70 who make up more than half of patients with colorectal cancer.

The ACCENT group pooled and analysed 11,953 patients age < 70 and 2,575 age ≥ 70 years from seven adjuvant therapy trials comparing IV FU with oral fluoropyrimidines (capecitabine, uracil, or tegafur) or combinations of fluoropyrimidines with oxaliplatin or irinotecan in stage 2/3 colon cancer. Endpoints were disease-free survival (DFS), overall survival (OS), and time to recurrence (TTR). They found that patients age ≥ 70 years seemed to experience reduced (rather than nil) benefit from adding oxaliplatin to fluoropyrimidines in the adjuvant setting, although statistically there was not a significant effect modification by age, and they also found that oral fluoropyrimidines retained their efficacy with increasing age.

We therefore conclude that chronological age should not be a barrier to adjuvant chemotherapy; that fluoropyrimidines bring about a similar proportional reduction in recurrence risk in older patients compared to younger patients; that oxaliplatin is not unreasonable in patients over the age of 70 but heed needs to be paid to physiological age, comorbidities, and explanation given that the benefit may be restricted to disease-free survival rather than overall survival (due to increasing frequency of other life-limiting diseases with age). Certainly, patients who are over the age of 70 and who have a stage 2 colorectal cancer are unlikely to gain extra benefit from the addition of oxaliplatin.

Optimal duration of adjuvant chemotherapy

When oxaliplatin was more routinely introduced into the adjuvant treatment for patients with stage 3 colon cancer, a six-month duration of a combination of this agent along with either infusional 5-FU/FA (FOLFOX) or with capecitabine (CAPOX) became adjuvant standard of care due to disease-free survival benefit observed, as outlined above, compared with 5-FU/FA alone. However, it was increasingly recognized that in the adjuvant setting, where potential life expectancy for these patients could be 30 years or more, that the main cumulative side effect of oxaliplatin, namely sensory neurotoxicity, was becoming a significant problem, affecting quality of life and draining healthcare resources. From the use of oxaliplatin in the advanced disease setting, it was clear that the incidence and severity of chronic neurotoxicity are largely related to the duration/cumulative dose exposure to the drug. Therefore, it was also clear that if we could reap the same relapse and survival benefits from three months of adjuvant oxaliplatin-based chemotherapy compared to six months, this would significantly reduce the chronic healthcare burden from this treatment.

The International Duration Evaluation of Adjuvant therapy (IDEA) collaboration was established to determine, in form of a pre-planned, pooled analysis of six independently conducted trials, whether a three-month duration of oxaliplatin-based therapy was non-inferior to six months. The IDEA Collaboration initially published results in the *New England Journal of Medicine* (Grothey et al., 2018) and these were further updated three years later (André et al., 2020). From June 2007 to December 2015 across 12 countries in CALGB/SWOG80702, IDEA France, SCOT, ACHIEVE, TOSCA, and HORG trials (sample sizes: 708 to 3,983), who started any treatment (modified intent-to-treat) were included. Fluoropyrimidine and oxaliplatin with 5-FU/folinic acid (FOLFOX) or capecitabine (CAPOX) were delivered every two and three weeks, respectively. The primary endpoint was disease-free survival (time to relapse, secondary colorectal primary tumour, or death due to all causes) and that overall survival (time to death due to all causes) was the pre-specified secondary endpoint. The overall survival NI margin was set to be HR = 1.11. Pre-planned subgroup analyses included regimen and risk group. In the initial publication, the authors detailed that non-interiority (NI) of the three-month regime could not be proven. However, they detected an unexpected interaction effect of the regimen used (FOLFOX versus CAPOX) in a pre-planned analysis. In patients treated with CAPOX, a longer duration of therapy did not provide additional benefit with NI demonstrated (74.8% vs 75.9%; HR 0.95; 95% CI 0.85–1.06), whereas six months of FOLFOX therapy was associated with moderate (73.6% vs 76%; HR 1.16; 95% CI, 1.06–1.26) but statistically improved three-year disease-free survival compared with three months. Of note, CAPOX versus FOLFOX was not randomly assigned in any of the IDEA trials, rather it was either that the regimen was dictated by the protocol or it was physician's choice per each patient; therefore, no direct outcomes comparison was possible between the two regimens. In the updated publication (André et al., 2020) with median follow-up of 72 months (IQR, 72.2–72.5), 2,584 deaths among 12,835 patients were observed. Of all patients, 39.5% received CAPOX and 60.5% FOLFOX. Comparing three vs six months across all patients irrespective of regimen, the five-year OS rate was 82.4% and 82.8% (HR) of 1.02; 95% CI 0.95–1.11; NI FDRadj $p = 0{\cdot}058$). For CAPOX, the three- vs six-months treatment five-year OS rates were 82.1% vs 81.2% (HR 0.96; 95% CI 0.85–1.08; NI FDRadj $p = 0.033$) and for FOLFOX the three- vs six-treatment five-year OS rates were 82.6% and 83.8%, estimated (HR 1.07; 95% CI 0.97–1.18; NI FDRadj p = 0.34) Updated disease-free survival results confirmed previous findings. The authors concluded that, while the NI for overall survival could not be confirmed after multiplicity adjustment, the absolute 0.4% difference in five-year overall survival should be placed in clinical context. And that overall the survival results support the use of three months of adjuvant CAPOX for the vast majority of stage 3 colon cancer patients. This conclusion is strengthened by the substantial reduction of toxicities, inconveniencies, and cost associated with a shorter treatment duration.

Improving prognostic and predictive profiling to personalize adjuvant treatment

Age of patient and histopathological stage of primary tumour are blunt instruments to use to define the optimal regimen and duration of adjuvant treatment and indeed, in terms of deciding whether any adjuvant treatment should be given at all. Every adjuvant treatment comes with costs; for the patient (time spent on treatment, costs of travel, toxicity morbidity, and risks of mortality), or even personal costs and of course in terms of financial and healthcare resources in the fast expanding field of oncology (where cancer incidence and the decision to treat are increasing exponentially).

The decision of when to offer adjuvant treatment should not be taken lightly and should be well balanced on the traditional risk vs benefit scale. The oncological community is moving towards improving the selection criteria for patients who might be best served by adjuvant treatment based on, novel biomarkers, including the molecular profiling of tumours as well as the dynamic changes in the circulating tumour cell DNA level. Traditionally, investigators have concentrated upon particular markers, for example the presence mutations in the *RAS* or *RAF* genes, and have then attempted to refine prognosis based on these alone. Due to the extreme complexity and interdependency of growth pathways within the cell, this kind of analysis is fraught with problems and does not stratify a patient accurately enough to guide therapy decisions. Indeed, one only has to look at the relationship between mismatch repair deficiency status (potentially better prognosis) and *BRAF* mutation (potentially worse prognosis) to see immediately that single factor prognostication can lead to very inaccurate prediction of outcome.

Pattern recognition profiling

More recently investigators have moved towards a broader fully encompassing pattern recognition predictor of prognosis. One publication describing such a process was published in the Lancet a couple of years ago (Skrede et al., 2020). The aim of the study was to develop a 'biomarker' of patient outcome after primary colorectal cancer resection by directly analysing scanned conventional haematoxylin and eosin (H&E)-stained sections using deep learning. In a hugely comprehensive analysis, more than 12 million image tiles from patients with a distinctly good or poor disease outcome from four cohorts were used to train a total of ten convolutional neural networks, purpose-built for classifying supersized heterogeneous images.

A prognostic biomarker integrating the 10 networks was determined using patients with a non-distinct outcome. The marker was tested on 920 patients initially, and then independently validated according to a predefined protocol in 1,122 patients treated with single-agent capecitabine. All cohorts included only patients with resectable tumours, and a formalin-fixed, paraffin-embedded tumour tissue block available for analysis. The primary outcome was cancer-specific survival.

The investigators reported that 828 patients from four cohorts had a distinct outcome and were used as a training cohort to obtain clear ground truth. A non-distinct outcome was found in 1,645 patients and was used for fine tuning. The biomarker provided a hazard ratio for poor vs good prognosis of 3.84 (95% CI 2.72–5.43; $p < 0.0001$) in the primary analysis of the validation cohort, and 3.04 (2.07–4.47; $p < 0.0001$) after adjusting for established prognostic markers significant in univariable analyses of the same cohort, which were pN stage, pT stage, lymphatic invasion, and venous vascular invasion. They therefore concluded that they had been able to develop a clinically useful prognostic marker using deep learning allied to digital scanning of conventional H&E-stained tumour tissue sections and that this could greatly improve prognostication in the adjuvant setting compared to using conventional H&E staining/TNM staging as assessed by individual pathologists. With the use of digital scanning etc., this also has the potential to decrease the intensive personnel resource required to determine prognosis. This technique is now being assessed in standard clinical practice across a range of centres to determine feasibility and deliverability.

Circulating tumour cell prognostication

Another potential method to refine prognostication that has been reported in the literature extensively over the last decade is the detection of circulating tumour cell (CTC) products in the systemic circulation of patients who have had their primary cancer recently resected (Fig. 16.1). More than 10 years ago, the term 'liquid biopsy' was coined by Pantel and Alix-Panabieres (Pantel et al., 2010) as a minimally invasive way for tissue sampling, allowing analysis of CTCs) or tumour cell products (e.g. ctDNA, cfRNA, extracellular vesicles, or proteins) released from primary tumours or metastatic deposits into the circulation (blood stream) or other body fluids.

In subsequent investigations, patients who underwent curative resection of colorectal cancer (stage 3) followed by FOLFOX chemotherapy, CTC count predicted relapse after chemotherapy (Murray et al., 2019). In non-metastatic CRC, pre-operative CTC detection was an independent prognostic marker. On multivariate analysis CTCs were the strongest prognostic factor in non-metastatic patients (hazard ratio (HR) 5.5; 95% confidence interval (CI) 2.3–13.6) and the result was surprising given that less than 300 patients were in the study (Bork et al., 2015).

In another study, CTC count correlated with reduced disease-free survival (Tsai et al., 2016). Again this study was small, with fewer than 100 patients. What was notably interesting is that CTC count correlated with distant recurrence of cancer but *not* with local/peritoneal recurrence, in keeping with the distinct modalities of spread to these distinct sites. Since then, there have been ongoing efforts in utilizing ctDNA as a valid biomarker to aid in decision-making around offering adjuvant treatment as well as in early detection. We have summarized four representative studies in Table 16.2.

For the reasons discussed above, CTC count may be much less relevant in T4 disease. Studies are now ongoing looking at much bigger cohorts, particularly in stage 2 colorectal cancer, to see if these prognostic projections are borne out, and also to see whether

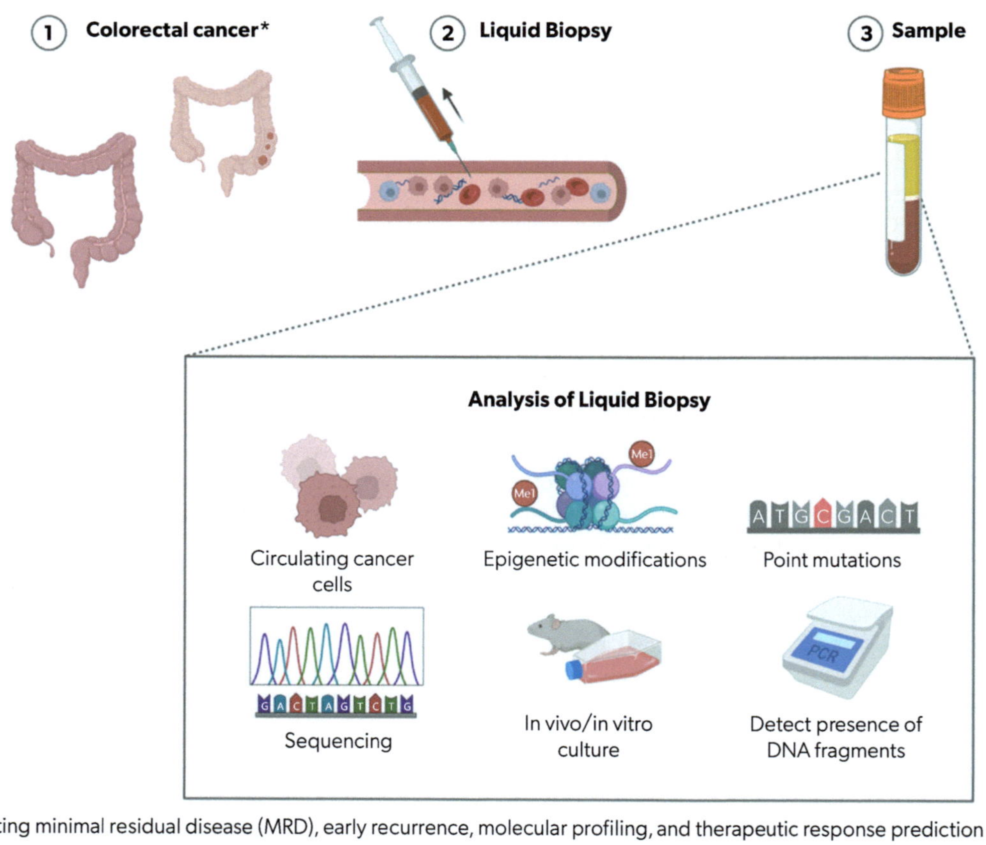

Figure 16.1 Created with BioRender.com.

Table 16.2 ctDNA in early CRC

Study name		Stage	Sample size	Outcome
ACTRN12615000381583 (Tie et al., 2022)	The role of ctDNA analysis in guiding Adjuvant therapy in Colon Cancer	2	455 patients	cdDNA guided decisions reduced the use of adjuvant ChT in stage II without compromising the recurrence free survival
ALGECOLS (Benhaim et al., 2021)	Role of ctDNA as a prognostic marker for recurrence	2 and 3	184 patients	Relevance of ctDNA as a recurrence risk factor in stage II and III CRC before surgery as well as a marker of MRD (minimal residual disease after surgery, which can predict recurrence months before imaging
Tarazona et al., 2019	ctDNA NGS to identify MRD	1–3	150	Postoperative ctDNA detected minimal residual disease and identified patients at higher risk of relapse. Detection of ctDNA follow-up preceded radiological recurrence by 11.5 months
ACTRN12612000345886 (Tie et al., 2021)	Role of ctDNA dynamics in patients undergoing curative resection of liver metastases	IV	54	Prognostic impact of post-surgery and post-treatment ctDNA in resected liver metastatic disease *limitations: small sample size and potential false positive findings

intervening with adjuvant chemotherapy based on these more differentiated profiles, will influence outcome.

Conclusions

Some commentators report that the last 10 years have been somewhat disappointing in the realm of adjuvant treatment for colorectal cancer, with the failure of bevacizumab, and the anti-EGFR antibody family to make any impact at all. There is truth in this perception to some extent. However, as can be seen earlier in this chapter, we have greatly built upon the foundations laid down by the early masters of adjuvant treatment, refining who we treat and how we treat them, and applying greater 'intelligence' to our prognostication (and this work is ongoing) and ensuring that all patients have access to appropriate information so that they can make an informed decision as to whether adjuvant chemotherapy is right for them, and what type and duration of adjuvant chemotherapy is most appropriate for their specific set of circumstances.

The next 10 years will be exciting as we refine prognostic profiling and perhaps even learn to retrospectively apply new prognostic profiling techniques to past trials and their collected tissue banks, to see if we can elucidate predictive profiles of potential responders to such agents as bevacizumab or cetuximab in the post resection setting. At the same time we will be processing data from large adjuvant trials of aspirin (Joharatnam-Hogan et al., 2019) and seeing if we can truly teach an 'old drug new tricks' in terms of improving colorectal cancer outcome with something very simple, cheap, and tolerable.

REFERENCES

André, T., Bensmaine, M. A., Louvet, C., et al. (1999). Multicenter phase II study of bimonthly high-dose leucovorin fluorouracil infusion, and oxaliplatin for metastatic colorectal cancer resistant to the same leucovorin and fluorouracil regimen. *Journal of Clinical Oncology, 17*, 3560–3568.

André, T., Boni, C., Mounedji-Boudiaf, L., et al. (2004). Oxaliplatin, fluorouracil, and leucovorin as adjuvant treatment for colon cancer. Multicenter International Study of Oxaliplatin/5-Fluorouracil/Leucovorin in the Adjuvant Treatment of Colon Cancer (MOSAIC) Investigators. *New England Journal of Medicine, 350*(23), 2343–2351.

André, T., Boni, C., Navarro, M., et al. (2009). Improved overall survival with oxaliplatin, fluorouracil, and LV as adjuvant treatment in stage II or III colon cancer in the MOSAIC trial. *Journal of Clinical Oncology, 27*(19), 3109–3116.

André, T., Quinaux, E., Louvet, C., et al. (2007). Phase III study comparing a semimonthly with a monthly regimen of fluorouracil and LV as adjuvant treatment for stage II and III colon cancer patients: final results of GERCOR C96.1. *Journal of Clinical Oncology, 25*(24), 3732–3738.

André, T., Meyerhardt, J., Iveson, T., et al. (2020). Effect of duration of adjuvant chemotherapy for patients with stage III colon cancer (IDEA collaboration): final results from a prospective, pooled analysis of six randomised, phase 3 trials. *Lancet Oncology, 21*(12), 1620–1629.

Benhaim, L., Bouche, O., Normand, C., et al. (2021). Circulating tumor DNA is a prognostic marker of tumor recurrence in stage II and III colorectal cancer: multicentric, prospective cohort study (ALGECOLS). *European Journal of Cancer, 159*, 24–33.

Bork, U., Rahbari, N. N., Schölch, S., et al. (2015). Circulating tumour cells and outcome in non-metastatic colorectal cancer: a prospective study. *British Journal of Cancer, 112*, 1306–1313.

Buyse, M., Zeleniuch-Jacquotte, A., & Chalmers, T. C. (1988). Adjuvant therapy of colorectal cancer: Why we still don't know. *JAMA, 259*, 3571–3578

de Gramont, A, Figer, A, Seymour, M, et al. (2000). Leucovorin and fluorouracil with or without oxaliplatin as first-line treatment in advanced colorectal cancer. *Journal of Clinical Oncology, 18*, 2938–2947.

Grothey, A., Sobrero, A. F., Shields, A. F., et al. (2018). Duration of adjuvant chemotherapy for stage III colon cancer. *New England Journal of Medicine, 378*(13), 1177–1188.

ONS 2017 Dataset: Cancer survival in England—adults diagnosed. Office for National Statistics <http://www.ons.gov.uk.

Haller, D. G., Catalano, P. J., Macdonald, J. S., et al. (2005). Phase III study of fluorouracil, LV, and levamisole in high-risk stage II and III colon cancer: final report of intergroup 0089. *Journal of Clinical Oncology, 23*(34), 8671–8678.

Joharatnam-Hogan, N., Cafferty, F., Hubner, R., et al. (2019). Aspirin as an adjuvant treatment for cancer: feasibility results from the Add-Aspirin randomised trial. *Lancet Gastroenterology & Hepatology, 4*(11), 854–862.

Kuebler, J. P., Wieand, H. S., O'Connell, M. J., et al. (2007). Oxaliplatin combined with weekly bolus fluorouracil and LV as surgical adjuvant chemotherapy for stage II and III colon cancer: results from NSABP C-07. *Journal of Clinical Oncology, 25*(16), 2198–2204.

Laurie, J. A., Moertel, C. G., Fleming, T. R., et al. (1989). Surgical adjuvant therapy of large-bowel carcinoma: An evaluation of levamisole and the combination of levamisole and fluorouracil: The North Central Cancer Treatment Group and the Mayo Clinic. *Journal of Clinical Oncology, 7*, 1447–1456.

Moertel, C. G., Fleming, T. R., Macdonald J. S., et al. (1990). Levamisole and fluorouracil for adjuvant therapy of resected colon carcinoma. *New England Journal of Medicine, 322*, 352–358.

Moertel, C., Fleming, T., Macdonald, J. S., et al. (1992). The intergroup study of 5-FU + levamisole and levamisole alone as adjuvant therapy for stage C colon cancer: A final report. *Proceedings of the American Society of Clinical Oncology, 11*, 161. Abstract.

Moertel, C. G., Fleming, T. R., Macdonald, J. S., et al. (1995). Intergroup study of fluorouracil plus levamisole as adjuvant therapy for stage II/Dukes' B2 colon cancer. *Journal of Clinical Oncology, 13*(12), 2936–2943.

Murray, N. P., Aedo, S., Villalon, R., et al. (2019). Effect of FOLFOX on minimal residual disease in Stage III colon cancer and risk of relapse. *Ecancermedicalscience, 13*, 935.

Pantel, K., & Alix-Panabières, C. (2010). Circulating tumour cells in cancer patients: challenges and perspectives. *Trends in Molecular Medicine, 16*, 398–406.

Quasar Collaborative Group, Gray, R., Barnwell, J., et al. (2007). Adjuvant chemotherapy versus observation in patients with colorectal cancer: a randomised study. *Lancet, 370*, 2020–2029.

Schmoll H. J., Cartwright, T., Tabernero, J., et al. (2007). Phase III trial of capecitabine plus oxaliplatin as adjuvant therapy for stage III colon cancer: a planned safety analysis in 1,864 patients. *Journal of Clinical Oncology, 25*(1), 102–109.

Schmoll, H. J., Tabernero, J., Maroun, A., et al. (2015). Capecitabine plus oxaliplatin (XELOX) versus bolus 5-fluorouracil/LV (5-FU/LV) as adjuvant therapy for stage III colon cancer: survival follow-up of study NO16968 (XELOXA). *Journal of Clinical Oncology, 33*(32), 3733–3740.

Skrede, O. J., De Raedt, S., Kleppe, A., et al. (2020). Deep learning for prediction of colorectal cancer outcome: a discovery and validation study. *Lancet, 395*(10221), 350–360.

Tarazona, N., Gimeno-Valiente, F., Gambardella, V., et al. (2019). Targeted next-generation sequencing of circulating-tumor DNA for tracking minimal residual disease in localized colon cancer. *Annals of Oncology, 30*(11), 1804–1812.

Tie, J., Cohen, J. D., Lahouel, K., et al. (2022). Circulating tumor DNA analysis guiding adjuvant therapy in stage II colon cancer. *New England Journal of Medicine, 386*(24), 2261–2272.

Tie, J., Wang, Y., Cohen, J., et al. (2021). Circulating tumor DNA dynamics and recurrence risk in patients undergoing curative intent resection of colorectal cancer liver metastases: a prospective cohort study. *PLoS Medicine, 18*(5), e1003620.

Tsai, W.-S., Chen, J.-S., Shao, H.-J., et al. (2016). Circulating tumor cell count correlates with colorectal neoplasm progression and is a prognostic marker for distant metastasis in non-metastatic patients. *Science Reports, 6*, 24517.

Twelves, C., Scheithauer, W., McKendrick, J., et al. (2015). Capecitabine versus 5-fluorouracil/folinic acid as adjuvant therapy for stage III colon cancer: final results from the X-ACT trial with analysis by age and preliminary evidence of a pharmacodynamic marker of efficacy. *Annals of Oncology, 23*(5), 1190–1197.

Wolmark, N., Rockette, H., Mamounas, E., et al. (1999). Clinical trial to assess the relative efficacy of fluorouracil and LV, fluorouracil and levamisole, and fluorouracil, LV, and levamisole in patients with Dukes' B and C carcinoma of the colon: results from National Surgical Adjuvant Breast and Bowel Project C-04. *Journal of Clinical Oncology, 17*(11), 3553–3559.

Yothers, G., O'Connell, M. J., Allegra, C. J., et al. (2011). Oxaliplatin as adjuvant therapy for colon cancer: updated results of NSABP C-07 trial, including survival and subset analyses. *Journal of Clinical Oncology, 29*(28), 3768–3774.

17

The precision medicine approach for advanced and metastatic colorectal cancer

Josep Tabernero, Elena Élez, Javier Ros, and Nadia Saoudi-Gonzalez

Introduction

Colorectal cancer (CRC) is the second cause of cancer-related death worldwide and the third most common cancer worldwide, accounting for approximately 900,000 deaths annually (Sung et al., 2021). Despite major efforts over recent decades, five-year relative survival in the metastatic setting is approximately 15% for these patients (Siegek et al., 2020). The historic backbone of standard treatment for metastatic CRC (mCRC) is based on chemotherapy combinations of fluoropyrimidines with oxaliplatin or irinotecan. More recent advances have seen the addition of biological treatments to the therapeutic armamentarium, notably the anti-epithelial growth factor receptor (EGFR) agents, cetuximab and panitumumab, as well as anti-vascular endothelial growth factor (VEGF)/VEGF receptor (VEGFR) inhibitors, such as bevacizumab and aflibercept (Van Cutsem et al., 2014).

Metastatic CRC presents a paradigm of heterogeneity in oncology, representing a challenge for personalized therapeutic approaches (Grady & Carethers, 2008). The goal of precision medicine is to identify personalized treatment for individual patients by taking into consideration the singular molecular and clinical characteristics of both the patient and the tumour. Since the first steps towards personalized medicine were made in the early 2000s, when *KRAS* was identified as a negative biomarker for response to EGFR inhibitors, dramatic improvements in the landscape of molecular characterization of CRC have been achieved (Misale et al., 2014), with meaningful improvements in specific mCRC molecular subtypes, notably with immunotherapy for patients with microsatellite instability (MSI) (André et al., 2020). The development and implementation of next-generation sequencing (NGS) techniques has led to the identification of a wide spectrum of molecular alterations, most of them suitable to be targeted with novel drugs; for example *NTRK* fusions or *KRAS* G12C mutations (Ros et al., 2022).

To address these disease complexities, preclinical models reproducing the genomic heterogeneity of mCRC have been developed. They range from molecularly selected cell lines to patient-derived models that assist the rapid translation of promising preclinical findings into clinical trials. Patient-derived xenograft (PDX) models (in which patient-derived tumour material is transplanted into an immunosuppressed mouse) can provide personalized patient avatars allowing specific treatments to be tested. The analysis of circulating free tumour DNA (ctDNA) obtained from patient plasma is a minimally invasive method that can capture the complex spatial and temporal heterogeneity of mCRC. ctDNA has proven to be a reliable means of identifying mCRC patients who could benefit from rechallenging with anti-EGFR therapies, and may furthermore be useful for detecting minimal residual disease in the adjuvant setting (Tie et al., 2016; Sartore-Bianchi et al., 2021).

The process of selecting patients for therapy based on genomic alterations is complex and imperfect due to the heterogeneity of mCRC, clonal cancer evolution, and the existence of intrinsic therapeutic resistance. This complexity is further confounded by the ongoing availability of new biomarkers and novel and expensive molecular tests that can introduce misinterpretation of the data and inappropriate treatment selection. Molecular tumour boards (MTB) are multidisciplinary teams of clinicians and scientists who review each patient's unique characteristics to assist in the interpretation and application of new data, and determine the personalized therapeutic plan for individual patients. In this chapter, we summarize current state-of-the-art precision medicine approaches in the field of mCRC.

Precision medicine technology tools in mCRC

In molecularly selected patients with mCRC, targeted therapy has proven to be both safer and more effective compared with conventional chemotherapy (Kopetz et al., 2019; André et al., 2020). In the context of personalized medicine, these promising therapies make tumour molecular profiling an early priority in the treatment management plan. International guidelines for CRC management include mandatory analysis of *RAS* (*KRAS* and *NRAS*) and *BRAF* status prior to anti-EGFR treatment in metastatic patients (Van Cutsem et al., 2016).

Biomarker technologies are also being continuously improved in parallel with the development of targeted therapies. Sequencing methods have evolved considerably since the 2000s when they focused on specific genes (gene panels), and now implicate whole-exome sequencing (WES) and whole-genome sequencing (WGS). This technological evolution, occurring at a tremendous speed, has allowed us to implement the findings of genetic diagnostics into the therapeutic arena. Current commercial and academic oncogenic panel testing can vary substantially in size from a small number of actionable genes (hotspot panels) to hundreds of genes. However, the harmonization, standardization, economic impact, and interpretation of these new techniques and results remains challenging. Table 17.1 presents the advantages and disadvantages of a single gene vs a multi-gene approach. Although NGS can identify infrequent targetable alterations in mCRC, such as fusions in *NTRK*, *ALK*, *ROS*, or *RET*, the current number of actionable driver events in mCRC remains modest. Clinicians should consider the patient's clinical context (first-line vs refractory), and the available treatments, when choosing the appropriate testing strategy. A number of relevant clinical trials evaluating targeted therapies based on molecular alterations in mCRC have been performed, as summarized in Table 17.2.

Blood-based ctDNA analysis is a minimally invasive and practical tool enabling precision medicine. It can capture tumour heterogeneity more effectively compared to DNA isolated from a biopsy collected from a single tumour site, offering a better representation of the patient's overall disease. Recent data suggest that ctDNA-guided treatment can benefit patients, as demonstrated by the retrospective analysis of the CRICKET trial and the prospective results of the CRONOS trial, showing that re-challenge with an anti-EGFR-containing regimen provides a significant progression-free survival (PFS) benefit to patients with no detected *RAS* mutations at the time of re-challenge (Cremolini et al., 2019; Sartore-Bianchi et al., 2021). Plasma ctDNA can also be used as a tool to detect genomic alterations of interest with a low prevalence in mCRC patients, offering these patients the option to be included in a clinical trial.

Table 17.1 Benefits and challenges of digital PCR vs NGS

	Digital PCR	Next-Generation Sequencing
Pros	Straightforward data interpretation More cost-effective to sequence a low number of targets Short turnaround time Hight sensitivity for genes with low VAF (0.1-0.001%)	Higher discovery power Higher sample throughput No required prior knowledge of mutations Absolute quantification of VAF
Cons	Interrogation of a limited set of variants Almost no discovery power	Time-consuming for sequencing low numbers of targets Extensive bioinformatic support for data interpretation Low sensitivity for genes with low VAF (5-0.1%)

VAF, variant allele frequency.

Table 17.2 Principal molecular biomarkers in mCRC and clinical trials with targeted agents

Biomarker	Clinical trial	Phase	Clinical setting	Description	Outcomes
***KRAS* G12C**	AMG-510 (Hong et al., 2020)	I	Refractory mCRC	42 mCRC patients treated with AMG 510	DCR: 31/42 (74%)
	KRYSTAL-1 (Weiss et al., 2021)	I/II	Refractory mCRC	Adagrasib (46 mCRC patients) +/- cetuximab (32 mCRC patients)	Adagrasib: DCR: 39/45 (87%)/ORR 10/45 (22%) Adagrasib + C: DCR 28/28(100%)/ORR 12/28 (43%)
***BRAF*-V600E**	BEACON (Tabernero et al., 2021)	III	Refractory mCRC	1:1:1 EBC (224 patients) / EC (220 patients) / Control (221 patients): FOLFIRI + C or C + irinotecan	EBC: mOS 9.3 months / EC: mOS 9.3 months Control: mOS 5.9 months
	ANCHOR (Van Cutsem et al., 2021)	II	First-line	Single-arm: E-B-C (41 patients)	mPFS 4.9 months
HER2	HERACLES A (Sartore-Bianchi et al., 2016)	II	HER-2 positive, refractory mCRC	Trastuzumab + lapatinib (27 patients)	ORR 28%, mPFS 4.7 months, mOS 10 months
	DESTINY-CRC01 (Siena et al., 2021)	II	HER-2 positive, refractory mCRC	Cohort A: Trastuzumab-deruxtecan *HER2* IHC3/2+ and ISH+ (53 patients) Cohort B: Trastuzumab-deruxtecan IHC 2+ and ISH - (7 patients) Cohort C: IHC 1+ (18 patients)	Cohort A: ORR 45%/ DCR 83%; Cohort A: mPF and mOS not reached. No responses in cohorts B and C
MSI	KEYNOTE-177 (André et al., 2020)	III	First-line	Pembrolizumab (153 patients) / control (154 patients) chemotherapy standard	mPFS 16.5 months (pembrolizumab) vs 8.2 months (control)
MGMT methylated and MGMT loss by IHC	MAYA (Morano et al., 2022)	II	Refractory mCRC	2 months priming with temozolomide followed by low dose ipilimumab plus nivolumab	mPFS 7.1 months, mOS 18.4 months

DCR: disease control rate. ORR: overall response rate. EBC: encorafenib, cetuximab and binimetinib. EC: encorafenib and cetuximab. C: cetuximab. Wt: wild-type. mPFS: median progression-free survival. mOS: median overall survival. IHC: immunochemistry. ISH: *in situ* hybridization. MGMT: O6-methylguanine-DNA methyltransferase.

Established precision treatments in metastatic colorectal cancer

As precision medicine treatment options expand, clinicians increasingly need to focus on the patient's clinical context (first-line vs refractory), the available targeted treatments, investigational clinical studies, and available resources for genomic testing, when choosing the optimal treatment strategy. Several relevant clinical trials evaluating targeted therapies based on molecular alterations in mCRC have been performed, as summarized in Table 17.2, and the list continues to grow. Below we review the biology and clinical trials of the main areas of targeted therapy development in mCRC precision medicine.

Microsatellite instability

DNA mismatch repair (MMR) is a highly conserved biological system composed of four proteins (MSH2, MSH6, MLH1, and PMS2) that form heterodimers able to recognize and repair erroneous insertion, detection, and misincorporation of bases arising during DNA replication. Defects are associated with genome-wide instability, leading ultimately to cancer. They encompass a wide range of tumours, and account for 15% of all primary CRCs and 5% of mCRC (Cortes-Ciriano et al., 2017). Germline alterations in MMR genes form the basis of Lynch syndrome, which in turn increases the risk of various cancers such as endometrial and colorectal tumours (Li, 2008). Somatic alterations in the MMR system can also be present in sporadic mCRC due to epigenetic silencing of the *MLH1* gene promoter, and are more frequent in *BRAF-V600E* mutated patients (Fang et al., 2014). A deficient MMR (dMMR) system results in the persistence of DNA mismatches in microsatellites and can lead to development of MSI, with the expansion or reduction in the length of repetitive sequences in tumour DNA (Li & Martin, 2016). MSI is thus a phenotypic consequence of dMMR proteins and can be used as an equivalent biomarker for dMMR, together with immunochemistry of MMR proteins (Ma et al., 2018). The accumulation of DNA errors due to dMMR proteins leads to a high accumulation of neoantigens, resulting in stimulation of the immune system, thereby forming the basis for evaluating immunotherapy in MSI mCRC patients (Llosa et al., 2015). Several trials have shown the benefit of immunotherapy in the refractory mCRC setting. The KEYNOTE-164 trial enrolled 124 MSI-H pre-treated mCRC patients, and treatment with pembrolizumab showed an overall response rate (ORR) of 32% and median PFS of 4.1 months, while median overall survival (OS) has not been reached (Le et al., 2020). In the CheckMate-142 study, 74 patients with refractory dMMR mCRC received nivolumab, achieving a 31% ORR and median PFS of 14.3 months (Overman et al., 2017). Combined treatment with nivolumab and ipilimumab gave a higher ORR (55%) but this came at the cost of a higher rate of immune-related adverse events (André et al., 2018). Based on these results, immunotherapy was evaluated in earlier treatment lines. The phase III KEYNOTE-177 trial compared pembrolizumab with standard of care chemotherapy in the first-line setting for MSI mCRC. Pembrolizumab demonstrated superiority over chemotherapy with a median PFS of 16.5 months (vs 8.2 months; hazard ratio (HR) 0.60; 95% confidence interval [CI], 0.45—0.80; $p = 0.0002$), with a non-significant trend towards better OS, albeit in the context of 36% of patients crossing over from chemotherapy to pembrolizumab (André et al., 2020). Based on these results, pembrolizumab is currently recommended as first-line therapy for MSI-H/dMMR mCRC, and the determination of microsatellite status by immunochemistry or PCR is recommended as part of the routine workup of all mCRC patient to detect those who could benefit from immunotherapy (Sepulveda et al., 2017).

RAS mutational status

The *RAS* gene family includes the *HRAS*, *KRAS*, and *NRAS* genes. These cytoplasmic proteins with GTPase activity transfer extracellular stimuli through tyrosine kinase receptors leading to the hydrolysis of GDP (Guanosine 5'-diphosphate) to GTP (Guanosine 5'-triphosphate) on *RAS*, activating the mitogen-activated protein kinase (MAPK) pathway, thus promoting cell growth, differentiation, proliferation, and survival (Prior et al., 2014). *KRAS* is mutated in 40% of mCRC cases, mostly in exon 2, and confers a worse prognosis compared to wild-type tumours (Yokota, 2012; Schirripa et al., 2015). *RAS* mutations play a critical role in clinical practice due to their status as a negative predictive biomarker for response to the EGFR inhibitors cetuximab and panitumumab. Several clinical trials involving cetuximab and panitumumab have shown that not only mutations in *KRAS* exon 2 but also mutations in exons 3 and 4, and also exons 2, 3, and 4 of *NRAS* (expanded *RAS* analysis) are associated with a poor response to anti-EGFR monoclonal antibodies (Bokemeyer et al., 2015; Douillard et al., 2013; Van Cutsem et al., 2019). International guidelines thus recommend up front *RAS* mutational status testing (Van Cutsem et al., 2016), and both panitumumab and cetuximab are currently restricted by the European Medicines Agency (EMA) to patients with *RAS* wild-type mCRC. Of note, *RAS* mutations do not systematically lead to anti-EGFR resistance. An optimal allele fraction (AF) cut-off has been established to identify those tumours harbouring mutations more prone to respond to an anti-EGFR therapy. In a retrospective analysis of the CRYSTAL trial, patients with a *RAS* AF $< 5\%$ who received cetuximab benefited in terms of OS compared with patients with AF $\geq 5\%$ (Van Cutsem et al., 2019). Other studies suggest that patients with low AF could obtain clinical benefit if the anti-EGFR is combined with chemotherapy, in both the first-line and refractory scenarios (Santos et al., 2019). ctDNA analyses have shown that *KRAS* mutant clones, originally present at subclonal levels, increase under anti-EGFR pressure and decline after anti-EGFR withdrawal in cases of acquired resistance to anti-EGFR agents (Siravegna et al., 2015).

Despite significant efforts, *RAS* mutations have remained an undruggable target for many years. In recent breakthroughs, a few targeted agents have demonstrated clinical activity against *KRAS* G12C mutations, which represents 3% of mCRC. The mutant cysteine of *KRAS* G12C is located close to a pocket related to the inactive GDP-bound form of KRAS. Sotorasib (AMG 510) is a first-in-class small molecule that specifically and irreversibly blocks the kinase by locking it in an inactive GDP-bound site. Interestingly, in the phase I trial with sotorasib monotherapy, four out of 15 patients achieved response (Hong et al., 2020). Acquired mechanisms of resistance to *KRAS* G12C inhibitors include *KRAS* G12C and *MET* amplification, activating mutations (*NRAS*, *BRAF*, *MAP2K1*, and *RET*), oncogenic fusions (*ALK*, *RET*, *BRAF*, *RAF1*, and *FGFR3*), loss-of-function mutations in *NF1* and *PTEN*, and the *KRAS* switch-II pocket mutation

(Awad et al., 2021; Tanaka et al., 2021). However, with EGFR signalling mutations being the dominant mechanism of CRC resistance to *KRAS* G12C inhibitors, the concomitant inhibition of both EGFR and *KRAS* G12C signalling has overcome intrinsic resistance to *KRAS* G12C blockade in monotherapy CRC.

KRSTYAL-1 is a multicohort phase I/II study that evaluated the *KRAS* G12C inhibitor adagrasib (MRTX849) (Weiss et al., 2021a). In this trial, 78 patients with previously treated CRC received adagrasib as monotherapy (46 patients) or in combination with cetuximab (32 patients). Among patients who received adagrasib monotherapy, the ORR was 22%, disease control rate (DCR) was 87%, and median PFS was 5.6 months. For the 28 evaluable patients treated with the combination of adagrasib and cetuximab, the ORR was 43%, the DCR was 100%, and median PFS has not yet been reached (Weiss et al., 2021a). The ORR with sotorasib-panitumumab was 17% with a DCR of 83% (Canon et al., 2019; Weiss et al., 2021b). KRYSTAL-10 is a phase III trial in the second-line setting comparing the combination of adagrasib-cetuximab with FOLFOX or FOLFIRI, and is currently recruiting (NCT04793958). Other trials targeting *KRAS* G12C that are currently recruiting include the phase I/Ib trial combining adagrasib plus BI1701963 (pan-KRAS SOS1 inhibitor; NCT04975256), and a phase I/II trial combining adagrasib with or without pembrolizumab, cetuximab, or afatinib for all solid tumours (NCT03785249).

BRAF-V600E mutational status

The *BRAF-V600E* mutation represents more than 90% of mutations in *BRAF* mutated tumours (Cantwell-Dorris et al., 2011), and has been described in up to 15% of patients with mCRC (Loupakis et al., 2009; Tie et al., 2011). This exon 15 mutation causes a valine amino acid substitution (V600E), conferring a significantly worse prognosis than wild-type patients. *BRAF-V600E* tumours are characterized by a particular phenotype including older age at diagnosis, female sex, proximal colon tumours, poorer differentiation, and mucinous histology (Ogino et al., 2006; Clancy et al., 2013; Gonsalves et al., 2014). Molecularly, *BRAF* mutations are almost always mutually exclusive with *RAS* mutations and approximately 20% of patients with *BRAF-V600E* mutant mCRC are MSI-high (MSI-H)/dMMR (Venderbosch et al., 2014). Prior to the current target therapy scenario, subgroup analyses suggested benefit is seen with aggressive frontline triplet-based chemotherapy in combination with anti-VEGF therapies (Cremolini et al., 205; Van Cutsem et al., 2012). Despite this benefit from triplet-based chemotherapy in combination with an anti-VEGF, data from the TRIBE-2 trial evaluating up-front exposure to the three cytotoxic drugs compared with a pre-planned sequential strategy of doublets, demonstrated that the *BRAF* subgroup does not benefit from the intensive approach. Furthermore, a meta-analysis of individual patient data with FOLFOXIRI-bevacizumab vs doublets plus bevacizumab showed no increased benefit in terms of OS among this subgroup (Cremolini et al., 2020). Thus, the use of FOLFOXIRI-bevacizumab should be individualized when considered for up-front therapy for *BRAF-V600E* tumours.

Unlike other tumoural types driven by a *BRAF-V600* mutation such as melanoma, BRAF inhibitors in monotherapy produced only marginal clinical activity in *BRAF-V600E* mutant colon cancer with response rates less than 5% (Hyman et al., 2015; Kopetz et al., 2015; Prahallad et al., 2012). *In vitro* studies demonstrated that inhibition of a single node in the MAPK pathway results in adaptive feedback reactivation of MAPK signalling mediated by EGFR activation, allowing sustained MAPK activation and continued cell proliferation. This supported that an anti-EGFR should be included together with a BRAF inhibitor to improve clinical activity. Subsequent studies combining BRAF inhibitors (vemurafenib or dabrafenib) with an EGFR monoclonal antibody, and a MEK inhibitor (trametinib) to achieve better MAPK suppression confirmed the synergic effect of these combinations (Gomez-Roca et al., 2014; Kopetz et al., 2015; Planchard et al., 2016; Corcoran et al., 2018). Indeed, confirmed response rates for dabrafenib plus trametinib, dabrafenib plus trametinib and panitumumab, and trametinib plus panitumumab were 10%, 21%, and 0%, respectively (Corcoran et al., 2010; Corcoran et al., 2018). These results suggested that the greater the inhibition of the MAPK pathway, the greater the anti-tumour activity achieved. Likewise, a triple pathway blockade phase Ib trial targeting *PIK3CA*, suggests that stronger inhibition of the pathway could produce deeper responses. This trial evaluated the combination of encorafenib and cetuximab with or without alpelisib. ORRs were 19% and 18% respectively, and median PFS was 3.7 and 4.2 months, respectively (Van Geel et al., 2017). BRAF inhibitors have also been tested in combination with chemotherapy in the SWOG1406 trial (Kopetzet al., 2021), where *BRAF*-mutant CRC patients were randomized to receive irinotecan plus cetuximab with or without vemurafenib. An ORR of 17% was reported with the triplet combination compared with 4% for the doublet. Double BRAF and EGFR inhibition using vemurafenib and panitumumab showed poor responses (Yaeger et al., 2015).

The BEACON trial has been the most meaningful step forward in the targeted therapy landscape of BRAF mCRC. This phase III trial compared double combination vs triple combination vs standard chemotherapy, and established a new standard of care. Refractory *BRAF-V600E* CRC patients were randomized to encorafenib plus cetuximab with or without binimetinib, or irinotecan/cetuximab-based chemotherapy (Kopetz et al., 2019). Updated results from the trial reported a median OS of 9.3 months for both the triplet and the doublet arms, compared with 5.9 months for patients who received chemotherapy (Tabernero et al., 2021). Based on this efficacy and a more tolerable toxicity profile, the doublet has been recommended as a new standard of care by both the US Food and Drug Administration (FDA) and the EMA. After the initial results from the safety lead-in of the BEACON trial, where the triplet appeared to be more effective than the doublet, the single-arm ANCHOR trial was designed, moving the triplet combination to the first-line. However, the results were disappointing with a confirmed ORR of 50% and median PFS of 4.9 months (Van Cutsem et al., 2021). Currently, the BREAKWATER trial (NCT04607421) is comparing the combination of encorafenib-cetuximab plus chemotherapy, encorafenib-cetuximab, or standard chemotherapy in the first-line setting. However, not all patients will respond and some responses are relatively short. These studies demonstrate that understanding mechanisms of resistance against BRAF inhibitor combinations is important for developing new therapies (Ros et al., 2021). In a small cohort of patients treated with a BRAF inhibitor plus an anti-EGFR with or without a MEK inhibitor, polysomy of chromosome 7 (which includes the *EGFR*, *MET*, and *BRAF* genes) was significantly associated with clinical benefit under BRAF-targeted therapy. *RNF43* somatic mutations were enriched in responders to BRAF inhibitor combination therapies, suggesting that differential activation of the

Wtn/beta-catenin pathway might underlie differential sensitivity to BRAF inhibitors (Élez et al., 2021). Finally, in an effort to improve response and overcome resistance, a phase II study evaluated dual BRAF and MEK inhibition with dabrafenib and trametinib respectively, combined with the anti-PD-1 spartalizumab, giving an ORR of 35% and a DCR of 75% (Corcoran et al., 2020). This provided evidence that the combination of BRAF inhibitors and anti-EGFR plus immune checkpoint inhibitors has demonstrated promising results (Corcoran et al., 2020; Morris et al., 2022).

HER2 amplification

Amplification of the human epidermal growth factor receptor 2 (*HER2, ERBB2*) gene has been observed in approximately 3% to 4% of all mCRC patients, and is enriched in the *RAS* wild-type population, where it has been reported in up to 8% of patients (Valtorta et al., 2015). Interestingly, it has been demonstrated that the *HER2* pathway is more commonly amplified in distal tumours compared to proximal tumours (Seo et al., 2014). Despite the lack of prospective clinical trials, evidence suggests that *HER2* amplification represents a negative predictive biomarker to response for anti-EGFR therapies (Bertotti et al., 2011), while evidence from diverse prospective clinical trials supports the positive predictive value of targeting *HER2*. The single-arm phase II HERACLES trial evaluated the combination of trastuzumab plus lapatinib in refractory HER2 amplified mCRC, showing a response rate of 30% (Sartore-Bianchiet al., 2016b). In the non-randomized phase IIa multiple basket MyPathway study, patients with refractory mCRC harbouring *HER2* amplification received pertuzumab plus trastuzumab, achieving a meaningful ORR of 38% (Meric-Bernstam et al., 2019). The MOUNTAINEER trial explored the combination of tucatinib (a selective anti-*HER2* tyrosine kinase inhibitor) plus trastuzumab, presenting a preliminary ORR of 55% (Strickler et al., 2019). Due to this impressive result in a molecularly selected refractory mCRC population, novel agents are being tested in this setting. The DESTINY-CRC01 trial is evaluating the role of trastuzumab-deruxtecan in *HER2* -amplified, *RAS/BRAF* wild-type refractory mCRC. The trial included patients previously treated with anti-*HER2* combinations. Among patients with *HER2* -positive immunohistochemistry (IHC) 3+ or IHC2+ with *in situ* hybridization (ISH)-positive tumours, the ORR was 45%, with a median PFS of 4.1 months while median OS was not reached (Siena et al., 2021). These data support evaluation of *HER2* inhibition in mCRC, particularly among patients with left-sided, *RAS/BRAF* wild-type tumours.

PI3KCA mutations

Phosphatidylinositol 3-kinase (PI3K) is a member of the intracellular lipid kinase family. PI3K and its downstream effectors, AKT and mTOR, are involved in the regulation of cellular proliferation, differentiation, and survival (Vanhaesebroeck et al., 2012). Over-expression of the PI3K/Akt/mTOR signalling pathway has been reported in various indications, especially in mCRC (Slattery et al., 2018). Due to the known driver role of PIK3CA in the initiation and progression events of CRC, PI3K is recognized as a key therapeutic target. The first in-human phase Ia trial of alpelisib as monotherapy included 35 patients with mCRC, presenting a DCR of 34% (Juric et al., 2018). In a phase I basket study, monotherapy with the PI3K inhibitor taselisib in patients with *PIK3CA*-mutated mCRC resulted in one partial response among 10 patients (Jhaveri et al., 2018). The predictive role of *PIK3CA* mutations for outcome in anti-EGFR treated patients with mCRC is unclear. *PIK3CA* and *KRAS* mutations have been described as predictive primary resistance markers for EGFR inhibition, where *PIK3CA* mutations explain a lack of response in 17% of *KRAS* wild-type mCRC patients (Sartore-Bianchi et al., 2009). Furthermore, emerging *PIK3CA* mutations in mCRC patients treated with cetuximab have been detected using ctDNA (Khan et al., 2018). Notwithstanding, clinical results from the CALGB 80405 trial showed that *RAS* and *BRAF* mutations, but not *PIK3CA* mutations, were associated with worse outcome in cetuximab-treated patients (Innocenti et al., 2019). Clinical trials evaluating the combination of PI3K and EGFR inhibitors are ongoing (NCT04929223, NCT04495621).

Other biomarkers

RET rearrangements

RET rearrangements have been described in a wide variety of solid tumours (Li et al., 2019). In CRC, *RET* fusions are described in a small percentage of patients (0.2%), mostly in right-sided, *RAS* and *BRAF* wild-type tumours, and confer a worse prognosis compared with patients without *RET* fusions (14 vs 38 months) (Pietrantonio et al., 2018). Primary resistance to anti-EGFR blockade in *RAS* and *BRAF* wild-type CRC over-expressing RET has been observed in preclinical models (Medico et al., 2015) and selective therapies for this subpopulation, such as the VEGFR-sparing RET inhibitors BLU-667 and LOXO-292, are currently under development. Enrolment in trials with RET inhibitors for patients with tumours harbouring *RET* alterations is highly encouraged when possible.

NTRK fusions

NTRK fusions have been reported at a low frequency in a wide range of tumours, including CRC tumours (< 0.5%) (Stransky et al., 2014). Molecularly driven therapy with the selective TRK inhibitor larotrectinib and multikinase inhibitors with activity against these fusion proteins (BAY2731954, entrectinib, repotrectinib, crizotinib, cabozantinib, altiratinib, foretinib, ponatinib, nintedanib, merestinib, BAY2731, MGCD516, PLX7486, DS-6051b, and TSR-011) have been tested in selected populations with *NTRK* fusions, including patients with mCRC (Demetri et al., 2018; Drilon et al., 2017; Drilon et al., 2018; Siena et al., 2019; Sartore-Bianchi et al., 2016a). Subgroup analyses of data from patients with gastrointestinal cancers receiving either larotrectinib or entrectinib showed a lower response rate than in the global population, although CRC-specific statistical analyses cannot be performed due to the modest number of patients (four for each pooled analysis). In November 2018, the FDA granted accelerated tissue-agnostic approval to larotrectinib for solid tumours with *NTRK* gene fusions.

MGMT methylation

Since O6-methylguanine–DNA methyltransferase (MGMT) promoter methylation is a key enzyme involved in DNA damage repair induced by alkylating agents, epigenetic MGMT silencing represents a mechanism of synthetic lethality after exposure to temozolomide. MGMT methylation is found in around 40% of CRC cases, however dacarbazine and its oral analogue temozolomide yielded modest activity in selected patients with MGMT-methylated mCRC, with an ORR of 10% (Amatu et al., 2013; Hochhauser et al., 2013; Pietrantonio et al., 2014). Acquired resistance to temozolomide may be associated with the onset of hypermutation. Thus, the induction of hypermutation by a temozolomide-priming treatment provides the rationale for immune-sensitization of pMMR/MSS, MGMT-silenced mCRC. The MAYA trial included patients with mCRC MSS and MGMT silencing tumours (Morano et al., 2022). Patients received two priming cycles of oral temozolomide followed, in the absence of progression, by its combination with ipilimumab and nivolumab. Overall, 24% of the patients did not progress after temozolomide induction and therefore received subsequent nivolumab plus ipilimumab. The ORR was 45% with a median PFS of 7.0 months and median OS of 18.4 months suggesting that a sequence of temozolomide priming followed by immune checkpoint inhibitors may induce durable clinical benefit in MSS and MGMT-silenced mCRC.

Conclusions and future directions

Our rapidly increasing genomic understanding of the heterogenic complexity of CRC has led to major advances in the last few years, with the definition of the main drivers responsible for intrinsic and acquired resistance to standard and biological treatments. These advances in the genomic landscape underlying CRC biology have translated into clinical benefit for our patients. Undoubtedly, many issues remain to be addressed, such as inter- and intra-tumour heterogeneity across various CRC subgroups, that limit the translation of clinical transcriptomic classification into predictive biomarkers.

Although the number of biomarker-based treatment options has seen impressive increases over the last decade, a high percentage of patients are still excluded from this personalized approach. In this regard, preclinical models of CRC tumours are of capital importance to help identify new biomarkers and new targeted agents. This bidirectional flow of information between preclinical models and patients has proven successful in the development and optimization of targeted therapies for patients with CRC.

The precision medicine approach provides an effective paradigm that should guide the development of the next generation of clinical trials, and will ultimately lead to better treatments for more patients with CRC. Although biomarker-guided treatment options for patients with primary CRCs remain limited, this field is continuously evolving. Most established biomarkers are found at a low prevalence, however the number of biomarkers is increasing and in this respect, CRC could be considered an 'umbrella diagnosis' encompassing numerous rare disease subtypes. Balancing this, the range of treatment options based on biomarker selection needs to be extended to a larger number of patients (e.g. immunotherapy strategies for 'cold tumours' not only for MSI tumours) and analysis of the principal drivers of resistance to treatment is critical at the time of the diagnosis of metastatic disease and throughout the subsequent disease course to personalize the treatment approach as the patient's disease history evolves.

When feasible, comprehensive genomic tests should be performed to identify rare fusions, known to be enriched in *RAS/BRAF* wild-type MSI right-sided tumours. Likewise, NGS analysis for a multitarget approach is more widely used and allows better tumour characterization which may lead to either personalized therapies or enrolment in a clinical trial. However, the future revolution in mCRC treatment will be not only to expand the use of accurate genome tests but also to integrate genomic, transcriptomic, and immune-stromal characteristics of the tumour to eliminate meaningless biomarkers and guarantee innovative effective therapeutic strategies.

REFERENCES

Amatu, A., Sartore-Bianchi, A., Moutinho, C., et al. (2013). Promoter CpG island hypermethylation of the DNA repair enzyme MGMT predicts clinical response to dacarbazine in a phase II study for metastatic colorectal cancer. *Clinical Cancer Research*, *19*(8), 2265–2272.

André, T., Lonardi, S., Wong, M., et al. (2018). Nivolumab + ipilimumab combination in patients with DNA mismatch repair-deficient/microsatellite instability-high (dMMR/MSI-H) metastatic colorectal cancer (mCRC): first report of the full cohort from CheckMate-142. *Journal of Clinical Oncology*, *36*(4_suppl), 553–553.

André, T., Shiu, K.-K., Kim, T. W., et al. (2020). Pembrolizumab in microsatellite-instability-high advanced colorectal cancer. *New England Journal of Medicine*, *383*(23), 2207–2218.

Awad, M. M., Liu, S., Rybkin, I. I., et al. (2021). Acquired resistance to KRAS G12C inhibition in cancer. *New England Journal of Medicine*, *384*(25), 2382–2393.

Bertotti, A., Migliardi, G., Galimi, F., et al. (2011). A molecularly annotated platform of patient-derived xenografts ('xenopatients') identifies HER2 as an effective therapeutic target in cetuximab-resistant colorectal cancer. *Cancer Discovery*, *1*(6), 508–523.

Bokemeyer, C., Köhne, C.-H., Ciardiello, F., et al. (2015). FOLFOX4 plus cetuximab treatment and RAS mutations in colorectal cancer. *European Journal of Cancer*, *51*(10), 1243–1252.

Canon, J., Rex, K., Saiki, A. Y., et al. (2019). The clinical KRAS(G12C) inhibitor AMG 510 drives anti-tumour immunity. *Nature*, *575*(7781), 217–223.

Cantwell-Dorris, E. R., O'Leary, J. J., & Sheils, O. M. (2011). BRAFV600E: implications for carcinogenesis and molecular therapy. *Molecular Cancer Therapeutics*, *10*(3), 385–394.

Clancy, C., Burke, J. P., & Kalady, M. F. (2013). BRAF mutation is associated with distinct clinicopathological characteristics in colorectal cancer: a systematic review and meta-analysis. *Colorectal Disease*, *15*(12), e711–718.

Corcoran, R. B., André, T., Atreya, C. E., et al. (2018). Combined BRAF, EGFR, and MEK inhibition in patients with BRAF V600E-mutant colorectal cancer. *Cancer Discovery*, *8*(4), 428–443.

Corcoran, R. B., Dias-Santagata, D., Bergethon, K., et al. (2010). BRAF gene amplification can promote acquired resistance to MEK inhibitors in cancer cells harboring the BRAF V600E mutation. *Science Signalling*, *23*, *3*(149), ra84.

Corcoran, R., Giannakis, M., Allen, J., et al. (2020). SO-26 clinical efficacy of combined BRAF, MEK, and PD-1 inhibition in BRAFV600E colorectal cancer patients. *Annals of Oncology*, *31*(226–227), S226–227.

Cortes-Ciriano, I., Lee, S., Park, W. Y., et al. (2017). A molecular portrait of microsatellite instability across multiple cancers. *Nature Communication*, *8*(1), 1–12.

Cremolini, C., Antoniotti, C., Stein, A., et al. (2020). Individual patient data meta-analysis of FOLFOXIRI plus bevacizumab versus doublets plus bevacizumab as initial therapy of unresectable metastatic colorectal cancer. *Journal of Clinical Oncology*,.

Cremolini, C., Loupakis, F., Antoniotti, C., et al. (2015). FOLFOXIRI plus bevacizumab versus FOLFIRI plus bevacizumab as first-line treatment of patients with metastatic colorectal cancer: Updated overall survival and molecular subgroup analyses of the open-label, phase 3 TRIBE study. *Lancet Oncology*, *16*(13), 1306–1315.

Cremolini, C., Rossini, D., Dell'Aquila, E., et al. (2019). Rechallenge for patients with RAS and BRAF wild-type metastatic colorectal cancer with acquired resistance to first-line cetuximab and irinotecan: a phase 2 single-arm clinical trial. *JAMA Oncology*, *5*(3), 343–350.

Demetri, G. D., Paz-Ares, L., Farago, A. F., et al. (2018). LBA17 efficacy and safety of entrectinib in patients with NTRK fusion-positive (NTRK-fp) tumors: pooled analysis of STARTRK-2, STARTRK-1 and ALKA-372-001. *Annals of Oncology*, *29*(suppl_8).

Drilon, A., Laetsch, T. W., Kummar, S., et al. (2018). Efficacy of larotrectinib in TRK fusion–positive cancers in adults and children. *New England Journal of Medicine*, *378*(8), 731–739.

Drilon, A., Siena, S., Ou, S.-H. I., et al. (2017). Safety and antitumor activity of the multitargeted pan-TRK, ROS1, and ALK inhibitor entrectinib: combined results from two phase I trials (ALKA-372-001 and STARTRK-1). *Cancer Discovery*, *7*(4), 400–409.

Élez, E., Ros, J., Martini, G., et al. (2021). LBA-3 Integrated analysis of cell-free DNA (cfDNA) BRAF mutant allele fraction (MAF) and whole exome sequencing in BRAFV600E metastatic colorectal cancer (mCRC) treated with BRAF-antiEGFR +/– MEK inhibitors. *Annals of Oncology*, *32*, S226–227.

Fang, M., Ou, J., Hutchinson, L., & Green, M. R. (2014). The BRAF oncoprotein functions through the transcriptional repressor MAFG to mediate the CpG island methylator phenotype. *Molecular Cell*, *55*(6), 904–915.

Gomez-Roca, C. A., Delord, J., Robert, C., et al. (2014). Encorafenib (Lgx818), an oral BRAF inhibitor, in patients (Pts) with BRAF V600E metastatic colorectal cancer (MCRC): results of dose expansion in an open-label, phase 1 study. *Annals of Oncology*, *25*:iv182.

Gonsalves, W. I., Mahoney, M. R., Sargent, D. J., et al. (2014). Patient and tumor characteristics and BRAF and KRAS mutations in colon cancer, NCCTG/Alliance N0147. *Journal of the National Cancer Institute*, *106*(7), 1–8.

Grady, W. M., & Carethers, J. M. (2008). Genomic and epigenetic instability in colorectal cancer pathogenesis. *Gastroenterology*, *135*(4), 1079.

Hochhauser, D., Glynne-Jones, R., Potter, V., et al. (2013). A phase II study of temozolomide in patients with advanced aerodigestive tract and colorectal cancers and methylation of the O 6-methylguanine-DNA methyltransferase promoter. *Molecular Cancer Therapeutics*, *12*(5), 809–818.

Hong, D. S., Fakih, M. G., Strickler, J. H., et al. (2020). KRAS G12C inhibition with sotorasib in advanced solid tumors. *New England Journal of Medicine*, *383*(13), 1207–1217.

Hyman, D. M., Diamond, E. L., Baselga, J., et al. (2015). Vemurafenib in multiple nonmelanoma cancers with BRAF V600 mutations. *New England Journal of Medicine*, *373*(8), 726–736.

Innocenti, F., Ou, F.-S., Qu, X., et al. (2019). Mutational analysis of patients with colorectal cancer in CALGB/SWOG 80405 identifies new roles of microsatellite instability and tumor mutational burden for patient outcome. *Journal of Clinical Oncology*, *37*(14), 1217–1227.

Jhaveri, K., Juric, D., Saura, C., et al. (2018). Abstract CT046: A phase I basket study of the PI3K inhibitor taselisib (GDC-0032) in PIK3CA-mutated locally advanced or metastatic solid tumors. *Cancer Research*, *78*(13_Supplement), CT046.

Juric, D., Rodon, J., Tabernero, J., et al. (2018). Phosphatidylinositol 3-kinase α-selective inhibition with alpelisib (BYL719) in PIK3CA-altered solid tumors: results from the first-in-human study. *Journal of Clinical Oncology*, *36*(13), 1291–1299.

Khan, K. H., Cunningham, D., Werner, B., et al. (2018). Longitudinal liquid biopsy and mathematical modeling of clonal evolution forecast time to treatment failure in the prospect-c phase ii colorectal cancer clinical trial. *Cancer Discovery*, *8*(10), 1270–1285.

Kopetz, S., Desai, J., Chan, E., et al. (2015). Phase II pilot study of vemurafenib in patients with metastatic BRAF-mutated colorectal cancer. *Journal of Clinical Oncology*, *33*(34), 4032–4038.

Kopetz, S., Grothey, A., Yaeger, R., et al. (2019). Encorafenib, binimetinib, and cetuximab in BRAF V600E-mutated colorectal cancer. *New England Journal of Medicine*, *381*(17), 1632–1643. https://doi.org/101056/NEJMoa1908075

Kopetz, S., Guthrie, K. A., Morris, V. K., et al. (2021). Randomized trial of irinotecan and cetuximab with or without vemurafenib in BRAF-mutant metastatic colorectal cancer (SWOG S1406). *Journal of Clinical Oncology*, *39*(4), 285–294.

Le, D. T., Kim, T. W., Van Cutsem, E., et al. (2020). Phase II open-label study of pembrolizumab in treatment-refractory, microsatellite instability-high/mismatch repair-deficient metastatic colorectal cancer: KEYNOTE-164. *Journal of Clinical Oncology*, *38*(1), 11–19.

Li, A. Y., McCusker, M. G., Russo, A., et al. (2019). RET fusions in solid tumors. *Cancer Treatment Reviews*, *81*, 101911.

Li, G.-M. (2008). Mechanisms and functions of DNA mismatch repair. *Cell Research*, *18*, 85–98.

Li, S. K. H., & Martin, A. (2016). Mismatch repair and colon cancer: mechanisms and therapies explored. *Trends in Molecular Medicine*, *22*(4), 274–289.

Llosa, N. J., Cruise, M., Tam, A., et al. (2015). The vigorous immune microenvironment of microsatellite instable colon cancer is balanced by multiple counter-inhibitory checkpoints. *Cancer Discovery*, *5*(1), 43–51.

Loupakis, F., Ruzzo, A., Cremolini, C., et al. (2009). KRAS codon 61, 146 and BRAF mutations predict resistance to cetuximab plus irinotecan in KRAS codon 12 and 13 wild-type metastatic colorectal cancer. *British Journal of Cancer*, *101*(4), 715–721.

Ma, J., Setton, J., Lee, N. Y., et al. (2018). The therapeutic significance of mutational signatures from DNA repair deficiency in cancer. *Nature Communication*, *9*(1), 1–12.

Medico, E., Russo, M., Picco, G., et al. (2015). The molecular landscape of colorectal cancer cell lines unveils clinically actionable kinase targets. *Nature Communication*, *6*(1), 7002.

Meric-Bernstam, F., Hurwitz, H., Raghav, K. P. S., et al. (2019). Pertuzumab plus trastuzumab for HER2-amplified metastatic colorectal cancer (MyPathway): an updated report from a multicentre, open-label, phase 2a, multiple basket study. *Lancet Oncology*, *20*(4), 518–530.

Misale, S., Di Nicolantonio, F., Sartore-Bianchi, A., et al. (2014). Resistance to anti-EGFR therapy in colorectal cancer: from heterogeneity to convergent evolution. *Cancer Discovery*, *4*(11), 1269–1280.

Morano, F., Raimondi, A., Pagani, F., et al. (2022). Temozolomide followed by combination with low-dose ipilimumab and nivolumab in patients with microsatellite-stable, O 6 -Methylguanine–DNA methyltransferase–silenced metastatic colorectal cancer: the MAYA trial. *Journal of Clinical Oncology*, *8*, 1–13.

Morris, V. K., Parseghian, C. M., Escano, M., et al. (2022). Phase I/II trial of encorafenib, cetuximab, and nivolumab in patients with microsatellite stable, BRAF V600E metastatic colorectal cancer. *Journal of Clinical Oncology*, *40*(4_suppl), 12–12.

Ogino, S., Brahmandam, M., Cantor, M., et al. (2006). Distinct molecular features of colorectal carcinoma with signet ring cell component and colorectal carcinoma with mucinous component. *Modern Pathology*, *19*(1), 59–68.

Overman, M. J., McDermott, R., Leach, J. L., et al. (2017). Nivolumab in patients with metastatic DNA mismatch repair-deficient or microsatellite instability-high colorectal cancer (CheckMate 142): an open-label, multicentre, phase 2 study. *Lancet Oncology*, *18*(9), 1182–1191.

Pietrantonio, F., Di Nicolantonio, F., Schrock, A. B., et al. (2018). RET fusions in a small subset of advanced colorectal cancers at risk of being neglected. *Annals of Oncology*, *29*(6), 1394–1401.

Pietrantonio, F., Perrone, F., de Braud, F., et al. (2014). Activity of temozolomide in patients with advanced chemorefractory colorectal cancer and MGMT promoter methylation. *Annals of Oncology*, *25*(2), 404–408.

Planchard, D., Besse, B., Groen, H. J. M., et al. (2016). Dabrafenib plus trametinib in patients with previously treated BRAFV600E-mutant metastatic non-small cell lung cancer: an open-label, multicentre phase 2 trial. *Lancet Oncology*, *17*(7), 984–993.

Prahallad, A., Sun, C., Huang, S., et al. (2012). Unresponsiveness of colon cancer to BRAF(V600E) inhibition through feedback activation of EGFR. *Nature*, *483*(7387), 100–103.

Prior, I. A., Lewis, P. D., & Mattos, C. (2012). A comprehensive survey of RASs mutations in cancer. 2457–2468.

Ros, J., Saoudi, N., Salvà, F., et al. (2022). Ongoing and evolving clinical trials enhancing future colorectal cancer treatment strategies. *Expert Opinion on Investigational Drugs, Feb*, 1–13.

Ros, J., Baraibar, I., Sardo, E., et al. (2021). BRAF, MEK and EGFR inhibition as treatment strategies in BRAF V600E metastatic colorectal cancer. *Therapeutic Advances in Medical Oncology*, *13*:175883592199297.

Santos, C., Azuara, D., Viéitez, J. M., et al. (2019). Phase II study of high-sensitivity genotyping of KRAS, NRAS, BRAF and PIK3CA to ultra-select metastatic colorectal cancer patients for panitumumab plus FOLFIRI: the ULTRA trial. *Annals of Oncology*, *30*(5), 796–803.

Sartore-Bianchi, A., Ardini, E., Bosotti, R., et al. (2016a). Sensitivity to entrectinib associated with a novel LMNA-NTRK1 gene fusion in metastatic colorectal cancer. *Journal of the National Cancer Institute*, *108*(1).

Sartore-Bianchi, A., Martini, M., Molinari, F., et al. (2009). PIK3CA mutations in colorectal cancer are associated with clinical resistance to EGFR-targeted monoclonal antibodies. *Cancer Research*, *69*(5), 1851–1857.

Sartore-Bianchi, A., Pietrantonio, F., Lonardi, S., et al. (2021). Phase II study of anti-EGFR rechallenge therapy with panitumumab driven by circulating tumor DNA molecular selection in metastatic colorectal cancer: The CHRONOS trial. *Journal of Clinical Oncology*, *39*(15_suppl), 3506–3506.https://doi.org/101200/JCO20213915_suppl3506

Sartore-Bianchi, A., Trusolino, L., Martino, C., et al. (2016b). Dual-targeted therapy with trastuzumab and lapatinib in treatment-refractory, KRAS codon 12/13 wild-type, HER2-positive metastatic colorectal cancer (HERACLES): a proof-of-concept, multicentre, open-label, phase 2 trial. *Lancet Oncology*, *17*(6), 738–746.

Schirripa, M., Cremolini, C., Loupakis, F., et al. Role of NRAS mutations as prognostic and predictive markers in metastatic colorectal cancer. *International Journal of Cancer*, *136*(7), 83–90.

Seo, A. N., Kwak, Y., Kim, D. W., et al. (2014). HER2 status in colorectal cancer: its clinical significance and the relationship between HER2 gene amplification and expression. *PLoS One*, *9*(5), e98528.

Sepulveda, A. R., Hamilton, S. R., Allegra, C. J., et al. (2017). Molecular biomarkers for the evaluation of colorectal cancer: guideline from the American Society for Clinical Pathology, College of American Pathologists, Association for Molecular Pathology, and the American Society of Clinical Oncology. *Journal of Clinical Oncology*, *35*(13), 1453–1486.

Siegel, R. L., Miller, K. D., & Jemal, A. Cancer statistics, 2020. (2020). *CA Cancer Journal for Clinicians*, *70*(1), 7–30.

Siena, S., Di Bartolomeo, M., Raghav, K., et al. (2021). Trastuzumab deruxtecan (DS-8201) in patients with HER2-expressing metastatic colorectal cancer (DESTINY-CRC01): a multicentre, open-label, phase 2 trial. *Lancet Oncology*, *22*(6), 779–789.

Siena, S., Doebele, R. C., Shaw, A. T., et al. (2019). Efficacy of entrectinib in patients (pts) with solid tumors and central nervous system (CNS) metastases: Integrated analysis from three clinical trials. *Journal of Clinical Oncology*, *37*(15_suppl), 3017–3017.

Siravegna, G., Mussolin, B., Buscarino, M., et al. (2015). Clonal evolution and resistance to EGFR blockade in the blood of colorectal cancer patients. *Nature Medicine*, *21*(7), 795–801.

Slattery, M. L., Mullany, L. E., Sakoda, L. C., et al. (2018). The PI3K/AKT signaling pathway: Associations of miRNAs with dysregulated gene expression in colorectal cancer. *Molecular Carcinogenesis*, *57*(2), 243–261.

Stransky, N., Cerami, E., Schalm, S., et al. (2014). The landscape of kinase fusions in cancer. *Nature Communication*, *5*(1), 4846.

Strickler, J. H., Zemla, T., Ou, F.-S., et al. (2019). Trastuzumab and tucatinib for the treatment of HER2 amplified metastatic colorectal cancer (mCRC): initial results from the MOUNTAINEER trial. *Annals of Oncology*, *30*, v200.

Sung, H., Ferlay, J., Siegel, R. L., et al. (2021). Global Cancer Statistics 2020: GLOBOCAN estimates of incidence and mortality worldwide for 36 cancers in 185 countries. *CA Cancer Journal for Clinicians*, *71*(3), 209–249.

Tabernero, J., Grothey, A., Van Cutsem, E., et al. (2021). Encorafenib plus cetuximab as a new standard of care for previously treated BRAF V600E–mutant metastatic colorectal cancer: updated survival results and subgroup analyses from the BEACON study. *Journal of Clinical Oncology*, *39*(4), 273–284.

Tanaka, N., Lin, J. J., Li, C., et al. (2021). Clinical acquired resistance to KRAS G12C inhibition through a novel KRAS Switch-II pocket mutation and polyclonal alterations converging on RAS–MAPK reactivation. *Cancer Discovery*, *11*(8), 1913–1922.

Tie, J., Gibbs, P., Lipton, L., et al. (2011). Optimizing targeted therapeutic development: analysis of a colorectal cancer patient population with the BRAFV600E mutation. *International Journal of Cancer*, *128*(9), 2075–2084.

Tie, J., Wang, Y., Tomasetti, C., et al. (2016). Circulating tumor DNA analysis detects minimal residual disease and predicts recurrence in patients with stage II colon cancer. *Science Translational Medicine*, *8*(346), 346ra92.

Valtorta, E., Martino, C., Sartore-Bianchi, A., et al. (2015). Assessment of a HER2 scoring system for colorectal cancer: Results from a validation study. *Modern Pathology*, *28*(11), 1481–1491.

Van Cutsem, E., Cervantes, A., Nordlinger, B., et al. (2014). Metastatic colorectal cancer: ESMO Clinical Practice Guidelines for diagnosis, treatment and follow-up. *Annals of Oncology*, *25* Suppl 3, iii1–9.

Van Cutsem, E., Cervantes, A., Adam, R., et al. (2016). ESMO consensus guidelines for the management of patients with metastatic colorectal cancer. *Annals of Oncology*, *27*(8), 1386–1422.

Van Cutsem, E., Lenz, H., Köhne, C., et al. (2019). Fluorouracil, leucovorin, and irinotecan plus cetuximab treatment and RAS mutations in colorectal cancer. *33*(7).

Van Cutsem, E., Taieb, J., Yaeger, R., et al. (2021). O-10 ANCHOR CRC: Results from a single-arm, phase 2 study of encorafenib, binimetinib plus cetuximab in previously untreated BRAF V600E–mutant metastatic colorectal cancer. *Annals of Oncology*, *32*, S222.

Van Cutsem, E., Tabernero, J., Lakomy, R., et al. (2012). Addition of aflibercept to fluorouracil, leucovorin, and irinotecan improves survival in a phase III randomized trial in patients with metastatic colorectal cancer previously treated with an oxaliplatin-based regimen. *Journal of Clinical Oncology*, *30*(28), 3499–4506.

Van Geel, R. M. J. M., Tabernero, J., Elez, E., et al. (2017). A phase Ib dose-escalation study of encorafenib and cetuximab with or without alpelisib in metastatic BRAF-mutant colorectal cancer. *Cancer Discovery*, *7*(6), 610–619.

Vanhaesebroeck, B., Stephens, L., & Hawkins, P. (2012). PI3K signalling: the path to discovery and understanding. *Nature Reviews Molecular Cell Biology*, *13*(3), 195–203.

Venderbosch, S., Nagtegaal, I. D, Maughan, T. S, et al. (2014). Mismatch repair status and BRAF mutation status in metastatic colorectal cancer patients: a pooled analysis of the CAIRO, CAIRO2, COIN, and FOCUS Studies. *Clinical Cancer Research*, *20*(20), 5322–5330.

Weiss, J., Yaegar, R. D., Johnson, M. L., et al. (2021a). KRYSTAL-1: Adagrasib (MRTX849) as monotherapy or combined with cetuximab (Cetux) in patients (Pts) with colorectal cancer (CRC) harboring a KRASG12C mutation. *Annals of Oncology*,.

Weiss, J., Yaegar, R. D., Johnson, M. L., et al. (2021b). Colorectal cancer LBA6 KRYSTAL-1: Adagrasib (MRTX849) as monotherapy or combined with cetuximab (Cetux) in patients (Pts) with colorectal cancer (CRC) harboring a KRASG12C mutation. *Annals of Oncology*, *32*, S1294.

Yaeger, R., Cercek, A., O'Reilly, E. M., et al. (2015). Pilot trial of combined BRAF and EGFR inhibition in BRAF-mutant metastatic colorectal cancer patients. *Clinical Cancer Research*, *21*(6), 1313–1320.

Yokota, T. (2012). Are KRAS/BRAF mutations potent prognostic and/or predictive biomarkers in colorectal cancers? *Anticancer Agents in Medicinal Chemistry*, *12*(2), 163–171.

18

The expanding landscape of immunotherapy in colorectal cancer

Sarah Chamberlain and Rachel Kerr

Introduction

As discussed in previous chapters, overall survival in patients with metastatic colorectal cancer (CRC) remains quite poor, with less than 20% surviving beyond five years (Biller & Schrag, 2021). Successful use of immunotherapy is currently restricted to a small subset of patients with metastatic CRC who are either mismatch repair deficient (dMMR) or have high microsatellite instability (MSI-H) who constitute 4-5% of the metastatic cohort. Even within this group there is evidently a significant degree of tumour heterogeneity, with only approximately half of all patients responding to single agent immunotherapy treatments.

Evolving evidence supports the need for a more comprehensive understanding of the immunological profiles and tumour microenvironment (TME) of both primary and metastatic tumours to effectively identify patients who would gain most benefit from such treatments and also how to render mismatch repair proficient (pMMR) and microsatellite stable CRC responsive. The enthusiasm surrounding the potential to achieve this is founded in the sustained durable responses to the novel immunotherapeutics, immune checkpoint inhibitors (ICIs) that is seen in other tumour types. In this chapter we will discuss the current understanding of the interaction between the immune system and colorectal tumours, immunotherapeutic biomarkers, an overview of the data that support current ICI use in clinical practice, and we will evaluate potential future applications to unlock the benefit of immunotherapy for a greater patient population.

Rationale for immunotherapy: the immune system and CRC

There is a growing body of data which evidences the importance of the interplay between the host immune system and colorectal tumour cells in several key stages of carcinogenesis. It was established in the 1980s that CRC, and to a lesser degree colonic adenomas, had reduced expression or complete loss of major histocompatibility complex (MHC) class I molecules which has a fundamental impact on antigen presentation pathways (Smith et al., 1989). This has been attributed to various different mutations in both the MHC machinery itself as well as associated transporter molecules. In 2006 Galon et al. demonstrated that high levels of lymphocytic infiltration into primary tumours (high TILs) in CRC patients showed a strong negative correlation with the risk of relapse and subsequent positive correlation of the chances of overall survival; that is, they described specific immune signatures high in TILs which were associated with good prognosis (Galon et al., 2006).

How tumours exploit the natural phenomenon of self-tolerance

Self-tolerance in the gastrointestinal tract is important in the avoidance of autoimmunity, as the lining cells come into contact with such a varied range of antigens within the gut microenvironment. Normal colorectal cellular secretion of immunosuppressive cytokines such as TGF-β, IL-10, and prostaglandins, a natural phenomenon which helps to prevent such autoimmunity, is pathologically increased in colonic carcinomas and, in this situation, this augmented secretion dampens any nascent immune responses to the developing tumour.

A host global immunosuppression has been observed with an *in situ* CRC, which subsequently reverses on the resection of the primary tumour. IL-6 has been shown in *in vitro* studies to promote growth of malignant cells within the colon and clinically has been associated with poor prognosis in metastatic CRC (mCRC) (Toyoshima et al., 2019). An IL-6 surge has been shown to occur in the immediate post-operative period which may facilitate immune escape of micrometastatic disease during the recovery period. In 2000, Heriot and colleagues evidenced the presence of monocyte/macrophage cells from CRC patients, which had attenuated responses to lipopolysaccharide (LPS)-induced cytokine production; this attenuation was proportional to the stage of cancer and was reversible on tumour resection, again demonstrating that sometimes there may be a tumour-induced 'break on the immune system' that can be released when the primary tumour is resected (Heriot et al., 2000). It is clearly a complex and ever-evolving interplay between the tumour and the immune system which needs increased understanding in order for us to effect the best outcomes for patients.

The tumour microenvironment (TME) is a complex and dynamic system composed of multiple interacting cellular and extracellular factors including immune cells, tumour cells, blood vessels, stroma, and extracellular matrix. The TME forms an important interface between cells of the tumour and of the host immune system. An appreciation of colorectal tumour biology, components of the TME, and their interaction with the host immune system is vital to understanding the principles of immunotherapeutics in treating CRC. Recent data suggest that the TME is likely to be just as important as tumour genetic variability between cancer cells, in terms of determining prognosis, and our burgeoning understanding of the TME will help us guide new drug development in the field of immunotherapy.

Certain features of the TME have been found to correlate with the risk of developing metastases from CRC and these include low density of TILs, low activity of T_H1 type helper cells. and increased TGF-β levels (Tauriello et al., 2018). Furthermore, mounting evidence highlights the important of differences between the TME of a primary colorectal tumour and distant metastatic disease at various anatomical locations (Kamal et al., 2020), meaning that immunotherapeutic strategies may have a tougher job dealing with metastases compared to primary tumours.

For example, we know that peritoneal metastases, which develop in up to a quarter of patients with metastatic disease, remain extremely challenging to treat as the peritoneum is a relative 'sanctuary site' when it comes to chemotherapy, and metastases to the peritoneum are associated with significant morbidity and mortality (see Chapter 13). Notably, a significant proportion of the normal peritoneum is comprised of tissue-resident macrophages (Narasimhan et al., 2019). These macrophages can actually be exploited by cancer cells which use them to help propagate themselves and promote disseminated disease within the abdomen.

Tumour cell hijacking of the host immune cells to propagate metastatic disease has been evidenced in other common metastatic sites, such as liver and lung, using a variety of mechanisms involving stellate macrophages in the liver, alveolar macrophages in the lung, exclusion of NK cells, and influx of regulatory T-cells. An appreciation of these differences is vital to further the development of successful immunotherapeutic agents, especially in the metastatic setting.

Components of the immune system relevant to tumours

Innate immune system: TAMs and NK cells

In essence, the role of the innate immune system in cancer, including tumour-associated macrophages (TAMs) and natural killer (NK) cells, is to induce tumour cell lysis and production of antigens for presentation and recognition of the cells of the adaptive arm of the immune system. TAMs have been associated with poor prognosis in many solid tumours, however their role in CRC appears to more complex and not always a marker of poorer outcome (Wang et al., 2021). Overall, TAMs in CRC are best considered anti-inflammatory cells that secrete specific patterns of cytokines and chemokines within the TME. These factors, when orchestrated, can promote invasion, support angiogenesis, and contribute to an immunosuppressive milieu that actively fosters metastatic progression.

Current studies further assessing the role of macrophages in CRC have, however, been somewhat contradictory. Several reasons for this finding have been postulated including the variable spatial locations of TAMs and the phenotypic diversity of macrophages within tumours. Furthermore studies have also shown that TAMs can express PD-1 and PD-L1 and therefore may actually represent interesting future targets for novel immunotherapy treatments.

NK cells play a particularly important role in immune surveillance and are able to recognize cells which have lost MHC class I, a mechanism used by many tumour cells to evade cytotoxic T-cell-mediated killing, and therefore specifically harnessing NK activity may actually be incredibly useful as an immunotherapeutic strategy. Reduced levels of circulating NK cell activity have been associated with increased risk of developing cancer including CRC (Jobin et al., 2017) and activated NK cells have been shown to recognize and kill CRC cells efficiently *in vitro* (Lanuza et al., 2018).

Adaptive immune system: dendritic cells and T-lymphocytes and immune checkpoints

The observation that T-cell immunosuppression in patients post organ transplant and in Acquired Immunodeficiency Syndrome (AIDS) can increase susceptibility to develop both haematological and solid cancers illustrates the principle that the adaptive, cellular component of the immune system may be most important in anti-tumour surveillance and responses (Midgley & Kerr, 2003). Although interestingly, unlike cancers such as Kaposi's sarcoma, CRC is not found to be more prevalent in this group.

Within the TME, dendritic cells function to process tumour antigens and once mature have the ability to present these peptides to CD8+ cytotoxic T-cells via MHC class I or to CD4+ T cells via MHC class II. Subsequent activation of specific T-cells occurs via this antigen recognition pathway, alongside activation of costimulatory molecules such as CD80 and CD40 (both present in high amounts on dendritic cells), and also in concert with cytokine release including interleukin-1 (IL-1), IL-2, IL-6, and interferon (IFN) γ.

Tumour-infiltrating lymphocytes (TILs) have been shown as key players in the host immune response to facilitate tumour cell death and prevention of anergy. The T-cell-mediated anti-tumour response includes CD8+ cytotoxic T lymphocytes (CTL) which are able to lyse tumour cells, and a subset of CD4+ T lymphocytes-T-cell helper 1 (T_H1), which facilitate the production of anti-tumour cytokines involved in cancer cell destruction including IL-2, IFN-γ, and tumour necrosis factor (TNF)-α.

Currently approved immunotherapies (mainly immune checkpoint inhibitors (ICIs)), utilized in solid tumours, rely on the principle that cancer cells predominantly evade recognition via the host immune system via regulatory T-lymphocyte immunosuppressive mechanisms (Golshani & Zhang, 2020), and that the specific agents may reverse this anergy.

Mechanisms by which cancers may evade the host immune system can include:

- Upregulation of cytokines that promote regulatory T-lymphocyte activation
- Deletion mutations in MHC class genes to prevent T-lymphocyte recognition
- Upregulation of checkpoint molecules which induces exhaustion of peripheral T-lymphocytes

Current established immunotherapeutic agents exploit this complex interaction between T-cells and tumour cells by inhibiting the

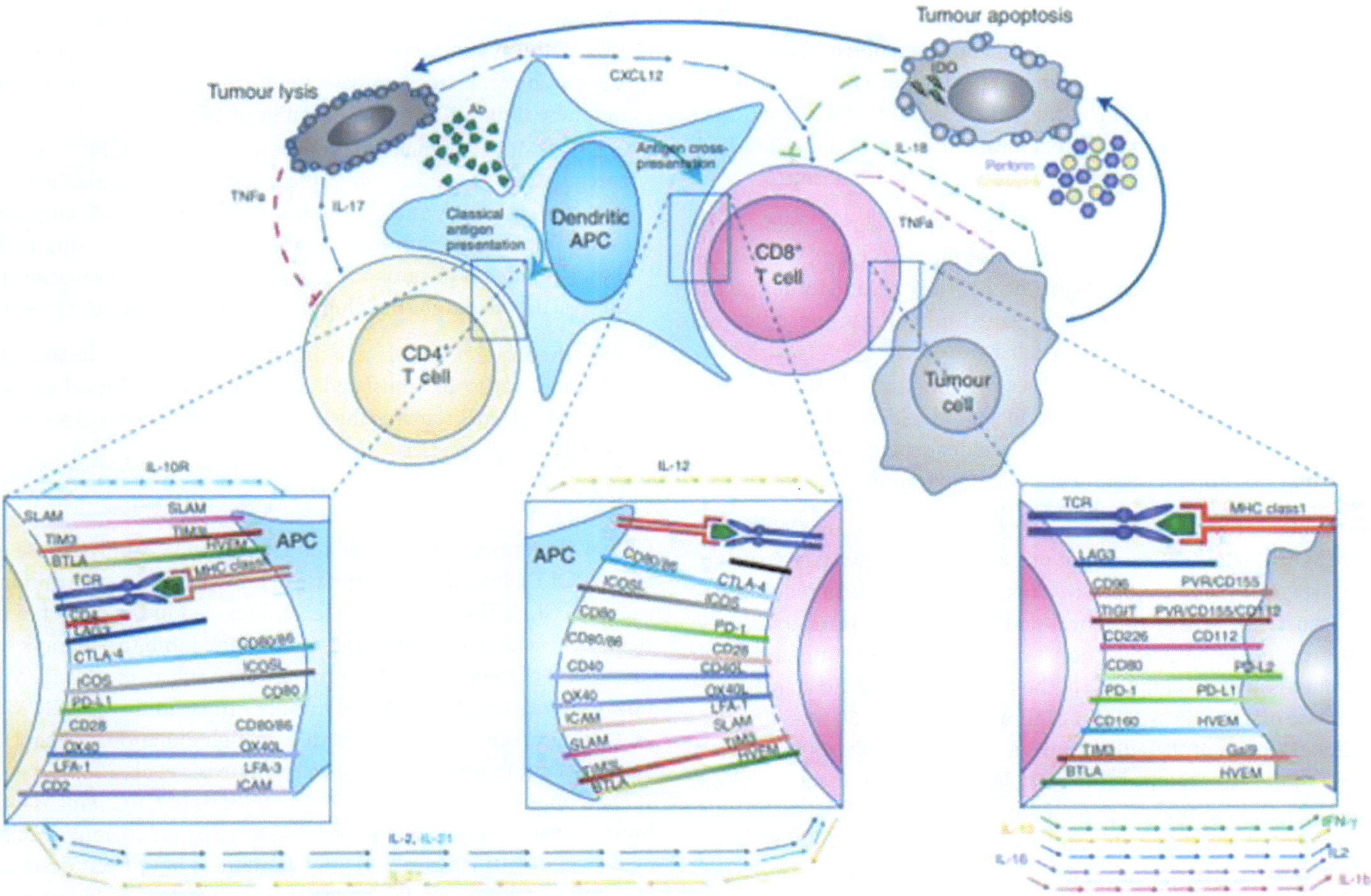

Figure 18.1 Immune checkpoint interface.
Demonstrates the immense complexity of the interface between tumour cells, APC cells, and T-cells involving a multitude of immune checkpoints with both activating and inhibitory receptors. The numerous depicted in the inset boxes and influence of cytokines and chemokines shown by the arrowed lines (adapted from A. P. Cogdill et al. (2017). Hallmarks of response to immune checkpoint blockade. *British Journal of Cancer*, *117*(1), 1–7. doi: 10.1038/bjc.2017.136. Epub 2017 May 18. PMID: 28524159; PMCID: PMC5520201.

immune checkpoint proteins that usually function to promote anergy within the TME. These immune checkpoint molecules include programmed cell death 1 (PD-1), (PD-L1), cytotoxic T lymphocyte-associated protein 4 (CTLA-4), and lymphocyte activation gene-3 (LAG-3) (Fig. 18.1).

PD-1 is a transmembrane protein expressed on a number of different haematopoietic cell lineages within the TME, most notably activated T-cells and myeloid-derived dendritic cells. PD-1 functions as an inhibitory receptor at the immune checkpoint interface, binding to PD-L1 on tumour cells to block downstream signalling, and as such, suppress immune recognition and response.

CTLA-4 is a co-inhibitory molecule at the immunological synapse which binds CD80 and CD86 on antigen-presenting cells, and downregulates activation of tumour directed T cells. LAG3 is a surface co-inhibitory receptor which is expressed on a wide range of immune cells within the TME and functions to suppress T-cell activation and subsequent cytokine secretion (Long et al., 2018).

LAG3 interacts with MHC class II on APCs and as such prevents binding with the T-cell receptor (TCR) to suppress downstream signal which would allow recognition of tumour associated antigens presented by this pathway. We will later discuss the agents currently available which inhibit these immune inhibitory checkpoints, which then allows the immune system to recognize aberrant malignant cells and remove them.

CRC classifications and their relation to immunotherapy

Colorectal cancer can be segregated into different types through a variety of classification systems, such as mismatch repair deficient versus mismatch repair proficient, or consensus molecular subtypes (CMS). These classifications and their relation to the immune system and anti-tumour immunity are described below.

Mismatch repair deficiency and microsatellites

Microsatellites are sections of coding or non-coding DNA regions with repeats of 1 to 10 nucleotides of variable length, typically 5 to 50 repeats in length, for example AAAAAAA or GTGTGT. These sections of DNA are particularly susceptible to mutations as during replication DNA polymerase is liable to slip resulting in mismatched sequences (Sun, 2021). The role of the mismatch repair (MMR) system in a healthy cell is to identify DNA base-base mismatches and correct them to maintain genomic stability. Where this protective mechanism fails, errors are translated into protein mutations and new alleles, which are inherited in subsequent generations. Microsatellite instability (MSI-H) is a consequence of MMR deficiency due to inactivation of ≥ 1 MMR genes including MLH1, MSH2, MSH6, and PMS2 and can be seen in several different tumour types including CRC. Loss of expression of MMR genes can occur via two mechanisms:

- *Germline* mutation in one of the four MMR genes, followed by a subsequent somatic inactivation of the wild-type (WT) allele, which predisposes patients to a large variety of solid tumours. The associated syndrome is often termed hereditary non-polyposis colon cancer (HNPCC) or Lynch syndrome.
- *Somatic* mutations or epigenetic silencing of both alleles of one of the MMR genes. This occurs in sporadic MMR-deficient CRC. These tumours generally occur in older patients and frequently display poor differentiation and *BRAF* mutations.

In general terms, MMR-deficient or MSI-H colorectal cancer (dMMR/MSI-H CRC) when it presents in the early stage (particularly stage 2) is associated with a better prognosis with reduced risk of recurrence. These tumours tend to have certain characteristic features including predilection to present as poorly differentiated mucinous adenocarcinomas of the proximal colon and an observed increase in TILs. dMMR/MSI-H tumours have 10–50 times the mutational load of proficient tumours and consequently respond better to immune checkpoint inhibitors (ICIs) (Llosa et al., 2021). More detail of clinical trials is given below. There are, however, key differences between sporadic and Lynch-associated germline MMR deficiency including clinical features, immune reactivity, and prognosis. Liu et al. assessed tumours in 67 patients with sporadic MMR deficiency and 85 patients with germline MMR deficiency. Lynch-associated germline dMMR tumours had statistically significant higher scores for immunoreactions, denser immunological infiltrates, more somatic mutations, and higher neoantigen burden than those patients in the sporadic dMMR group, a result which correlates with real-world clinical responses to immunotherapy that many GI oncologists are observing in clinical practice (Liu et al., 2018).

Consensus molecular subtypes

Four consensus molecular subtypes (CMS) of CRC have been described, representing an international collaborative effort using a transcriptome-based approach to improve our understanding of the heterogeneity in CRCs (Fig. 18.2). The aim of this system is to allow for a more representative comparison of data across clinical trials, inform prognosis, and improve identification of the most appropriate therapeutic agents (Becht et al., 2016). The four sub-types are as follows:

- CMS1 MSI Immune: Characterized by a hypermutated genotype and immune cell infiltration. This group is enriched in tumours that are dMMR/MSI-high, *BRAF* mutated, and those with CpG-island methylator phenotype (CIMP). Expectantly this subgroup contains tumours most likely to respond to ICI.
- CMS2 Canonical: A sub-type with high chromosomal instability and marked upregulation of downstream targets of the Wnt and MYC signalling pathways as described in the adenoma–carcinoma sequence model for chromosomal instability in colorectal cancer (Walther et al., 2009). They comprise the largest group of CRC with metastatic disease to the liver.
- CMS 3 Metabolic: A group with prominent disruption of metabolic pathways and enriched with *KRAS*-mutated tumours. This sub-group comprises the majority of colorectal adenomas (73%) and these tumours have low densities of TILs.
- CMS4 Mesenchymal: Tumours which exhibit marked upregulation of genes and protein expression fundamental to epithelial–mesenchymal transition, TGF-β activation, angiogenesis, complement pathways, and stromal invasion. This group shows a tendency towards late-stage presentation and worse overall survival despite exhibiting a high expression of immune signatures.

Despite the academic interest in the application of this classification system, it is yet to be translated into mainstream clinical use and the dMMR/pMMR remains the biggest differentiator that we use in standard clinical practice

POLE/POLD1 mutations

CRC with germline or somatic mutations in DNA polymerase epsilon (POLE) and DNA polymerase delta 1 (POLD1) are a minority group of CRC. They are not currently included in the cohort of patients who can access immune checkpoint inhibitor therapies in most parts of the world. However, they are a subset of pMMR/MSI-Low tumours which are phenotypically similar to the dMMR/MSI-High tumours in that they also exhibit a high mutational phenotype and dense infiltrates of immune cells (Bourdais et al., 2017).

Data on the prevalence of POLE mutations in CRC remain fairly limited but is likely to be around 1–8% based on current available evidence. Whilst germline POLD1 mutations have been described in familial CRC, somatic mutations are yet to be documented. Germline mutations in POLD1 and POLE are inherited in an autosomal dominant fashion and seem to have a high penetrance. DNA polymerases play important roles in DNA synthesis and repair during replication and contain a proofreading exonuclease domain to enable correction of errors. Mutations have a tendency to cluster in or in close proximity to the proofreading domain and result in deficient DNA repair, with base substitutions and genomic instability during replication (Palles et al., 2013). In combined datasets from three CRC cohorts (TCGA, Genetech, and DFCI), 77% of tumours with mutations associated with the exonuclease domain were pMMR (Bourdais et al., 2017).

In the Cancer Genome Atlas (TCGA) group, which included 224 resected CRC, all the tumour samples that were observed to be hypermutated but which were pMMR were found to have a *POLE* gene mutation ($n = 7$) (TCGA, 2012).

In a retrospective analysis of 6,517 patients with resected stage 2 or 3 CRC, 66 had a somatic *POLE* mutation (about 1%) and all were pMMR. These would be missed on our routine mutational profiling after biopsy or resection of CRC. Similar to dMMR tumours, they exhibited upregulation of genes encoding immune checkpoints as well as high densities of TIL. Data presented at the American Society of Clinical Oncology Meeting 2020 showed disease control rate (DCR) of 53.8% in patients with *POLE/POLD1* mutations treated with PD-1/PDL-1 agents (Garmezy et al., 2020). Whilst *POLE/POLD1*-mutated tumours comprise a relatively small subset of CRC patients, they clearly represent another patient group that are highly likely to benefit from immunotherapeutics, and it is likely that, given the frequency and duration of such responses, there will be increasing pressure for tumours to undergo POLE and POLD1 assessment

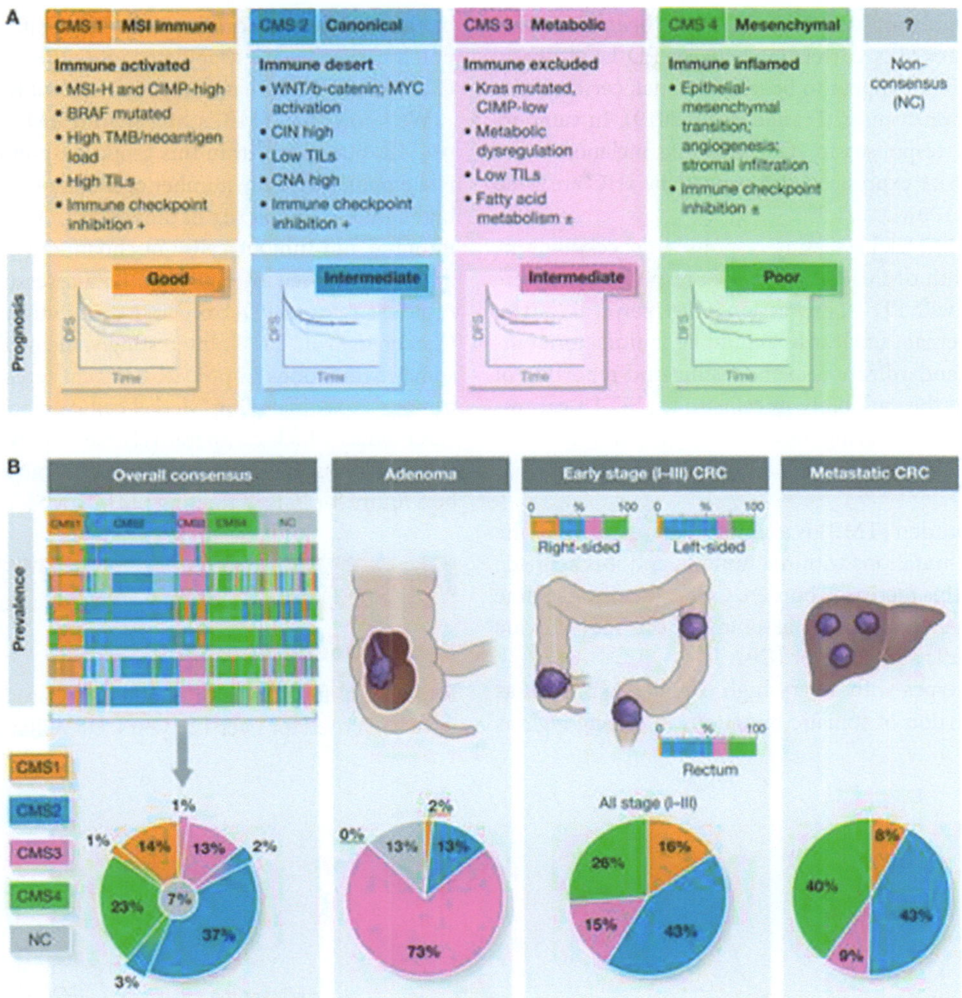

Figure 18.2 Consensus molecular subtypes in CRC.
A. The main features of the four subtypes described including prognosis. **B.** Prevalence and distribution across disease stages (adapted from A. Kanani et al. (2021). Neoadjuvant immunotherapy in primary and metastatic colorectal cancer. *British Journal of Surgery*, *108*(12), 1417–1425 https://doi.org/10.1093/bjs/znab342. Used under the terms of the Creative Commons Attribution License (<https://creativecommons.org/licenses/by/4.0/>), no alterations made.

routinely. At the time of publication there are several ongoing early phase clinical trials including patients with POLE/POLD1-mutated colorectal tumours testing immunotherapy in the neoadjuvant, adjuvant and metastatic settings.

Biomarkers for immunotherapy response in CRC

It is important to understand what features and molecular profiles have been tested for their predictive capability in terms of determining response to immunotherapy, and to differentiate those which do or do not appear to be important for selection in CRC.

MMR and MSI status: MMR status as assessed by immunohistochemistry (IHC) and MSI assessed by polymerase chain reaction (PCR) are currently the only available biomarkers used to select patients with CRC who are most likely to respond to ICI therapy.

The KEYNOTE-016 trial highlighted the superior response to immunotherapy in patients with dMMR/MSI-H disease compared to pMMR/MSI-low (MSI-L) disease (Le et al., 2015; see later in this chapter). Patients with dMMR/MSI-H CRC comprise only ~5% of mCRC cases and not all of them respond to immune checkpoint inhibitors. Through retrospective tumour analysis, a variety of mechanisms of intrinsic and acquired resistance have been suggested, including genetic loss of β2-microglobulin which is key to antigen presentation and MHC class I expression as well as NK cell and macrophage infiltration (Gurjao et al., 2019). At present, the molecular and immunological characteristics of resistant dMMR/MSI-H tumours are not well understood and further evaluation is required.

PD-L1 expression

A wide range of different solid tumours overexpress PD-L1 as part of the complex process of establishing an immunosuppressive environment (Patel et al., 2015). PD-L1 is one of the most investigated biomarkers in efforts to try and predict responses to ICI in solid tumours, but its application remains contentious.

Whilst PD-L1 upregulation within the TME has been associated with increased density of TILs, correlation between PD-L1 positivity and ICI response does not appear to be proportional, certainly not in terms of CRC responsiveness (Franke et al., 2019). In tumours known to have good responses to ICI, including melanoma and NSCLC, levels of PD-L1 expression determined by IHC are wide ranging, from 14% to 100%.

In the CheckMate-142 trial assessing response to checkpoint inhibition in patients with dMMR/MSI-H CRC, response rates were not found to correlate with PD-L1 expression (Overman et al., 2018). The reasons for this remain unclear but could be multifactorial including the lack of standardization in the testing and reporting of PD-L1 'positivity', and the variability in cell surface PD-L1 expression at different time points during the carcinogenic pathway.

Tumour mutational burden

Tumour mutational burden (TMB) is a simplistic assessment of the frequency of tumour mutations within a tumour, and it is agnostic about the pathway to this increased burden. Consequently, for some investigators, it has been tempting to assume that this may provide the broadest 'therapeutic audience' for ICIs.

In certain tumour types with a very high overall TMB, such as melanoma, the proportion of somatic mutations in coding regions has been shown to correlate with ICI treatment response. This has not, however, been extrapolated into other tumour types, including CRC, where results have been inconsistent (Kamal et al., 2020).

We know that TMB is higher in dMMR tumours compared to pMMR, but even within this group, response rates to ICI can correlate poorly with the number of mutations present. This is likely to highlight the complexity of the interactions at the interface between immune and tumour cells. Yarchoan and colleagues performed a systematic review of published data assessing TMB and objective response rates to PD-1 or PD-L1 inhibition as shown in Fig. 18.3 (Yarchoan et al., 2017). Interestingly, the median number of coding somatic mutations in pMMR CRC clustered in a similar region to tumour types including Merkel cell carcinoma and hepatocellular carcinomas which comparatively have shown much better ORR to ICI therapies. This undoubtedly gives some hope that there may yet be a future for ICIs in treating pMMR/MSI-L CRC.

Immunotherapeutic agents in CRC

Early 'immunotherapeutic' agents

Rudimental forms of immunotherapy-based treatments for cancer have been used for over 120 years. Dr William Coley, often referred

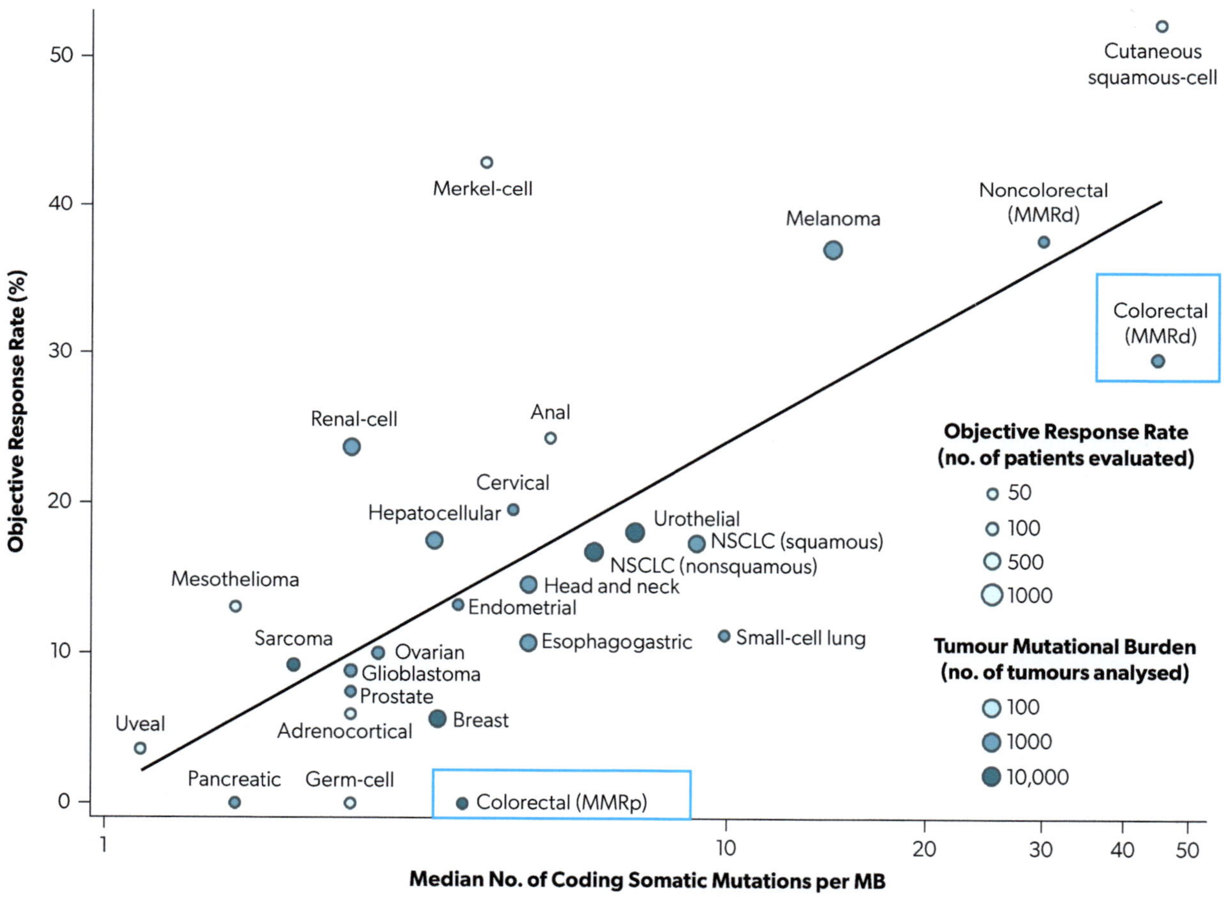

Figure 18.3 Graph depicting the correlation between tumour mutational burden (TMB) and objective response rate (ORR) with anti-PD-1 or -PD-L1 therapy.

Twenty-seven different tumour types are shown with results based on published studies where data on coding somatic mutations and ORR were available. The number of patients evaluated for the ORR is shown by the size of the circle and the degree of shading represents the number of tumours analysed to calculate the TMB (adapted from M. Yarchoan et al. (2017). Tumor mutational burden and response rate to PD-1 inhibition. *New England Journal of Medicine*, *377*(25), 2500–2501. doi: 10.1056/NEJMc1713444. PMID: 29262275; PMCID: PMC6549688.

to as the 'father' of immunotherapy, was an American orthopaedic surgeon who observed complete regression of an inoperable osteosarcoma in a patient who developed an associated *Streptococcal* skin infection. His insightful observation highlighted the importance of the host immune system and its potential to destroy malignant cells (Carlson et al., 2020). Coley went on to inject *Streptococcal* organisms (later termed 'Coley's toxins') into patients with inoperable sarcomas, reporting excellent results over a period of 40 years. Understandably, Coley's work was met with a great deal of criticism and scepticism in the medical community, predominantly because his colleagues simply did not believe the results.

In CRC, the early history of immunotherapy treatments is somewhat complex and its utility has faced a significant degree of scepticism. This was to be expected, as studies evaluating immunotherapeutics in CRC indiscriminately, often among heavily treated patients with very different forms of CRC and at very different stages, produced largely underwhelming results. These included the use of intraperitoneal Bacillus Calmette Guérin (BCG) vaccine, Levamisole anti-helminthic drug, and cytokine therapies such as IL-2 and IFN-α (QUASAR Collaborative Group, 2007).

Below we describe succinctly some of these first generation immunotherapies.

Autologous cancer cell vaccines

Some of the earliest modern age trials in CRC attempting to harness the immune system to destroy cancer cells focused on the development of autologous cancer cell vaccines. These vaccines were produced using whole tumour cell preparations which were then treated to render the cells in a non-proliferative state but still metabolically active (Chiang et al., 2015). The cell preps were subsequently combined with adjuvants such as BCG or bacterial cell wall products. The principle behind this approach is to increase the presence of circulating tumour-specific antigens and thereby drive a targeted anti-cancer response from the host immune system (Uyl-de Groot et al., 2005). The broad potential of such treatment lies in the broad range of tumour-associated antigens that can be generated, in comparison to the more limited repertoire with other approaches that are therefore liable to the development of resistance. One of the key challenges to this approach has been the technical complications in the production of autologous cancer cell vaccines and hence the paucity of randomized clinical trials in this area to date.

Oncovax® is an autologous cancer cell vaccine that has been tested in a multicentre, randomized, controlled phase 3 clinical trial in the adjuvant setting for stage 2 and 3 CRC (Uyl-de Groot et al., 2005). The trial randomized 254 patients post resection of their primary colorectal tumour to either the control group or to the Oncovax® group where they received four autologous tumour cell vaccinations between 28–35 day post-operatively. The group reported favourable rates of five-year PFS in the Oncovax® group of 69.5% ($n = 128$) compared to 61.1% ($n = 126$) in the control group ($p = 0.073$) as well as for overall survival rates of 75% compared to 71.4% respectively ($p = 0.100$). The benefit was most marked and statistically significant in the stage 2 colon group. This presents an interesting consideration for adjuvant treatments in patient with stage 2 colon cancer in whom the role of adjuvant chemotherapy is more controversial. However, most people accept that the technological confines of this 'not off-the-shelf' treatment strategy are likely to prevent it from being rolled out in any useful form.

Dendritic cell-based cancer vaccine therapies

As mentioned above, dendritic cells (DCs) are powerful antigen-presenting cells (APCs) which play a fundamental role in the host T-lymphocyte mediated anti-tumour immune response. Interest in DC-based vaccines began in the late 1980s when preclinical studies showed anti-tumour effects of tumour lysate-pulsed DCs (Wooster et al., 2021). Alternative approaches to DC priming have been explored including priming with autologous tumour cell lysates, with the benefit of providing a broad repertoire of both known and unknown tumour-associated antigens versus priming with specific tumour-associated peptides known to be over-expressed. CRC is an attractive candidate for DC-based immunotherapeutics as its cells express a range of potentially targetable antigens including carcinoembryonic antigen (CEA) and Wilm's tumour gene-1 (WT-1). CEA is a particularly attractive option as it is known to be produced at high levels in the majority of patients with colorectal adenocarcinoma.

In 1999, Morse et al. reported the first phase 1 trial of DCs primed with HLA-A2-restricted CEA peptide in 21 patients with advanced CEA-producing cancers, including 11 patients with CRC (Morse et al., 1999). Whilst the treatment was found to have a pleasing safety profile, none of the CRC patients in the trial exhibited an objective response to treatment. In 2001, Fong et al. treated 12 patients with HLA-A2+ cancers, 10 mCRCs and two NSCLCs, with HLA-A2-restricted DCs primed with altered CEA peptides, given concurrently with a haematopoietic growth factor, Flt3, to facilitate DC expansion (Fong et al., 2001). Immunization induced production of antigen-specific CTLs that were able to recognize tumour-associated CEA. The group reported two of the patients with CRC achieved objective disease response in metastatic lesions post vaccination; one had a mixed response and two had stable disease.

Overall, whilst DC-based vaccine therapies can stimulate CTL activation and responses to CRC-specific antigen targets, this has not yet been translated into significant clinical improvements for patients. It is likely this is due to the immunosuppressive barriers presented by the TME. Given the pivotal role that DCs play in antigen presentation and anti-tumour responses there remains great interest in this immunotherapeutic field with ongoing clinical trials of DC-based vaccines yet to report, including combination approaches with ICIs.

Immune checkpoint inhibitors

A complex array of activating ligands, inhibitory ligands, and reciprocal receptors form an interface called the immunological synapse between the host immune system and tumour cells (Fig. 18.1). The inhibitory interactions in this 'synapse' are called immune checkpoints and their overactivity plays an essential role in regulating/suppressing T-cell function within the TME, as already described. Therapeutic agents targeting these checkpoints (including PD-1, PD-L1, CTLA-4, and LAG-3) comprise the mainstay of current immunotherapy treatment in solid tumours (see Table 18.1). Initial trials evaluating ICIs in CRC recruited patients, irrespective of biological and molecular characteristics, and produced negative results.

One of the first ICI trials published in 2010, which delivered a disappointing response to tremelimumab, an anti-CTLA-4 monoclonal antibody (mAb), was trialling the therapeutic in a cohort of patients with heavily pre-treated mCRC ($n = 47$). Only one participant

Table 18.1 Immune checkpoint inhibitors in CRC (2022)

Therapeutic agent	Checkpoint target	Current Applications
Atezolizumab	*PD-L1*	Phase 3 clinical trials in combination approaches including with chemotherapy and cobimetinib (MAPK inhibitor)
Avelumab	*PD-L1*	Early phase clinical trials including combination approaches with chemotherapy and cetuximab, anti EGFR
Durvalumab	*PD-L1*	Early phase clinical trials in combination with tremelimumab
Favezelimab	*LAG-3*	Early phase trials in combination with pembrolizumab in MSS mCRC
Ipilimumab	*CTLA-4*	NICE approved in UK for use in combination with nivolumab in pre-treated dMMR-MSI-H mCRC
Nivolumab	*PD-1*	NICE approved in UK for use in combination with ipilimumab in pre-treated dMMR-MSI-H mCRC. FDA approval as single agent therapy.
Pembrolizumab	*PD-1*	NICE approval in the UK for upfront use in patients with dMMR-MSI-H mCRC
Relatlimab	*LAG-3*	Early phase clinical trials in combination with nivolumab in dMMR-MSI-H mCRC resistant to PD-1/PD-L1 inhibition
Tremelimumab	*CTLA-4*	Early phase clinical trials in combination with durvalumab

achieved an objective response, which was partial, most likely due to (unknown at the time) MMR deficiency (Chung et al., 2010).

Several subsequent trials investigating the efficacy of pembrolizumab, a humanized anti-PD-1 mAb, in a range of advanced solid tumours showed no objective responses in small groups of patients recruited with unselected mCRC, in contrast to the positive results seen in patients with melanoma, renal cell cancer, and NSCLC. However, in 2013 a complete radiological response following six months of anti-PD-1 therapy with nivolumab was reported in one elderly patient with relapsed heavily pre-treated CRC (Lipson et al., 2013). Subsequent retrospective IHC analysis of the patient's primary tumour revealed dMMR disease with cell surface expression of PD-L1 on both immune and tumour cells within the sample.

What was especially exciting was that following nine months of treatment with nivolumab, this individual remained in complete remission for three years, a durability of response never before seen in this mCRC cohort. This single patient was the driving factor behind the KEYNOTE-016 study, which was the first to clearly evidence an objective response to immune checkpoint inhibition in patients with dMMR tumours, including CRC (Le et al., 2015).

In the KEYNOTE-016 phase 2 study, investigators reported a 40% ORR (n = 10, 95% CI 12–74) to pembrolizumab (10 mg/kg every 14 days) in dMMR CRC previously exposed to ≥ two lines of chemotherapy. Disease control rate (DCR) was 90%, two-year progression-free survival (PFS) 61%, and two-year overall survival (OS) was 66% in this small patient group. This was in sharp contrast to 0% ORR (n = 18) and 11% PFS in the cohort with pMMR CRC.

Several subsequent phase 1 and 2 studies of pembrolizumab in patients with solid tumours collectively demonstrated that dMMR/MSI-H status is a fundamental biomarker of patients with CRC who are most likely to respond to ICI. In May 2017, the US Food and Drug Administration (FDA) granted accelerated approval for the use of pembrolizumab in the treatment of metastatic dMMR/MSI-H CRC that has progressed despite chemotherapy treatment with a fluoropyrimidine, oxaliplatin, and irinotecan.

KEYNOTE-164 was a confirmatory phase 2, multicentre study designed to evaluate the activity of pembrolizumab in previously treated advanced or metastatic dMMR/MSI-H CRC (Le et al., 2019). Eligible patients were assigned to cohort A or B depending on whether they had received ≥ two or ≥ one previous lines systemic anti cancer therapy (SACT) of respectively and were given intravenous (IV) pembrolizumab dosed at 200 mg every three weeks for up to 35 cycles (n = 124). Results demonstrated an ORR of 33% in both cohorts and DCR of 51% and 57% in cohorts A and B, respectively. Complete responses were seen in two patients from cohort A and five patients from cohort B. Not only did the KEYNOTE-164 add to the existing evidence in support of ICI treatment in dMMR/MSI-H CRC but it also suggested that treatment earlier in the therapeutic pathway was associated with better outcomes, in keeping with results seen in other solid tumours.

Following on from the results of KEYNOTE-164, the next unanswered question was whether immunotherapy should replace chemotherapy in the first-line setting for dMMR/MSI-H CRC. KEYNOTE-177, a phase 3 study which randomized 307 participants from this patient group 1:1 to receive first-line treatment with either pembrolizumab (n = 153) given as 200 mg every three weeks for up to two years or standard of care (SOC) 5-fluorouracil-based chemotherapy (n = 154) every two weeks (Andre et al., 2020). This showed a statistically significant superior PFS with pembrolizumab compared to SOC chemotherapy (median PFS of 16.5 months vs 8.2 months respectively (95% CI 0.45–0.80, p = 0.0002)) and this was achieved with a lower rate of Grade 3+ adverse events (AEs).

Somewhat disappointingly, the mature OS data released in May 2021 did not meet the predefined statistical significance in support of pembrolizumab over SOC chemotherapy (Andre et al., 2021). However, a striking 60% of patients given cytotoxic treatment on trial crossed over to immunotherapy at the time of disease progression. Based on this high volume of crossover it is therefore unsurprising that whilst pembrolizumab showed a marked improvement in PFS and trend towards improved OS, the significance point was not met for OS. In June 2021, pembrolizumab was approved by the UK's National Institute for Health and Care Excellence (NICE) for treatment naïve metastatic CRC with high MSI or mismatch repair deficiency (TA709).

In parallel to these findings pembrolizumab's sister anti-PD-1 agent, nivolumab, has produced similarly successful results in the dMMR / MSI-H CRC cohort. CheckMate-142 is a phase 2, open-label, multicentre study. Within this trial, 74 patients with dMMR/MSI-H CRC which had progressed following ≥ one previous line of chemotherapy were given nivolumab at a dose of 3 mg/kg every two weeks until PD, unacceptable toxicity or death (Overman et al.,

2017). At the median follow-up time of 12 months, 31.1% of participants had an objective response to nivolumab and 69% of participants had disease control which lasted for ≥ 12 weeks, including 8 patients whose responses were ≥ 12 months. In July 2017, just two months behind pembrolizumab, the US FDA granted accelerated approval for nivolumab in patients with dMMR/MSI-H CRC which had progressed following chemotherapy.

In one of the combination treatment arms of the CheckMate-142 study, 45 patients with advanced or metastatic dMMR/MSI-H CRC were given nivolumab in combination with low-dose ipilimumab, an anti-CTLA-4 agent, dosed at 1 mg/kg every six weeks (Overman et al., 2018). This approach was based on the biological principle that synergistic dual immune checkpoint inhibition can produce superior responses, as already evidenced in other solid tumours such as melanoma. Echoing this, ORR in advanced or metastatic dMMR/MSI-H CRC with median follow-up of 13.4 months was superior with combination ICI therapy at 55% with a DCR for ≥ 12 weeks of 80%. Twelve-month PFS was 71% and OS 85%, alongside clinically and statistically significant improvement in patient-reported outcomes on treatment. At longer-term follow-up (median 25.4 months), 119 patients had been treated with combination immunotherapy following ≥ two previous lines of chemotherapy, with ORR 58%, DCR 81%, PFS 60%, and OS 74%, including 6% of patients with a complete response (Overman et al., 2019).

Evidently, the responses seen with combination therapy were superior and durable. Whilst we have to bear in mind that CheckMate-142 is a phase 2, non-randomized study design, and therefore direct comparison of treatment arms must be interpreted with caution, withstanding such caveats the suggestion of improved responses with combination ICI was quite clear, but it must be borne in mind that the autoimmune toxicity may also be amplified.

Moving forward in the treatment pathway, results from the front-line combination arm of the CheckMate-142 study published in October 2021. In this cohort of 45 patients with previously untreated dMMR/MSI-H metastatic CRC received nivolumab and low-dose ipilimumab (Lenz et al., 2021). The primary end point of ORR at a median follow-up time of 29.0 months was 69% with a DCR of 84% and CR seen in 13% of patients. The durability of response was again notable, with median duration of response, PFS, and OS not reached; an unprecedented achievement in the treatment of metastatic CRC patients.

In 2025, final results of the confirmatory phase 3 study, CheckMate 8HW, were published. Here, patients were randomly assigned to receive single agent nivolumab, combination nivolumab with low-dose ipilimumab or investigators' choice SOC chemotherapy. A total of 303 patients were recruited to the dual agent immunotherapy versus SOC chemotherapy comparison. In the first publication, which documented the comparison between dual agent immunotherapy and SOC chemotherapy: 24-month PFS was 72% (95% CI, 64–79) with nivolumab plus ipilumimab and 14% (95% CI, 6–25) with chemotherapy, a very radical difference (Andre et al., 2024).

Subsequently in 2025, the same group has published the results of the dual immunotherapy versus single agent immunotherapy comparison: 707 patients were randomized to dual agent immunotherapy versus nivolumab alone. At the data cut-off of August 2024, median follow-up was 47 months. The dual combination showed clinically meaningful improvement in PFS with the combination compared to nivolumab alone (hazard ratio 0.62, 95% CI 0.48 to 0.81, p = 0.0003). The authors suggest that the combination of nivolumab plus ipilumimab should become the new standard of care treatment in the first-line therapy of metastatic dMMR/MSI-H CRC (Andre et al., 2025). In May 2025, NICE approved this doublet immunotherapy combination for the management of untreated unresectable or metastatic dMMR/MSI-H CRC in the UK (TA1065). One month prior the Medicines and Healthcare products Regulatory Agency (MHRA) approved a subcutaneous formulation of nivolumab enabling the drug to be administered within a few minutes as opposed to 30-60 minutes intravenously; a notable reduction in treatment burden for both the patient and cancer treatment units.

The future of immunotherapeutics in CRC

Translation into the neoadjuvant and adjuvant setting

As we develop our underlying knowledge of the activity of immunotherapy in CRC, the landscape and scope for use in this tumour site continue to expand and change. As with all anti-cancer treatment modalities, beyond the proof of efficacy in the advanced setting, we then question the most beneficial timing for treatment.

Approximately 10–20% of early stage CRCs are dMMR/MSI-H (Lumish & Cercek, 2021). Evidence of neoadjuvant ICI in other tumour types suggests that response rates are higher with a deeper tumour-specific T-cell response when used in this earlier stage of disease. Consequently there is interest in understanding how ICI may work in the neoadjuvant as well as adjuvant settings. At present the SOC for operable stage 1–3 CRC remains up-front surgical resection followed by adjuvant chemotherapy in patients with high-risk stage 2 and stage 3 disease.

Emerging evidence from several studies supports the use of neoadjuvant chemotherapy in preference to adjuvant chemotherapy for patients with locally advanced colon cancer with a trend towards superior DFS and OS when combining available data in this field (Cheong et al., 2020). In the large, multicentre FOXTROT trial response rates to neoadjuvant chemotherapy in dMMR tumours were poor and therefore assessment of neoadjuvant immunotherapy is warranted.

The NICHE trial was an exploratory study which assessed the feasibility of administering neoadjuvant combination ICI therapy in patients with early stage operable, but high-risk colon cancers irrespective of MMR status (Chalabi et al., 2020). Forty patients received a single low-dose of ipilimumab and two doses of nivolumab preoperatively. Of note, stage 3 tumours comprised the majority in this study at 81% in the dMMR group and 40% in the pMMR group. In the pMMR cohort ($n = 19$), patients were also randomized to receive celecoxib from D1 of treatment until the day before their operation, based on the principle that this group tend not to respond to ICI and some evidence of a potential synergistic effect in combination with COX-2 inhibition. All (100%) patients went on to have radical resections with formation of a primary anastomosis within 6 weeks of study inclusion. Neoadjuvant immunotherapy produced pathological responses in all patients with dMMR tumours with 19 major pathological responses (MPR, ≤ 10% visible residual tumour) and 12 pathological complete responses (CRs). In addition 27% (four out of 15) patients with pMMR tumours responded with three MPRs and one partial response. Median follow-up time was limited at nine months but found all patients with dMMR tumours to be alive with no evidence of disease relapse. In the pMMR tumour cohort one patient had died of an unrelated disease and another who did not respond to neoadjuvant ICI was alive but had relapsed.

Whilst the numbers of participants treated in this exploratory study was small, co-expression of both CD8 and PD-1 in T-cell populations was identified as the single biomarker in pMMR tumours predictive of response. The value of this potential biomarker requires further evaluation. Notably, increases in CD8+ T-lymphocytes, TCR clonality, IFNγ score and CXCL13 expression *irrespective* of response. This suggests that ICI can induce modulation of the TME which does not result in a biological response in the tumour. Of further interest, results in this study evidenced a step-wise accumulation of CD8+ T-lymphocytes at the peripheral tumour margins, which then went on to infiltrate the tumour core in pMMR tumours which exhibited delayed responses to treatment, but not seen in non-responding tumours.

Tumours which are dMMR/MSI-H have a favourable prognosis in early stage disease with 90% patients with stage 2 disease cured with surgery alone (Cohen et al., 2020). However, this is in contrast to patients with stage 3 disease where one in three will relapse, and at relapse their outcome with chemotherapy is poor. Determining patients within this group who are most likely to relapse and therefore gain most benefit from adjuvant systemic therapy remains an unmet medical need. We know that patients with dMMR/MSI-H CRC have poorer responses to cytotoxic agents, therefore it is likely in principle that adjuvant exposure to ICIs would be superior in this cohort. At the time of writing we await the results of a number of clinical trials evaluating the utility of ICIs in this setting.

Immunotherapy for pMMR/MSI-L CRC

Around 95% of mCRC patients have pMMR-MSI-L tumours which currently gain no significant clinical benefit from immunotherapy (Baraibar et al., 2021). This has been clearly evidenced in trials inclusive of this cohort, including KEYNOTE-028 and KEYNOTE-016, both reporting ORRs of 0% in pMMR/MSI-L tumours. Consequently the focus of a significant proportion of current research in this area is assessing potential combination approaches to turn immunologically 'cold' colorectal tumours 'hot'. In the field of immunotherapeutics the terms 'hot' and 'cold' tumours have been coined to represent the degree of immune cell infiltration and consequent likely responsiveness to immunotherapy. Undoubtedly to consider the immunological profile of tumours as a binary entity is a huge oversimplification of a complex spectrum of varying degrees of immunogenicity.

In order to devise effective combination immunotherapeutic approaches for pMMR-MSI-L tumours it is important that we continue to investigate and further our understanding of the mechanisms of both intrinsic and acquired resistance. Here we will discuss some of the combinations under investigation, which have been explored to varying degrees through past and current clinical trials.

ICIs with chemotherapy +/− VEGF inhibition

Chemotherapy with ICI agents is one of the most analysed combinations to date. It is hypothesized that chemotherapy will increase the exposure of tumour neoantigens and mutational burden, which in turn could prime pMMR/MSI-L CRC to respond to checkpoint inhibition. There have been a number of studies in support of this principle in both the pre-clinical and clinical setting. In 2017, Wang et al., showed in a mouse xenograft model of colon cancer that oxaliplatin in combination with ICI treatment exhibited a synergistic anti-tumour response (Wang et al., 2017).

The rationale for combining vascular endothelial growth factor (VEGF) inhibitors with ICI is based on the hypothesis that VEGF acts as a mediator of immunosuppression in the TME through compromise of dendritic cell function in antigen presentation pathways (Ohm & Carborne, 2001). VEGF inhibition can support normalization of vasculature within the TME, increased T-cell infiltration, and stimulate maturation of dendritic cells. In a phase 1b trial where patients with CRC were given anti-PDL1 with bevacizumab +/− FOLFOX chemotherapy, combination bevacizumab with ICI showed activity in both groups, although greater in the chemotherapy combination cohort (ORR 8% vs 36% respectively) and increased CD8+ T-cell infiltration and PD-L1 expression compared to FOLFOX alone (Bendell et al., 2015).

The phase 2 AtezoTRIBE trial evaluated FOLFOXIRI chemotherapy with bevacizumab alone (Arm A) or in combination with Atezolizumab (Arm B) in the first-line setting in unresectable or metastatic CRC patients followed by maintenance treatment with bevacizumab and 5-FU/leucovorin +/− atezolizumab (Cremolini et al., 2021). In 218 patients treated within this trial a modest but statistically significant improvement in PFS with the addition of atezolizumab was seen (13.1 vs 11.5 months, HR 0.69, 80% CI 0.56–0.85, $p = 0.012$). Overall response rates (ORR) did not reach statistical significance (59% vs 64%, $p = 0.412$). Expectantly the benefit was higher in patients with MSI-H CRC, with PFS 12.9 months in the combination cohort versus 11.4 months in the control cohort with MSS disease. We await results of the translational analysis and subsequent phases of this trial at the time of writing.

ICIs with chemotherapy + anti-EGFR mAbs

Anti-EGFR treatment of metastatic *RAS/BRAF* WT colorectal tumours with monoclonal antibody (mAb) inhibitor agents has been shown to modify tumour gene expression inducing antibody-dependant cytotoxicity and a marked increase in the density of T-cells in the core of metastatic lesions (Van den Eynde et al., 2018). This supports the rationale behind combination approaches with ICIs and EGFR inhibitors in priming immunologically cold tumours.

Results of trials with these combinations to date have been somewhat mixed but with many positive aspects to work from going forward. The single-arm phase 2 AVETUX trial investigated the benefit of adding avelumab to mFOLFOX6 chemotherapy with cetuximab in the front-line metastatic setting for *RAS/BRAF* WT CRC irrespective of microsatellite status (Stein et al., 2020). Whilst secondary end point ORR of the 39 patients included in the intention-to-treat (ITT) analysis was reported to be 79.5% (including six CR (complete responses), 25 PRs (partial responses) and five with SD (stable disease), the study did not meet its primary endpoint of improvement in PFS at 12 months which was 40% (57% target).

In the third-line setting, the phase 2 single-arm CAVE trial assessed the efficacy of combining avelumab with cetuximab in patients with *RAS/BRAF* WT mCRC who had previously responded to anti-EGFR treatment and also irrespective of microsatellite status (Martinelli et al., 2021). This study in a group with advanced and heavily pre-treated CRC was designed based on the evidence that patients with chemotherapy-refractory disease rechallenged with anti-EGFR agents following previous exposure can respond again.

In a cohort of 77 participants, 92% of whom has MSS disease, showed a median OS of 11.6 months and median PFS of 3.6 months. Interestingly, this study also used baseline ctDNA evaluation and found that in subgroup analysis participants with detectable *RAS/BRAF* WT ctDNA prior to treatment had longer OS and PFS; 17.3 months versus 10.4 months ($p = 0.02$) and 4.1 versus 3.0 months ($p = 0.04$) respectively. Evidently there is a degree of efficacy which can be achieved in combining EGFR inhibitors with ICI therapies, but when and how we combine these agents to glean the most benefit is yet to be elucidated.

ICIs plus radiotherapy

The potential benefit from combining ICI therapies with radiotherapy (RT) is very interesting but remains unclear. Initially, trial results when using a single ICI agent with RT, whilst well tolerated, showed limited anti-tumour responses (Franke et al., 2019). The principle of synergism of these treatment modalities is based predominantly on preclinical data which suggests an increase in tumour neoantigens and antigen presentation following RT. The rationale behind this approach in treating *metastatic* disease hinges predominantly on the principle of harnessing the abscopal effect where responses are induced in distant, non-irradiated lesions thereby extending the anti-tumour effect beyond the treatment field. The impact of true abscopal responses remains controversial and widely debated.

In a single-arm, non-randomized, phase 2 trial (NCT03104439) patients with pancreatic ductal adenocarcinoma and MSI-L mCRC were treated with combination low-dose ipilimumab (1 mg/kg) and nivolumab at a dose of 240 mg followed by nivolumab alone every two weeks on day 15 and 29 of a 42-day cycle (Parikh et al., 2021). Providing there was no evidence of clinical or radiological progression and ICI treatment was not limited by toxicity, RT was then commenced at cycle 2 with a total dose of 24 Gy given as 8 Gy in 3 fractions. Disease control was reported in 10 out of 40 patients with MSS mCRC (DCR 25%, 95% CI 13–41%). There are several clinical trials assessing the efficacy of dual agent ICI with radiation in larger cohorts yet to report at the time of writing (e.g. NCT02888743). Whilst such results present promise for the pMMR-MSI-L cohort, there is still a great deal of knowledge to be gained in understanding how these treatments may function in a synergistic manner in terms of radiation doses, fractionation, and timing alongside checkpoint inhibition.

Conclusions and future directions

The history of immunotherapy treatments in CRC has been turbulent. From a molecular perspective there is good evidence to support ongoing assessment of immunotherapeutics in this group, but there is a significant degree of both intra- and inter-tumoural heterogeneity which hampers progress. Furthermore our ability to select patients correctly who will respond to these treatments is suboptimal. The advent of immune checkpoint inhibition has revolutionized the landscape of treatment for patients with dMMR/MSI-H CRC. There remain however many significant ongoing challenges, both in treating intrinsic resistance in pMMR/MSI-L disease and acquired resistance in dMMR/MSI-H disease. How to overcome this resistance and turn immunologically 'cold' tumours 'hot' is yet to be established. In patients with dMMR-MSI-H CRC there are further questions regarding correct timing of immunotherapy in a cohort known to respond poorly to conventional chemotherapy agents at disease relapse.

Whilst immunotherapy treatment is generally well tolerated in comparison to chemotherapy, the toxicity profile remains idiosyncratic and unpredictable, especially when using combination ICIs. The identification and management of immunotherapy toxicity present ongoing clinical challenges and their underpinning mechanisms remain quite poorly understood.

A further level of complexity is presented in the interpretation of responses to immunotherapy both clinically and radiologically,

Table 18.2 Noteworthy clinical trials of immune checkpoint inhibitors in CRC

Trial Identifier	Therapeutic agent(s)	Year	Phase	Study Population	Outcomes
NCT00313794	Tremelimumab anti-CTLA-4	2010	2	Treatment refractory mCRC	< 1% ORR (1/45 with partial response)
First-in-human phase 1 trial of the anti-PD-1 antibody	BMS-936558 (nivolumab) anti-PD-1	2013	1	Treatment refractory solid tumours	1 patient with complete response for 3 years
KEYNOTE-016 (NCT01876511)	Pembrolizumab anti-PD-1	2016	2	MSI-H/dMMR mCRC	ORR 50%
KEYNOTE-164 (NCT02460198)	Pembrolizumab anti-PD1	2018	2	MSI-H/dMMR mCRC with $\geq$ 1 line or previous therapy	ORR 33% 2 years OS 63%
KEYNOTE-177 (NCT02563002)	Pembrolizumab anti-PD-1	2020	3	Treatment naïve MSI-H mCRC	ORR 43.8% (vs 33.1% with standard chemotherapy)
CheckMate-142 (NCT02060188)	Nivolumab anti-PD-1	2017	2	MSI-H/dMMR mCRC with $\geq$ 1 line of previous therapy	ORR 31% 1 year OS 73%
CheckMate-142 Combination Arm (NCT02060188)	Nivolumab and ipilimumab anti-PD-1 and anti-CTLA-4	2020	2	Treatment naïve MSI-H-dMMR mCRC	ORR 69% 2 year PFS 74% 2 year OS 79%

which can be quite distinct from those seen with other therapies. Pseudoprogression in response to ICI was first described in advanced melanoma patients treated with anti-CTLA4 agent ipilimumab (Di Giacomo et al., 2009), but has subsequently been observed in multiple other solid tumours treated with immunotherapy including CRC. The term 'pseudoprogression' refers to the observation of transient tumour flare in response to treatment and subsequent delayed tumour regression, which can be durable. This change has been attributed to the dense infiltration of immune cells that occurs during treatment response, as confirmed on histological samples. In the NICHE neoadjuvant study of combination immunotherapy treatment in patients with early-stage colon cancers, correlation between the radiological assessment of response post treatment and pre-operatively was poor, especially amongst patients with major pathological responses (≤ 10% visible residual tumour) who were often assessed as having gross residual disease on computed tomography (CT) (Chalabi et al., 2020).

This clearly creates an additional layer of complexity in the assessment of treatment efficacy for clinicians treating patients with immunotherapy and in the accurate reporting clinical trial outcomes. Withstanding the challenges that new treatments inevitably present, immunotherapy has undoubtedly had an unprecedented impact on the treatment landscape for many solid tumours and a welcome addition to our treatment armoury in CRC. Expanding its utility to help a wider scope of patients with CRC to gain clinically meaningful and durable responses remains possible, but is yet to be achieved.

REFERENCES

André, T., Shiu, K. K., Kim, T. W., et al. (2021). Final overall survival for the phase III KN177 study: Pembrolizumab versus chemotherapy in microsatellite instability-high/mismatch repair deficient (MSI-H/dMMR) metastatic colorectal cancer (mCRC). *Journal of Clinical Oncology*, *39*(15), suppl. 3500.

André, T., Elez, E., Van Cutsem, E., et al. (2024). Nivolumab plus ipilumumab in microsatellite-instability-high metastatic colorectal cancer. *New England Journal of Medicine*, *391*(21), 2014–2026.

André, T., Elez, E., Lenz, H. J., et al. (2025). Nivolumab plus ipilumumab versus nivolumab in microsatellite instability-high metastatic colorectal cancer (Checkmate 8HW): A randomised open-label, phase 3 trial. *Lancet*, *405*, 383–395.

Baraibar, I., Mirallas O., Saoudi, N., et al. (2021). Combined treatment with immunotherapy-based strategies for MSS metastatic colorectal cancer. *Cancers (Basel)*, *13*(24), 6311.

Becht, E., de Reyniès, A., Giraldo, N. A., et al. (2016). Immune and stromal classification of colorectal cancer is associated with molecular subtypes and relevant for precision immunotherapy. *Clinical Cancer Research*, *22*(16), 4057–4066.

Bendell, J. C., Powderly, J. D., Lieu, C. H., et al. (2015). Safety and efficacy of MPDL3280A (anti-PDL1) in combination with bevacizumab (bev) and/or FOLFOX in patients (pts) with metastatic colorectal cancer (mCRC). *Journal of Clinical Oncology*, *33*(3_suppl), 704–704.

Biller, L. H., & Schrag, D. (2021). Diagnosis and treatment of colorectal cancer. A review. *JAMA*, *325*(7), 669–685.

Bourdais, R., Rousseau, B., Pujals, A., et al. (2017). Polymerase proofreading domain mutations: New opportunities for immunotherapy in hypermutated colorectal cancer beyond MMR deficiency. *Critical Reviews in Oncology/Hematology*, *113*, 242–248.

Cancer Genome Atlas. (2012). Comprehensive molecular characterization of human colon and rectal cancer. *Nature*, *487*, 330–337.

Carlson, R. D., Flickinger, J. C. Jr., & Snook, A. E. (2020). Talkin' toxins: from Coley's to modern cancer immunotherapy. *Toxins (Basel)* *12*(4), 241.

Chalabi, M., Fanchi, L. F., Dijkstra, K. K., et al. (2020). Neoadjuvant immunotherapy leads to pathological responses in MMR-proficient and MMR-deficient early-stage colon cancers. *Nature Medicine*, *26*(4), 566–576.

Cheong, C. K., Nistala, K. R. Y., Ng, C. H., et al. (2020). Neoadjuvant therapy in locally advanced colon cancer: a meta-analysis and systematic review. *Journal of Gastrointestinal Oncology*, *11*(5), 847–857.

Chiang, C. L. L., Coukos, G., & Kandalaft, L. E. (2015). Whole tumor antigen vaccines: where are we?' *Vaccines*, *3*, 344–372.

Chung, K. Y., Gore, I., Fong, L., et al. (2010). Phase II study of the anti-cytotoxic T-lymphocyte-associated antigen 4 monoclonal antibody, tremelimumab, in patients with refractory metastatic colorectal cancer. *Journal of Clinical Oncology*, *28*(21), 3485–3490.

Cohen, R., Shi, Q., & André, T. (2020). Immunotherapy for early stage colorectal cancer: a glance into the future. *Cancers (Basel)* *12*(7), 1990.

Cremolini, C., Rossini, D., Antoniotti, C., et al. (2021). FOLFOXIRI plus bevacizumab (bev) plus atezolizumab (atezo) versus FOLFOXIRI plus bev as first-line treatment of unresectable metastatic colorectal cancer (mCRC) patients: Results of the phase II randomized AtezoTRIBE study by GONO. *Annals of Oncology*, *32*(5), S1294–S1295.

Di Giacomo, A. M., Danielli, R., Guidoboni, M., et al. (2009). Therapeutic efficacy of ipilimumab, an antiCTLA-4 monoclonal antibody, in patients with metastatic melanoma unresponsive to prior systemic treatments: clinical and immunological evidence from three patient cases. *Cancer Immunology, Immunotherapy*, 58, 1297–1306.

Fong, L., Hou, Y., Rivas, A., et al. (2001). Altered peptide ligand vaccination with Flt3 ligand expanded dendritic cells for tumor immunotherapy. *Proceedings of the National Academy of Sciences of the USA*, *98*, 8809–8814.

Franke, A. J., Skelton, W. P., Starr, J. S., et al. (2019). Immunotherapy for colorectal cancer: a review of current and novel therapeutic approaches. *Journal of the National Cancer Institute*, *111*(11), 1131–1141.

Galon, J., Costes, A., Sanchez-Cabo, F., et al. (2006). Type, density and location of immune cells within human colorectal tumours predict clinical outcome. Science, *313*(5795), 1960–1964.

Garmezy, B., Gheeya, J. S., Thein, K. Z., et al. (2020). Correlation of pathogenic POLE mutations with clinical benefit to immune checkpoint inhibitor therapy. *Journal of Clinical Oncology*, *38*(15), suppl 3008.

Golshani, G., & Zhang, Y. (2020). Advances in immunotherapy for colorectal cancer: a review. *Therapeutic Advances in Gastroenterology*, *13*, 1756284820917527.

Gurjao, C., Liu, D., Hofree, M., et al. (2019). Intrinsic resistance to immune checkpoint blockade in a mismatch repair-deficient colorectal cancer. *Cancer Immunology Research*, *7*(8), 1230–1236.

Heriot, A. G., Marriott, J. B., Cookson, S., Kumar, D., & Dalgleish, A. G. (2000). Reduction in cytokine production in colorectal cancer patients: association with stage and reversal by resection. *British Journal of Cancer*, *82*(5), 1009–12.

Jobin, G., Rodriguez-Suarez, R., & Betito, K. (2017). Association between natural killer cell activity and colorectal cancer in high-risk subjects undergoing colonoscopy. *Gastroenterology*, *153*(4), 980–987.

Kamal, Y., Schmit, S. L., Frost, H. R., & Amos, C. I. (2020). The tumor microenvironment of colorectal cancer metastases: opportunities in cancer immunotherapy. *Immunotherapy*, *12*(14), 1083–1100.

Lanuza, P. M., Vigueras, A., Olivan, S., et al. (2018). Activated human primary NK cells efficiently kill colorectal cancer cells in 3D spheroid cultures irrespectively of the level of PD-L1 expression. *Oncoimmunology*, *7*(4), e1395123.

Le, D. T., Uram, J. N., Wang, H., Bartlett, B. R., Kemberling, H., & Eyring, A. D. (2015). PD-1 blockade in tumors with mismatch-repair deficiency. *New England Journal of Medicine*, *372*(26), 2509–2520.

Lenz, H. J., Van Cutsem, E., Luisa Limon, M., et al. (2022). *Journal of Clinical Oncology*, *40*(2), 161–170.

Lipson, E. J., Sharfman, W. H., Drake, C. G., et al. (2013). Durable cancer regression off-treatment and effective reinduction therapy with an anti-PD-1 antibody. *Clinical Cancer Research*, *19*(2), 462–468.

Liu, G. C., Liu, R. Y., Yan, J. P., et al. (2018). The heterogeneity between Lynch-associated and sporadic MMR deficiency in colorectal cancers. *Journal of the National Cancer Institute*, *110*(9), 975–984.

Llosa, N. J., Cruise, M., Tam, A., et al. (2021). The vigorous immune microenvironment of microsatellite instable colon cancer is balanced by multiple counter-inhibitory checkpoints. *Cancer Discovery*, *5*(1), 43–51.

Long, L., Zhang, X., Chen, F., et al. (2018). The promising immune checkpoint LAG-3: from tumor microenvironment to cancer immunotherapy. *Genes & Cancer*, *9*(5-6), 176–189.

Lumish, M. A., & Cercek, A. (2021). Immunotherapy for the treatment of colorectal cancer. *Journal of Surgical Oncology*, *123*(3), 760–774.

Martinelli, E., Martini, G., Famiglietti, V., et al. (2021). Cetuximab rechallenge plus avelumab in pretreated patients with RAS wild-type metastatic colorectal cancer: the phase 2 single-arm clinical CAVE trial. *JAMA Oncology*, *7*(10), 1529–1535.

Midgley, R., & Kerr, D. J. (2003). Immunotherapy for colorectal cancer. *Expert Review of Anticancer Therapy*, *3*(1), 63–78.

Morse, M. A., Deng, Y., et al (1999). A Phase I study of active immunotherapy with carcinoembryonic antigen peptide (CAP-1)- pulsed, autologous human cultured dendritic cells in patients with metastatic malignancies expressing carcinoembryonic antigen. *Clinical Cancer Research*, *5*, 1331–1338.

Narasimhan, V., Toan, P., Wilson, K., et al. (2019). Colorectal peritoneal metastases: exploring the immune landscape and the potential of immunotherapy using organoid models,' *Cancer Research*, *79*(13), 2.

Ohm, J. E., & Carborne, D. P. (2001). VEGF as a mediator of tumor-associated immunodeficiency. *Immunologic Research*, *23*, 263–272.

Overman, M. J., Lonardi, S., Wong, K. Y. M., et al. (2018). Durable clinical benefit with nivolumab plus ipilimumab in DNA mismatch repair-deficient/microsatellite instability-high metastatic colorectal cancer. *Journal of Clinical Oncology*, *36*(8), 773–779.

Overman, M. J., Lonardi, S., Wong, K. Y. M., et al. (2019). Nivolumab (NIVO) + low-dose ipilimumab (IPI) in previously treated patients (pts) with microsatellite instability-high/mismatch repair-deficient (MSI-H/dMMR) metastatic colorectal cancer (mCRC), Long-term follow-up. *Journal of Clinical Oncology*, *37*(4), suppl. 635.

Overman, M. J., McDermott, R., Leach, J. L., et al. (2017). Nivolumab in patients with metastatic DNA mismatch repair-deficient or microsatellite instability-high colorectal cancer (CheckMate 142), an open-label, multicentre, phase 2 study. *Lancet Oncology*, *18*(9), 1182–1191.

Palles, C., Cazier, J. B., Howarth, K., et al. (2013). Germline mutations in the proof-reading domains of *POLE* and *POLD1* predispose to colorectal adenomas and carcinomas. *Nature Genetics*, *45*(2), 136–144.

Parikh, A. R., Szabolcs, A., Allen, J. N., et al. (2021). Radiation therapy enhances immunotherapy response in microsatellite stable colorectal and pancreatic adenocarcinoma in a phase II trial. *Nature Cancer*, *2*, 1124–1135.

Patel, S. P., & Kurzrock, R. (2015). PD-L1 expression as a predictive biomarker in cancer immunotherapy. *Molecular Cancer Therapeutics*, *14*(4), 847–856.

Quasar Collaborative Group; Gray, R., Barnwell, J., et al. (2007). Adjuvant chemotherapy versus observation in patients with colorectal cancer: a randomised study. *Lancet*, *370*(9604), 2020–2029.

Smith, M. E. F., Bodmer, J. G., Kelly, A. P., et al. (1989). Variation in HLA expression on tumors: an escape from immune response. *Cold Spring Harbor Symposia on Quantitative Biology*, *54*, 581–586.

Stein, A., Binder, M., Goekkurt, E., et al. (2020). Avelumab and cetuximab in combination with FOLFOX in patients with previously untreated metastatic colorectal cancer (MCRC): final results of the phase II AVETUX trial (AIO-KRK-0216). *Journal of Clinical Oncology*, *38*(4), suppl. 96–96.

Sun, B. L. (2021). Current microsatellite instability testing in management of colorectal cancer. *Clinical Colorectal Cancer*, *20*(1), e12–20.

Tabernero, J., Grothey, A., Van Cutsem, E., et al. (2021). Encorafenib plus cetuximab as a new standard of care for previously treated *BRAF* V600E-mutant metastatic colorectal cancer: updated survival results and subgroup analyses from the BEACON study. *Journal of Clinical Oncology*, *39*(4), 273–284.

Tauriello, D., Palomo-Ponce, S., Stork, D., et al. (2018). TGFβ drives immune evasion in genetically reconstituted colon cancer metastasis. *Nature*, *554*, 538–543.

TCGA. (2012). Comprehensive molecular characterization of human colon and rectal cancer. *Nature*, *18*, **487**(7407), 330–337.

Toyoshima, Y., Kitamura, H., Xiang, H., et al. (2019). IL6 modulates the immune status of the tumor microenvironment to facilitate metastatic colonization of colorectal cancer cells. *Cancer Immunology Research*, **7**, 1944–1957.

Uyl-de Groot, C. A., Vermorken, J. B., Hanna, M. G. Jr., et al. (2005). Immunotherapy with autologous tumor cell-BCG vaccine in patients with colon cancer: a prospective study of medical and economic benefits. *Vaccine*, *23* (17–18), 2379–2387.

Van den Eynde, M., Mlecnik, B., Bindea, G., et al. (2018). The link between the multiverse of immune microenvironments in metastases and the survival of colorectal cancer patients. *Cancer Cell*, *34*(6), 1012–1026.

Walther, A., Johnstone, E., Swanton, C., et al. (2009). Genetic prognostic and predictive markers in colorectal cancer. *Nature Reviews Cancer*, *9*, 489–499.

Wang, H., Tian, T., & Zhang, J. (2021). Tumor-associated macrophages (TAMs) in colorectal cancer (CRC): from mechanism to therapy and prognosis. *International Journal of Molecular Sciences*, *22*(16), 8470.

Wang, S., Sun, J., Chen, K., et al. (2018). Perspectives of tumor-infiltrating lymphocyte treatment in solid tumors. *BMC Medicine*, *19*, 140.

Wang, W., Wu, L., Zhang, J., et al. (2017). Chemoimmunotherapy by combining oxaliplatin with immune checkpoint blockades reduced tumor burden in colorectal cancer animal model. *Biochemical and Biophysical Research Communications*, *487*(1), 1–7.

Wooster, A. L., Girgis, L. H., Brazeale, H., et al. (2021). Dendritic cell vaccine therapy for colorectal cancer. *Pharmacological Research*, *164*, 105374.

Yarchoan, M., Hopkins, A., & Jaffee, E. M. (2017). Tumor mutational burden and response rate to PD-1 inhibition. *New England Journal of Medicine*, *377* (25), 2500–2501.

19

Novel targets for drug development

Jesus Garcia-Foncillas

Molecular sub-types in colorectal cancer

Three major pathways are involved in colorectal cancer (CRC) origin and progression: (a) chromosomal instability (CIN); (b) microsatellite instability (MSI); (c) CpG island methylation phenotype (CIMP). CIN is the most common (85% of total CRCs) genetic mechanism occurring in CRC (Testa et al., 2020).

CIN is characterized by the acquisition of a consistent karyotypic variability, aneuploidy, chromosomal and subchromosomal aberrations, gene amplifications, and loss of heterozygosity. MSI involves several recurrent alterations in the microsatellite zone, approximately 15% of all CRCs due to germline mutations in mismatch repair (MMR) system or somatic inactivation by promoter hypermethylation of MLH1 gene. CIMP pathway is responsible for 20–30% of total CRCs and is predominantly observed in the proximal colon (30–40%) and more rarely in distal colon (3–12%) (Müller et al., 2016).

The CMS transcriptional classification was implemented through the analysis of microenvironment signatures, showing consistent correlation between these two classification systems: the CMS1 subgroup was characterized by elevated expression of genes specific to cytotoxic T lymphocytes; the CMS4 subgroup was characterized by several microenvironmental features, including expression of monocytic markers and a combined angiogenesis and inflammatory and immunosuppressive signature; at pathologic level, CMS4 tumours display numerous infiltrating fibroblasts, producing cytokines and chemokines inducing the angiogenetic and inflammatory phenotypes; CMS2 and CMS3 subgroups exhibit low inflammatory and immune signatures (Becht et al., 2016).

Currently the management of metastatic colorectal cancer is based on three biomarkers that are well established: RAS status, to select a treatment based on chemotherapy plus anti-EGFR; BRAF to use BRAF inhibitors alone or in combination with MEK inhibitors; and dMMR/MSI-H to identify candidates to be treated with immunotherapy. In this chapter, new targets for drug development will be reviewed.

Targets on cell membrane

Claudin 18.2

Alterations in claudin expression can impair tight junction function, influence signalling pathways, and act as a tumour-promoting event in some epithelial cancers. In total, 4.1% from a total of 414 were claudin 18.2-positive, including colorectal with a frequency of 0.9%. In the whole group, no significant difference was found in overall survival between patients with and without claudin 18.2 expression (Hong et al., 2020).

CLDN18 was assessed in colitis-associated colorectal adenocarcinomas (CAC) and it was reported positive in 27% of CACs vs 5% in sporadic CRCs. CLDN18-positive CACs were more likely to have lymph node metastasis than CLDN18-negative CACs (67% versus 36%; $P = 0.017$) (Iawaya et al., 2021).

CEACAM5

Carcinoembryonic antigen (CEA, CEACAM5, CD66) is a promoter of metastasis in epithelial cancers that is widely used as a prognostic clinical marker of metastasis. The Molecular analysis identified significantly enriched pathways: cytokine–cytokine receptor interaction, MAPK signalling pathway, TGF-beta signalling pathway, and pyrimidine metabolism. These data suggest that CEA production by colorectal cancer cells triggers colorectal cancer progression by inducing the epithelial–mesenchymal transition, increasing tumour cell invasiveness into the surrounding tissues and suppressing stress and apoptotic signalling (Bajenova et al., 2016).

The T-cell bispecific antibody cibisatamab (CEA-TCB) binds carcino-embryonic antigen (CEA) on cancer cells and CD3 on T-cells, which triggers T-cell killing of cancer cell lines expressing moderate to high levels of CEA at the cell surface. Cell surface CEA expression was up-regulated by inhibitors of the Wnt/β-catenin pathway. Based on these preclinical findings, heterogeneity and plasticity of CEA expression appear to confer low cibisatamab sensitivity in PDOs. Pharmacological inhibition of the WNT/β-catenin pathway may be a rational combination to sensitize CRCs to cibisatamab (Gonzalez-Exposito et al., 2019).

Labetuzumab govitecan is an antibody-drug conjugate targeting carcinoembryonic antigen-related cell adhesion molecule 5 (CEACAM5) for tumour delivery of 7-ethyl-10-hydroxycamptothecin (SN-38). Monotherapy with labetuzumab govitecan demonstrated a manageable safety profile and therapeutic activity in heavily pretreated patients with metastatic colorectal cancer, all with prior irinotecan therapy (Dotan et al., 2017).

CXCR4

Chemokines are chemotactic cytokines that promote cancer growth, metastasis, and regulate resistance to chemotherapy. Stromal cell-derived factor 1 (SDF1) also known as C-X-C motif chemokine 12 (CXCL12), a prognostic factor, is an extracellular homeostatic chemokine that is the natural ligand for chemokine receptors C-X-C chemokine receptor type 4 (CXCR4), also known as fusin or cluster of differentiation 184 (CD184) and chemokine receptor type 7 (CXCR7). CXCR4 is the most widely expressed rhodopsin-like G protein coupled chemokine receptor (GPCR). The CXCL12-CXCR4 axis is involved in tumour growth, invasion, angiogenesis, and metastasis in colorectal cancer (CRC) (Khare et al., 2021).

A meta-analysis reported High CXCR4 expression is clearly associated with increased risk of death and progression in CRC. However, strong methodologic heterogeneity in CXCR4 assessment hinders direct translation into clinical practice (Ottaiano et al., 2021).

CXCR4 plays an important role in the metastatic potential resulting in a poorer prognosis and disease recurrence in solid tumours. In colon cancer, CXCR4 expression is associated with advanced Union for International Cancer Control (UICC) stages and lymphatic or hematopoietic metastases. In our study, CXCR4 was associated with mucinous adenocarcinomas, advanced T-stage, and high MSI. Whether CXCR4 over-expression explains the need for prolonged adjuvant treatment in T4 colon cancer patients (Maderer et al., 2021).

FGFR

Fibroblast growth factor receptor (FGFR) genetic alterations are frequently observed in cancer, suggesting that FGFR inhibition may be a promising therapy in patients harbouring these lesions (Karkera et al., 2017). Karkera et al. (2017) did not find FGFR family gene amplifications in colon cancer. In a series published by Sun et al. (2020) the overall prevalence of FGFR aberrations was 7.0%. FGFR1 amplification was the most common genetic alteration in colorectal cancer, breast cancer, and lung cancer, while FGFR2 amplification was more commonly observed in gastric cancer (Su et al., 2020).

Rogaratinib, an FGFR inhibitor, was tested in human colorectal cancer cell line-derived models showing a significant efficacy with FGFR2 amplifications (Grünewald et al., 219).

HER2

Amplification of *ERBB2* (formerly referred to as HER2) is present in nearly 3% of patients with metastatic colorectal cancer overall and 5% of patients with *KRAS* and *NRAS* wild-type tumours (Strickler et al., 2022).

It has been compared the addition of trastuzumab to chemotherapy versus chemotherapy alone or in combination to cetuximab or bevacizumab. The study revealed a significant difference in median PFS in favour for those patients treated with anti-HER therapy (Yang et al., 2022).

In the Heracles clinical trial, *KRAS* exon 2 wild-type and HER2-positive metastatic colorectal cancer refractory to standard of care (including cetuximab or panitumumab) were enrolled and treated with trastuzumab and lapatinib until evidence of disease progression. The primary endpoint was the proportion of patients with objective response; 30% achieved an objective response: 4% complete response and 26% partial responses; 44% stable disease. Grade 3 adverse events were reported in 22% (Sartore-Bianchi et al., 2016).

Following this study, HERACLES-B trial assessed the efficacy of the combination of pertuzumab and trastuzumab-emtansine (T-DM1) in metastatic colorectal cancer; 48% with ≥ four lines of previous therapies were included. Objective response rate was 9.7% and stable disease 67.7%. Objective response or stable disease with a duration longer or equal to four months was associated with higher HER2 immunohistochemistry score (3+ vs 2+, $p = 0.03$). Median PFS was 4.1 months.

In a phase 2 trial evaluating the efficacy of pertuzumab plus trastuzumab for metastatic colorectal cancer (mCRC), HER2 amplification was confirmed in tissue and/or ctDNA. This study confirmed an objective response rate of 30% in tissue HER2-positive patients and 28% in ctDNA HER2-positive, as compared to an objective response rate of 0% in a matched real-world reference population treated with standard-of-care salvage therapy. Decreased ctDNA fraction three weeks after treatment initiation associated with therapeutic response. Pertuzumab plus trastuzumab showed similar efficacy in patients with mCRC with HER2 amplification in tissue or ctDNA, showing that ctDNA genotyping can identify patients who benefit from dual-HER2 blockade as well as monitor treatment response (Nakamura et al., 2021). Pyrotinib has also demonstrated in HER2-positive non-breast advanced solid tumours has good antitumor activity and acceptable safety (Wang et al., 2022).

Trastuzumab deruxtecan showed promising and durable activity in HER2-positive metastatic colorectal cancer refractory to standard treatment, with a safety profile consistent with that reported in previous trastuzumab deruxtecan trials. Interstitial lung disease and pneumonitis are important risks requiring careful monitoring and prompt intervention (Siena et al., 2021).

cMET mutation

Probably the most comprehensive assessment of cMET was done by Caris Life Sciences with a frequency of positivity by immunohistochemistry in colorectal cancer of 38.8% and a rate of mutations of 2.7%. Concordance was poor based on kappa coefficients, with calculated values of 0.012 (between IHC and FISH/CISH) and 0.007 (between FISH/CISH and NGS). Also, of 2938 cases where all three tests were performed, 904 cases (31%) had only one of three positive tests (Arguello et al., 2013).

Currently three inhibitors have been evaluated: capmatinib, savolitinib, and tepotinib.

In the dose escalation of the phase 1 study of capmatinib in MET-positive solid tumour patients eight colorectal cancer patients were recruited. In one of these cases, a near-complete p-MET shutdown by immunohistochemistry was reached 15 days after the first dose (Bang et al., 2022).

TROP2

TROP2 is a calcium signal transducer and is highly expressed in several types of tumours. The cases with high TROP2 expression showed a higher frequency of liver metastasis, deeper depth of invasion, and more lymph node metastasis. Patients with high TROP2 expression tumours had poorer prognosis (Ohmachi et al., 2006).

TROP2 expression in primary tumours and liver oligometastases was significantly positively correlated ($r = 0.758$, $p < 0.001$). This subsetting of patients with high TROP2 expression had worse three-year relapse-/recurrence-free survival (RFS) (44.2% vs 66.4%, $p = 0.007$) and three-year overall survival (OS) rates (70.3% vs 85.4%, $p = 0.035$) than did those with low TROP2 expression. Gene expression profile analysis indicated that high TROP2 expression was associated with TNFα signalling via NF-κB, the inflammatory response, and epithelial–mesenchymal transition (Peng et al., 2019).

Sacituzumab govitecan (SG), a trophoblast cell surface antigen-2 (TROP-2)-directed antibody-drug conjugate, has demonstrated anti-tumour efficacy and acceptable tolerability in a phase 1/2 multicentre trial (NCT01631552) in patients with advanced epithelial cancers. In colorectal cancer it has been reported a response rate of 3.2% and a stable disease rate of 51.6% (Bardia et al., 2021).

Signalling transduction

KRAS G12C

Osterlund et al. described that KRAS-G12C frequency was 2–4% of all colorectal cancer samples and 4–8% of KRAS mutated tumours in the cohorts (mean 7%) (Osterlund et al., 2022).

Giamperi et al. reported 12% KRAS G12C mutated of all KRAS mutant colorectal cancer (Giamperi et al., 2021). In KRAS G12C patients when treated with standard chemotherapy doublet + bevacizumab, 27% had partial response and 40% stable disease. In patients with other KRAS mutations, 52% had partial response and 35% stable disease. The difference in response rate between the two groups of patients was statistically significant ($p = 0.017$). On the other hand, no difference in PFS ($p = 0.76$) and OS ($p = 0.56$) was observed. KRAS G12C mutations were not associated with differences in sites of metastatic involvement, sex, and ECOG PS. On the other hand, synchronous vs metachronous metastatic disease, age > 75 years, and mucinous histology were more frequent in G12C mutated tumours (Giamperi et al., 2021).

In the CodeBreaK100 clinical trial, sotorasib was assessed in previously treated colorectal cancers with KRAS(G12C) mutation. Sixty-two patients were enrolled. Objective response was observed in 9.7%, all with partial response. Treatment-related adverse events at grade 3 occurred in 10% patients, the most common of which was diarrhoea (3%), and at grade 4 occurred in 2% (blood creatine phosphokinase increase). This overall response rate did not reach the benchmark, so new combinations with sotorasib are under evaluation to increase potential activity (Fakih et al., 2022).

Adagrasib, an oral small-molecule inhibitor of the mutant KRAS protein has shown clinical activity in pretreated metastatic CRC. In the KRYSTAL-1 trial adagrasib plus cetuximab was administered to patients who had previously received fluoropyrimidines, oxaliplatin, and irinotecan; the combination gave a confirmed overall response rate of 34% and a disease control rate of 85% (Yeager et al., 2024). Because of the usual poor prognosis of this mutated G12C patient population, the US Food and Drug Administration (FDA) granted accelerated approval to this combination in this setting of metastatic CRC in 2024.

PI3K

Mutations in the alpha catalytic subunit (PI3KCA) of the enzyme phosphatidylinositol-3 kinase (PI3K) were found in 20% to 25% of colorectal cancers. Mutations in PIK3CA are associated with higher rates of mutations in other genes such as the tyrosine kinase receptors/K-Ras/BRAF/MAPK and the Wnt/β-catenin pathway. In addition, PIK3CA mutated colorectal cancers display a higher TMB than non-mutated cancers (Voutsadakis, 2021).

Immunotherapy targeting the CD274 (PD-L1)/PDCD1 (PD-1) axis has been raised as a promising treatment strategy. Different evidence suggests that PI3KCA signalling may upregulate CD274 expression (Ugai et al., 2021). Ugai et al. have reported that PIK3CA-mutated PTEN-lost tumours showed higher prevalence of CD274-positivity (82%) than PIK3CA-wild-type PTEN-lost tumours (70% CD274-positivity) and PTEN-expressed tumours (50% CD274-positivity) (Ugai et al., 2021). Low TMBs and PTEN mutations, especially mutations in the phosphatase domain associated with an immunosuppressive environment, were mutually exclusive and might be negative predictors of PD-1 blockade responses in patients with MSI-H/dMMR gastrointestinal (GI) tumours (Chida et al., 2021).

Dumbrava et al. (2021) reported in a clinical series of different tumour types including colorectal cancer 85% harbouring PIK3CA mutations in tumour tissue and 74% PIK3CA mutations in ctDNA with an overall concordance of 72%. PIK3CA-mutated ctDNA VAF of ≤ 8.5% showed a longer median survival compared with patients with a higher VAF (15.9 vs 9.4 months; $P = 0.014$). Longitudinal analysis of ctDNA showed that those with a decrease in PIK3CA VAF had a longer time to treatment failure (TTF) compared with patients with an increase or no change (10.7 vs 2.6 months; $P = 0.048$) (Dumbrava et al., 2021).

In a phase 1 trial of the oral PI3K inhibitor BKM120 plus mFOLFOX6 were evaluated in GI malignancies including colorectal cancer, cholangiocarcinoma, pancreatic cancer, and hepatocellular carcinoma. DLT (dose-limiting toxicity) included grade 3 hyperglycaemia, grade 3 AST/ALT elevation, grade 4 neutropenia, and grade 4 thrombocytopenia. One patient demonstrated an unconfirmed partial response and three patients had stable disease (McRee et al., 2015).

Resistance to epidermal growth factor inhibition in patients with KRAS wild-type colorectal cancer may occur because of PI3K/AKT/mTOR signalling. Patients with chemotherapy refractory KRAS wild-type who were EGFRi naive were enrolled. One patient (5.9%) who was PTEN and PIK3CA negative by IHC had a partial response, seven had stable disease, and nine had disease progression (Goodwin et al., 2020).

PX-866 is an oral, irreversible, pan-isoform inhibitor of PI3K. Patients with anti-EGFR-naive KRAS codon 12 and 13 wild-type were randomized to cetuximab with or without PX-866. The median PFS was 59 days versus 104 days for arms A (cetuximab + PX-866) and B (cetuximab alone), respectively. OS between the two arms (266 vs 333 days for arm A vs B) were similar. PIK3CA mutations and PTEN loss by immunohistochemistry were infrequently seen. The combination arm had greater toxicity and may have been harmful in this study (Bowles et al., 2016).

In a phase-1 clinical trial PI3K/mTOR inhibitor gedatolisib (PF-05212384) in combination with the MEK inhibitor PD-0325901 or irinotecan were tested in different arms in patients with advanced solid tumours. In colorectal cancer gedatolisib plus irinotecan produced a response rate of 5% and clinical benefit in 16% of patients with advanced colorectal cancer (progression-free survival, 2.8 months) (Wainberg et al., 2017).

SH2P

The SH2 domain-containing phosphatase 2 (SHP2) is a widely expressed protein tyrosine phosphatase, and it is proposed to act as an oncogenic protein (Yu et al., 2021). SRC homology region 2 domain-containing phosphatase 1 (SHP-1) has been implicated as a potential cancer therapeutic target by its negative regulation of immune cell activation (Kundu et al., 2010). SHP2 is also engaged in drug resistance of a variety of cancers. Yu et al. reported that SHP2 contributes oxaliplatin resistance through AKT and ERK and suggested that SHP2-targeting is a potential strategy for overcoming oxaliplatin resistance in colon cancer (Yu et al., 2021).

In this way, Cruz-Duarte et al. (2022) described a novel resistance mechanism involving a noncatalytic role of PLCγ1 SH2 tandem domains in the propagation of downstream signalling via SH2-containing protein tyrosine phosphatase 2 (SHP2). Accordingly, SHP2 inhibition sensitizes PLCγ1-resistant cells to cetuximab (Cruz-Duarte et al., 2022).

DNA repair and gene expression control

Homologous recombination deficiency (HRD)

In a large series of colorectal cancer samples, 13.6% were homologous recombination deficient (HRD). HRD tumours were more frequent among MSI-H/dMMR than MSS/pMMR tumours (73.4% vs 9.5%; $p < .001$). In MSS/pMMR group, HRD tumours were more frequently tumour mutational burden high (8.1% vs 2.2%; $p < .001$) and PD-L1 positive (5.0% vs 2.4%; $p < .001$; $q = 0.001$), enriched in all immune cell and fibroblast populations and genomic loss of heterozygosity-high (16.2% vs 9.5%; $p = .03$). In the TRIBE2 study, patients with MSS/pMMR and HRD tumours (10.7%) showed longer overall survival compared with MSS/pMMR and HRP tumours (40.2 vs 23.8 months; $p = .04$) (Moretto et al., 2022).

Defects in the homologous recombination (HR) repair pathway are of clinical interest due to sensitivity of HR-deficient cells to PARP inhibitors. Arena et al. (2020) assessed multiple colorectal cancer cell lines and found 13% highly sensitive to clinically active concentrations of olaparib and displayed functional deficiency in homologous recombination. These authors outlined that as mCRC patients receive very often therapies based on oxaliplatin, maintenance treatment with PARP inhibitors could be an option to be explored (Arena et al., 2020).

A phase 1 study of olaparib and irinotecan in patients with colorectal cancer was conducted by the Canadian Cancer Trials Group (IND 187). Twenty-five patients with advanced colorectal cancer whose disease progressed after at least one systemic therapy regimen were enrolled. Intermittent olaparib administration was better tolerated than continuous, and the recommended phase 2 doses were olaparib 50 mg p.o. (orally) twice daily days 1 to 5 and irinotecan 125 mg/m^2 intravenously (IV) every two weeks. Common toxicities included fatigue, anorexia, diarrhoea, nausea, vomiting, neutropenia, thrombocytopenia, and abdominal pain. The efficacy was low with nine patients with stable disease as the best response. Both olaparib and irinotecan required significant dose reductions (Chen et al., 2016).

In a phase 2 trial olaparib was evaluated for patients with metastatic CRC failing standard therapies with confirmed tumour MSI status. The primary endpoint was the tumour response. Thirty-three patients (20 microsatellite stable (MSS), 13 MSI-H) were enrolled. All patients received at least one 28-day cycle of olaparib. No patient had a complete or partial response. Nausea (48%), fatigue (36%), and vomiting (33%) were the most reported treatment-related adverse events. The median PFS for all patients was 1.84 months. No statistically significant differences were found in the median PFS or OS for the MSS group compared with the MSI-H group. In this trial, single agent olaparib failed to elicit responses in patients with MSI-H colorectal tumours. It is possible that by adding olaparib to radiation therapy, or to a systemic DNA damaging agent, tumour lethality could be obtained (Leichman et al., 2016).

LSD1

Epigenetic mechanisms are known to play a key role in cancer progression. Specifically, histone methylation involves reversible post-translational modification of histones that govern chromatin structure remodelling, genomic imprinting, gene expression, DNA damage repair, and meiotic cross-over recombination, among other chromatin-based activities. Demethylases are enzymes that catalyse the demethylation of their substrate using a flavin adenine dinucleotide-dependent amine oxidation process. Lysine-specific demethylase 1 (LSD1) and its homolog, lysine-specific demethylase 2 (LSD2), are over-expressed in a variety of human cancer types and, thus, regulate tumour progression (Malagraba et al., 2022).

Peng et al. reported overexpression of LSD1 as a potential marker for 5-FU resistance in colorectal cancer suggesting that could be a promising target to overcome this lack of response to fluoropyrimidines. These authors described the combination of ZY0511, a novel LSD1 inhibitor, and 5-FU synergistically reduced CRC cells viability and migration *in vitro*. It also suppressed Wnt/β-catenin signalling and DNA synthesis pathways, which finally induced apoptosis of CRC cells. In addition, the combination of ZY0511 with 5-FU significantly reduced CRC xenograft tumour growth, along with lung and liver metastases *in vivo* (Peng et al., 2020).

Lysine-specific demethylase 1 has been described as upregulated in colon cancer tissues, and the high LSD1 expression was significantly associated with tumour-node-metastasis stages and distant metastasis. The LSD1 physically interacted with the promoter of CDH-1 and decreased dimethyl histone H3 lysine 4 (H3K4) at this region, downregulated CDH-1 expression, and consequently contributed to colon cancer metastasis (Ding et al., 2013).

Ly6G6d

Human microsatellite-stable colorectal cancers are immunologically cold tumour sub-types characterized by reduced immune cytotoxicity. Giordano et al. identified the lymphocyte antigen 6 complex, locus G6D (LY6G6D) as significantly over-expressed in colorectal cancer when compared with its relatively low expression in other human solid tumours (Giordano et al., 2019).

Lymphocyte antigen 6 (Ly-6) superfamily members are cysteine-rich, generally GPI-anchored cell surface proteins, which have definite or putative immune related roles. There are 27 members of this family described so far in the human genome and 37 in the mouse. Five of them are clustered in the class III region of the human and mouse MHCs (Mallya et al., 2006).

LY6G6D upregulation was predominant in microsatellite stable characterized by an enrichment of immune suppressive regulatory T-cells and a limited repertoire of PD-1/PD-L1 immune checkpoint receptors. Coexpression of LY6G6D and CD15 increases the risk of metastatic relapse in response to therapy. Both JAK-STAT5 and RAS-MEK-ERK cascades act in concert as key regulators of LY6G6D and fucosyltransferase 4 (FUT4), which direct CD15-mediated immune-resistance. Momelotinib, an inhibitor of JAK1/JAK2, consistently abrogated the STAT5/LY6G6D axis *in vitro*, sensitizing MSS cancer cells with an intact JAK-STAT signalling, to efficiently respond to trametinib, an MEK inhibitor used in clinical setting. Notably, colon cancer cells can evade JAK2/JAK1-targeted therapy by a reversible shift of the RAS-MEK-ERK pathway activity, which explains the treatment failure of JAK1/2 inhibitors in refractory CRC (Giordano et al., 2019).

Wang et al. (2022) developed a novel T cell-dependent bispecific antibody (TDB) targeting tumour-associated antigen LY6G6D for the treatment of colorectal cancer. Expression analyses reveal limited expression of LY6G6D in normal human tissues and in non-colorectal tumour types; meanwhile, significant LY6G6D upregulation in colorectal cancer was observed with high prevalence in microsatellite stable and microsatellite unstable colorectal cancer. The optimized anti-LY6G6D/CD3 TDB, which targets a membrane-proximal epitope of LY6G6D and binds to CD3 with high affinity, exhibited potent anti-tumour activity both *in vitro* and *in vivo*. *In vitro* functional assays showed that LY6G6D-TDB-mediated T-cell activation and cytotoxicity were conditional and target-dependent. In mouse xenograft tumour models, LY6G6D-TDB demonstrated anti-tumour efficacy as a single agent against established CRC tumours, and enhanced efficacy can be achieved when LY6G6D-TDB is combined with PD-1 blockade (Wang et al., 2022).

Gene fusions

NTRK

In a large collection of 1012 specimens of colorectal cancer only two NTRK-positive cases (0.2%) were identified whereas no ALK- or ROS1-positive cases were found. Reverse transcription polymerase chain reaction (RT-PCR) detected an LMNA-NTRK1 fusion in a case of adenosquamous carcinoma and a TPM3-NTRK1 fusion in a case of tubular adenocarcinoma. Both NTRK1 fusion-positive cases lacked activating mutations in KRAS and BRAF and were mismatch repair-deficient with loss of MLH1 and PMS2 expression and MLH1 promoter methylation (Yonemaru et al., 2021).

In a greater clinical series (4,569 samples) pan-Trk IHC was positive in 0.2% of colorectal cancer. 89% IHC positive cases were both MMRd (all showing MLH1/PMS2 loss) and lacked BRAFV600E mutation; that is, IHC was positive in 5.3% MLH1/PMS2/BRAFV600E triple negative CRCs. All IHC positive CRCs demonstrated gene rearrangements (LMNA-NTRK1, TPR-NTRK1, STRM-NTRK1, MUC2-NTRK2, and NTRK1 with an unknown partner), suggesting close to 100% specificity for IHC in this sub-population. NTRK fusions were associated with right-sided ($p = 0.02$), larger tumours ($p = 0.029$) with infiltrative growth ($p = 0.021$) (Chou et al., 2020). The authors concluded that performing pan-Trk IHC on this pre-selected subgroup of MLH1/PMS2/BRAFV600E triple negative CRCs (only 3.3% of all CRC patients) is a resource effective approach to identify most colorectal cancer patients with NTRK gene fusions (Chou et al., 2020).

Kim et al. reported that NTRK-rearranged colorectal tumours are developed through the serrated neoplasia pathway and can be initiated from non-dysplastic sessile serrated lesions without BRAF/KRAS mutations prior to full occurrence of microsatellite instability-high/CpG island methylator phenotype-high (Kim et al., 2021).

In the Navigate clinical trial, 10 patients with metastatic colorectal cancer were recruited and treated with larotrectinib. Objective response rate was 50%, 10% complete response, 40% partial response, and 50% stable disease. Median duration of response was 15.5 months (95% CI 3.7–27.3), median PFS 5.5 months (95% CI 2.2–29.4), and a median OS that reached 29.4 months (95% CI 2.8–36.5) (Boni, 2020).

NRG1

NRG1 gene fusions which activate ErbB signalling are rare but potentially actionable oncogenic drivers that are present in some solid tumours (Jonna et al., 2019). Chimeric transmembrane proteins encoded by NRG1 fusions are predicted to maintain this extracellular domain-activating ERBB3 (Drilon et al., 2018).

Out of 21,858 tumour specimens profiled 41 cases (0.2%) harboured an NRG1 fusion. The greatest incidence was in non-small cell lung cancer (NSCLC, 25), though this represented only 0.3% of NSCLC cases tested. Other tumour types harbouring an NRG1 fusion included gallbladder cancer, renal cell carcinoma, bladder cancer, ovarian cancer, pancreatic cancer, breast cancer, neuroendocrine tumour, sarcoma, and colorectal cancer (Jonna et al., 2019).

In a short clinical series of patients NRG1 fusion (+), one patient with colorectal cancer and harbouring a novel POMK-NRG1 fusion and a KRAS mutation was treated with afatinib, a pan-ErbB family inhibitor, showing a significant clinical benefit in terms a longer stable disease (Cadranel et al., 2021).

In the first-in-human study of GSK2849330, an anti-HER3 monoclonal antibody conducted in HER3-expressing solid tumours, seven patients with colorectal cancer were enrolled. Patients with various tumour types were prospectively selected for HER3 expression by immunohistochemistry and a subset was also screened for NRG1 mRNA expression. The best response in the group of colorectal cancer was two stable diseases. Interestingly, the only confirmed durable response achieved was in a patient with CD74-NRG1-rearranged lung cancer. This highlights the potential utility of screening for NRG1 fusions prospectively across tumour types to enrich potential responders to these new anti-HER3 agents (Gan et al., 2021).

RET

Colorectal carcinoma harbouring oncogenic fusions has been reported to be highly enriched in mismatch repair deficient (dMMR) tumours with MLH1 hypermethylation (MLH1(me+)) and wild-type BRAF and RAS. Using RNA NGS in this sub-setting of patients (dMMR MLH1(me+) BRAF/RAS wild-type), Wang et al. revealed a proportion of fusion-positive tumours of 56% (Wang et al., 2021).

Clifton et al. (2019) described as potential mechanism of resistance to anti-EGFR in colorectal cancer 1.1% of gene fusions detected in circulating tumour DNA detected: *RET* 36% of all fusions detected, FGFR3 27%, ALK 23%, NTRK1 7%, ROS1 5%, and FGFR2 2%. Mutations associated with a previously reported anti- EGFR resistance signature (RAS or EGFR mutations) were found with fusions in FGFR3 (83% of all FGFR3 fusions detected), *RET* (56%), and ALK (70%) (Clifton et al., 2019).

According to Pietrantonio et al. (2018), *RET* fusions were more frequent in older patients with ECOG PS 1-2, RAS and BRAF wild-type and MSI-high. These patients with *RET* fusion-positive tumours showed a significantly worse OS when compared with *RET*-negative ones (median OS 14.0 versus 38.0 months, HR: 4.59; 95% CI, 3.64–32.66; $P < 0.001$) (Pietrantonio et al., 2018).

On the other hand, Yang et al. (2021) studied the incidence of *RET* mutations and the clinicopathological features of this group. These authors found an incidence of 2.7% of *RET* mutations. Males comprised most cases with *RET* mutations (93.8%). Furthermore, all patients with *RET* mutations were younger than 60 years (100%). Individuals with tumours positive for *RET* mutations more frequently exhibited mucinous histology (31.2%), a lower incidence of liver metastasis, and higher incidence of peritoneal metastasis. Patients with *RET* mutations had a higher median TMB (Yang et al., 2021).

Ponatinib, an *RET* inhibitor, has been evaluated in PDX models of colorectal cancer harbouring *RET* fusions (*NCOA4-RET* and *CCDC6-RET*). Mice with subcutaneous PDX tumours were dosed with ponatinib or the standard of care agent 5-flourouracil (5-FU). Ponatinib displayed 79% tumour growth inhibition in the *NCOA4-RET* model and near complete regression in the *CCDC6-RET* model. In both cases, ponatinib's efficacy was greater than 5-FU. Ponatinib's efficacy in these *RET* fusion-positive PDXs was also associated with the expected pharmacodynamic suppression of *RET* phosphorylation (Gozgit et al., 2018).

Conclusions

Today decision-making in the clinical routine of the metastatic colorectal cancer is based on RAS, BRAF, and dMMR/MSI-H. However, the scenario which has been outlined in this chapter describes a broad spectrum of new potential actionable targets that likewise will be available soon to be incorporated in the therapeutic armamentarium of the metastatic colorectal cancer. Therefore, these new targeted therapies require a very precise identification of candidates to provide the maximum benefit for each patient; in this way, the molecular analysis should be not only the first step in the initial workup of any patient of metastatic colorectal cancer and at the progression of disease for a better decision-making.

REFERENCES

Arena, S., Corti, G., Durinikova, E., et al. (2020). A subset of colorectal cancers with cross-sensitivity to olaparib and oxaliplatin. *Clinical Cancer Research, 26*, 1372–1384.

Arguello, D., Feldman, R., Xiu, J., et al. (2013). Distribution of cMET by IHC, FISH, and next generation sequencing in cancer a large cohort analysis. <https://www.carislifesciences.com/publications/distribution-of-cmet-by-ihc-fish-and-next-generation-sequencing-in-cancer-a-large-cohort-analysis/>.

Bajenova, O., Gorbunova, A., Evsyukov, I., et al. (2016). The genome-wide analysis of carcinoembryonic antigen signaling by colorectal cancer cells using RNA sequencing. *PLoS One, 11*, e0161256.

Bang, Y. J., Su, W. C., Schuler, M., et al. (2020). Phase 1 study of capmatinib in MET-positive solid tumor patients: dose escalation and expansion of selected cohorts. *Cancer Science, 111*, 536–547.

Bardia, A., Messersmith, W. A., Kio, E. A., et al. (2021). Sacituzumab govitecan, a Trop-2-directed antibody-drug conjugate, for patients with epithelial cancer: final safety and efficacy results from the phase I/II IMMU-132-01 basket trial. *Annals of Oncology, 32*, 746–756.

Becht, E., de Reyniès, A., Giraldo, N. A., et al. (2016). Immune and stromal classification of colorectal cancer is associated with molecular subtypes and relevant for precision immunotherapy. *Clinical Cancer Research, 22*, 4057–4066.

Boni, V. (2020). Efficacy and safety of larotrectinib in patients with TRK fusion-positive gastrointestinal cancer: an expanded dataset. *Annals in Oncology, 32*(3), 5214–5215.

Bowles, D. W., Kochenderfer, M., Cohn, A., et al. (2016). A randomized, phase II trial of cetuximab with or without PX-866, an irreversible oral phosphatidylinositol 3-kinase inhibitor, in patients with metastatic colorectal carcinoma. *Clinical Colorectal Cancer, 15*(337), 344.e2.

Cadranel, J., Liu, S. V., Duruisseaux, M., et al. (2021). Therapeutic potential of afatinib in NRG1 fusion-driven solid tumors: a case series. *Oncologist, 26*, 7–16.

Chen, E. X., Jonker, D. J., Siu, L. L., et al. (2016). A Phase I study of olaparib and irinotecan in patients with colorectal cancer: Canadian Cancer Trials Group IND 187. *Investigational New Drugs, 34*, 450–457.

Chida, K., Kawazoe, A., Kawazu, M., et al. (2021). A low tumor mutational burden and PTEN mutations are predictors of a negative response to PD-1 blockade in MSI-H/dMMR gastrointestinal tumors. *Clinical Cancer Research, 27*, 3714–3724.

Chou, A., Fraser, T., Ahadi, M., et al. (2020). NTRK gene rearrangements are highly enriched in MLH1/PMS2 deficient, BRAF wild-type colorectal carcinomas-a study of 4569 cases. *Modern Pathology, 33*, 924–932.

Clifton, K., Rich, T. A., Parseghian, C., et al. (2019). Identification of actionable fusions as an anti-EGFR resistance mechanism using a circulating tumor DNA assay. *JCO Precision Oncology, 3*, 10.1200/PO.19.00141. eCollection 2019.

Cruz-Duarte, R., Rebelo de Almeida, C., Negrão, M., et al. (2022). Predictive and therapeutic implications of a novel PLCγ1/SHP2-driven mechanism of cetuximab resistance in metastatic colorectal cancer. *Clinical Cancer Research, 28*, 1203-1216.

Ding, J., Zhang, Z. M., Xia, Y., et al. (2013). LSD1-mediated epigenetic modification contributes to proliferation and metastasis of colon cancer. *British Journal of Cancer, 109*, 994–1003.

Dotan, E., Cohen, S. J., Starodub, A. N., et al. (2017). Phase I/II trial of labetuzumab govitecan (anti-CEACAM5/SN-38 antibody-drug conjugate) in patients with refractory or relapsing metastatic colorectal cancer. *Journal of Clinical Oncology, 35*, 3338–3346.

Drilon, A., Somwar, R., Mangatt, B. P., et al. (2018). Response to ERBB3-directed targeted therapy in NRG1-rearranged cancers. *Cancer Discoveries, 8*, 686–695.

Dumbrava, E. E., Call, S. G., Huang, H. J., et al. (2021). PIK3CA mutations in plasma circulating tumor DNA predict survival and treatment outcomes in patients with advanced cancers. *ESMO Open, 6*, 100230.

Fakih, M. G., Kopetz, S., Kuboki, Y., et al. (2022). Sotorasib for previously treated colorectal cancers with KRAS(G12C) mutation

(CodeBreaK100): a prespecified analysis of a single-arm, phase 2 trial. *Lancet Oncology*, *23*, 115–124.

Gan, H. K., Millward, M., Jalving, M., et al. (2021). A phase I, first-in-human study of GSK2849330, an anti-HER3 monoclonal antibody, in HER3-expressing solid tumors. *Oncologist*, *26*, e1844–1853.

Giampieri, R., Lupi, A., Ziranu, P., et al. (2021). Retrospective comparative analysis of KRAS G12C vs. other KRAS mutations in mCRC patients treated with first-line chemotherapy doublet + bevacizumab. *Frontiers in Oncology*, *11*, 736104.

Giordano, G., Parcesepe, P., D'Andrea, M. R., et al. (2019). JAK/Stat5-mediated subtype-specific lymphocyte antigen 6 complex, locus G6D (LY6G6D) expression drives mismatch repair proficient colorectal cancer. *Journal of Experimental Clinical Cancer Research*, *38*, 28–35.

Gonzalez-Exposito, R., Semiannikova, M., Griffiths, B., et al. (2019). CEA expression heterogeneity and plasticity confer resistance to the CEA-targeting bispecific immunotherapy antibody cibisatamab (CEA-TCB) in patient-derived colorectal cancer organoids. *Journal of Immunotherapy Cancer*, *7*, 101–103.

Goodwin, R., Jonker, D., Chen, E., et al. (2020). A phase Ib study of a PI3Kinase inhibitor BKM120 in combination with panitumumab in patients with KRAS wild-type advanced colorectal cancer. *Investigational New Drugs*, *38*, 1077–1084.

Gozgit, J. M., Chen, T. H., Song, Y., et al. (2018). RET fusions observed in lung and colorectal cancers are sensitive to ponatinib. *Oncotarget*, *9*, 29654–29664.

Grünewald, S., Politz, O., Bender, S., et al. (2019). Rogaratinib: a potent and selective pan-FGFR inhibitor with broad antitumor activity in FGFR-overexpressing preclinical cancer models. *International Journal of Cancer*, *145*, 1346–1357.

Hong, J. Y., An, J. Y., Lee, J., et al. (2020). Claudin 18.2 expression in various tumor types and its role as a potential target in advanced gastric cancer. *Translational Cancer Research*, *9*, 3367–3374.

Iwaya, M., Hayashi, H., Nakajima, T., et al. (2021). Colitis-associated colorectal adenocarcinomas frequently express claudin 18 isoform 2: implications for claudin 18.2 monoclonal antibody therapy. *Histopathology*, *79*, 227–237.

Jonna, S., Feldman, R. A., Swensen, J., et al. (2019). Detection of NRG1 gene fusions in solid tumors. *Clinical Cancer Research*, *25*, 4966–4972.

Karkera JD, Cardona GM, Bell K, et al. (2017). Oncogenic characterization and pharmacologic sensitivity of activating fibroblast growth factor receptor (FGFR) genetic alterations to the selective FGFR inhibitor erdafitinib. *Molecular Cancer Therapeutics*, *16*, 1717–1726.

Khare, T., Bissonnette, M., & Khare, S. (2021). CXCL12-CXCR4/CXCR7 axis in colorectal cancer: therapeutic target in preclinical and clinical studies. *International Journal of Molecular Sciences*, *22*, 7371. doi: 10.3390/ijms22147371

Kim, J. H., Hong, J. H., Choi, Y. L., et al. (2021). NTRK oncogenic fusions are exclusively associated with the serrated neoplasia pathway in the colorectum and begin to occur in sessile serrated lesions. *Journal of Pathology*, *255*, 399–411.

Kundu, S., Fan, K., Cao, M., et al. (2010). Novel SHP-1 inhibitors tyrosine phosphatase inhibitor-1 and analogs with preclinical antitumor activities as tolerated oral agents. *Journal of Immunology*, *184*, 6529–6536.

Leichman, L., Groshen, S., O'Nei,l B. H., et al. (2016). Phase II study of olaparib (AZD-2281) after standard systemic therapies for disseminated colorectal cancer. *Oncologist*, *21*, 172–177.

Maderer, A., Fiteni, F., Tanis, E., et al. (2021). CXCR4 and hif-1α as prognostic molecular markers for stage 3 colon cancer patients: post hoc analysis of the randomized, multicenter phase 3 PETACC-2 trial dataset. *Acta Oncologica*, *60*, 1543–1547.

Malagraba, G., Yarmohammadi, M., Javed, A., et al. (2022). The role of LSD1 and LSD2 in cancers of the gastrointestinal system: an update. *Biomolecules*, *12*, 462. doi: 10.3390/biom12030462

Mallya, M., Campbell, R. D., & Aguado, B. (2006). Characterization of the five novel Ly-6 superfamily members encoded in the MHC, and detection of cells expressing their potential ligands. *Protein Science*, *15*, 2244–2256.

McRee, A. J., Sanoff, H. K., Carlson, C., et al. (2015). A phase I trial of mFOLFOX6 combined with the oral PI3K inhibitor BKM120 in patients with advanced refractory solid tumors. *Investigational New Drugs*, *33*, 1225–1231.

Moretto, R., Elliott, A., Zhang, J., et al. (2022). Homologous recombination deficiency alterations in colorectal cancer: clinical, molecular, and prognostic implications. *Journal of the National Cancer Institute*, *114*, 271–279.

Müller, M. F., Ibrahim, A. E., & Arends, M. J. (2016). Molecular pathological classification of colorectal cancer. *Virchows Archive*, *469*, 125–134.

Nakamura, Y., Okamoto, W., Kato, T., et al. (2021). Circulating tumor DNA-guided treatment with pertuzumab plus trastuzumab for HER2-amplified metastatic colorectal cancer: a phase 2 trial. *Nature Medicine*, *27*, 1899–1903.

Ohmachi, T., Tanaka, F., Mimori, K., et al. (2006). Clinical significance of TROP2 expression in colorectal cancer. *Clinical Cancer Research*, *12*, 3057–3063.

Osterlund, E., Ristimäki, A., Kytölä, S., et al. (2022). KRAS-G12C mutation in one real-life and three population-based Nordic cohorts of metastatic colorectal cancer. *Frontiers in Oncology*, *12*, 826073.

Ottaiano, A., Santorsola, M., Del Prete, P., et al. (2021). Prognostic significance of CXCR4 in colorectal cancer: an updated meta-analysis and critical appraisal. *Cancers (Basel)*, *13*, 3284. doi: 10.3390/cancers13133284

Peng, J., Ou, Q., Deng, Y., et al. (2019). TROP2 overexpression in colorectal liver oligometastases is associated with poor prognosis after liver resection. *Therapeutic Advances in Medical Oncology*, *11*, 1758835919897543.

Peng, W., Zhang, H., Tan, S., et al. (2020). Synergistic antitumor effect of 5-fluorouracil with the novel LSD1 inhibitor ZY0511 in colorectal cancer. *Therapeutic Advances in Medical Oncology*, *12*, 1758835920937428.

Pietrantonio, F., Di Nicolantonio, F., Schrock, A. B., et al. (2018). RET fusions in a small subset of advanced colorectal cancers at risk of being neglected. *Annals of Oncology*, *29*, 1394–1401.

Sartore-Bianchi, A., Trusolino, L., Martino, C., et al. (2016). Dual-targeted therapy with trastuzumab and lapatinib in treatment-refractory, KRAS codon 12/13 wild-type, HER2-positive metastatic colorectal cancer (HERACLES): a proof-of-concept, multicentre, open-label, phase 2 trial. *Lancet Oncology*, *17*, 738–746.

Siena, S., Di Bartolomeo, M., Raghav, K., et al. (2021). Trastuzumab deruxtecan (DS-8201) in patients with HER2-expressing metastatic colorectal cancer (DESTINY-CRC01): a multicentre, open-label, phase 2 trial. *Lancet Oncology*, *22*, 779–789.

Strickler, J. H., Yoshino, T., Graham, R. P., et al. (2022). Diagnosis and treatment of ERBB2-positive metastatic colorectal cancer: a review. *JAMA Oncology*, *8*(5), 760–769.

Sun, Y., Li, G., Zhu, W., et al. (2020). A comprehensive pan-cancer study of fibroblast growth factor receptor aberrations in Chinese cancer patients. *Annals of Translational Medicine*, *8*, 1290–5118.

Testa, U., Castelli, G., & Pelosi, E. (2020). Genetic alterations of metastatic colorectal Cancer. *Biomedicines*, *8*, 414.

Ugai, T., Zhao, M., Shimizu, T., et al. (2021). Association of PIK3CA mutation and PTEN loss with expression of CD274 (PD-L1) in colorectal carcinoma. *Oncoimmunology*, *10*, 1956173.

Voutsadakis, I. A. (2021). The landscape of PIK3CA mutations in colorectal cancer. *Clinical Colorectal Cancer*, *20*, 201–215.

Wainberg, Z. A., Alsina, M., Soares, H. P., et al. (2017). A multi-arm phase I study of the PI3K/mTOR inhibitors PF-04691502 and gedatolisib (PF-05212384) plus irinotecan or the MEK inhibitor PD-0325901 in advanced cancer. *Target Oncology*, *12*, 775–785.

Wang, J., Li, R., Li, J., et al. (2021). Comprehensive analysis of oncogenic fusions in mismatch repair deficient colorectal carcinomas by sequential DNA and RNA next generation sequencing. *Journal of Translational Medicine*, *19*, 433–436.

Wang, J., Zhang, B., Cheng, X., et al. (2022). Retrospective study on the efficacy and safety of pyrotinib-based therapy for HER2-positive nonbreast advanced solid tumors. *Journal of Oncology*, *2022*, 4233782.

Yang, L., Li, W., Lu, Z., et al. (2022). Clinicopathological features of HER2 positive metastatic colorectal cancer and survival analysis of anti-HER2 treatment. *BMC Cancer*, *22*, 355–x.

Yang, Y. Z., Hu, W. M., Xia, L. P., et al. (2021). Association between somatic RET mutations and clinical and genetic characteristics in patients with metastatic colorectal cancer. *Cancer Medicine*, *10*, 8876–8882.

Yeager, R., Uboha, N., Pelster, M., et al (2024). Efficacy and safety of adagrasib plus cetuximab in patients with KRASG12C-mutated metastatic colorectal cancer. *Cancer Discoveries*, *14*(6), 982–993.

Yonemaru, J., Hashimoto, T., Takayanagi, D., et al. (2021). NTRK fusion-positive colorectal cancer in Japanese population. *Pathology International*, *71*, 355–3359.

Yu, M., Xu, C., Zhang, H., et al. (2021). The tyrosine phosphatase SHP2 promotes proliferation and oxaliplatin resistance of colon cancer cells through AKT and ERK. *Biochemical and Biophysical Research Communications*, *563*, 1–7.

Wang, P., Sun, L. L., Clark, R., et al. (2022). Novel anti-LY6G6D/CD3 T cell-dependent bispecific antibody for the treatment of colorectal cancer. *Molecular Cancer Therapeutics*, *21*(6), 974–985.

20

Support for the colorectal cancer patient before, during, and after treatment

Vanessa Shearwood and Alexandra Poole

Introduction

With so many individual healthcare professionals being involved in a single patient's cancer pathway, it is imperative that a keyworker helps the patient navigate this complex time of their life and signposts them along the whole journey, acting as an advocate, throughout diagnosis and pre-treatment, treatment (surgery/chemotherapy/radiotherapy/novel therapies), and post treatment. The Clinical Nurse Specialist (CNS) stands at the interface of multiple specialties and frequently sits on multiple multidisciplinary teams and so is in a pivotal position to be able to fulfil this role.

This chapter will discuss the importance of prehabilitation in preparing patients for treatment, assessment of their needs, consequences and side effects of treatment, dietary support, and finally ongoing personalized support once treatment has been completed. This is not exhaustive and further reading is advised.

Colorectal Cancer Nurse Specialist role

As mentioned, the role of the Colorectal Cancer Nurse Specialist is an essential component of the colorectal cancer patient journey. Although it is not universally utilized, in countries where this role exists it is multifaceted and it has expanded greatly over time. Whatever its guise in a specific nation, the core elements of acting as the patient's advocate, and the provision of emotional and practical support, remain the same basic principles across the globe.

As a highly trained expert in their field, the CNS works closely alongside other key professionals with whom the patient will have contact, bridging gaps which may occur between services, and providing continuity across the patient's pathway. The CNS team members provide a 'familiar face', often attending multiple specialist clinics from surgery to oncology, and even providing initial guidance and advice in the endocscopy suite, when a patient has received their initial provisional diagnosis. CNSs will use their specialist detailed knowledge of colorectal cancer and the individual treatments to help patients navigate the complex decision-making that is required when considering their treatment options.

It is important for the CNS to have a good understanding of multiple aspects of colorectal cancer, including but not exclusively, cancer biology, disease staging, surgical interventions and complications, oncological treatment and toxicities, and identifying relapse/progression.

It is expected the CNS is recognized as a core member of the multidisciplinary team (MDT), attending all MDT meetings to provide clear patient centre information, ensuring the patient's voice is heard during treatment discussions and patient wishes are clearly represented.

CNSs can manage complex needs, identifying patient concerns early; they can put in place interventions to prevent unnecessary hospital admissions and enable patients to self-manage their cancer pathway. Utilizing assessment tools, the CNS will develop care plans, enhance recovery from treatments, and provide prehabilitation through health promotion, dietary, and exercise advice.

Often inefficiencies in health services are due to lack of coordination and no centralized point of contact. The CNS becomes that point of contact for not only patients but also their relatives, allowing open communication between the patient and hospital team. This open communication is vital, especially when dealing with side effects of oncological treatments, as it is known to enhance prompt interventions and improve patient outcomes.

Significant changes have seen the CNS develop nurse-led clinics, often relieving pressures on specialist services. Correctly used, a highly experienced nurse specialist team has been shown to make a significant difference to patients, improving the quality and experience of the care they receive.

Prehabilitation

On average, cancer patients have been identified as having poorer background physical health, making them more vulnerable to the side effects of cancer treatments. This can lead to a high frequency of long-term health problems with treatment, irrespective of the cancer type or stage of disease.

The concept of prehabilitation is to optimize a cancer patient before their planned treatments, and to prevent or reduce functional decline during and following treatment (Crevenna et al., 2021). It not only focuses on the physical improvements but also nutritional, psychological, and comorbidities of an individual.

The last 10 to 20 years have seen some improvements for colorectal patients undergoing surgery in the form of prehabilitation programmes, such as changes to diet and exercise. However, improving the health and well-being of patients undergoing more chronic systemic oncological treatments such as chemotherapy or radiotherapy have lagged behind, in terms of taking this more holistic approach. However, it is imperative that health professionals do consider these ancillary aspects to treatment as, not only do they allow the patients to withstand better the impact of the treatments they receive, and improve morbidity outcomes, but in optimizing the patient's health, potentially a wider spectrum of treatment options can be offered. All prehabilitation interventions should start as early as possible and in advance of each and any cancer treatment (not just the first cancer treatment). Any prehabilitation programme must incorporate and have access to all appropriately trained professions; for example dietitians, occupational therapists, physiotherapists, psychologists, as well as other health and well-being services to help with smoking cessation and alcohol abstinence.

Dietz (1969) described four rehabilitation stages for cancer as follows. Preventive (at diagnosis); Restorative (recovery phase); Supportive (enabling patients who have progressive disease); and Palliative (improving quality of life when in terminal phase). Prehabilitation should be seen as part of this cancer continuum and introduced with clear guidance, giving patients a degree of control and a sense of empowerment to improve their quality of life and health and well-being.

The three key principles of prehabilitation (Minnella & Carli, 2018) are:

1. Screening:
   - Use validated tools to lead onto more detailed assessment based on nutrition, psychological aspects, physical activity
2. Assessment:
   - Individualized assessments based on the screening results
3. Interventions:
   - Based on the assessment interventions can be specialist/targeted/universal

A key document is the 'Principles and Guidance for Prehabilitation within the Management and Support of People with Cancer' developed in the United Kingdom by Macmillan cancer support in conjunction with the Royal College of Anaesthetists, National Institute for Health Research Cancer, and Nutrition Collaboration (Macmillan, 2020).

Assessment of needs and care planning

As discussed in the previous section, people who have had a diagnosis and treatment for cancer experience ongoing poorer health and well-being than the wider population (Jefford et al., 2017). A study by Sodergren et al. (2019) as part of the ColoREctal Wellbeing (CREW) study looking into unmet needs of colorectal cancer patients found that 43% of patients who underwent colorectal cancer surgery still had unmet needs at 15 months following treatment.

Interventions developed to try to address unmet needs can be grouped under the umbrella term 'survivorship', and there are several well-recognized assessment tools available: the Supportive Care Needs Survey (SCNS) (Boyes et al., 2009), the Distress Thermometer (Roth et al., 1998), and the Hospital Anxiety and Depression Scale (HADS). The most widely used tool within the English National Health Service (NHS) is the Macmillan Holistic Needs Assessment Tool.

The aim of any intervention is to improve a patient's quality of life and to do this, the patient must be fully assessed, focusing on the whole patient and not just on individual symptoms or diagnosis. NHS England (NHSE, 2016) believe the assessment process should cover:

- Physical health
- Emotional well-being
- Spiritual needs
- Psychological status
- Social needs
- Environmental issues

Within the United Kingdom these assessments are most often undertaken by the Cancer specialist nurse, however they can be completed by any appropriately qualified health professional. These tools can aid conversations which may be difficult to start for both patients/relatives and care professionals. Once patients have completed an assessment, a care plan is developed. This sets out a plan to address concerns or any needs raised. The specialist nurses may provide information, guidance, signposting for support or referral on to specialist services. The patient should receive a copy of the care plan to enable self-management. Further copies are stored in the medical records and can be sent to their General Practitioner (GP) or family doctor to ensure ongoing support. Ultimately, the aim is to empower patients to live well and take control of their follow-up.

Physical consequences of treatment

This section will focus on the physical side effects of treatments, common treatment options, and advice and support for patients.

Bowel dysfunction

Unfortunately, persistent poor bowel symptoms following treatment for colorectal cancer are common. The patient may experience symptoms such as faecal urgency and frequency, irregular or incomplete emptying, loose stools, clustering, fragmented stools, incontinence (of flatus and/or stool), excessive flatus, and abdominal bloating.

Poor bowel function is distressing; it can be unrelenting, impactful, and restricting on all aspects of daily life (Peiri & Patton, 2020) due to repeated, urgent trips to the toilet and disrupted sleep patterns. Different symptoms are more troublesome to different patients. Coping with and managing these unpredictable symptoms can have a significant impact on patient's relationships and social and working lives; for example, by having to reduce or change working hours, changing how they travel, reducing social contact, and not being able to continue with preferred hobbies or exercise (Lim et al., 2021).

In patients who have undergone rectal surgery, up to 90% of patients experience poor bowel function (Pieri & Patton, 2020). This is regardless of whether they have had a temporary stoma formed or not. Rectal symptoms are further exacerbated if the patient has received neoadjuvant and adjuvant therapies. Together these symptoms are commonly referred to as Low Anterior Resection Syndrome (LARS), and they impact on a person's physical and emotional wellbeing significantly and negatively, due to toilet dependence and preoccupation with bowel function (Burch, 2021).

It is vital that before surgery, patients are informed and counselled about the risks of LARS, and that this is personalized to take into account whether the patient has received neoadjuvant treatment with chemotherapy, radiotherapy, or chemoradiotherapy. The likely severity of symptoms and their possible duration should be discussed, as well as possible interventions to help with the symptoms.

If symptoms are apparent post-operatively these should be assessed and an individualized management strategy planned (Burch, 2021). Part of the specialist nurse's role is to assess the severity of the symptoms at this point, and to provide a consistent management strategy which will enable patients to improve their quality of life.

Symptoms can be assessed using a validated tool, such as the LARS score (Emmertsen & Laurberg, 2012). Patients are asked to score their symptoms by answering five questions.

1. Do you have occasions when you cannot control your flatus (wind)?
2. Do you ever have accidental leakage of liquid stool?
3. How often do you open your bowels?
4. Do you ever have to open your bowels again within one hour of the last bowel opening?
5. Do you ever have such a strong urge to open your bowels that you have to rush to the toilet?

The higher the score the higher the severity of LARS is, and appropriate management can be planned.

The following conservative treatment options for LARS should be considered. These can also be used to help with other bowel symptoms:

Dietary management

- Food diary/bowel diary to measure symptoms
- Low fibre diet
- Dietary modifications: e.g. avoid foods which cause gas (carbonated drinks, calciferous vegetables, and chewing gum) and avoid spices/spicy foods.
- Ensure regular mealtimes and snacks. Chew food thoroughly.
- Increase fluid intake.

Physiotherapy

- Advice on toilet positioning.
- Pelvic floor exercises to strengthen the muscles used for bowel control.

Pharmacotherapy

- Laxatives
- Anti-diarrhoeal medication—loperamide slows colonic motility and may increase internal anal sphincter tone.
- Bulking agents—e.g. ispaghula/psyllium husk and sterculia. They work by absorbing water in the bowel and increasing the bulk of the stool.
- Anti-spasmodic medication.

In severe cases of LARS, referral can be made to a specialist team to consider:

- Biofeedback or pelvic floor muscle retraining
- Sacral nerve stimulation
- Trans-anal irrigation
  - Enhances colonic emptying more so than enemas or suppositories
  - Requires motivation
- Stoma formation
  - Surgery to create stoma (colostomy or ileostomy)
  - Antegrade Continence Enema (ACE)

Bowel dysfunction tends to be more common for survivors of rectal cancer rather than colon cancer, due to the lower join and the increased likelihood of neoadjuvant treatment having been implemented. However, colon cancer surgery can also result in changes to bowel function, such as loose stools and increased frequency (Hope et al., 2020). The right colon is the main site of water reabsorption so the loss of this with a right hemicolectomy may contribute to looser stools. Removal of the ileocaecal valve, terminal ileum, and right colon can result in prolonged malabsorption, resulting in more bile acids entering the colon. This also can cause diarrhoea, bloating, abdominal pain, and excessive offensive wind.

The ileocaecal valve also plays a part in preventing the entry of colonic bacteria into the small bowel and its removal can promote the development of small bowel bacterial overgrowth. The symptoms of this include abdominal bloating and discomfort, belching and flatulence, and a change in bowel habit. Usually, symptoms will gradually improve over time post-operatively.

The following may be helpful in the assessment and management of symptoms.

- Bacterial overgrowth
  - Stool specimen
  - Treatment with a course of antibiotics
  - Probiotics
- Bile acid malabsorption
  - Selenium homocholic acid taurine test (SeHCAT)
  - Blood tests
  - Manage with low fat diet and bile acid sequestrants, e.g. cholestyramine or colesevelam.

Radiotherapy can also cause inflammation and ischaemia of the lining of the rectum, called radiation proctitis. This can cause rectal bleeding, increase mucous discharge, and can lead to tenesmus, diarrhoea or constipation, and cramping in the rectum or anus when opening the bowels. Radiation proctitis can occur during treatment, after treatment, or years later.

Mild cases may not need treatment, but if patients have acute pain and bleeding which is affecting quality of life, then treatment is recommended.

- Medication: the aim of this is to manage inflammation and decrease bleeding' e.g. corticosteroid or sucralfate enemas, antibiotics, and stool softeners (to optimize bowel function).

- Argon plasma coagulation (APC): this is performed with an endoscope. The aim is to coagulate the thinned and fragile blood vessels (telangectasias).

Urinary function

Urinary dysfunction is common after radiotherapy and/or surgery for rectal cancer. Symptoms include incontinence, frequency, urinary retention, incomplete bladder emptying, haematuria, and dysuria. This is caused by nerve damage during pelvic surgery, weakening of the pelvic floor muscles, and fibrosis of the bladder caused by radiotherapy.

Long-term urinary dysfunction can have a huge impact on daily life and on confidence and mental well-being. Patients should be offered support and assessment and management options by their healthcare professional.

Management:

- Medication
  - to relax the bladder
  - to reduce bleeding
- Prompt treatment of urinary tract infections
- Changes in diet
  - Drink plenty of fluids (at least 2 litres per day)
  - Avoid caffeine
  - Avoid acidic drinks
  - Healthy diet and avoid becoming constipated
- Pelvic floor exercises: referral to pelvic physiotherapist if necessary
- Bladder retraining
- Referral to community continence team
- Referral to urologist if symptoms severe

Adhesions and herniae

Chronic pain after abdominal surgery can be caused by abdominal adhesions or hernias. Adhesions don't often cause any problems but can cause occasional abdominal pain or discomfort. In a small number of cases adhesions can cause bowel strangulation or intermittent small bowel obstruction requiring hospitalization and surgery.

An incisional hernia or a parastomal hernia is a common complication following colorectal surgery. Most occur in the first year following surgery, but they can occur later. Most are caused by weakness or thinning of the surgical scar tissues. Symptoms include sharp pain that occurs during sneezing or coughing, while exercising or lifting heavy objects. Surgical repair of the hernia can be offered but recurrence is frequent. If the hernia becomes strangulated, then emergency surgery is necessary.

Patients should be informed of the risks pre-operatively and given advice on reducing these risks. This includes doing gentle exercises to strengthen abdominal muscles, keeping to a healthy body mass index (BMI), stopping smoking, avoiding heavy lifting and strenuous housework in the immediate post-operative period, and avoiding becoming constipated/straining at stool.

Sexual dysfunction

Although sex may not be a priority for all patients, as they are usually more concerned about treating their cancer, it is imperative that clinical teams do discuss and offer counselling to patients, particularly younger patients, or those not yet in a long-term relationship. They are then prepared for potential sexual dysfunction caused by their upcoming oncological treatments.

Pelvic surgery, radiotherapy, and systemic chemotherapy for colorectal cancer can all contribute to sexual problems (Milbury et al., 2013). This may be due to the psychological effects of a cancer diagnosis leading to changes in sexual desire, or physical changes such as nerve damage, as a direct consequence of treatment.

There is a variety of symptoms that can comprise sexual dysfunction. They include erectile or ejaculatory dysfunction for men, and vulvovaginal atrophy, vaginal dryness, and dyspareunia for women. Loss of sexual desire can be due to factors such as treatment related fatigue, changes in body image (e.g. stoma and/or hair loss), and fear of faecal incontinence. Milbury et al. (2013) found that sexual dysfunction in colorectal cancer survivors was high in both men and women. Worse outcomes were reported in those treated for rectal cancer rather than colon cancer, clearly related to more destructive treatments (pelvic radiotherapy and surgery) for this patient group.

Information and specialist counselling on sexual problems following treatment is crucial. Following treatment, it is imperative to carry out an assessment of sexual function and sexual quality of life during follow-up by questioning patients either face to face or in the form of a questionnaire, and then referring to appropriate services. The use of patient reported outcome questionnaires are helpful.

Female sexual dysfunction

Female sexual problems that may be encountered include:

- Vaginal dryness
- Shortening of the vagina
- Pain during sex (dyspareunia)
- Vaginal bleeding
- Vaginal narrowing
- Sensitivity changes
- Vaginal infection
- Low libido
- Early menopause or premature ovarian insufficiency (POI)

Treatments that may be offered include:

- Counselling with trained therapist
- Vaginal lubricants: help with vaginal dryness during sex
- Vaginal dilators: used daily to help gently stretch and widen the vagina and it may help with painful sex
- Hormone therapy: hormones help boost libido and restore vaginal health Hormones can be given in a cream, vaginal ring, or patch
- Pelvic floor exercises: retrain and strengthen pelvic floor muscles

Male sexual problems that may be encountered include:

- Erectile dysfunction
- Painful ejaculation
- Dry ejaculation
- Low libido

Treatments that may be offered include:

- Counselling with a trained therapist
- Ensure good lifestyle choices: reduce alcohol, stop smoking, good control of diabetes

- Phosphodiesterase 5 (PDE5) inhibitors, e.g. Viagra
- Vacuum erection devices
- Intraurethral creams or pellets
- Penile injections
- Penile implants

Ultimately, for a significant proportion of patients, sexual quality of life and body image are compromised after colorectal cancer treatments. It is therefore vital that sexual concerns are addressed as early as possible to limit broader-reaching psychosocial effects (Reese et al., 2018), and clinicians should be honest, at the outset of treatment, about the impact that patients may experience.

Fertility

The potential loss of fertility is recognized as a devastating long-term side effect of cancer treatment for many patients. As health providers we must discuss fertility preservation options with patients and should not make any prejudicial assumptions based on age, gender, relationship status, or whether patients have children already. Conversations need to be honest and straightforward and must be done before any treatment begins, although it is recognized that this is often difficult in a very pressurized system.

Although most of the drugs used in colorectal cancer treatment do not necessarily lead to complete infertility, they may reduce fertility, or, if a patient is nearing menopause, they may precipitate the menopause. Radiotherapy can also lead to infertility by causing the ovaries to stop releasing eggs and reducing or stopping the release of hormones such as oestrogen and progesterone (ovarian failure) and so initiating an early menopause (Mariani et al., 2019). Furthermore, radiation can damage the uterus, and therefore the ability to carry a pregnancy to term may be compromised.

Fertility preservation in women with colorectal cancer is feasible prior to starting treatment. The options for doing this includes freezing embryos, freezing eggs, or ovarian tissue cryopreservation. These are complicated procedures and are not always successful and may delay the start of any treatment. Careful counselling of patients regarding the options and potential risks is crucial. Other options which could be considered if fertility is affected include using donor eggs, donated sperm, surrogacy, or adoption.

Cancer treatments can affect the reproductive ability of male patients by damaging spermatogenesis, although again, the evidence that the standardly used chemotherapy drugs in CRC causes this is very limited. Many men recover full sperm production after treatment, but some have a reduced sperm count or none in their semen (Frankel Kelvin, 2015). Pelvic surgery and radiation can also cause injury resulting in erectile or ejaculatory dysfunction and these patients may therefore be producing sperm but are unable to pass it to their female partner through intercourse. Cryopreservation of ejaculated semen, or sperm banking, is the standard fertility preservation option for adult males undergoing cancer treatment. This is a simple, non-invasive way for male patients to preserve their ability to have biological children in the future without delaying any treatment.

The National Institute for Health and Care Excellence (NICE) recommends that doctors should offer sperm banking to any man having cancer treatment that may affect their fertility. In some areas of the United Kingdom, sperm banking is available free on the NHS. In other areas you need to pay for it.

Peripheral neuropathy

Oxaliplatin is a chemotherapy drug that is used commonly in CRC, both in the metastatic phase of treatment but also as a standard component of adjuvant treatment. These patients may therefore have many more years of life ahead of them and chronic side effects need to be considered carefully. Oxaliplatin-induced peripheral neuropathy is common and is thought to be due to the accumulation of oxaliplatin in the dorsal root ganglia (Denlinger & Barsevick, 2009).

Symptoms include numbness, pain, paraesthesia, and dysesthesias in the hands and feet. For most patients, the symptoms will improve over time, but for a small group of patients (up to 12%) it can remain as a chronic and debilitating condition. Chronic symptoms include persistent numbness, tingling, and cold-induced pain. These can affect fine motor skills and therefore the ability to hold and pick up small objects, fasten buttons, writing, and walking, and so affect confidence and quality of life.

It is not possible to reverse the nerve damage caused by oxaliplatin. Medications such as gabapentin or pregabalin can be used to help manage nerve pain. Referral to physiotherapy and occupational therapy teams can be helpful to assess patients who have difficulty managing activities of daily living.

With the movement towards using shorter courses of adjuvant treatment (three versus six months), the frequency of chronic neuropathy in 'potentially cured' patients has been radically reduced, but it does remain an issue for patients with metastatic disease.

Psychological impact of treatment and diagnosis

The effects of psychological distress in cancer care have been well researched. It increases the risk of developing depression and anxiety, as well as impacting negatively on overall quality of life, marital/family relationships, compliance with treatments, prolonging hospitalization, and it can even effect overall survival. As patients adjust to their diagnosis and progress through treatment into follow-up, they will have many different emotions; uncertainty, grief, shock, anger, confusion, and difficulty concentrating are all common. to name but a few.

Cancer patients and their families will have many needs which will vary at the different stages of their pathway. Acknowledgment and understanding the psychological impact of a cancer diagnosis and the consequences of treatments is a requirement of all health professionals.

Hoon et al. (2013) identified that psychosocial intervention programmes can improve colorectal patient outcomes with regards to length of hospital stay, number of days it took a patient to learn to care for their stoma, a reduction in hospital anxiety and depression, and overall, improvements in their quality of life.

Where possible, access to a psychological medicine team who can assess and screen patients thoroughly is valuable, not only to the individual but it also has added value for hospital systems by a reduction in the use of and burden on services. Screening allows for the expected levels of distress, worries, and fears to be identified which can be managed by the clinical teams involved, and for those patients with significant and morbid distress to be referred to and be treated by more specialist services.

The types of outcomes which can be measured are guided by a definition of 'distress' from the National Comprehensive Cancer Network (Holland et al., 2010, pp. 450), which is:

> Distress is a multi-determined unpleasant emotional experience of a psychological (cognitive, behavioural, emotional), social, and/or spiritual nature that may interfere with the ability to cope effectively with cancer, its physical symptoms, and its treatment. Distress extends along a continuum, ranging from common normal feelings of vulnerability, sadness and fears to problems that can become disabling, such as depression, anxiety, panic, social isolation, and existential and spiritual crisis.

It is important to recognize that distress does not necessarily end when treatment has been completed. For many patients, either because they have ongoing symptoms from their treatment, or because they have not fully come to terms with their diagnosis, the distress can be prolonged and very intrusive. Identifying this, and acting upon it, during follow-up is crucial.

Body image

Body image and body confidence issues are prevalent among colorectal cancer survivors. These changes are particularly noted post-surgery due to changes in body shape, scarring, weight changes, and stoma formation. Laparoscopically assisted surgery compared to open surgery offers better cosmetic results but scarring and skin changes obviously cannot be completely avoided.

Stoma formation and all its sequela obviously has a significant impact on body image. Stomas may be permanent or temporary and they are most often needed for those having surgery for rectal cancer, or those undergoing surgery in an emergency situation, or where neoadjuvant treatment is planned.

A stoma changes how the body looks and functions (Taylor, 2015). Higher rates of negative body image have been found in patients who have had surgery requiring a permanent stoma, such as abdominoperineal resection (APR) (Lawday et al., 2021). For the patients, there is no control over when the stoma 'works', and leaks from the stoma bag can be very distressing and humiliating for the patient. A stoma often causes changes and difficulties in social interactions, may impact upon occupational considerations, and can significantly derail daily activities. Parastomal hernias can also occur and can be difficult to manage.

Body image and confidence can also be affected by unwanted and embarrassing changes in the way the body functions because of treatments such as unpredictable bowel control or increased flatulence, even when a stoma has been avoided. This can significantly change the way a patient feels about themselves, and they can feel 'betrayed' by their own bodies. This in turn can lead to reduced self-confidence and anxiety, and can disrupt social functioning and quality of life. If these changes are persistent then they can severely impact the way survivors view themselves (Benedict et al., 2016).

Targeting body image problems will lead to an improved quality of life and so psychological support should be offered. Psychological interventions can decrease a patient's distress and so improve their quality of life. Nurses play a key role in identifying body image concerns and ameliorating those concerns by helping patients strengthen their self-image (Taylor, 2015). Reassurance and good communication to enable patients to achieve a good quality of life. Nurses need to be aware of the psychological needs of patients with stomas and offer supportive programmes. Training for nurses in psychological support is important.

Thankfully, most consequences of chemotherapy which can affect body image such as loss of hair and weight loss/weight gain are temporary and usually reversible once chemotherapy has stopped, but the patient may need increased psychological support for the period that they are suffering these changes.

Moving forward to better diet and nutrition

It is well documented that colorectal cancer is more prevalent in people with a raised BMI, higher adiposity, and in the presence of diabetes (Amadou et al., 2021; Pang et al., 208; Zheng et al., 2018). Dietary factors also affect risk, with a lower incidence of CRC in diets that are high in fibre (particularly from grains, cereals, vegetables, and fruits (Kunzmann et al., 2016; Peters et al., 2003)), and low in red and processed meats, as well as sugar (Zoltick et al., 2021). It is therefore critical that we take diet seriously when we are counselling our patients.

Danish Dietary Guidelines were also associated with a lower risk of colorectal cancer (Zhang et al., 2021) and have been updated as follows:

- Eat a variety of foods, but not too much, and be physically active
- Eat fruits and lots of vegetables
- Eat more fish
- Choose whole grains
- Choose lean meats and cold meats
- Choose low-fat dairy products
- Eat less saturated fat
- Eat foods with less salt
- Eat less sugar
- Drink water

Side effects of treatment can reduce appetite causing weight loss and loss of muscle mass. Malnutrition can impede cancer treatment, making it less effective or difficult to endure. The proactive implementation of nutritional screening and assessment is essential to identify this early (Reber et al., 2021) using validated screening tools such as the Malnutrition Universal Screening Tool, the Subjective Global Assessment (Duerkson et al., 2021), or Nutrition Risk Screening. Prompt input from a Registered Dietitian with a dietetic care plan and ongoing support can then greatly ease the nutritional burden of disease.

Following treatment, the importance of adhering to a balanced healthy diet and weight remains important, especially as a healthy diet has been associated with a decrease in disease recurrence and improved survival. However, as there is no definitive evidence-based guidance on diet following treatment, the Danish Dietary guidelines could be utilized.

Dietary intake can influence and exacerbate unwanted side effects, and therefore adjustments will need to be made depending on an individual's disease state, treatment, surgical procedures, tolerances, and symptoms. Often a trial-and-error approach is the only way for patients to identify foods which they can tolerate. 'Healthy' foods such as fruit and vegetables can sometimes be difficult to tolerate. Keeping a food and symptom diary and looking for a trend can sometimes help to identify a food which may be causing a problem.

Specific dietary advice for common problems

Colostomy and ileostomy

After the initial reintroduction of solids and fibre post-surgery, a healthy balanced diet can be resumed. Some long-term food adjustments may be required depending on digestive changes. It is important for patients to take their time and chew foods thoroughly as blockages can happen. Foods such as nuts and uncooked skins on fruit and vegetables can increase this risk.

Due to absorption issues, ileostomy patients should be monitored long term for deficiencies in vitamin B12 and iron (Phipps et al., 2021); they are also more susceptible to dehydration. Fluid intake and stoma output should be closely monitored to ensure good hydration status, with advice given on hypotonic drinks if output is high. If dehydration persists, admission to hospital may be required for subcutaneous or parenteral saline, and added magnesium may be given. Monitoring of serum urea, electrolytes, magnesium, and a random urine sodium concentration should be conducted (Nightingale, 2022).

Wind

Adjustments can be made to the amounts of food containing resistant starch, artificial sweeteners, beer, and fizzy drinks, as well as behaviour changes such as eating regularly, chewing food well, and avoiding chewing gum. Drinking peppermint drinks such as cordial or tea can be helpful.

Diarrhoea

Reducing the intake of very spicy foods, lagers and beer, pure fruit juices, and some fruit and vegetables can show some benefit.

Constipation

Advice should be given to eat more fibre-containing foods by choosing wholemeal and whole-grain carbohydrates and increasing intake of fruit and vegetables. This is in addition to drinking plenty of fluids: at least six to eight cups a day. If patients wish to avoid medications, natural laxatives such as prunes or prune juice may be helpful as a first step.

Advice about physical activity

Often patients may feel apprehensive about undertaking physical activity. Commonly there is a concern that cancer treatments and outcomes can be negatively impacted. However, not only it is well documented that physical activity improves the functional capacity of patients at various stages of their treatment but it also appears to reduce the risk of cancer recurrence and mortality (Meyerhardt et al., 2006). It is vital that patients are aware of this positive impact physical activity can have on both their physical and psychological well-being.

It is important to remember that physical activity can comprise many forms of activity from gardening and cleaning to more aerobic activities such as running and dancing. Encouraging patients to remain active or to become active during or after treatment should be discussed alongside other treatment discussions. Types of activity will depend on the ability of the patient pre-treatment, current physical status, and considering side effects of treatment such as peripheral neuropathy caused by oxaliplatin-based chemotherapy, which may mean some exercises cannot be undertaken.

Positive consequences of activity:

- Improved quality of life
- Better tolerance of treatments
- Reduction in side effects of treatments, e.g. fatigue
- Mental health benefits
- Recovery of physical strength fitness post treatment

It is important that our patients are provided with the guidance and support which is personalized to them, identifying and assessing the level of activity they can undertake safely, and a package of rehabilitation tools made available to them.

Chronic cancer-related fatigue

Cancer-related fatigue (CRF) is one of the most common and debilitating side effects of cancer and its treatment. Even simple tasks can leave a patient feeling exhausted, with fatigue persisting for many years following completion of treatment (Husson et al., 2015). There are different reasons a patient may be suffering with CRF, and they may include physiological and/or psychological problems. It is important that patients are screened appropriately to assess CRF and its impact on their quality of life. As well as taking a history, thorough blood work is needed to ensure there are no reversible reasons.

Common reasons for CRF include:

- Anaemia: iron deficiency, myelosuppression
- Endocrine disorder/electrolyte imbalance: hypomagnesaemia, thyroid issues, calcium
- Infection: post surgery, urinary tract
- Nutritional deficiency: high output stoma, malabsorption
- Uncontrolled pain: adhesions
- Medications: opioids
- Psychological effects: altered sleep, stress, depression, anxiety, altered body image, work problems, relationship problems

Treatment-related fatigue is important to assess prior to each cycle of treatment while a patient is on active treatment. Patients who have other health problems, or who have multiple treatments, are more likely to be affected by CRF.

In terms of chemotherapy, patients may start to feel fatigue after about a week of treatment which will peak and then start to wane, becoming better until just before the next cycle starts. This can slowly build up or accumulate as cycles progress and may be a cause for some patients to end their treatment early, if CRF is becoming debilitating.

In terms of radiotherapy, although used for localized management of cancer, CRF is common, building up as treatment progresses and continuing for several months post-treatment before a patient will return to a pre-treatment level of function.

In terms of surgery, depending on the patient's pre-surgical energy levels, it is expected that patients will be able to return to work approximately six to eight weeks after surgery, however to return completely to pre-surgical levels can take up to around six months, depending on the complexity of surgery.

Practical advice for patients to help them with CRF include:

- Prioritize what they need to do/deal with what is most important first
- Conserve energy by breaking big tasks into smaller ones
- Ask friends and family for help getting through your daily responsibilities
- Exercise: although patients may not feel like this, it is important to keep moving, even just taking short walks each day
- Sleep: encourage regular sleep patterns, use relaxation techniques can be helpful
- Good nutritional foods that give energy: fresh fruits, vegetables, whole grains, and lean protein, and drinking plenty of water
- Patient diary: to identify episodes times/triggers of CRF

Work and financial impact

Unfortunately, job loss and financial distress amongst cancer patients happens, especially during treatment when side effects and hospital appointments take over. It is important we are aware of the financial situation of patients to prevent non-adherence to treatments and provide them with information on how and where to access financial advice.

Cancer patients can also incur additional costs with travelling to hospital for treatment or follow-up appointments, and costs related to medication and stoma supplies. We should therefore be aware of any local support services available to them to alleviate financial pressures. Within the United Kingdom organizations such as Macmillan and the Citizens Advice Bureau have information and helplines for support, help, and advice to assess financial situations in order to gain access to grants and benefits.

Once patients are post-treatment, physical symptoms can become barriers to retuning to the workplace. These symptoms include poor unpredictable bowel function, neuropathy, and fatigue which can all affect performance (Lim et al., 2021) and may necessitate the need to change working hours. For some, however, this is not possible due to their financial situation.

It is important for health professionals to be aware of laws which may afford protection to patients. Within the United Kingdom, the law considers patients who have had or have cancer as having a disability. Employers cannot treat people with cancer less favourably than other people who do not have cancer or for reasons connected to the cancer. This is covered within the Equality Act 2010.

Personalized follow-up

Following cancer treatment, it is important to offer patients an effective personalized stratified follow-up. This allows health professionals to effectively follow-up patients while adapting to care needs and improving outcomes for people living with and beyond cancer.

The implementation of these pathways tailored to individual needs offers benefits not only to patients but also healthcare services and it considers differing patient needs by varying the intensity, setting, and professionals involved, thus making services more efficient and cost-effective.

Providing these self-management tools to our patients so they are better informed about their disease, treatment, signs of recurrence, and any longer-term effects ensures that patient concerns are identified in a timely manner. It also allows for an increased focus on health and well-being and improving patients' quality of life, and patients are supported to make healthier lifestyle choices and manage their own care.

There are several healthcare models are available but most incorporate key elements including: patient education, emotional and psychosocial support, treatment summaries, care plans, surveillance, long-term side effects of treatment, and primary care support.

The Recovery Package (NHSE, 2016) is a set of essential interventions designed to deliver a person-centred approach to care for people affected by cancer, including:

1) Holistic Needs Assessment (HNA) and care planning
2) Treatment summary
3) Health and well-being events
4) Cancer care review: GP questionnaire

Summary

This brief chapter has covered the different areas of patient care which should be considered at various points of their treatment pathway. Of course, there are many more topics to discuss but the aim was to identify some of the key issues colorectal cancer patients may face, before, during, and after their treatment.

What is clear is that the interventions we offer today may have an ongoing life-long impact on patients and their families' quality of life long after they leave our care. Patients must be aware of these potential impacts, and a personalized approach to giving the right information at the right time is a balance we must reach. We must offer them opportunities to improve their quality of life through health and well-being services, and ensure the support remains into the follow-up phase of their care and not just during their treatment.

Acknowledgements

We would like to acknowledge the contribution to this chapter made by Natasha Guildford (Macmillan Hepato-Pancreato-Biliary Dietitian at Oxford University Hospitals NHS Foundation Trust) for her input on dietary advice for this patient group.

REFERENCES

Amadou, A., Freisling, H., Jenab, M., et al (2021). Prevalent diabetes and risk of total, colorectal, prostate and breast cancers in an ageing population: meta-analysis of individual participant data from cohorts of the CHANCES consortium. *British Journal of Cancer, 124*(11), 1882–1890. https://doi.org/10.1038/s41416-021-01347-4

Benedict, C., Rodriguez, V. M., Carter, J., et al. (2016). Investigation of body image as a mediator of the effects of bowel and GI symptoms on psychological distress in female survivors of rectal and anal cancer. *Supportive Care in Cancer, 24*(4), 1795–1802. https://doi.org/10.1007/s00520-015-2976-2

Boyes, A., Girgis, A., & Lecathelinais, C. (2009). Brief assessment of adult cancer patients' perceived needs: development and validation of the 34-item Supportive Care Needs Survey (SCNS-SF34). *Journal of Evaluation in Clinical Practice*, *15*(4), 602–606. https://doi.org/10.1111/j.1365-2753.2008.01057.x

Burch, J. (2021). Improving bowel function after colorectal cancer surgery. How to assess and treat the symptoms of low anterior resection syndrome (LARS). *Gastrointestinal Nursing*, *19*(2) https://doi.org/10.12968/gasn.2021.19.2.8

Burch, J. (2021). Low anterior resection syndrome: impact on quality of life and nurse-led management. *Gastrointestinal Nursing*, *19*(Sup4a) https://doi.org/10.12968/gasn.2021.19.2.8

Crevenna, R., Palma, S., & Licht, T. (2021). Cancer prehabilitation—a short review. *Memo*, *14*, 39–34. https://doi.org/10.1007/s12254-021-00686-5

Denlinger, C. S., & Barsevick, A. M. (2009) The challenges of colorectal cancer survivorship. *Journal of the National Comprehensive Cancer Network*, *7*(8) 883–894. https://doi.org/10.6004/jnccn.2009.0058

Dietz J. H., Jr. (1969). Rehabilitation of the cancer patient. *Medical Clinics of North America*, *53*(3), 607–624.

Duerksen, D. R., Laporte, M., & Jeejeebhoy, K. (2021). Evaluation of nutrition status using the subjective global assessment: malnutrition, cachexia, and sarcopenia. *Nutrition in Clinical Practice*, *36*(5), 942–956. https://doi.org/10.1002/ncp.10613

Emmertsen, K. J., & Laurberg, S. (2012). Low anterior resection syndrome score: development and validation of a symptom-based scoring system for bowel dysfunction after low anterior resection for rectal cancer. *Annals of Surgery*, *255*(5), 922–928. https://doi.org/10.1097/SLA.0b013e31824f1c21

Frankel Kelvin, J. (2015). Sperm banking: fertility preservation for male patients with cancer. *Clinical Journal of Oncology Nursing*, *19*(1), 108–110. https://doi.org/10.1188/15.CJON.108-110

Holland, J. C., Andersen, B., Breitbart, W. S., et al. (2010). Distress management. *Journal of the National Comprehensive Cancer Network*, *8*(4), 448–485. https://doi.org/10.6004/jnccn.2010.0034

Hoon, L. S., Chi Sally, C. W., & Hong-Gu, H. (2013). Effect of psychosocial interventions on outcomes of patients with colorectal cancer: a review of the literature. *European Journal of Oncology Nursing*, *17*(6), 883–891. https://doi.org/10.1016/j.ejon.2013.05.001

Hope, C., Reilly, J., Lund, J., et al. (2020). Systematic review: the effect of right hemicolectomy for cancer on postoperative bowel function. *Supportive Care in Cancer*, *28*(10), 4549–4559. https://doi.org/10.1007/s00520-020-05519-5

Husson, O., Mols, F., van de Poll-Franse, L. V., et al. (2015). The course of fatigue and its correlates in colorectal cancer survivors: a prospective cohort study of the PROFILES registry. *Supportive Care in Cancer*, *23*(11), 3361–3371. https://doi.org/10.1007/s00520-015-2802-x

Jefford, M., Ward, A. C., Lisy, K., et al. (2017). Patient-reported outcomes in cancer survivors: a population-wide cross-sectional study. *Supportive Care in Cancer*, *25*(10), 3171–3179. https://doi.org/10.1007/s00520-017-3725-5

Kunzmann, A. T., Coleman, H. G., Huang, W. Y., et al. (2016). Fruit and vegetable intakes and risk of colorectal cancer and incident and recurrent adenomas in the PLCO cancer screening trial. *International Journal of Cancer*, *138*(8), 1851–1861. https://doi.org/10.1002/ijc.29922

Lawday, S., Flamey, N., Fowler, G. E., et al. (2021). Quality of life in restorative versus non-restorative resections for rectal cancer: systematic review. *BJS Open*, *5*(6), zrab101. https://doi.org/10.1093/bjsopen/zrab101

Lim, C., Laidsaar-Powell, R. C., Young, J. M., et al. (2021). Colorectal cancer survivorship: A systematic review and thematic synthesis of qualitative research. *European Journal of Cancer Care*, *30*(4), e13421. https://doi.org/10.1111/ecc.

Macmillan. (2020). Principles and Guidance for Prehabilitation Within the Management and Support of People with Cancer. https://cdn.macmillan.org.uk/dfsmedia/1a6f23537f7f4519bb0cf14c45b2a629/1532-source/prehabilitation-for-people-with-cancer-tcm9-353994?_ga=2.148926644.38321043.1647189532-673761543.1642778261 accessed 13 March 2021.

Mariani, S., Chiloiro, G., Villa, P., et al. (2019). Fertility preservation in chemo-radiotherapy for rectal cancer: a combined approach. *Clinical and Translational Radiation Oncology*, *19*, 77–79. https://doi.org/10.1016/j.ctro.2019.09.002

Meyerhardt, J. A., Giovannucci, E. L., Holmes, M. D., et al. (2006). Physical activity and survival after colorectal cancer diagnosis. *Journal of Clinical Oncology*, *24*(22), 3527–3534. https://doi.org/10.1200/JCO.2006.06.0855

Milbury, K., Cohen, L., Jenkins, R., et al. (2013). The association between psychosocial and medical factors with long-term sexual dysfunction after treatment for colorectal cancer. *Supportive Care in Cancer*, *21*(3), 793–802. https://doi.org/10.1007/s00520-012-1582-9

Minnella, E. M., & Carli, F. (2018). Prehabilitation and functional recovery for colorectal cancer patients. *European Journal of Surgical Oncology*, *44*(7), 919–926. https://doi.org/10.1016/j.ejso.2018.04.016

NHSE. (2016). Implementing the cancer taskforce recommendations: Commissioning person centered care for people affected by cancer. <http://www.england.nhs.uk> accessed 15 March 2022.

Nightingale J. (2021). How to manage a high-output stoma. *Frontline Gastroenterology*, *13*(2), 140–151. https://doi.org/10.1136/flgastro-2018-101108

Pang, Y., Kartsonaki, C., Guo, Y., et al. (2018). Adiposity and risks of colorectal and small intestine cancer in Chinese adults: a prospective study of 0.5 million people. *British Journal of Cancer*, *119*(2), 248–250. https://doi.org/10.1038/s41416-018-0124-8

Peiri, C., & Patton, V. (2020). Clinical nursing management of low anterior resection syndrome - a practical guide to understanding and managing symptoms. *Journal of Stomal Therapy Australia*, *40*(2), 8–13 https://doi.org/10.33235/jsta.40.2.8-13

Peters, U., Sinha, R., Chatterjee, N., et al. (2003). Dietary fibre and colorectal adenoma in a colorectal cancer early detection programme. *Lancet*, *361*(9368), 1491–1495. https://doi.org/10.1016/S0140-6736(03)13173-X

Phipps, O., Brookes, M. J., & Al-Hassi, H. O. (2021). Iron deficiency, immunology, and colorectal cancer. *Nutrition Reviews*, *79*(1), 88–97. https://doi.org/10.1093/nutrit/nuaa040

Reber, E., Schönenberger, K. A., Vasiloglou, M. F., et al. (2021). Nutritional risk screening in cancer patients: the first step toward better clinical outcome. *Frontiers in Nutrition*, *8*, 603936. https://doi.org/10.3389/fnut.2021.603936

Reese, J. B., Handorf, E., & Haythornthwaite, J. A. (2018). Sexual quality of life, body image distress, and psychosocial outcomes in colorectal cancer: a longitudinal study. *Supportive Care in Cancer*, *26*(10), 3431–3440. https://doi.org/10.1007/s00520-018-4204-3

Roth, A. J., Kornblith, A. B., Batel-Copel, L., et al. (1998). Rapid screening for psychologic distress in men with prostate carcinoma: a pilot study. *Cancer*, *82*(10), 1904–1908. https://doi.org/10.1002/(sici)1097-0142(19980515)82:10<1904::aid-cncr13>3.0.co;2-x

Sodergren, S. C., Wheelwright, S. J., Permyakova, N. V., et al. (2019). Supportive care needs of patients following treatment for colorectal cancer: risk factors for unmet needs and the association between unmet needs and health-related quality of life-results from the ColoREctal Wellbeing (CREW) study. *Journal of Cancer*

Survivorship: Research and Practice, 13(6), 899–909. https://doi.org/10.1007/s11764-019-00805-6

Taylor, C. (2015). Body image concerns after colorectal cancer surgery. *British Journal of Nursing, 24*(10), S8–14. https://doi.org/10.12968/bjon.2015.24.Sup10.S8

Zhang, J., Nyvang, D., Ibsen, D. B., et al. (2021). Adherence to the Danish food-based dietary guidelines and risk of colorectal cancer: a cohort study. *British Journal of Cancer, 125*(12), 1726–1733. https://doi.org/10.1038/s41416-021-01556-x

Zheng, R., Du, M., Zhang, B., et al. (2018). Body mass index (BMI) trajectories and risk of colorectal cancer in the PLCO cohort. *British Journal of Cancer, 119*(1), 130–132. https://doi.org/10.1038/s41416-018-0121-y

Zoltick, E. S., Smith-Warner, S. A., Yuan, C., et al. (2021). Sugar-sweetened beverage, artificially sweetened beverage and sugar intake and colorectal cancer survival. *British Journal of Cancer, 125*(7), 1016–1024. https://doi.org/10.1038/s41416-021-01487-7

Index

For the benefit of digital users, indexed terms that span two pages (e.g., 52–53) may, on occasion, appear on only one of those pages.

Note: Tables and figures are indicated by an italic *t* and *f* following the page number.